Designed for the maintenance of good nutrition of practically
all healthy people in the United States

Water-Soluble Vitamins

Vitamin C (mg)	Thiamin (mg)	Riboflavin (mg)	Niacin (mg NE)[f]	Vitamin B₆ (mg)	Folate (µg)	Vitamin B₁₂ (µg)
30	0.3	0.4	5	0.3	25	0.3
35	0.4	0.5	6	0.6	35	0.5
40	0.7	0.8	9	1.0	50	0.7
45	0.9	1.1	12	1.1	75	1.0
45	1.0	1.2	13	1.4	100	1.4
50	1.3	1.5	17	1.7	150	2.0
60	1.5	1.8	20	2.0	200	2.0
60	1.5	1.7	19	2.0	200	2.0
60	1.5	1.7	19	2.0	200	2.0
60	1.2	1.4	15	2.0	200	2.0
50	1.1	1.3	15	1.4	150	2.0
60	1.1	1.3	15	1.5	180	2.0
60	1.1	1.3	15	1.6	180	2.0
60	1.1	1.3	15	1.6	180	2.0
60	1.0	1.2	13	1.6	180	2.0
70	1.5	1.6	17	2.2	400	2.2
95	1.6	1.8	20	2.1	280	2.6
90	1.6	1.7	20	2.1	260	2.6

Minerals

Calcium (mg)	Phosphorus (mg)	Magnesium (mg)	Iron (mg)	Zinc (mg)	Iodine (µg)	Selenium (µg)
400	300	40	6	5	40	10
600	500	60	10	5	50	15
800	800	80	10	10	70	20
800	800	120	10	10	90	20
800	800	170	10	10	120	30
1,200	1,200	270	12	15	150	40
1,200	1,200	400	12	15	150	50
1,200	1,200	350	10	15	150	70
800	800	350	10	15	150	70
800	800	350	10	15	150	70
1,200	1,200	280	15	12	150	45
1,200	1,200	300	15	12	150	50
1,200	1,200	280	15	12	150	55
800	800	280	15	12	150	55
800	800	280	10	12	150	55
1,200	1,200	300	30	15	175	65
1,200	1,200	355	15	19	200	75
1,200	1,200	340	15	16	200	75

[c] Retinol equivalents. 1 retinol equivalent = 1 µg retinol or 6 µg ß-carotene.

[d] As cholecalciferol. 10 µg cholecalciferol = 400 IU of vitamin D.

[e] α-Tocopherol equivalents. 1 mg d-α tocopherol = 1 α-TE.

[f] 1 NE (niacin equivalent) is equal to 1 mg of niacin or 60 mg of dietary tryptophan.

Estimated Safe and Adequate Daily Dietary Intakes of Selected Vitamins and Minerals[a]

Category	Age (years)	Vitamins	
		Biotin (µg)	Pantothenic Acid (mg)
Infants	0–0.5	10	2
	0.5–1	15	3
Children and adolescents	1–3	20	3
	4–6	25	3–4
	7–10	30	4–5
	11 +	30–100	4–7
Adults		30–100	4–7

Category	Age (years)	Trace Elements[b]				
		Copper (mg)	Manganese (mg)	Fluoride (mg)	Chromium (µg)	Molybdenum (µg)
Infants	0–0.5	0.4–0.6	0.3–0.6	0.1–0.5	10–40	15–30
	0.5–1	0.6–0.7	0.6–1.0	0.2–1.0	20–60	20–40
Children and adolescents	1–3	0.7–1.0	1.0–1.5	0.5–1.5	20–80	25–50
	4–6	1.0–1.5	1.5–2.0	1.0–2.5	30–120	30–75
	7–10	1.0–2.0	2.0–3.0	1.5–2.5	50–200	50–150
	11 +	1.5–2.5	2.0–5.0	1.5–2.5	50–200	75–250
Adults		1.5–3.0	2.0–5.0	1.5–4.0	50–200	75–250

[a] Because there is less information on which to base allowances, these figures are not given in the main table of RDA and are provided here in the form of ranges of recommended intakes.

[b] Since the toxic levels for many trace elements may be only several times usual intakes, the upper levels for the trace elements given in this table should not be habitually exceeded.

Nutrition Throughout the Life Cycle

NUTRITION THROUGHOUT THE LIFE CYCLE

Edited by

SUE RODWELL WILLIAMS, Ph.D., M.P.H., R.D.

President, SRW Productions, Inc., and Director, The Berkeley
Nutrition Group, Berkeley, California; Metabolic Nutrition Consultant,
Kaiser-Permanente Northern California Regional Newborn Screening and
Metabolic Program, Kaiser-Permanente Medical Center, Oakland, California

BONNIE S. WORTHINGTON-ROBERTS, Ph.D., R.D.

Professor and Director, Nutritional Sciences, Chief Nutritionist,
Child Development and Mental Retardation Center, Clinical Training Unit,
University of Washington, Seattle, Washington

Coauthors

ELEANOR D. SCHLENKER, Ph.D., R.D.

Professor and Department Head, Human Nutrition and Foods,
The College of Human Resources,
Virginia Polytechnic Institute and State University, Blacksburg, Virginia

PEGGY PIPES, M.S., R.D.

Assistant Chief, Nutrition Section, Child Development and Mental Retardation Center,
Clinical Training Unit, University of Washington, Seattle, Washington

JANE M. REES, M.S., R.D.

Director, Nutrition Services and Education, Child Development and Mental Retardation Center,
Clinical Training Unit, Teaching Associate, Department of Pediatrics,
University of Washington, Seattle, Washington

SECOND EDITION

With 102 Illustrations

**Mosby
Year Book**

St. Louis Baltimore Boston Chicago London Philadelphia Sydney Toronto

Mosby
Year Book
Dedicated to Publishing Excellence

Acquisitions Editor: Vicki Malinee
Assistant Editor: Cathy Waller
Project Manager: Linda J. Daly
Book Design: Gail Morey Hudson
Cover & Chapter Opener Illustrations: Molly Babich

SECOND EDITION

Printed in the United States of America

Mosby–Year Book, Inc.
11830 Westline Industrial Drive, St. Louis, MO 63146

Library of Congress Cataloging in Publication Data

Nutrition throughout the life cycle / edited by Sue Rodwell Williams
and Bonnie S. Worthington-Roberts; co-authors, Eleanor D.
Schlenker, Peggy Pipes, Jane M. Rees.—2nd ed.
    p.   cm.
    "Mosby life cycle series"—Pref.
    Includes bibliographical references and index.
    ISBN 0-8016-6477-2
    1. Nutrition. I. Williams, Sue Rodwell. II. Worthington
-Roberts, Bonnie S., 1943- III. Schlenker, Eleanor D. IV. Pipes,
Peggy L. V. Rees, Jane Mitchell.
    [DNLM: 1. Nutrition. QU 145 N97606]
TX354.N87   1992
613.2—dc20
DNLM/DLC
for Library of Congress
91-46281
CIP

92 93 94 95 96 GW/VH 9 8 7 6 5 4 3 2 1

Preface

The second edition of *Nutrition Throughout the Life Cycle* is in a real sense a *new* book. With strengthened focus on its title, this new edition begins the life cycle with young adults who conceive and sustain new life, building upon a fundamental nutrition foundation in its redesigned and reorganized format and content to meet expanded needs of a broader range of students and practitioners alike.

Here the authors of the highly successful Mosby Life Cycle Series books bring together in this newly designed and developed edition unique backgrounds and working knowledge of each stage of human development. In this project we continue our goal to provide for students, teachers, and practitioners a unified view of the life cycle as one whole, supported in each stage by the nutrition foundation that is essential for this development.

This underlying developmental concept of human life remains the unifying thread throughout the life cycle. It has become increasingly significant in today's modern world as lifespan has lengthened but for many persons has not improved in quality. We recognize anew that the quality of this lengthened life, genetically programmed from conception but dependent upon a nourishing environment for fulfillment of this genetic potential, builds at each stage upon a complex of all past and present life experiences.

We also recognize that our environment is rapidly changing and affecting individual lives in many ways, some of which are not always beneficial. In the midst of these changes, we are made increasingly aware that nutritional needs—so fundamental to human growth and development—do not exist in a vacuum. At each life stage they are always interwoven with many other personal, socioeconomic, and cultural factors that make up the whole of life and influence positive growth and development and health in both subtle and obvious ways.

This new edition of our book reflects these far-reaching changes. Its guiding principle continues to be the commitment, along with that of our publisher, to the integrity of each of our individual books. Our expanded goal here is to produce an even stronger book for today's needs, with new design and format and sound content to meet the expectations and changing needs of a broader range of students, faculty, and practitioners in nutrition and health promotion for all ages.

OBJECTIVES OF THE BOOK

This new text is designed to meet the expanded needs of a broad spectrum of students, with varying degrees of nutrition backgrounds, in courses in life cycle nutrition and for health professionals working in both individual and community health programs. It approaches nutrition from a basic developmental approach, maintaining a person-centered view of individual integrity. It seeks to build nutritional needs as growth proceeds on the basis of both physical growth and psychosocial development. It focuses throughout on positive health for which nutrition provides a fundamental foundation.

MAJOR CHARACTERISTICS OF THE NEW EDITION

In a very real sense, then, this second edition is indeed a new book for our new times and needs. To accommodate the demands of our rapidly developing science and society, yet retain a clearly understood writing style, we have largely rewritten the text, including new chapters, and have made major changes throughout to increase its usefulness.

New chapters. To set direction and lay a fundamental nutrition foundation for the age-group chapters of the life cycle, we have created three new chapters:

- Chapter 1, *Introduction to the Life Cycle: The Role of Nutrition,* provides an overview of the essential nature of nutrition, nutrients and food plans to provide students, in the process of human growth and development throughout the life cycle, with a focus on health maintenance and disease prevention.
- Chapter 2, *Nutrition and Assessment Basics,* develops the theme, laying a nutrition foundation to cover wide ranges of entering students' knowledge base in a succinct application of the nature of nutrients and their roles in health care, and the parallel role of nutritional status assessment in determining individual and group needs.
- Chapter 3, *Nutrition and the Adult: Planning for a Healthy Lifestyle,* has been included at the beginning of the life cycle to focus on the role of this nutrition foundation to young adults and their building of healthy lifestyles to start and nurture the new generation. Special focus is given to the needs of young women, who must conceive and nourish the new life, and the continuing health issues of women as their life cycle continues.

New format and design. A new chapter format enhances the appeal of this text and encourages its use. Definitions of key terms have been drawn out of the text into the margin to clarify meaning. Many illustrations, tables, charts, topic headings, and sub-headings make the text easier to understand and more interesting to read.

New illustrations. We have expanded the number and diversity of illustrations, including artwork, graphs, charts, and photographs, to help both students and practitioners better understand the concepts and health care practices we are presenting.

Enhanced readability and student interest. We have rewritten our text in a style that helps "unfold" the material. We want to make developmental nutrition *come alive* in real situations. We want to create new interest and help students understand basic concepts better by expanded definitions and explanations to "flesh out" the human development and needs at each life stage discussed.

LEARNING AIDS THROUGHOUT THE TEXT

As indicated, the second edition is especially significant in its stronger use of many learning aids throughout the text.

Basic concepts. To immediately draw students into the topic for study, each chapter opens with a concise list of the basic concepts involved, and a brief chapter overview leading into the topic to "set the stage."

Chapter headings. Throughout each chapter, the major headings and subheadings in special type indicate the organization of the chapter material. This makes for easy reading and understanding of the key ideas. Main concepts and terms are also brought out with bold type and italics.

Definitions of terms. Key terms important to the student's understanding and application of the material in nutritional care are now presented in three ways. First, as they are discussed in the text they are identified in bold type. Second, they are brought out of the text into the margins for emphasis and developed meaning, often with interesting derivation and description of the words. Finally, all of the boldface terms are listed alphabetically in a glossary at the back of the book for quick reference.

One Step Further boxes. At different places in the text special related material is placed in boxes to provide further explanation or application. These boxes contain expanded material that takes students a step further to increase their understanding of a key concept.

Case Study boxes. Case studies have been highlighted in separate boxes throughout the text to focus the student's attention on related health needs or problems. Each case is accompanied by challenging questions for case analysis. Students can use these examples for similar situations in their individual or community learning experiences.

Chapter summaries. Brief summary paragraphs review chapter highlights and help students see the "big picture." Then they can return to any part of the material for repeated study and clarification of details as needed.

Review questions. To help the student understand and think through key parts of the chapter or apply it to health care problems, questions are given after the summary for each chapter for review and analysis of the material presented.

Cited references. Carefully researched and updated background references throughout the text strengthen the material presented and provide resources for students who may want to "dig further" into a particular topic of interest.

Further annotated readings. To encourage further reading of useful materials for expanding knowledge of key concepts or applying the material in practical ways for nutritional care and education, a brief list of annotated resources is provided at the end of each chapter.

Appendixes. An expanded set of appendixes supplies key reference tools for individual study or group projects. For example, nutrition assessment reference standards include anthropometric age-sex norms for body measures and weight-height tables for all ages, as well as developmental growth charts from infancy through childhood, and including an additional weight-height-age table for older adults. Other new assessment references include normal values for biochemical assessment, clinical signs and symptoms for evaluating clinical findings. References for dietary assessment include tables for normal body levels of nutrients or related measurements, as well as new Recommended Nutrient Intakes for Canadians, and the current food exchange lists for nutrient-energy calculations and meal-planning. The standard Recommended Dietary Allowances (RDA) tables have been placed inside the book covers for easy quick reference.

SPECIAL FEATURES OF THIS NEW TEXT

Throughout all its chapters, this newly organized text is distinctive in its breadth of topics discussed, especially in its comprehensive research base, and its many practical and helpful applications to meet individual and group situations. Its major references bring current scientific knowledge to a variety of modern situations and problems. Students can then further apply this up-to-date comprehensive knowledge to needs they discover for themselves. We provide a basis for students to weigh pros and cons and understand why the scientific method is important to decision making, because often there are no "cookbook" answers to complex life problems and basic principles must be the guiding light. Such principles and concepts are highlighted here in many ways to help students see just how nutrition "works" in the lives of people at all ages.

The Core Life Cycle Chapters: The Developmental Concept

Chapters 3 through 9, the life cycle chapters, continue to provide the strong core of this text. We strengthen our discussions of the cycle in this new edition, however, by starting it where it naturally begins, with the young adult, especially the young woman, who conceives and nurtures the new life to its birth. As a whole unit, these chapters show clearly the overall developmental concept of life itself—constant dynamic change and balance. To the discussion of each life stage, the authors bring their unique knowledge and experience, their caring and sensitivity to meet human needs. In-depth reviews of early fetal growth and development during pregnancy and breastfeeding of the newborn infant probe fundamental relationships of nutrition to maternal health and the outcome of pregnancy, and to the following process of lactation. A clear foundation is laid for the varying nutritional needs of rapid infant growth and the slowed erratic growth of young children, revealing the lifetime importance of these early family and cultural food experiences and learned behaviors. An especially sensitive discussion of the volatile nature of rapid adolescent growth and sexual maturation displays the increased nutritional and personal needs of these teenagers "coming of age" in an increasingly complex modern society. The important theme of health promotion through the strengthening of a healthy life style continues through the middle and older adult years and provides the basis for helping persons through these later years of adulthood to reduce their risks of health problems, those that affect food intake and use and thus nutritional status, as well as those leading to chronic disease.

Throughout the life cycle chapters, we weave the common human threads of both physiologic and psychosocial needs that build positive health, without which strengths nutrition and health problems develop and disease risks increase. Also, we have integrated material on body composition and nutrition assessment with each life cycle stage to focus on changing status and needs of emerging growth and development.

Finally, Chapter 10, *Nutrition Education,* completely updated and revised, relates nutrition knowledge, motivation, and food behavior to the learning process, food guides, and nutrition education. Here, then is the crux of the matter. We are reminded anew that all the nutrient needs crucial to each stage of human growth and development, as well as the healthful and enjoyable food habits we have discussed, will never come to pass unless individuals *want* them to, until they are motivated to change food habits toward these positive health directions. To this end, this chapter is packed with down-to-earth practical insights and suggestions for helping persons make these behavioral changes. It provides guidance for developing and evaluating nutrition education programs based on sound communications theory, and suggests principles for selecting appropriate materials and resources. A number of current strategies in nutrition education are described, as well as ways that realistic nutrition education may be involved in food assistance programs such as school lunch, WIC, and meals for the aged.

Acknowledgments

A realistic and useful college textbook is never the work of one person or even a team of authors as in this case. It develops into the planned product through the committed hands and hearts of a number of persons. It would be impossible to name all the individuals involved here, but several groups deserve special recognition.

First, we are indebted to Mosby–Year Book, and the many persons there, new and old friends, who have had a part in this project. Especially do we thank our publisher and editorial staff, including Ed Murphy, Vicki Malinee, Cathy Waller, and Linda Daly. All of these skilled persons have helped shape the manuscript and support our efforts and goals. We also thank Leslie Tinsley, marketing manager, for her patience and skill in helping to guide the result of our efforts to its ultimate users.

Second, we are grateful to the reviewers who gave their valuable time and skills to help us strengthen the final manuscript:

Leta Aljadir
University of Delaware

Patsy Brannon
University of Arizona

Mike Keenan
Louisiana State University

Bernice Kopel
Oklahoma State University

Karen Kubena
Texas A&M University

Marsha Read
University of Nevada–Reno

Joanne Spaide
University of Iowa

Third, as the overall coordinating editor on this writing team, responsible for producing the full manuscript through its several production stages, I, Sue Williams, am grateful to my own production staff, especially to my expert systems analyst and business manager, Jim Williams, who has developed and set up my expanded computer system, a true joy to work with. And to Tony Rinella, friend and computer expert, who has responded with grace to my calls for help at all sorts of odd hours, I give special thanks for being there when I needed him.

Fourth, to our many students and interns, colleagues, clients, and patients over the years who have enriched our professional and personal lives, we give our thanks. Each one has taught us something about human experience and we are grateful for these opportunities for personal growth.

Finally, but most of all, we want to thank our families—our "home teams." These beautiful people never cease to provide loving support for all our work, and to each one we are eternally grateful.

Sue Rodwell Williams
Bonnie S. Worthington-Roberts

Contents

3 NUTRITION AND THE ADULT: PLANNING FOR A HEALTHY LIFESTYLE, 50

Sue Rodwell Williams
Eleanor D. Schlenker

4 MATERNAL NUTRITION: THE COURSE AND OUTCOME OF PREGNANCY, 86

Bonnie S. Worthington-Roberts

5 LACTATION AND HUMAN MILK, 148

Bonnie S. Worthington-Roberts

6 NUTRITION DURING INFANCY, 214

Peggy Pipes

7   NUTRITION IN CHILDHOOD, 252

Peggy Pipes

8　NUTRITION IN ADOLESCENCE, 284

Jane M. Rees

9   NUTRITION FOR AGING AND THE AGED, 344

Eleanor D. Schlenker

10 NUTRITION EDUCATION, 384

Eleanor D. Schlenker

APPENDIXES

NUTRITION THROUGHOUT THE LIFE CYCLE

1

Introduction to the Life Cycle: The Role of Nutrition

Bonnie S. Worthington-Roberts

Basic Concepts

- ✔ *Each stage of the life cycle is associated with a distinct set of nutritional priorities.*
- ✔ *All persons throughout life need the same nutrients but in varying amounts.*
- ✔ *Health promotion and disease prevention are underlying lifetime goals.*
- ✔ *At times, especially in the later years, disease management may impact significantly on dietary planning.*

*F*rom beginning to end, the human life cycle is a fascinating sequence of events. From the moment of fertilization through the stages of growth, development, maturation, and aging, the interaction between genes and environment determine the details of the process. The importance of the genetic base cannot be ignored but it is clear that an assortment of environmental factors have the potential of significantly modifying the course of events. Nutrition is one of those influential factors demanding special attention.

This text considers in some depth the contributions that diet and nutrition make to support the growth and developmental process throughout the life cycle. Each chapter illustrates that in this health promotion process our food and its nutrients are essential factors to prevent deviations from the normal state or the establishment of acute or chronic disease.

THE NUTRIENTS: A BRIEF REMINDER

Survival requires not only oxygen and water but food as well. Food provides the energy required to support the body's life-sustaining processes; it also contains the materials needed to build and maintain all body cells. These materials are referred to as *nutrients;* each plays a role in assuring that the biochemical machinery of the human body runs smoothly.

Nutrients are classified in six categories (Table 1-1), including the energy-yielding **macronutrients** carbohydrates, fats, and proteins, the **micronutrients** vitamins and minerals, and water. Their basic features include the following:

1. *Carbohydrates* contain carbon, hydrogen, and oxygen combined in small molecules called sugars and large molecules represented mainly by starch.
2. **Lipids** (fats and oils) contain carbon, hydrogen, and oxygen as do carbohydrates, but the amount of oxygen is much less. **Triglyceride** is the main form of food fat.
3. *Proteins* contain carbon, hydrogen, and oxygen, plus nitrogen and sometimes sulfur atoms arranged in small compounds called **amino acids.** Chains of amino acids make up dietary proteins.
4. *Vitamins* are organic compounds that serve to catalyze or support a number of biochemical reactions in the body.
5. *Minerals* are inorganic elements or compounds that play important roles in metabolic reactions and serve as structural components in body tissues such as bone.
6. *Water* is vital to the body as a solvent and lubricant and as a medium for transporting nutrients and waste.

Triglyceride
(Gr *treis,* three; L *glycerinum,* glycerol) Chemical name for fat; a compound of three fatty acids esterified to glycerol base. A neutral fat, synthesized from carbohydrate, stored in adipose tissue. It releases free fatty acids into the blood when hydrolyzed by enzymes.

Amino acids
(*amino,* the monovalent chemical group NH_2) Carriers of essential element nitrogen; structural units of protein; specific amino acids being linked in specific sequence by peptide chains to form specific proteins.

TABLE 1-1   **Essential Nutrients in the Human Diet**

	Energy Nutrients				
Carbohydrate	Fat (Lipid)	Protein (Amino Acid)	Vitamins	Minerals	Water
Glucose (or a carbohydrate that yields glucose)	Linoleic acid (omega-6) α-Linolenic acid (omega-3)	Histidine Isoleucine Leucine Lysine Methionine Phenylalanine Threonine Tryptophan Valine	A D E K Thiamin Riboflavin Niacin Pantothenic acid Biotin B-6 B-12 Folate C	Arsenic Boron Calcium Chloride Chromium Cobalt Copper Fluoride Iodide Iron Magnesium Manganese Molybdenum Nickel Phosphorus Potassium Selenium Silicon Sodium Sulfur Zinc	Water

From Wardlaw GM and Insel PM: Perspectives in nutrition, St Louis, 1990, Mosby–Year Book, Inc.

DIET: INFLUENCES DURING THE LIFE CYCLE

While food likes and dislikes probably determine largely what people eat, food choices also reflect socioeconomic status and budget, cultural experiences, religious beliefs, time constraints, health-related concerns, susceptibility to advertising, and other such factors. As one expert stated, "Food symbolizes much of what we think about ourselves."

Childhood Experiences

The food environment in which we are raised has a significant effect on food choices later in life. Environment reflects social and cultural preferences, which in turn are influenced by monetary constraints, limitations in the food supply, parental decisions about introduction of new foods to children, and an array of other variables. Innate food preferences do exist, such as the universal enjoyment of sweet foods and the dislike of sour or bitter substances. It is possible, however, to modify these preferences through the process of conditioning or learning. Some people learn, for example, to like very hot and spicy foods or foods that are very salty.

Social Situations

Special occasions are associated with the serving of specific foods. Foods often represent long established traditions within a family or cultural group. Also, family schedules dictate the family mealtime group. The traditional family meal occurs less frequently now than in times past and busy schedules often lead to eating outside the home. Some Americans have developed a pattern of **"grazing"** as opposed to "meal-eating." Negative nutritional effects may follow.

Grazing
Informal descriptive label for food pattern of frequent small snacks throughout the day rather than more formal regular meals. Term taken from animal pattern of constant eating in a pastureland.

Financial Resources

Family income certainly determines the kinds of foods selected. More affluent people tend to purchase more fresh vegetables and fruits and more meat, poultry, and fish. Income also dictates in most families the pattern of eating away from home. However, since cost of food in the United States is *relatively* inexpensive, differences in food choices of Americans are less than one might suspect.

Advertising

Billions of dollars are spent annually to entice the public to choose certain foods. While the impact of such efforts was minimal at one time, the sophistication of modern advertising has markedly affected our pattern of product selection today. While some of the advertising may promote important nutrition considerations, emphasis is often placed on sweets and other "goodies." Whatever the case, the force of advertising is now recognized to be substantial. This is true not only in the supermarket but also in the fast-food restaurant industry.

Daily Routine

While we think of America as a society with much variation, a close look at any individual often discloses that the patterns of daily living include a rather limited food menu. People become locked into food choices that they enjoy, are readily available and affordable, and don't test their limited wishes to stray from "what is familiar." Children raised in an environment in which trying new foods is encouraged may very well accept the challenges of new food experiences better than children exposed to limited options.

Health Concerns

A growing number of Americans are concerned enough about health that they select foods in part based upon this factor. Some surveys indicate that half of the U.S. population considers health maintenance important when shopping for or ordering food. Real attention to proper food choices for promotion of health was sparked in the late 1960s by the "back to nature" movement, along with the recommendations of the American Heart Association that fat and cholesterol may contribute to coronary heart disease. Recent years have seen the publication of evidence that some cancers may also be "preventable" with choice of a good diet. These findings have not gone unnoticed by the general public. The food industry recognizes this and is now providing an array of products that are specifically of low-calorie low-fat composition. Also, government regulatory agencies are in the process of reforming food labeling to present sound nutrition information for the consumer. These directions are very likely to continue to the year 2000 and beyond.

LIFE CYCLE NUTRITIONAL NEEDS

From the moment of conception, the human organism depends on nutrition for growth, development, and long term survival. Prior to birth, the fetus must draw from maternal nutrient supplies and this process may continue after birth if the mother chooses to breastfeed her baby. Ultimately, an outside food supply provides the ongoing nutritional support for life. This nutritional support may come from both animal and plant food sources. An unlimited number of food combinations are known to satisfy nutrient needs. Consequently, peoples of the world consuming vastly different foods and food mixtures demonstrate satisfactory growth and health.

Stages of the Life Cycle

Fetal and maternal needs. The **mammalian** fetus is completely dependent on nutritional support from the mother. The quantitative requirements are very small in the beginning but increase gradually until birth. During this time it is absolutely essential that a correct equilibrium be maintained among the various nutrients circulating in the maternal blood. This required biochemical **milieu** depends entirely on the mother's diet, her nutritional stores, and her metabolic idiosyncrasies. The adverse effects of nutritional-biochemical imbalance during **gestation** have been examined most frequently in animal models. Fortuitous observations of human experience, however, have contributed to our slowly growing knowledge base in this field. In general, the repercussions of abnormal nutrition depend on the stage at which a given nutrient factor acts, the nature of the nutrient considered, the intensity of the disequilibrium, and the species or strain of the animal studied. The types of repercussion are very different. They include death, tissue alterations, delayed growth, alterations of cellular differentiation, and malformations. Improvement in pregnancy outcome depends in part on motivating the pregnant woman to establish satisfactory diet and supplementation practices.[1]

Lactation. Establishment of **lactation** and continued production of sufficient high-quality milk also demands that the mother consume an adequate diet. While lactation is a high-priority physiologic process maintained even in the face of serious nutritional deprivation, without continuing nutritional support the quantity of milk production is generally hampered and milk quality eventually deteriorates. In either case, the nutritional well-being of the mother will be compromised as will eventually her health and preparedness for "mothering."[1,2]

Infancy. The first year after birth is a time in the life cycle when many changes occur in relation to food and nutrient intake. A number of factors influence these dramatic changes: (1) a rapid then gradually declining rate of physical growth, (2) maturation of oral structures and functions, (3) development of fine and gross motor skills, and (4) establishment of relationships with parents and family. As a result of these tremendous changes, infants prepared at birth to suck liquids from a nipple are at 1 year of age making attempts to feed themselves table foods with culturally defined utensils. The need for

Milieu
(Fr *milieu,* surroundings) Environment, social or physical. An important concept in nutrition, referring to both external socio-physical setting and internal biochemical environments, and the interacting balances between them.

Gestation
(L *gestare,* to bear) Intrauterine fetal growth period from conception to birth.

Neuromotor
(Gr *neuron*, nerve; L *motorium*, movement center) Movement involving nerve impulses to muscles.

nutrients and energy depends on the infant's requirement for physical growth, maintenance, and energy expenditure. The foods offered to infants reflect culturally accepted practices. Infants' acceptance of food is influenced by **neuromotor** maturation and by their interactions with their parents. Well-nourished children at any month during infancy will consume a variety of food combinations.[3]

Preschool years. During the preschool years, the decreased rates of growth bring decreased appetites. Children learn to understand language and to talk and ask for food. Development of gross motor skills permits them to learn to feed themselves and to prepare simple foods such as cereal and milk and sandwiches. They learn about food and the way it feels, tastes, and smells. Preschool children learn to eat a wider variety of textures and kinds of food, give up the bottle, and drink from a cup. They demand independence and refuse help in many tasks, such as self-feeding, in which they are not yet skillful. As they grow older, they become less interested in food and more interested in their environment. They test and learn the limits of acceptable behavior.[3]

School age children. Between preschool and adolescence, children continue to grow slowly and demonstrate maturation of fine and gross motor skills. Individual personality develops and degree of independence increases. All of these changes influence the amounts of food consumed, the manner in which it is eaten, and the acceptability of specific foods. Food habits, likes, and dislikes are established, some of which are transient, but many of which form the base for a lifetime of food experiences. Environmental influences and parental behaviors reinforce or extinguish food-related behaviors. Parents need to provide appropriate foods and supportive guidance so that appropriate food patterns develop. The nutrition knowledge of the parents and other care providers positively influences children's requests for and acceptance of various foods. School feeding programs provide an opportunity for nutrition education.[3]

Adolescence. The adolescent period is a unique stage in the process of growth and development. It is characterized by a wide variability in norms of growth, increasingly independent behavior, and the testing of adult roles. This critical period of human development occurs at physiologic, psychologic, and social levels. These tumultuous changes do not occur simultaneously but at varying rates. Although adolescence may be defined as the teenage years between 12 and 20, physical maturation and changes in nutrient requirements actually begin at younger years and sometimes extend into the third decade.[3,4]

Teenagers assume greater responsibility for decision-making in their own lives. In contrast to younger children, adolescents themselves most often determine their food intake. Their food choices reflect various factors including family eating patterns, peer influence, media, appetite, and food availability. Some of these factors can be positive for nutritional quality and others may leave a lot to be desired. Body image plays a very important role in the eating behaviors of adolescents. Eating disorders account for a large number of nutritional concerns during adolescence.[3,4]

Adulthood. The adult years span a number of decades during which nutritional needs change very little, but family circumstances and lifestyle often undergo substantial change. Marital status, living environment, job setting and responsibilities, income, and a variety of other factors significantly impact upon specific food choices and long term dietary patterns. Ideally, a major focus during these years is health promotion and disease prevention. This goal entails, among other things, establishing nutritional practices that will maximize health and minimize risk for developing preventable chronic diseases. Appropriate practices vary somewhat among individuals due in large part to differences in genetic bases. Of primary concern, however, is maintaining desirable body fatness by eating moderate amounts of a wide variety of wholesome foods.[5-7]

Older adults. Persons who are 65 years of age or older comprise the fastest growing segment of the population in most developed countries (Fig. 1-1). Of these older indi-

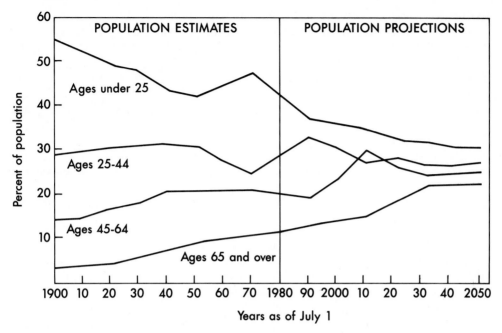

FIG. 1-1   Trend in age distribution of U.S. population (including Armed Forces overseas).
From Insel PM and Roth WT: Core concepts in health, ed 5, Mountain View, Calif, 1988, Mayfield Publishing.

viduals, 95% live within the community, many of them on incomes barely sufficient for survival. Financial limitations adversely affect food purchasing power. However, an assortment of other factors also contribute to the increased prevalence of malnutrition in this age group. Important contributors to the problem include loneliness, depression, oral discomfort, and chronic diseases, all of which lead to poor appetite. Physical and mental handicaps may limit the ability to shop for food or to prepare it. Use of an assortment of drugs, both prescription and over-the-counter, may further interfere with the maintenance of satisfactory nutritional status. The aging process itself may reduce nutrient absorption, increase urinary loss, and interfere with normal pathways of nutrient utilization.[8]

GUIDELINES FOR HEALTH MAINTENANCE AND DISEASE PREVENTION

During the past 10 years, understanding of the role of nutrition in health promotion and disease prevention has improved. Relationships between specific nutrient deficiencies and inferior health status have long been recognized. But in recent years, diet has been associated with a number of chronic diseases, such as cardiovascular disease, cancer, and diabetes. The focus of concern about human nutrition has moved from the issues of nutritional deficiencies toward increased emphasis on chronic disease prevention and health maintenance in all phases of the life cycle.

The American public has been presented with a variety of dietary recommendations for health maintenance and disease prevention. The federal government of the United States has provided the Recommended Dietary Allowances, the most recent issue of which is shown in Table 1-2.[9] This famous directive, now in its tenth edition, specifies its

TABLE 1-2 *Food and Nutrition Board, National Academy of Sciences: National Research Council Recommended Dietary Allowances,[a] Revised 1989*

Category	Age (years)	Weight[b] (kg)	Weight[b] (lb)	Height[b] (cm)	Height[b] (inches)	Protein (g)	Fat-Soluble Vitamins Vita-min A (µg RE)[c]	Vita-min D (µg)[d]	Vita-min E (mg α-TE)[e]	Vita-min K (µg)
Infants	0.0-0.5	6	13	60	24	13	375	7.5	3	5
	0.5-1.0	9	20	71	28	14	375	10	4	10
Children	1-3	13	29	90	35	16	400	10	6	15
	4-6	20	44	112	44	24	500	10	7	20
	7-10	28	62	132	52	28	700	10	7	30
Males	11-14	45	99	157	62	45	1000	10	10	45
	15-18	66	145	176	69	59	1000	10	10	65
	19-24	72	160	177	70	58	1000	10	10	70
	25-50	79	174	176	70	63	1000	5	10	80
	51+	77	170	173	68	63	1000	5	10	80
Females	11-14	46	101	157	62	46	800	10	8	45
	15-18	55	120	163	64	44	800	10	8	55
	19-24	58	128	164	65	46	800	10	8	60
	25-50	63	138	163	64	50	800	5	8	65
	51+	65	143	160	63	50	800	5	8	65
Pregnant						60	800	10	10	65
Lactating										
1st 6 months						65	1300	10	12	65
2nd 6 months						62	1200	10	11	65

[a]The allowances, expressed as average daily intakes over time, are intended to provide for individual variations among most normal persons as they live in the United States under usual environmental stresses. Diets should be based on a variety of common foods in order to provide other nutrients for which human requirements have been less well defined. See text for detailed discussion of allowances and of nutrients not tabulated.

[b]Weights and heights of Reference Adults are actual medians for the US population of the designated age, as reported by NHANES II. The use of these figures does not imply that the height-to-weight ratios are ideal.

[c]Retinol equivalents. 1 retinol equivalent = 1 µg retinol or 6 µg β-carotene.

[d]As cholecalciferol. 10 µg cholecalciferol = 400 IU of vitamin D.

[e]α-Tocopherol equivalents. 1 mg d-α tocopherol = 1 α-TE.

[f]1 NE (niacin equivalent) is equal to 1 mg of niacin or 60 mg of dietary tryptophan.

TABLE 1-2   *Food and Nutrition Board, National Academy of Sciences: National Research Council Recommended Dietary Allowances,[a] Revised 1989—cont'd*

Water-Soluble Vitamins							Minerals						
Vita-min C (mg)	Thiamin (mg)	Ribo-flavin (mg)	Niacin (mg NE)[f]	Vita-min B$_6$ (mg)	Folate (µg)	Vita-min B$_{12}$ (µg)	Calcium (mg)	Phos-phorus (mg)	Mag-nesium (mg)	Iron (mg)	Zinc (mg)	Iodine (µg)	Sele-nium (µg)
30	0.3	0.4	5	0.3	25	0.3	400	300	40	6	5	40	10
35	0.4	0.5	6	0.6	35	0.5	600	500	60	10	5	50	15
40	0.7	0.8	9	1.0	50	0.7	800	800	80	10	10	70	20
45	0.9	1.1	12	1.1	75	1.0	800	800	120	10	10	90	20
45	1.0	1.2	13	1.4	100	1.4	800	800	170	10	10	120	30
50	1.3	1.5	17	1.7	150	2.0	1200	1200	270	12	15	150	40
60	1.5	1.8	20	2.0	200	2.0	1200	1200	400	12	15	150	50
60	1.5	1.7	19	2.0	200	2.0	1200	1200	350	10	15	150	70
60	1.5	1.7	19	2.0	200	2.0	800	800	350	10	15	150	70
60	1.2	1.4	15	2.0	200	2.0	800	800	350	10	15	150	70
50	1.1	1.3	15	1.4	150	2.0	1200	1200	280	15	12	150	45
60	1.1	1.3	15	1.5	180	2.0	1200	1200	300	15	12	150	50
60	1.1	1.3	15	1.6	180	2.0	1200	1200	280	15	12	150	55
60	1.1	1.3	15	1.6	180	2.0	800	800	280	15	12	150	55
60	1.0	1.2	13	1.6	180	2.0	800	800	280	10	12	150	55
70	1.5	1.6	17	2.2	400	2.2	1200	1200	320	30	15	175	65
95	1.6	1.8	20	2.1	280	2.6	1200	1200	355	15	19	200	75
90	1.6	1.7	20	2.1	260	2.6	1200	1200	340	15	16	200	75

guidelines in gram and milligram amounts. For professionals, this series of recommendations is useful in evaluating the quality of diets of groups of people. More understandable directions are presented by the U.S. Department of Agriculture (USDA) and the U.S. Department of Health and Human Services (USDHHS) in the Dietary Guidelines for Americans listed in Table 1-3, and by the National Academy of Sciences in their publication *Diet and Health,* summarized in Table 1-4.[10,11]

In 1980, the Surgeon General of the United States included specific nutrition objectives in his recommendations for the health promotion of Americans.[12] In 1990, these objectives have been updated to define the nation's goals for the year 2000, as shown in the box on p. 11.[13] Among the broad goals to be achieved by 2000 are:

- Increase the number of healthy years for Americans.
- Reduce health disparities among segments of Americans.
- Achieve equal access to preventive health services for all Americans.

Among the major nutrition objectives identified are reducing overweight and dietary fat intake. Just how each of these objectives should be addressed during the various stages of the life cycle will be examined throughout this text.

TABLE 1-3 *Dietary Guidelines for Americans*

Eat a variety of foods
Maintain desirable body weight
Choose a diet low in fat, saturated fat, and cholesterol
Choose a diet with plenty of vegetables, fruits, and grain products
Use sugars in moderation
Use salt and sodium in moderation
If you drink alcoholic beverages, do so in moderation

From Report of the Dietary Guidelines Advisory Committee for Americans, Washington, DC, 1990, USDA.

TABLE 1-4 *1989 National Academy of Sciences Recommendations (Diet and Health)*

- Reduce total *fat* intake to 30% or less of kcalories. Reduce saturated fatty acid intake to less than 10% of kcalories, and the intake of cholesterol to less than 300 mg daily.
- Increase intake of starches and other *complex carbohydrates.*
- Maintain *protein* intake at moderate levels.
- Balance food intake and physical activity to maintain appropriate *body weight.*
- For those who drink *alcoholic beverages,* limit consumption to the equivalent of less than 1 oz of pure alcohol in a single day. Pregnant women should avoid alcoholic beverages.
- Limit total daily intake of *salt* (sodium chloride) to 6 g or less.
- Maintain adequate *calcium* intake.
- Avoid taking dietary *supplements* in excess of the RDA in any one day.
- Maintain an optimal intake of *fluoride,* particularly during the years of primary and secondary tooth formation and growth.

Reprinted with permission from Diet and health, © 1989 by the National Academy of Sciences. Published by National Academy Press, Washington, DC.

ONE STEP FURTHER

The Public Health Service National Nutrition Objectives for 2000

Looking to the year 2000, the U.S. Surgeon General has identified 21 specific nutrition-related objectives to improve the nation's health.

1. Reduce coronary heart disease to no more than 100 per 100,000 people.
2. Reverse the rise in cancer deaths to achieve a rate of no more than 130 per 100,000 people.
3. Reduce overweight to a prevalence of no more than 20% among people aged 20 and older and no more than 15% among adolescents aged 12 through 19.
4. Reduce growth retardation among low-income children aged 5 and younger to less than 10%.
5. Reduce dietary fat intake to an average of 30% of calories or less, and average saturated fat intake to less than 10% of calories among people aged 2 and older.
6. Increase complex carbohydrates and fiber-containing foods in the diets of adults to five or more daily servings for vegetables and fruits, and to six or more daily servings for grain products.
7. Increase to at least 50% the proportion of overweight people aged 12 and older who have adopted sound dietary practices combined with regular physical activity to attain an appropriate weight.
8. Increase calcium intake so at least 50% of youth aged 12 through 24 and 50% of pregnant and lactating women consume three or more servings daily of foods rich in calcium, and at least 50% of people aged 25 and older consume two or more servings daily.
9. Decrease salt and sodium intake so at least 65% of home meal preparers prepare foods without adding salt, at least 80% of people avoid using salt at the table, and at least 40% of adults regularly purchase foods modified or lower in sodium.
10. Reduce iron deficiency to less than 3% among children aged 1 through 4 and among women of childbearing age.
11. Increase to at least 75% the proportion of mothers who breastfeed their babies in early postpartum period and to at least 50% the proportion who continue breastfeeding until their babies are 5 to 6 months old.
12. Increase to at least 75% the proportion of parents and caregivers who use feeding practices that prevent baby bottle tooth decay.
13. Increase to at least 85% the proportion of people aged 18 and older who use food labels to make nutritious food selections.
14. Achieve useful and informative labeling for virtually all processed food and at least 40% of fresh meats, poultry, fish, fruits, vegetables, baked goods, and ready-to-eat carry-away food.
15. Increase to at least 5,000 brand names the availability of processed food products that are reduced in fat and saturated fat.
16. Increase to at least 90% the proportion of restaurants and institutional food service operations that offer identifiable low-fat, low-calorie food choices, consistent with the *Dietary Guidelines for Americans*.
17. Increase to at least 90% the proportion of school lunch and breakfast services and child care foodservices with menus that are consistent with the nutrition principles in the *Dietary Guidelines for Americans*.
18. Increase to at least 80% the receipt of home foodservices by people aged 65 and older who have difficulty in preparing their own meals or are otherwise in need of home-delivered meals.
19. Increase to at least 75% the proportion of the nation's schools that provide nutrition education from preschool through 12th grade.
20. Increase to at least 50% the proportion of worksites with 50 or more employees that offer nutrition education and/or weight management programs for their employees.
21. Increase to at least 75% the proportion of primary care providers who provide nutrition assessment and counseling and/or referral to qualified nutritionists or dietitians.

From US Public Health Service: Healthy people 2000—national health promotion and disease prevention objectives, Washington, DC, 1990, USDHHS-PHS, US Government Printing Office.

DIET THERAPY AS A COMPONENT OF DISEASE MANAGEMENT

While the maintenance of health and prevention of disease is a priority focus throughout the life cycle, circumstances arise in every stage of life when dietary interventions are required to treat disease, trauma, or other undesirable situations. The basic principles governing diet therapy are simple: meet nutritional needs while modifying the diet to satisfy the health problem under treatment. Some changes in diet may be easily implemented, but others require special planning and in some cases major changes from established food habits. The degree to which an individual—with the help of family, friends, health care providers, and others—is able to follow short term or permanent changes in diet varies in each case. The needed diet changes may impact significantly on quality of life and in some cases even on chances of survival. While the focus of this book is health maintenance and disease prevention, some discussion of necessity will include selected problems that require diet and nutrition intervention.

Summary

Growth, development, reproduction, and the maintenance of health require that the human organism satisfy basic biologic needs. Nutrition is a basic need that can be met minimally to prevent death or optimally to help achieve maximum genetic potential. The goal of this book is to approach the issue of optimum nutrition from the developmental framework of specific stages of the life cycle. Attention to normal needs and feeding practices will predominate but management strategies for selected special problems will be addressed. For more detailed coverage of special problems requiring diet therapy, the reader is referred to other available clinical texts.

Review Questions

1. Outline key functions of the basic nutrients.
2. Describe major influences on food choices of Americans.
3. Define key nutritional concerns at each stage of the life cycle.
4. Summarize the National Nutrition Objectives for the year 2000.

References

1. Worthington-Roberts B and Williams SR: Nutrition in pregnancy and lactation, ed 4, St Louis, 1989, Times Mirror/Mosby College Publishing.
2. Lawrence RA: Breastfeeding: a guide for the medical profession, ed 3, St Louis, 1989, Times Mirror/Mosby College Publishing.
3. Pipes P: Nutrition in infancy and childhood, ed 4, St Louis, 1989, Times Mirror/Mosby College Publishing.
4. Mahan LK and Rees JM: Nutrition in adolescence, St Louis, 1984, Times Mirror/Mosby College Publishing.
5. Pennington JAT: Dietary patterns and practices, Clin Nutr 5(1):17, Jan/Feb, 1986.
6. Crosetti AF and Guthrie HA: Alternate eating patterns and the role of age, sex, selection, and snacking in nutritional quality, Clin Nutr 5(1):34, Jan/Feb, 1986.
7. Lecos C: America's changing diet, FDA Consumer, p. 4, October 1985.
8. Schlenker ED: Nutrition in aging, St Louis, 1984, Times Mirror/Mosby College Publishing.

9. National Research Council: Recommended dietary allowances, ed 10, Washington, DC, 1989, National Academy Press.
10. US Departments of Agriculture and Health and Human Services: Dietary Guidelines for Americans, Washington, DC, 1990, US Government Printing Office.
11. National Research Council: Diet and health: implications for reducing chronic disease risk, Washington, DC, 1989, National Academy Press.
12. US Department of Health and Human Services, Public Health Service: Promoting health/preventing disease: objectives for the nation, Washington, DC, 1980, US Government Printing Office.
13. US Department of Health and Human Services, Public Health Service: Healthy people 2000: national health promotion and disease prevention objectives, Washington, DC, 1990, US Government Printing Office.

CHAPTER

2

Nutrition and Assessment Basics

Sue Rodwell Williams

Basic Concepts

✦✦✦

✔ *An integral component of health promotion for all persons throughout the life cycle is optimal personal and community nutrition.*

✔ *Through their specific and interdependent physiologic roles, certain nutrients in the food we eat are essential to life, health, and well-being.*

✔ *Changing nutrient needs throughout the life cycle relate to normal growth and development and resulting changes in body composition.*

✔ *The overall process of nutrition assessment reflects individual and community nutritional status and provides an important basis for personal health care plans and public nutrition intervention programs.*

*W*e live in a rapidly changing world, one of changing environment, food supply, scientific knowledge, and population. Our numbers are increasing not only in total population and age distribution, but also in ethnic diversity. Then within individual environments and communities, with physical growth and development through the life cycle come personality changes and with them come changing personal needs and goals. These *constant changes* of life must be in *balance* to produce healthy living at any age.

Thus to be realistic, within these life concepts of change and balance our study of life-cycle nutrition focuses on health promotion through good food and its basic nutrients and an on-going assessment of nutritional status and health needs. Because the background knowledge of students using this book concerning nutrition varies widely and to set the overall learning focus, we provide a brief overview of nutrient and assessment basics in terms of the three most fundamental physiologic components that must be present for the human body to survive and remain healthy: (1) *energy* to do its work, (2) *building materials* to maintain its form and functions, and (3) *control agents* to regulate these processes efficiently.

NUTRIENTS: PHYSIOLOGIC ROLES
Macronutrients and Energy

Carbohydrate: basic fuel source. All three of the macronutrients in our food—carbohydrate, fat, and protein—can be **metabolized** to yield body **energy.** However, the body uses carbohydrate as its basic fuel supply, along with fat, and reserves protein mainly for its unique tissue-building role. In the human energy system, this major carbohydrate fuel comes from the two forms of carbohydrate foods we eat—starches and sugars. To produce energy from a basic fuel supply, a successful energy system must be able to do three things: (1) change the basic "raw" fuel to a refined fuel form that the system is designed to use, (2) carry this refined fuel to the places that need it, and (3) burn this refined fuel at these energy production sites in the special equipment set up to do it. Far more efficient than any man-made machine, the body easily does these three things. It digests its basic food fuel, carbohydrate, changing it to the refined fuel **glucose,** then absorbs this refined fuel and transports it through blood circulation to the cells that constantly need it. There glucose is broken down in the cell's highly specific equipment, releasing energy through its intricate biochemical pathways, **glycolysis** and the **citric acid cycle,** of cell metabolism. In this overall process, glucose is broken down to its basic carbon and hydrogen atoms and combined with oxygen, yielding energy as the cell's energy currency compound **adenosine triphosphate (ATP),** with its high-energy phosphate bonds, and releasing carbon dioxide and water as end products.

Metabolism
(Gr *metaballein,* to change) Sum of all the various biochemical and physiologic processes by which the body grows and maintains itself (anabolism) and reshapes tissues (catabolism), transforming energy to do its work.

Glycolysis
Initial energy production pathway by which 6-carbon glucose is changed to active 3-carbon fragments of acetyl CoA, the fuel ready for final energy production.

Citric acid cycle
Final energy production pathway in the cell mitochrondria that transforms the ultimate fuel acetyl CoA from carbohydrate and fat, capturing energy for cell metabolism in high-energy phosphate bonds.

Adenosine triphosphate (ATP)
The energy currency of the cell, binding energy in its high-energy phosphate bonds for release as these bonds are split.

TABLE* 2-1   *Summary of Carbohydrate Classes

Chemical Class Name	Class Members	Sources

Polysaccharides
  Multiple sugars, complex carbohydrates
	Starch	Grains and grain products
		  Cereal, bread, crackers, and other baked goods
		  Pasta
		  Rice, corn, bulgar
		Legumes
		Potatoes and other vegetables

	Glycogen	Animal tissues, liver and muscle meats
	Dietary fiber	Whole grains Fruits Vegetables Seeds, nuts, skins
Disaccharides Double sugars, simple carbohydrates	Sucrose	"Table" sugar: sugar cane, sugar beets Molasses
	Lactose	Milk
	Maltose	Starch digestion, intermediate Sweetener in food products
Monosaccharides Single sugars, simple carbohydrates	Glucose (dextrose)	Starch digestion, final Corn syrup (large use in processed foods)
	Fructose	Fruits, honey
	Galactose	Lactose (milk)

From Williams SR: Basic nutrition and diet therapy, ed 8, St Louis, 1988, Times Mirror/Mosby College Publishing.

The classes of food carbohydrates vary from simple to complex structures and thus differ in the speed with which they yield energy (Table 2-1). **Simple carbohydrates**—sugars—made up of only one or two sugar (saccharide) units are broken down easily releasing energy quickly. On the other hand, **complex carbohydrates**—polysaccharides—are large complex compounds of many saccharide units. For example, starch, the most significant polysaccharide in human nutrition, is made up of both straight-chained coiled structure (amylose, 15% to 20% of the molecule) and many branching chains (amylopectin, 80% to 85% of the molecule). Each of the multiple branching chains is composed of 24 to 30 sugar units of glucose, which are gradually split off in digestion to supply a steady source of energy over a period of time. **Glycogen,** the body's small amount of stored carbohydrate, sometimes called *animal starch,* has a similar structure and sustains energy during brief fasting periods such as sleep hours.

Certain other carbohydrate compounds, fibrous polysaccharides, are nondigestible because humans lack the necessary enzymes to split their particular saccharide links. However, these compounds, especially those that are soluble, contribute valuable **dietary fiber** essential to health (Tables 2-2 and 2-3).[1,2] A listing of some major food sources of dietary fiber is provided in the Appendix for reference.

Fat: concentrated energy. Fats supply a concentrated fuel source for the body's energy system, yielding over twice the energy value of carbohydrate. Because the body can easily convert carbohydrate to fat and store it in various body **adipose tissues,** fat is an important

Complex carbohydrates
Main dietary carbohydrate, the polysaccharide starch in varied foods such as legumes, grains, breads, cereals, and potatoes.

Glycogen
Briefly stored form of carbohydrate in the body cells, available for energy fuel during fasting periods of sleep; built up in larger amounts by high starch meals prior to endurance athletic events for sustained energy.

Dietary fiber
Nondigestible form of carbohydate; of nutritional importance in gastrointestinal disease such as diverticulosis and management of serum lipid and glucose levels in risk-reduction related to chronic conditions such as heart disease and diabetes.

Adipose tissue
Fat storage sites composed of adipocytes (fat cells).

TABLE 2-2 *Summary of Dietary Fiber Classes*

Class	Source	Function
Cellulose	Main cell wall constituent of plants	Holds water; reduces elevated colonic intraluminal pressure; binds zinc
Noncellulose polysaccharides		Slows gastric emptying; provides fermentable material for colonic bacteria with production of gas and volatile fatty acids; binds bile acids and cholesterol
Gums	Secretions of plants	
Mucilages	Plant secretions and seeds	
Algal polysaccharides	Algae, seaweeds	
Pectin substances	Intercellular cement plant material	
Hemicellulose	Cell wall plant material	Holds water and increases stool bulk; reduces elevated colonic pressure; binds bile acids
Lignin	Woody part of plants	Antioxidant; binds bile acids, cholesterol, and metals

From Williams SR: Basic nutrition and diet therapy, ed 8, St Louis, 1988, Times Mirror/Mosby College Publishing.

TABLE 2-3 *Summary of Soluble and Insoluble Fibers in Total Dietary Fiber*

Insoluble	Soluble
Cellulose	Gums
Most hemicelluloses	Mucilages
Lignin	Algal polysaccharides
	Most pectins

form of body fuel for energy reserves. Food fats from both animal and plant sources yield the same amount of energy, but have significantly different relationships to health. Excess dietary fat, especially fat from animal sources, and excess dietary cholesterol, which is synthesized only by animals and can only be supplied in the diet by animal food sources, are health risk factors.[1] The dietary guidelines for Americans recommend lowering our daily dietary fat intake to 30% of the total kilocalories.[3] Do you know how much fat you are eating? Try calculating it by the directions given in the box below.

Protein: available energy as needed. As indicated, carbohydrate and fat are primary fuel sources in the body's energy system. However, sometimes protein may furnish additional body energy, but it is a less efficient source. The fuel value of protein is the same as that of carbohydrate.

Measurement of nutrient energy value. The energy yielded by the macronutrients is measured in **kilocalories** (kcalories or kcal). Carbohydrate yields 4 kcal/g, fat 9 kcal/g, and protein 4 kcal/g. These values are called their respective fuel factors. The energy values of various foods, therefore, are based on their carbohydrate, fat, and protein composition. Any portion of these macronutrients not used for energy is restructured for body tissue storage as glycogen or fat for fuel use between meals, or for use in synthesizing other metabolic compounds needed in the body. Excess energy intake (kcalories) over energy use by the body to do its work results in weight gain. Insufficient energy intake to meet body needs results in weight loss. Any alcohol in beverages is also metabolized by the body to yield 7 kcal/g. Excess alcohol intake, therefore, is harmful in terms of both weight gain (when it is converted to fat and stored) and its toxic effects.

Kilocalorie (kcalorie, kcal)
Unit of measure of energy produced in the body by the energy-yielding macronutrients carbohydrate, fat, and protein.

Amino Acids and Protein Metabolism

Amino acids: basic building material. All protein, whether in our bodies or in the food we eat, is made up of its building units, the **amino acids.** These amino acids are joined by peptide linkages in unique chain sequence to form specific proteins. When we

Amino acids
Structural units of protein that supply essential nitrogen.

ONE STEP FURTHER

How Much Fat Are You Eating?

- Keep an accurate record of everything you eat or drink for 1 day. Be sure to estimate and add amounts of all fat or other nutrient seasonings used with your foods. (If you want a more representative picture and have a computer available with nutrient analysis programming, keep a 1-week record and calculate an average of the 7 days.)
- Calculate the total kilocalories (kcal) and grams of each of the energy nutrients (carbohydrate, fat, and protein) in everything you eat. Multiply the total grams of each energy nutrient by its respective fuel value:

$$\text{fat} \underline{\hspace{1cm}} \text{g} \times 9 = \underline{\hspace{1cm}} \text{kcal}$$
$$\text{protein} \underline{\hspace{1cm}} \text{g} \times 4 = \underline{\hspace{1cm}} \text{kcal}$$
$$\text{carbohydrate} \underline{\hspace{1cm}} \text{g} \times 4 = \underline{\hspace{1cm}} \text{kcal}$$

- Calculate the percentage of each energy nutrient in your total diet:

$$\frac{\text{Fat kcal}}{\text{Total kcal}} \times 100 = \% \text{ fat kcal in diet}$$

- Compare with fat in American diet (40% to 45%); with the U.S. dietary goals (25% to 30%).

From Williams SR: Basic nutrition and diet therapy, ed 8, St Louis, 1988, Times Mirror/Mosby College Publishing.

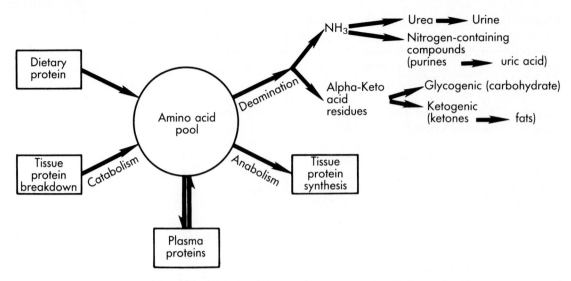

FIG. 2-1   Balance between protein compartments and amino acid pool.

eat protein foods, the protein (for example, casein in milk and cheese, albumin in egg white, or gluten in wheat products) is broken down into its constituent amino acids in the digestive process. According to need, from the body's overall metabolic "pool" of amino acids (Fig. 2-1), specific ones are then reassembled in the body in the *specific* order to form *specific* tissue proteins (for example, collagen in connective tissue, myosin in muscle tissue, hemoglobin in red blood cells [see Fig. 2-2 on p. 26], cell enzymes, or insulin) that are required by the body.

Role as nitrogen supplier. Amino acids are named for their chemical nature. The word *amino* refers to the monovalent chemical group—NH_2. Like carbohydrates and fats, proteins have a basic structure of carbon, hydrogen, and oxygen. But unlike fats and carbohydrates, which contain no nitrogen, protein is about 16% nitrogen. In addition, some proteins contain small but valuable amounts of minerals such as sulfur.

Essential amino acids. Nine amino acids are now classed as **essential amino acids** because the body cannot manufacture them, or cannot do so in sufficient amounts. Thus the term *essential* as used here means that they are necessary in the diet. In the strict physiologic sense, all amino acids are essential in overall body metabolism. Although the ninth amino acid added to the essential list, histidine, has previously been known as essential for infants, it was not demonstrated to be required by adults until recently.[4,5] The nine essential amino acids are histidine, isoleucine, leucine, lysine, methionine, phenylalanine, threonine, tryptophan, and valine (Table 2-4) (see the box on p. 19). Applying this concept of essentiality to our dietary food choices, we would need to obtain all of these nine essential amino acids in our diet to meet our protein needs for tissue growth and maintenance throughout the life cycle. A protein food that supplies all of these essential amino acids in sufficient quantities to meet human needs is called a **complete protein.** Since only foods of animal source—milk, cheese, egg, and meat—are complete proteins, a person following a vegetarian food pattern would need to plan carefully to obtain sufficient quantities of essential amino acids by using combinations of complementary plant proteins, as described in the box on p. 19. During the growth years, arginine is also essential to meet normal childhood growth demands. Although arginine is synthesized by the body, it may not be made in sufficient amounts to meet the rapid growth of infants, especially premature infants, and young children.[5]

Essential amino acid
An amino acid that the body cannot synthesize in sufficient amounts to meet body needs so it must be supplied by the diet, hence a *dietary* essential for nine such specific amino acids.

TABLE 2-4 *Amino Acids Required in Human Nutrition, Grouped According to Nutritional (Dietary) Essentiality*

Essential Amino Acids	Semiessential Amino Acids*	Nonessential Amino Acids
Histidine	Arginine	Alanine
Isoleucine	Cystine (cysteine)	Asparagine
Leucine	Tyrosine	Aspartic acid
Lysine		Glutamic acid
Methionine		Glutamine
Phenylalanine		Glycine
Threonine		Hydroxyproline
Tryptophan		Hydroxylysine
Valine		Proline
		Serine

*These are considered semiessential because the rate of synthesis in the body is inadequate to support growth; therefore these are essential for children.
From Williams SR: Nutrition and diet therapy, ed 6, St Louis, 1989, Times Mirror/Mosby College Publishing.

ONE STEP FURTHER

Essential Amino Acids—Nine or Eleven?—and Their Complementary Food Proteins

All of the nine essential amino acids must be supplied by the diet. But two of them, phenylalanine and methionine, have helpers as interactive backup. The body makes the amino acid tyrosine, which can spare some of the phenylalanine, and cystine, which can interact with methionine. So although there are only nine essential amino acids the body cannot make, some may speak of 11 when they add the two helpers tyrosine and cystine.

The real life concern in a vegetarian diet is to get a balanced amount of the essential amino acids to complement one another and make complete food combinations. Only three of these nine essential amino acids are critical, however, because if persons eat foods to supply enough of these three in a combined pattern, they will get sufficient amounts of the others too. These three amino acids are thus called the *limiting amino acids*—lysine, methionine, and tryptophan. Of these three, lysine is the most limiting.

The answer lies in mixing families of foods like grains, legumes, and milk products to make complementary food combinations to balance these needed amino acids. For example, grains are low in lysine and high in methionine, while legumes are just the opposite—low in methionine and high in lysine. Basically, grains and legumes will always balance one another and additions of milk products and eggs will enhance their adequacy. Here are a few sample food combination dishes to illustrate:

Rice + black-eyed peas—a Southern United States dish called "Hopping John"
Whole wheat or bulgur + soybeans + sesame seeds—protein enhanced by the addition of yogurt
Cornmeal + kidney beans—a combination in many Mexican dishes, protein enhanced by the addition of cheese
Soybeans + peanuts + brown rice + bulgur wheat—an excellent sauce dish served over the rice and wheat

Prepared with a variety of herbs, spices, onions, and garlic, to suit your taste, such dishes can supply needed nutrients and good eating.

Catabolism
Metabolic process by which tissue is broken down.

Anabolism
Metabolic process by which tissue is built up.

Deamination
Process by which the nitrogen radical (NH$_4$) is split off from amino acids, important in maintaining nitrogen balance.

Nitrogen balance
Metabolic balance between nitrogen intake in dietary protein and output in urinary nitrogen compounds such as urea and creatinine.

Nonessential amino acids. All amino acids have essential tissue-building and metabolic functions. However, as used here, the nonessential amino acids are 12 amino acids that the body can synthesize, so they are not essential in the diet.

Protein balance. The term *balance* refers to the relative intake and output of substances in the body to maintain normal levels needed for health in various circumstances during the life cycle. We can apply this concept of balance to life-sustaining protein and the nitrogen it supplies. The body's tissue proteins are constantly being broken down, a process called **catabolism,** and then resynthesized into tissue protein as needed, a process called **anabolism.** To maintain nitrogen balance, the nitrogen-containing amino part of the amino acid may be removed by a process called **deamination,** converted to ammonia (NH$_3$), and the nitrogen excreted as urea in the urine, as shown in Fig. 2-1. The remaining non-nitrogen residue can be used to make carbohydrate or fat, or reattached to an amino group ($-$NH$_2$) to make another amino acid according to need. The rate of this protein and nitrogen turnover varies in different tissues, according to their degree of metabolic activity. This process involves a continuous reshaping and rebuilding, adjusting as needed to maintain overall protein balance within the body. Also, the body maintains an internal balance between tissue protein and plasma protein. Then, in turn, these two body protein stores are further balanced with dietary protein intake. With this finely balanced system, a metabolic "pool" of amino acids from both tissue protein and dietary protein is always available to meet construction needs.

Nitrogen balance. The body's **nitrogen balance** indicates how well its tissues are being maintained. The intake and use of dietary protein is measured by the amount of nitrogen intake in the food protein and the amount of nitrogen excreted in the urine. Total 24-hour nitrogen excretion is used with calculated dietary nitrogen intake over the same 24-hour period to determine a person's nitrogen balance:

$$\text{Nitrogen balance} = \frac{\text{Protein intake}}{6.25} - (\text{Urinary urea nitrogen} + 4)$$

The formula factor of 4 in the equation represents the additional nitrogen loss through feces and skin. Urinary urea nitrogen excretion reflects metabolism of dietary protein, as the nitrogen balance formula indicates, and is a measure of the adequacy of protein nitriture. For example, 1 g of urinary nitrogen results from the digestion and metabolism of approximately 6.25 g of protein. Therefore, if for every 6.25 g of protein consumed 1 g of nitrogen is excreted in the urine, the body is said to be in nitrogen balance. This is the normal pattern in adult health, but at different times during the life cycle, or in states of malnutrition or illness, this balance may be either positive or negative.

1. **Positive nitrogen balance.** A positive nitrogen balance exists when the body takes in more nitrogen than it excretes. This means that the body is storing nitrogen by building more tissue than it is breaking down. This situation occurs normally during periods of rapid growth such as infancy, childhood, adolescence, and during pregnancy and lactation. It also occurs in persons who have been ill or malnourished and are being "built back up" with increased nourishment. In such cases protein is being stored to meet increased needs for tissue building and associated metabolic activity.

2. **Negative nitrogen balance.** A negative nitrogen balance exists when the body takes in less nitrogen than it excretes. This means that the body has an inadequate protein intake and is losing nitrogen by breaking down more tissue than it is building up. This situation occurs in states of malnutrition and illness. For example, this nitrogen imbalance is seen not only in underdeveloped countries but also in America in cases where specific protein deficiency exists, even when kcalories from carbohydrate and fat may be adequate, causing the classic protein deficiency disease

kwashiorkor.[6] Failure to maintain nitrogen balance may not become apparent for some time, but it will eventually cause loss of muscle tissue, impairment of body organs and functions, and increased susceptibility to infection. In children, negative nitrogen balance will cause growth retardation.

Primary tissue building. Protein is the fundamental structural material of every living cell in the body. In fact, the largest portion of the body, excluding the water content, is made up of protein. Body protein, mainly the lean mass of muscles, accounts for about three fourths of the dry matter in most tissues other than bone and adipose tissue.[1] Protein not only makes up the bulk of the muscles, internal organs, brain, nerves, skin, hair, and nails, but also is a vital part of regulatory substances such as enzymes, hormones, and blood plasma. All of these tissues must be constantly repaired and replaced. The primary functions of protein are to repair worn-out, wasted, or damaged tissue and to build up new tissue. Thus protein meets growth and development needs during early life and maintains tissue health during adult years.

Micronutrients and Metabolic Control

As indicated, the body uses the macronutrients carbohydrate, fat, and protein to solve its two major needs of energy production and tissue building and rebuilding to maintain life and health, processes that require thousands of interrelated physiologic and metabolic activities. However, meeting these two basic needs creates a major overall problem, that of how to establish metabolic regulation and control. To maintain life and health, all of these multiple physiologic tasks must proceed in a highly organized and orderly fashion, without which metabolic chaos, illness, and death would occur. Such order requires specific control agents. In harmony with hormones and specific partnerships with key cell enzymes, the remaining nutrients, the micronutrients vitamins and minerals, operate mainly in the key role of **coenzyme factors,** as is the case with some vitamins, or essential enzyme components, as with some minerals, required in a specific enzyme system for a particular metabolic reaction to occur.

Vitamins

From 1900 to 1950, as the discoveries of the **vitamins** occurred, two characteristics marked a compound for assignment to the vitamin group: (1) it must be a vital organic dietary substance, which is neither carbohydrate, fat, nor protein (hence noncaloric), and is necessary in only very small quantities to do special metabolic jobs or to prevent its deficiency disease; and (2) it cannot be manufactured by the body, and therefore must be supplied in food. With current knowledge, however, it has become evident that one of these organic substances—vitamin D—has been misassigned to the vitamin group. It is now known to behave as a hormone in its active form, now called vitamin D hormone, or *calcitriol,* but is still generally discussed with the vitamins in most source materials for the sake of convenience. Vitamins are usually grouped according to solubility in a medium. The fat-soluble vitamins—A, D, E, and K—are closely associated with lipids in their fate in the body. The water-soluble vitamins—B-complex and C—have fewer problems in absorption and transport throughout.

Fat-soluble vitamins. Vitamin A enters the body in two forms: (1) the preformed vitamin A from animal food sources, usually associated with lipids; and (2) the **precursor** beta-carotene pigment from plant food sources, which actually supplies about two thirds of the vitamin A necessary in human nutrition. Its major physiologic roles relate to the eye's vision cycle adaptation to light and dark and to a more generalized role in the formation and maintenance of healthy functioning epithelial tissue, the body's primary barrier to infections.

Vitamin D hormone is produced in the body, first by sunlight irradiation of a precursor

Kwashiorkor
Classic protein deficiency disease, frequently encountered in children in developing countries, but also seen in the United States in poverty areas and in metabolically stressed and debilitated hospitalized patients.

Coenzyme factors
Major metabolic role of the micronutrients vitamins and minerals as essential partners with cell enzymes in a variety of reactions in both energy and protein metabolism.

Vitamin
A non–energy-yielding micronutrient required in very small amounts for specific metabolic tasks that cannot be synthesized by the body so must be supplied in the diet.

Precursor
Substance from which another substance is produced.

cholesterol compound in the skin, intermediate product synthesis in the liver, and subsequent formation in the kidneys of the physiologically active form, *calcitriol*—1,25-dihydroxycholecalciferol [1,25($OH)_2D_3$]. Its major physiologic role is in regulation of bone and mineral metabolism, although more recent research suggests a more widespread function in controlling basic cell processes related to cellular proliferation and differentiation.[7,8]

Vitamin E has a vital physiologic role relating to its action in many tissues as an antioxidant, an agent that prevents tissue breakdown by oxygen—the process of oxidation. It acts as nature's most potent fat-soluble antioxidant, protecting the cell membrane fatty acids from damage. For example, vitamin E can protect fragile red blood cell membranes in premature infants from breaking down and causing **hemolytic anemia** (see box below).

Hemolytic anemia
(Gr *haima*, blood; *lysis*, dissolution) An anemia (reduced number of red blood cells) caused by breakdown of red blood cells and loss of their hemoglobin.

ONE STEP FURTHER

Vitamin E and Premature Infants

A medical problem found in infants, especially those born prematurely, has responded positively to vitamin E therapy. This problem is *hemolytic anemia.*

Anemia is a blood condition characterized by loss of mature functioning red blood cells. Different types of anemia are usually named according to cause, or to the nature of an abnormal nonfunctioning cell produced instead of the normal cell. In this case the name comes from the cause. The word *hemolysis* has two roots, *hemo* referring to blood and *lysis* meaning dissolving or breaking. Hemolysis is the bursting or dissolving of red blood cells and the resulting condition is hemolytic anemia.

Vitamin E can help prevent this destruction of red blood cells and the loss of their vital oxygen-carrying hemoglobin, because it is one of the body's foremost antioxidants. An oxidant is a compound, or oxygen itself, that oxidizes other compounds and in the process breaks them down or changes them. Vitamin E is readily oxidized. When there is plenty of vitamin E among other compounds exposed to an oxidant, it can take on the oxidative attack and thus protect the others. Vitamin E is fat soluble so it is found in fat-rich tissues of the body among the polyunsaturated fatty acids that make up the core of the cell membranes. The cell membranes of red blood cells are particularly rich in these polyunsaturated lipids and they are exposed to concentrated oxygen because they constantly circulate through the lungs. This would be a destructive situation were it not for the vitamin E present. It takes the oxygen itself, protecting the polyunsaturated fatty acids, and preserving the red blood cells intact to continue their life-sustaining journey throughout the body. Thus vitamin E acts as nature's most potent fat-soluble antioxidant. It interrupts the oxidative breakdown by free radicals (parts of compounds broken off by cell metabolism) in the cell, protecting the cell membrane fatty acids from the oxidative damage.

Infants fed formulas rich in polyunsaturated fatty acids and supplemented with iron (an oxidant) may develop hemolytic anemia as the fragile red blood cell membranes break down due to the high cell oxidative process and the induced deficiency of vitamin E. This protective need for increased vitamin E is especially great with small premature infants fed formulas containing iron, which acts as an oxidant, and high concentrations of polyunsaturated fatty acids, which are vulnerable to oxidative breakdown. To avoid this problem and comply with American Academy of Pediatrics recommendations, manufacturers have increased the vitamin E and lowered the iron in formulas for premature infants. Now the improved formula ratio of vitamin E, polyunsaturated fatty acids, and iron no longer makes additional supplement necessary to prevent hemolytic anemia.

Adapted from Bieri JG, et al: Medical uses of vitamin E, N Engl J Med 308(18):1063, 1983; and National Research Council, Food and Nutrition Board: Recommended dietary allowances, ed 10, Washington, DC, 1989, National Academy Press.

It is interesting that vegetable oils, the richest sources of vitamin E, are also the richest sources of polyunsaturated fatty acids, which vitamin E protects.

Vitamin K has a basic physiologic role relating to the body's vital blood-clotting process through its essential presence in the formation of several proteins involved, including *prothrombin*. In this role it can serve as an antidote for excess effects of anticoagulant drugs and is often used in the control and prevention of certain types of hemorrhages. Since intestinal bacteria usually synthesize adequate vitamin K, supporting food sources such as green leafy vegetables, a deficiency is unlikely except in clinical conditions related to blood clotting. For example, patients treated with antibiotics that kill intestinal bacteria and who are then placed on poor diets after surgery are susceptible to vitamin K deficiency with resulting blood loss and poor wound healing.[9] A more detailed summary of the fat-soluble vitamins is given in Table 2-5 for review.

Water-soluble vitamins. Nine vitamins, eight B-complex vitamins and vitamin C, comprise the water-soluble group. The letter name "B" remains loosely attached, from the initial name *water-soluble B* given to the food factor in rice polishings used by early investigators to cure beriberi. When an increasing number of water-soluble vitamins were discovered, however, their distinct and unique natures led to a new naming system, now in common use, based on individual chemical structure or function, and we now know that initial "water-soluble B" as *thiamin,* a name based on its ringlike chemical structure. These eight initial "B" vitamins are now recognized as unique individual compounds and so named (although the "B" is still commonly used for two of them): thiamin, niacin, riboflavin, pyridoxine (B_6), pantothenic acid, biotin, folate, cobalamin (B_{12}). Discovered later than the initial "B" vitamins, water-soluble vitamin C still carries its common letter

TABLE 2-5 *A Summary of Fat-Soluble Vitamins*

Vitamin	Functions	Results of Deficiency	Food Sources
A (retinol); provitamin A (carotene)	Vision cycle—adaption to light and dark; tissue growth, especially skin and mucous membranes; toxic in large amounts	Night blindness, xerophthalmia, susceptibility to epithelial infection, changes in skin and membranes	Retinol (animal foods): liver, egg yolk, cream, butter or fortified margarine, fortified milk; carotene (plant foods): green and yellow vegetables, fruits
D (chole-calciferol)	Absorption of calcium and phosphorus, calcification of bones; toxic in large amounts	Rickets, faulty bone growth	Fortified or irradiated milk, fish oils
E (tocopherol)	Antioxidant—protection of materials that oxidize easily; normal growth	Breakdown of red blood cells, anemia	Vegetable oils, vegetable greens, milk, eggs, meat, cereals
K (phylloquinone)	Normal blood clotting	Bleeding tendencies, hemorrhagic disease	Green leafy vegetables, milk and dairy products, meat, eggs, cereals, fruits, vegetables

From Williams SR: Basic nutrition and diet therapy, ed 8, St Louis, 1988, Times Mirror/Mosby College Publishing.

TABLE 2-6   A Summary of B-Complex Vitamins

Vitamin	Functions	Results of Deficiency	Food Sources
Thiamin	Normal growth; coenzyme in carbohydrate metabolism; normal function of heart, nerves, and muscle	Beriberi; GI: loss of appetite, gastric distress, indigestion, deficient hydrochloric acid; CNS: fatigue, nerve damage, paralysis; CV: heart failure, edema of legs especially	Pork, beef, liver, whole or enriched grains, legumes
Riboflavin	Normal growth and vigor; coenzyme in protein and energy metabolism	Ariboflavinosis; wound aggravation, cracks at corners of mouth, swollen red tongue, eye irritation, skin eruptions	Milk, meats, enriched cereals, green vegetables
Niacin (precursor: tryptophan)	Coenzyme in energy production; normal growth, health of skin, normal activity of stomach, intestines, and nervous system	Pellagra; weakness, lack of energy, and loss of appetite; skin: scaly dermatitis; CNS: neuritis, confusion	Meat, peanuts, legumes, enriched grains
Pyridoxine	Coenzyme in amino acid metabolism: protein synthesis, heme formation, brain activity; carrier for amino acid absorption	Anemia; CNS: hyperirritability, convulsions, neuritis	Grains, seeds, liver and kidney meats; milk, eggs, vegetables
Pantothenic acid	Coenzyme in formation of coenzyme A: fat, cholesterol, and heme formation and amino acid activation	Unlikely because of widespread occurrence	Meats, cereals, legumes; milk, vegetables, fruit
Biotin	Coenzyme A partner; synthesis of fatty acids, amino acids, purines	Natural deficiency unknown	Liver, egg yolk, soy flour, cereal (except bound form in wheat), tomatoes, yeast
Folic acid	Part of DNA, growth and development of red blood cells	Certain type of anemia: megaloblastic (large, immature red blood cells)	Liver, green leafy vegetables, legumes, yeast
Cobalamin	Coenzyme in synthesis of heme for hemoglobin, normal red blood cell formation	Pernicious anemia (B_{12} is necessary extrinsic factor that combines with intrinsic factor of gastric secretions for absorption)	Liver, kidney, lean meats, milk, eggs, cheese

GI, gastrointestinal; CNS, central nervous system; CV, cardiovascular.
From Williams SR: Basic nutrition and diet therapy, ed 8, St Louis, 1988, Times Mirror/Mosby College Publishing.

TABLE 2-7   A Summary of Vitamin C (Ascorbic Acid)

Functions	Clinical Applications	Food Sources
Intercellular cement substance; firm capillary walls and collagen formation Helps prepare iron for absorption and release to tissues for red blood cell formation	Scurvy (deficiency disease) Sore gums Hemorrhages, especially around bones and joints Tendency to bruise easily Stress reactions Growth periods Fevers and infections Wound healing, tissue formation Anemia	Citrus fruits, tomatoes, cabbage, leafy vegetables, potatoes, strawberries, melons, chili peppers, broccoli, chard, turnip greens, green peppers, other green and yellow vegetables

From Williams SR: Basic nutrition and diet therapy, ed 8, St Louis, 1988, Times Mirror/Mosby College Publishing.

name, although its true chemical name, *ascorbic acid* (based on its function in curing scurvy) is more precise.

Despite this remarkable diversity of chemical structure and physiologic roles, the water-soluble vitamins are alike in many ways. Aside from sharing enough likeness in chemical structure to have the common chemical characteristic of water solubility, all these vitamins—with one exception in each case—share three additional characteristics significant in human nutrition:

1. **Food source.** All are synthesized by plants and are supplied in the diet by plant foods (as well as by animal foods)—except *cobalamin (vitamin B$_{12}$)*.
2. **Storage.** All have no stable body "storage" form and must therefore be provided regularly in the diet—except *cobalamin (vitamin B$_{12}$)*.
3. **Function.** All serve as coenzyme factors in cell enzyme reactions—except *ascorbic acid (vitamin C)*, mainly as a structural agent in building connective tissue.

Tables 2-6 and 2-7 provide reviews of the water-soluble vitamins for reference.

Minerals

The remaining micronutrients, the minerals, are single inorganic elements that are widely distributed in nature. During the eons in which the earth was forming, shifting oceans and mountains deposited a large number of minerals into earth materials. Over time these minerals have moved from rocks to soil, then to plants, to animals, and to humans. As a result, the mineral content of the human body is quite similar to that of the earth. Of the 54 known earth elements in the periodic table of elements, 25 have been shown to be essential to human life. In comparison with the vitamins, which are large complex organic compounds, minerals—single inert elements—may seem very simple. However, in their activated form of **ions** (carrying a positive or negative electrical charge) they perform a fascinating variety of essential metabolic tasks. Minerals differ from vitamins in the variety of their physiologic roles and in the amounts, relatively large to exceedingly small, needed for these tasks.

Variety of physiologic roles. These seemingly simple, single elements, in comparison with the much larger organic structure of vitamins, perform an impressive variety of metabolic tasks. They build, activate, regulate, transmit, and control. For example, sodium and potassium control water balance. Calcium and phosphorus are building materials that

Ions
(Gr *ion*, wanderer) Activated form of certain minerals, such as sodium (NA$^+$), potassium (K$^+$), and chloride (Cl$^-$), that carry an electrical charge and perform a variety of essential metabolic tasks.

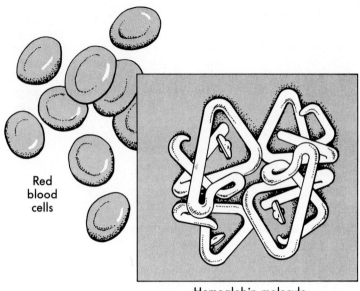

Red
blood
cells

Hemoglobin molecule

FIG. 2-2 Hemoglobin is an oxygen-carrying protein of red blood cells.

structure body framework. Iron helps build the vital oxygen carrier hemoglobin in red blood cells (Fig. 2-2). Cobalt is the central core of cobalamin (vitamin B_{12}). Iodine helps structure thyroid hormone, which in turn regulates the overall rate of all body metabolism. Thus, far from being static and inert, minerals are active essential participants, helping to control many of the body's overall metabolic processes.

Variety in amount needed. As indicated, all vitamins are required in very small amounts for their specific metabolic tasks. On the contrary, minerals occur in varying amounts in the body. For example, calcium forms a relatively large amount of the body weight— about 2%. Most of this amount is in bone tissue. An adult who weighs 150 lb has about 3 lb of calcium in the body. On the other hand, iron occurs in very small amounts. This same adult has only about 3 g (about $\frac{1}{10}$ oz) of iron in the body. In both cases, the amount of each mineral is essential for its specific task. This varying amount of individual minerals in the body provides the basis for classifying them into two main groups, major minerals and trace elements.

Major minerals
Minerals that occur in relatively large quantities in the body and hence have greater dietary requirements.

Trace elements
Minerals that occur in small amounts, or traces, in the body, and hence are required in very small amounts.

1. **Major minerals.** Elements are referred to as major minerals not because they are more important in metabolism, but simply because they occur in larger amounts in the body; thus their requirement is greater. On this basis, seven elements for which the requirement is greater than 100 mg/day are classified as **major minerals.** They contribute from 60% to 80% of the inorganic material in the human body. These seven major minerals are calcium, phosphorus, sodium, potassium, magnesium, chloride, and sulfur (Table 2-8). A review of their physiologic roles is given in Table 2-9. Our major food sources of calcium for bone growth through the life cycle (see p. 71) are milk and other dairy products (Fig. 2-3).

2. **Trace elements.** The remaining 18 elements in Table 2-8 make up the group of **trace elements.** These minerals are no less important, but they occur in very small traces or amounts in the body, contributing only 20% to 40% of all the inorganic material in the human body. For example, the human body contains only about

TABLE 2-8   Major Minerals and Trace Elements in Human Nutrition

| | Trace Elements | |
Major Minerals (Required Intake over 100 mg/day)	Essential (Required Intake under 100 mg/day)	Essentiality Unclear
Calcium (Ca)	Iron (Fe)	Silicon (Si)
Phosphorus (P)	Iodine (I)	Vanadium (V)
Sodium (Na)	Zinc (Zn)	Nickel (Ni)
Potassium (K)	Copper (Cu)	Tin (Sn)
Magnesium (Mg)	Manganese (Mn)	Cadmium (Cd)
Chlorine (Cl)	Chromium (Cr)	Arsenic (As)
Sulfur (S)	Cobalt (Co)	Aluminum (Al)
	Selenium (Se)	Boron (B)
	Molybdenum (Mo)	
	Fluorine (Fl)	

From Williams SR: Basic nutrition and diet therapy, ed 8, St Louis, 1988, Times Mirror/Mosby College Publishing.

FIG. 2-3   Milk is the major food source of calcium.
From The Image Bank.

45 mg of iron per kilogram body weight. Nonetheless, each of these trace elements is necessary for its specific metabolic task. A review of the main physiologic roles of the trace elements is given in Table 2-10.

The concept of essentiality. You will note in Table 2-8 that the trace elements are divided into two subgroups on the basis of essentiality in human nutrition. In the first subgroup labeled essential, 10 trace elements have been deemed definitely essential on the basis of defined function and requirement determined from research. The remaining group of eight elements is probably essential also, but a more complete understanding of their status requires finer means of analysis and tests for function.

Text continued on p. 32.

TABLE 2-9   A Summary of Major Minerals

Mineral	Metabolism	Physiologic Functions	Clinical Application	Requirements	Food Sources
Calcium (Ca)	Absorption according to body need, aided by vitamin D; hindered by binding agents (oxalates), or excessive fiber Parathyroid hormone controls absorption and mobilization	Bone formation Teeth Blood clotting Muscle contraction and relaxation Heart action Nerve transmission	Tetany – decrease in ionized serum calcium Rickets Osteoporosis	Adults: 1200 mg Pregnancy and lactation: 1200 mg Infants: 400-600 mg Children: 800-1200 mg	Milk Cheese Whole grains Egg yolk Legumes, nuts Green leafy vegetables
Phosphorus (P)	Absorption with calcium aided by vitamin D; hindered by excess binding agents (aluminum)	Bone and tooth formation Overall metabolism Energy metabolism (enzymes) Acid-base balance	Bone loss Poor growth	Adults: 1200-800 mg Pregnancy and lactation: 1200 mg Infants: 300-500 mg Children: 800-1200 mg	Milk Cheese Meat Egg yolk Whole grains Legumes, nuts
Sodium (Na)	Readily absorbed	Major extracellular fluid control Water balance Acid-base balance Muscle action; transmission of nerve impulse and resulting contraction	Fluid shifts and control Buffer system Losses in gastrointestinal disorders Dehydration	Limit to 2.4 g or less	Table salt (NaCl) Milk Meat Egg Baking soda Baking powder Carrots, beets, spinach, celery

Mineral	Absorption	Functions	Clinical applications	Requirement	Food sources
Potassium (K)	Secreted and reabsorbed in digestive juices	Major intracellular fluid control Acid-base balance Regulates nerve impulse and muscle contraction Glycogen formation Protein synthesis Energy metabolism	Fluid shifts Heart action—low serum potassium (cardiac arrest) Insulin release Blood pressure factor	About 2000-3500 mg Diet adequate in protein, calcium, and iron contains adequate potassium	Fruits Vegetables Meats Whole grains Legumes
Magnesium (Mg)	Absorption increased by parathyroid hormone	Aids thyroid hormone secretion, normal BMR Activator and coenzyme in carbohydrate and protein metabolism Muscle, nerve action	Tremor, spasm; low serum level following gastrointestinal losses or renal losses from alcoholism; convulsions	Adults: 280-350 mg Pregnancy and lactation: 320-355 mg Deficiency in humans unlikely	Whole grains Nuts Legumes Green vegetables (chlorophyll)
Chlorine (Cl)	Absorbed readily	Acid-base balance—chloride shift Gastric hydrochloric acid—digestion	Hypochloremic alkalosis in prolonged vomiting, diarrhea, tube drainage	Parallel requirement of sodium	Table salt
Sulfur (S)	Absorbed as such and as constituent of sulfur-containing amino acid methionine	Essential constituent of cell protein Hair, skin, nails Vitamin structure Collagen structure High-energy sulfur bonds in energy metabolism	General protein malnutrition	Diet adequate in protein contains adequate sulfur	Meat Egg Cheese Milk Nuts, legumes

From Williams SR: Basic nutrition and diet therapy, ed 8, St Louis, 1988, Times Mirror/Mosby College Publishing.

TABLE 2-10   A Summary of Selected Trace Elements

Element	Metabolism	Physiologic Functions	Clinical Application	Requirements	Food Sources
Iron (Fe)	Absorption according to body need; aided by vitamin C Heme and nonheme forms Excretion from tissue in minute quantities; body conserves then reuses	Hemoglobin formation Cellular oxidation of glucose Myoglobin in muscle Antibody production Drug detoxification Carotene conversion to vitamin A Collagen synthesis	Growth Pregnancy demands Deficiency — anemia	Men: 10 mg Women: 15 mg Pregnancy: 30 mg Lactation: 15 mg Children: 10-15 mg	Liver Meats Egg yolk Whole grains Enriched bread and cereal Dark green vegetables Legumes, nuts
Iodine (I)	Absorbed as iodides, taken up by thyroid gland under control of thyroid-stimulating hormone (TSH) Excretion by kidney	Synthesis of thyroxine, the thyroid hormone, which regulates cell oxidation BMR regulation	Deficiency — endemic colloid goiter; cretinism Hypothyroidism Hyperthyroidism	Men: 150 µg Women: 150 µg Infants: 35-45 µg Children: 70-150 µg	Iodized salt Seafood
Zinc (Zn)	Transported with plasma proteins Excretion largely intestinal Stored in liver, muscle, bone, and organs	Essential enzyme constituent Combined with insulin for storage of the hormone Immune system leukocytes	Wound healing Taste and smell acuity Retarded sexual and physical development	Men: 15 mg Women: 12 mg Children: 10-15 mg Infants: 5 mg	Meat Seafood, especially oysters Eggs Milk Whole grains Legumes
Copper (Cu)	Stored in muscle, bone, liver, heart, kidney, and central nervous system Iron twin	Associated with iron in Energy production Hemoglobin synthesis Absorption and transport of iron	TPN deficiency Anemia	Adults: 1.5-3.0 mg Children: 1.0-2.5 mg (estimated)	Liver Seafood Whole grains Legumes, nuts

Manganese (Mn)	Absorption limited. Excretion mainly by intestine	Activates reactions in Urea formation Protein metabolism Glucose oxidation Lipoprotein clearance and synthesis of fatty acids	Clinical deficiency in protein-energy malnutrition Inhalation toxicity in miners	Adults: 2-5 mg (estimated) Children: 1-5 mg	Cereals, whole grain Soybeans Legumes, nuts Tea Vegetables Fruits
Chromium (Cr)	Improves faulty uptake of glucose by body tissues as part of glucose tolerance factor	Associated with glucose metabolism; raises abnormally low fasting blood sugar levels	Possible link with cardiovascular disorders and diabetes	μg (estimated) Adults: 50-200 μg Children: 20-200 μg	Whole grains Cereal products
Cobalt (Co)	Absorbed chiefly as constituent of vitamin B_{12}	Constituent of vitamin B_{12}; essential factor in red blood cell formation	Deficiency associated with deficiency of vitamin B_{12} – pernicious anemia	Unknown	Supplied by preformed vitamin B_{12}
Selenium (Se)	Active as cofactor in cell oxidation enzyme systems	Associated with vitamin E as antioxidant; protects lipid in cell membrane	Keshan disease, heart muscle failure TPN deficiency	Men: 70 μg Women: 55 μg Children: 20 μg	Seafoods Kidney Liver Meats Whole grains
Molybdenum (Mo)	Minute traces in the body	Constituent of specific enzymes involved in Purine conversion to uric acid Aldehyde oxidation		Adults 75-250 μg (estimated)	Organ meats Milk Whole grains Leafy vegetables Legumes
Fluorine (Fl)	Deposited in bones and teeth	Associated with dental health	Small amount prevents dental caries Excess causes endemic dental fluorosis	Adults 1.5-4 mg (estimated) Children 0.5-2.5 mg	Fluoridated water (1 ppm Fl)

From Williams SR: Basic nutrition and diet therapy, ed 8, St Louis, 1988, Times Mirror/Mosby College Publishing.

By the simplest definition, an essential element is one required for the existence of life, and conversely, its absence brings death. However, for components that occur in very small amounts in the body, this determination of essentiality is not easy to make. Most living matter, as we know it, is made up of five fundamental elements, carbon (C), hydrogen (H), oxygen (O), nitrogen (N), and sulfur (S), which make up the macronutrients. We know these elements well because their concentrations are relatively large, hence more easily studied, and their requirements for human function can be expressed in multiples of gram per kilogram body weight. We have the means for analysis of such quantities and can easily see that these are essential elements. Also, the major minerals occur in respectable quantities in the body, and their essentiality has been more easily studied and determined. However, the much larger number of trace elements occur in biologic matter in very small amounts, and we know less about them. It is harder to determine essentiality of these trace elements because we require so little of them in the face of relatively large amounts found in our diet and environment. This makes it experimentally difficult to demonstrate essentiality, which of course requires removing it from the diet and the environment—an almost impossible task.

Essential function. Nonetheless, despite these difficulties in determining essentiality of these small amounts of trace elements in our bodies, studies have indicated that essentiality can be determined on the basis of function and deficiency effect. Mertz, a leading researcher in trace element metabolism, has indicated that an element is essential when a deficiency causes an impairment of function and when supplementation with that substance, but not with others, prevents or cures this impairment.[10] These early and continuing studies identify the function of trace elements in terms of **catalytic** and *structural* components of larger molecules:

Catalyst

(Gr *katalysis*, dissolution) A substance, such as enzymes and their component trace elements, that controls specific cell metabolism reactions but is not changed or consumed itself in the reaction as are the specific substances on which it works.

1. **Catalytic components.** Small amounts of various trace elements may function as an enzyme component in a catalytic manner in essential cell metabolic reactions.
2. **Structural components.** Additional elements act as a structural molecule component in building materials used in cell and tissue formation.

These trace elements carry out their function in three ways: (1) they may amplify the full function of the larger molecule of which they are a part, (2) they are specific to the particular function involved, and (3) they contribute to homeostatic regulation through their absorption-excretion balance and the degree of their carrier transport situation. Stages of research concerning trace element needs can be compared in terms of how far advanced our knowledge is: (1) long-standing knowledge, such as is the case with iron and iodine; (2) recent history and questions, as for elements such as chromium, copper, zinc, and selenium; and (3) newer but incomplete knowledge, such as exists for silicon, vanadium, nickel, and arsenic.

Water

The final basic nutrient, water, underlies all the functions of the other nutrients and, next to air, is the most essential substance to our survival. It creates the water-based environment necessary for the vast array of chemical actions and reactions that comprise body metabolism and sustain life. Also, it provides the means for maintaining a stable body temperature and helps give structure and form to our bodies through the turgor it provides for the tissues. We obtain this life-giving water in fluids we drink including water and other beverages, in foods we eat, and the water of oxidation created within from the end products of cell metabolism. The average adult metabolizes from 2.5 to 3 L of water/day in a constant turnover balanced between intake and output. This water enters and leaves the body by various routes, controlled by basic mechanisms such as thirst and hormonal activity.

THE HUMAN LIFE CYCLE AND CHANGING NUTRIENT NEEDS
Growth and Development

Physical growth. Growth may be defined as an increase in size, but it encompasses far more than that. Biologic growth of an organism occurs through cell multiplication. Development is the associated process in which growing tissues and organs take on an increased complexity of function. Both processes combine to form a unified whole in the many aspects of human growth and development throughout the life cycle. This dual concept indicates the magnitude and quality of maturational changes that establish early embryonic cells through cell multiplication and differentiation, set the pattern for subsequent rapid fetal growth and development, produce a fully formed small, dependent newborn, and transform this newborn infant through successive childhood growth periods into a fully functioning, independent adult.

Physiologic and psychosocial development. Physiologic growth depends on a variety of nutrients in the food a child eats. It also depends on the vast number of biochemical processes of metabolism that supply the right materials in the right place at the right time for forming and maintaining unique body tissues. Human growth and development, however, involves far more than the physical process alone. It takes in social and psychologic influences and relationships—indeed, the entire environment and culture that promotes individual growth potential. Food and feeding, especially during the early formative childhood years but also throughout the life cycle, do not and cannot exist apart from this broader, overall personal growth and development. Although we are concerned about necessary nutrients at any age, we do not eat nutrients; we eat food, with all the uniquely different social, cultural, and personal meanings it holds for each of us.

Changing nutrient needs. Through the successive age groups of the life cycle, changing nutrient needs reflect an increasing differentiation based on age and sex as the physical body grows and develops. There is a general steady increase in nutrient and energy needs through early age groups to about age 10 to 12 years, with individuals within any age group often having different needs according to individual growth patterns. With the onset of puberty and the differing sexual development of boys and girls, nutrient needs for the two sexes begin to vary. During this adolescent period, the final growth spurt of childhood occurs. Maturation during this period varies so widely that chronologic age as a reference point for discussing growth ceases to be useful (if indeed it ever was, for individual differences occur at all ages). **Physiologic age** becomes more important in dealing with individual adolescent boys and girls. It accounts for wide fluctuations in metabolic rates, food requirements, scholastic capacity, and even illness. These capacities can be more realistically viewed in individual physiologic growth terms. The profound growth period of adolescents requires increases in energy, protein, minerals, and vitamins. Boys usually eat well enough to receive all necessary nutrients, whereas girls often do not.

Body Composition

Individual variation. Throughout the life cycle the physical composition of the human body is changing. From conception and birth, throughout childhood growth and adult aging, to old age decline and death, the human body and its basic components change and adapt in a remarkable fashion to meet physiologic needs. Given the genetic imprint of its heritage and the physical and psychosocial nature of its environment, the human body, in the most literal sense, is the product of its nutrition throughout life. Through profound and fascinating transformations, food makes possible the living body and all its functions, and the varying mass of tissue it produces and maintains. There is no precise "ideal" or "standard" **body composition** except for purposes of study in the laboratory.

Physiologic age
Rate of biologic maturation in individual adolescents that varies widely and accounts for more than does chronologic age for wide and changing differences in their metabolic rates, nutritional needs, and food requirements.

Body composition
The relative sizes of the four body compartments that make up the physical body—lean body mass, fat, water, and mineral mass.

In reality this is a hazardous assumption, for within the limits of genetic potential, individuals differ widely. There is great variability among healthy persons in both body composition and body response to internal and external environmental influences and to disease. However, a general knowledge of body composition components and their interrelatedness provides an important basis for measuring and determining the nutritional status of specific individuals of all ages, as well as the many influences that shape it.

Basic concepts of compartments and balance. Using the two basic physiologic concepts of body compartments and balance for a foundation, we can identify and describe the gross components of body composition, especially in relation to body changes and nutritional needs through the life cycle. The concept of *balance* provides a dynamic view of the body, ever changing and adjusting to its internal and external environments. The biologic term **compartment** is used to describe the body's internal collection of a given vital substance. The concept of compartments gives a comprehensive view of the human body, not of static mechanical parts, but of **homeostasis,** a state of dynamic equilibrium within an interdependent whole. The nutritional needs of individuals throughout growth and development can be understood through the application of these two basic concepts.

Body Composition Compartments Based on Metabolic Activity

Nutritional scientists, who are interested in nutritional status as a means of determining nutritional needs throughout life, usually use the criterion of metabolic activity to define the gross components of body composition. On this basis many researchers commonly distinguish four main components in two divisions: (1) that part that is most active in energy metabolism—*lean body mass*—and (2) those parts that are relatively inactive—*body fat,* the *extracellular water,* and the *mineral mass of the bones and smaller structural parts*. The remaining body compartment most active in energy metabolism is the **lean body mass.**

Lean body mass compartment. The body's lean cell mass is the primary determinant of its energy requirements and thus its overall nutrient needs. Its relative size and metabolic activity, as well as its relation to weight changes, are important considerations.

1. **Compartment size and metabolic activity.** In various individuals the lean body mass, as a collective compartment of the body's active fat-free mass of cells, will account for anything from 30% to 65% of the total body weight. However, in any person it accounts for almost all the energy consumption. As a percentage of body weight, for example, the values for this lean cell mass will range from low levels in very fat, sedentary persons to higher levels in very muscular persons.

2. **Relation to weight changes.** When persons gain or lose weight due to diet changes, it is not merely a reflection of changes in the body fat mass but also in the lean body mass. Numerous studies have shown that the density of the tissue added or lost is never that of pure fat.[11] The density of the nonfat lean part also changes with nutritional status. Added exercise enhances its relative size.

Body fat compartment. The gross amount of the body fat compartment can vary widely and affect individual health status. In general, it reflects the number and size of fat cells—**adipocytes**—making up the adipose tissue. However, adipose tissue is not pure fat. It also contains parts of other compartments such as blood vessels, connective tissue, cell membranes, and water.

1. **Compartment size.** In relation to a standard "reference body" and from body water measurements, the body fat compartment has been variously estimated in healthy persons to range in an adult man, for example, from about 14% to 28% of the total body weight. The woman's "reference body" would have a somewhat larger fat compartment, about 15% to 29% of total body weight. These percentages vary with factors such as age, climate, exercise, and fitness. About half of the total body fat is in the subcutaneous fat layers, which serve the important task of helping to maintain body temperature.

Body compartment
The collective quantity of a particular vital substance in the body; for example, the mineral compartment, composed mainly of the skeletal bone mass.

Adipocytes
(L *adipis,* fat; Gr *kytos,* hollow vessel, cell) Fat cells.

2. **Relation to health.** Extremes in size of the body fat compartment can affect individual health status. For example, some athletes, especially compulsive runners, may strive for a very low level of body fat, even in some cases to an unhealthy deficit. Conversely, at the other extreme, massively obese sedentary persons carry increased health risks from an excessively large body fat mass. However, common beliefs that even moderate overweight brings poorer health and a shorter life span are unfounded. Population studies, such as those of Andres, show that it is the extremes of both underweight and obesity that increase health risks and contribute to higher mortality rates, concluding that moderate amounts of overweight, especially in older adults, may actually offer health protection.[12]

Body water compartment. The total body water content varies widely with relative body composition in terms of leanness and fatness, since lean muscle tissue contains more water than any other body tissue except blood. It also varies with age, being relatively higher in infants, and with hydration status, being lower in conditions causing dehydration and higher in conditions causing increased tissue fluid. In pregnancy the total maternal body water increases normally to support the increased metabolic work, and sometimes abnormally in complications of pregnancy-induced hypertension.

1. **Total body water compartments.** The total body water is divided into two sub-compartments—the collective water inside the cells and the remaining collective water outside of cells. The water inside of cells is part of the active cell mass or lean body mass. So it is the remaining collective water outside of cells, the **extracellular fluid (ECF),** that makes up this designated water compartment of gross body composition.

2. **ECF compartment.** Since the size of the ECF compartment varies with individual fatness or leanness, it is higher in thin persons and lower in fat persons. In average weight adults, the collective water outside cells makes up about 20% of the total body weight; in fat persons, about 15%; in thin persons, about 25%. The ECF consists of four parts: (1) *blood plasma,* which accounts for about 25% of the ECF and 5% of body weight; (2) *interstitial fluid,* the water surrounding the cells; (3) *secretory fluid,* the circulating secretions in transit; and (4) *dense tissue fluid,* the water in dense connective tissue, cartilage, and bone (Fig. 2-4).

Extracellular fluid (ECF) The total body water compartment composed of the collective water outside of cells.

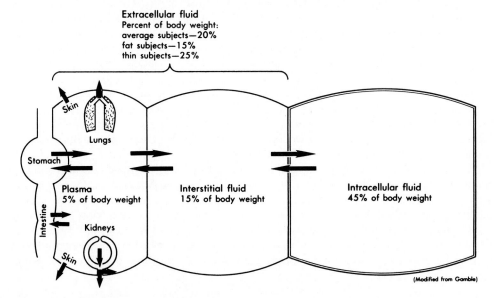

FIG. 2-4 Body fluid compartments. Note the relative total quantities of water in the intracellular compartment and in the extracellular compartment.

Mineral compartment
Smallest part of the body composition, found mainly in the skeletal bone mass.

Body mineral compartment. The body's major mineral content by far is found in its large skeletal mass, with much smaller amounts in teeth, nails, and hair. Of all the minerals in the human body, calcium is present in far greater amounts than any other, comprising about 2% of the total body weight.

1. **Skeletal mass.** The human skeleton is a relatively large structure, comprising in the living body about one sixth of the total body mass. Most of the body calcium—about 99%—is in the skeleton, accounting for most of the total body mineral compartment. Other minerals occur in varying lesser amounts.

2. **Mineral ash.** Only a small part of the skeletal mass, however, is comprised of mineral matter. The other components of bone—water, protein, and fat—are accounted for in their respective body composition compartments. In its dried defatted state, the skeleton represents only about 6% of the gross body weight. Bone mineral mass as estimated from bone ash values is about 5% of total body weight.

NUTRIENT NEEDS AND FOOD GUIDES FOR HEALTH PROMOTION
Nutrient Standards

Most of the developed countries of the world have set up nutrition standards for the major nutrients to serve as guidelines for maintaining healthy populations. These standards, however, are not intended to indicate individual requirements or therapeutic needs, but rather serve as a reference for levels of intake of the essential nutrients considered, on the basis of current scientific knowledge, to be adequate to meet the known nutritional needs of most healthy population groups. Although these standards are similar in different countries, they may vary somewhat according to the philosophy of scientists and practitioners in a particular country as to their purpose and use. In the United States these standards are called the **Recommended Dietary Allowances (RDA).**

Recommended Dietary Allowances (RDA)
U.S. nutrient standards for population groups by age and sex; updated every 4 to 5 years to reflect current research results.

U.S. nutrient standards: Recommended Dietary Allowances. The U.S. nutrient standards for population groups are outlined by age groups and sex. These standards are developed and maintained by groups of leading scientists and practitioners in the field of nutrition, working through the National Academy of Sciences in Washington, D.C. The Academy has numerous divisions of councils and is supported by the National Institutes of Health. The working group of nutrition scientists responsible for the RDAs make up the Food and Nutrition Board of the National Research Council. The U.S. RDA was first published in 1943, during World War II, as a guide for planning and obtaining food supplies for national defense and providing average population standards as a goal for good nutrition. The RDA has been revised and expanded over the years, with a revision usually coming out every 4 or 5 years. The current tenth edition issued in 1989 reflects increasing scientific knowledge as well as expanding social concerns about nutrition and health.[5,13] (See current tables inside book covers.)

Other nutrient standards. Canada and most European countries publish nutrient standards that are similar to the U.S. Recommended Dietary Allowances. (See Appendix I for the Canadian nutrient standards.) In less developed countries where factors such as quality of protein foods available must be considered, health workers look to standards such as those set by the Food and Agriculture Organization (FAO) of the World Health Organization (WHO). Nonetheless, all of these standards provide basic nutrient guidelines to help health workers in a variety of population groups promote good health through sound nutrition.

Food Guides for Diet Planning

To interpret and apply sound nutrient standards such as the RDA, persons need practical food guides to use in nutrition education and diet planning with individuals and families. Such tools include the familiar long-used guide, the basic four food groups, the food exchange groups, and the more recently developed health promotion guide, the U.S. dietary guidelines.

Basic food groups. The basic four food group system, first developed by the U.S. Department of Agriculture (USDA) in 1917, has reflected in its original and subsequent editions agricultural commodity concerns as well as nutritional ones.[14] In 1979 the basic four food groups system was revised by the USDA to include a fifth group—fats, sweets, and alcoholic beverages. This revision, published as *The Hassle-Free Daily Food Guide,* also noted the importance of specific vitamins and minerals within particular food groups, addressed the need for fiber, and encouraged the use of whole grains.

In 1991 the USDA revised *The Hassle-Free Daily Food Guide* to represent a total diet, rather than simply a foundation for a diet (Table 2-11). This current plan is called *A Pattern for Daily Food Choices*. The changes in this guide include an increase in fruit and vegetable servings from 4 per day to 5 to 9 per day, and bread and cereal servings from 4 per day to 6 to 11 per day. These changes provide the bulk of dietary energy intake from carbohydrate while limiting fat intake (Fig. 2-5).

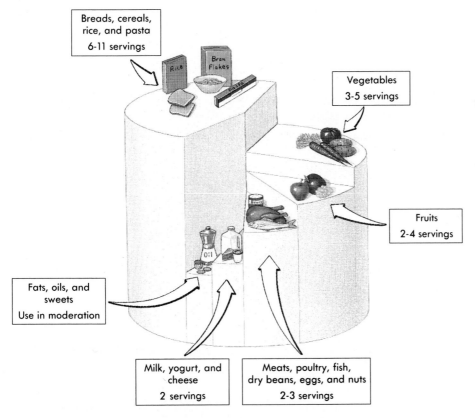

FIG. 2-5   *A Pattern for Daily Food Choices.* This plan forms the basis for a healthy diet if one follows the average American food pattern.

TABLE 2-11 **A Pattern for Daily Food Choices**

Food Group	Suggested Daily Servings	What Counts as a Serving?
Breads, cereals, and other grain products Whole-grain Enriched	6-11 servings from entire group (include several servings of whole-grain products daily)	1 slice of bread ½ hamburger bun or English muffin a small roll, biscuit, or muffin 3 to 4 small or 2 large crackers ½ cup cooked cereal, rice, or pasta 1 ounce of ready-to-eat breakfast cereal
Fruits Citrus, melon, berries Other fruits	2-4 servings from entire group	a whole fruit such as a medium apple, banana, or orange a grapefruit half a melon wedge ¾ cup of juice ½ cup of berries ½ cup cooked or canned fruit ¼ cup dried fruit
Vegetables Dark-green leafy Deep-yellow Dry beans and peas (legumes) Starchy Other vegetables	3-5 servings from entire group (include all types regularly; use dark-green leafy vegetables and dry beans and peas several times a week)	½ cup of cooked vegetables ½ cup of chopped raw vegetables 1 cup of leafy raw vegetables, such as lettuce or spinach
Meat, poultry, fish, and alternates (eggs, dry beans and peas, nuts, and seeds)	2-3 servings from entire group	Amounts should total 5 to 7 ounces of cooked lean meat, poultry, or fish a day. Count 1 egg, ½ cup cooked beans, or 2 tablespoons peanut butter as 1 ounce of meat.
Milk, cheese, and yogurt	2 servings from entire group (3 servings for women who are pregnant or breastfeeding and for teens and young adults to age 24)	1 cup of milk 8 ounces of yogurt 1½ ounces of natural cheese 2 ounces of process cheese
Fats, sweets, and alcoholic beverages	Avoid too many fats and sweets. If you drink alcoholic beverages, do so in moderation.	

From *Preparing Foods and Planning Menus* HG 232-8.

Food exchange groups. In 1950 the American Diabetes Association and the American Dietetic Association introduced a quite different food groups guide, the food exchange groups, as a meal-planning tool for managing diets for persons with diabetes. Over two revisions, the latest in 1986, the use of this food guide has been expanded to include any situation in which management of nutrient and energy values is needed. The major 1986 revisions reflect current nutrition and health-promotion guidelines and provide a practical tool for planning a healthy diet.[15] The basic six food groups have been completely reorganized: (1) starch/bread; (2) meat in three subgroups: lean, medium fat, and high fat; (3) vegetables; (4) fruits; (5) milk in three subgroups to reduce fat; and (6) fat in subgroups of unsaturated and saturated food sources. Three expanded lists were added: free foods and seasonings, combination foods, and foods for occasional use. In all groups, values for dietary fiber and sodium were identified and flagged. In addition to the revised meal planning booklet for use in diabetes management, the American Dietetic Association has issued a new companion booklet designed for use in general weight management.[16] The revised food exchange lists are included in Appendix J.

U.S. dietary guidelines. The U.S. dietary guidelines were issued as a result of growing public concerns beginning in the 1960s and subsequent Senate investigations studying hunger and nutrition in the United States. They are based on a developing concern about chronic health problems in an aging population and a changing food environment. From the beginning, they have encountered controversy, centering mainly on the broad issues of the roles of government and science in maintaining health. The U.S. Departments of Agriculture and Health and Human Services reissued this food guide in 1980 under the new title *Dietary Guidelines for Americans*. These statements relate current scientific thinking to America's leading health problems. Recent review by expert committees have led to only minimal updating changes over the past decade. The current 1990 issue is entitled *Nutrition and Your Health: Dietary Guidelines for Americans*.[3,17-19] It reflects a comprehensive evaluation of the scientific evidence of a relationship between diet and health, based on the extensive research findings in two important reports: (1) the Surgeon General's 1988 report *Nutrition and Health*, and (2) the National Academy of Sciences 1989 report *Diet and Health: Implications for Reducing Chronic Disease*.[1,20] The seven statements in the current guidelines, introduced briefly in Chapter 1 (Table 1-3, p. 10), are developed here in relation to their health promotion basis in the box on p. 40. They continue to serve as a useful general guide for a concerned public. Although no guidelines can guarantee health or well-being, and although people differ widely in their food needs, these general statements can lead individuals to evaluate their food habits and move toward general improvements. Many references are made to these guidelines throughout this book because they have wide application in our current national health goals for health promotion and disease prevention. Good food habits based on moderation and variety can help to build sound healthy bodies throughout the life cycle.

Individual needs. Whatever type of food guide is used, individual food patterns will vary with personal needs, living situations, energy demands, ethnic diversity, and the changing American food market. On the whole, however, within widely diverse individual situations and needs, Americans seem to be gradually learning that what they eat does influence their health. Even the fast-food restaurants, where Americans eat one in 12 meals, are beginning to respond to their customers' desires for less fat in fast foods, though some nutritional concerns still exist.[21,22] In any case, more than ever, people are being more selective about what they eat.

Food exchange groups
A meal planning system of six food exchange lists with indicated portion sizes for each food that are equivalent in food values and hence may be exchanged within a given group to maintain an appropriate individual food pattern with a variety of food choices. Used in diabetes control and weight management.

U.S. dietary guidelines
A set of seven statements to guide food choices that reflect current health promotion and disease prevention national health objectives.

ONE STEP FURTHER

Dietary Guidelines for Americans

Eat a variety of foods

About 40 different known nutrients, and probably additional as yet unknown factors, are needed to maintain health. No single food can supply all the essential nutrients in the amounts needed to maintain health. Thus the greater the variety of foods used, the less likely a person is to develop either a deficiency or an excess of any single nutrient. One way to ensure a varied balanced diet, is to select foods each day from all the major food groups.

Maintain healthy weight

Excessive fatness is associated with some chronic disorders such as hypertension and diabetes, which in turn relate to heart disease. The healthy body weight, however, must be determined individually because many factors are involved, such as body composition (muscle/fat ratio), body metabolism, genetics, and physical activity.

Choose a diet low in fat, saturated fat, and cholesterol

Americans have traditionally consumed a high-fat diet. In some persons, excess fat leads to high levels of blood fats and cholesterol. Elevated blood levels of these fats and cholesterol are associated with a higher risk of coronary heart disease. Thus it is wise to reduce intake of fats in general, using them only in moderation.

Choose a diet with plenty of vegetables, fruits, and grain products

Increasing use of these foods will help supply more of the needed starches (complex carbohydrates) for energy, many essential nutrients, and necessary dietary fiber. Research indicates that certain types of dietary fiber may help control chronic bowel diseases, contribute to improved blood glucose management for persons with diabetes mellitus, and bind dietary cholesterol.

Use sugars only in moderation

The major health hazard from eating too much sugar is tooth decay (dental caries). Contrary to popular opinion, however, too much sugar does not in itself cause diabetes. It can only contribute to poor control of diabetes in persons who have inherited the disease. Most Americans consume a relatively large amount of sugar, over 100 pounds per person each year, much of it in processed food products. Again, moderation is the key.

Use salt and sodium only in moderation

Our main source of dietary sodium is in ordinary table salt. Excessive salt is not healthy for anyone and certainly not for persons with hypertension. Many processed food products contain considerable amounts of salt and other sodium compounds, and many Americans use more salt in foods than they need. Thus it is wise to limit salt use in food preparation or at the table and to reduce the use of "salty" food products. This approach will lower individual salt tastes, which are learned habits and not biologic necessities. There is ample sodium as a natural mineral in foods to meet usual needs.

If you drink alcoholic beverages, do so in moderation

Alcoholic beverages tend to be high in kilocalories and low in other nutrients. Limited food intake may accompany excessive alcohol intake. Heavy drinking also contributes to chronic liver disease and some neurologic disorders, as well as some throat and neck cancers. Moreover, it is a major factor in highway deaths. Thus moderation is the key, if alcohol is used at all, and persons should *never* drink and drive.

From Williams SR: Basic nutrition and diet therapy, ed 9, St Louis, 1992, Mosby–Year Book.

ASSESSMENT OF NUTRITIONAL STATUS
Nutritional Status of Persons and Populations

Throughout the life cycle, in the health care of individuals or communities, **nutritional assessment** is the first step in developing nutritional care plans and programs. At both levels of care, individual clinical care plans and public health programs, although the scope of the work may vary from a simple conversation with a clinic patient or parent to a complex nationwide survey including all ages, the basic principles of the assessment process remain the same—to identify nutritional status and needs on which to base care plans and programs designed to meet these identified needs.

Person-Centered Clinical Care

Levels of care. Nutrition is essential to individual health on two levels:

1. **Tissue level.** Nutrients and energy from the food we eat build and maintain body tissues and it is on the integrity of these tissues that the physiologic functioning and health of the body depend.
2. **Personal level.** Food has many meanings that help fulfill personal needs and it is on the integrity of these personal psychosocial and cultural values that human health depends.

In personal health care or clinical nutrition, assessment of individuals helps health care providers, together with the patient or client, determine nutritional and health status on both physiologic tissue level and psychosocial personal level, and plan nutritional care according to personal needs and goals. The overall goal is health promotion and disease prevention, or treatment of disease. If an underlying chronic disorder such as diabetes mellitus is present, or if risk factors for potential health problems such as heart disease have begun to develop, the goal is healthy control of the disorder or prevention of the health problem by reduction of risk factors. All of these nutrition and health goals involve personal health and nutrition education and skills in self-care, as well as collaboration of a skilled and sensitive team of health care professionals, including the clinical nutritionist.

Phases of the clinical care process. Five distinct yet interactive phases are essential in the **clinical care process:**

1. **Assessment.** A broad base of information about the person's body composition, nutrition and health status, food habits, and personal living situation provides necessary knowledge for assessing initial nutritional status and needs. Useful background information will come from various sources, primarily the individual and family, as well as health-care records and other health care team members.
2. **Analysis.** The data collected must be analyzed carefully to determine specific needs. Some will be evident immediately. Others will develop as the situation unfolds. On the basis of this analysis, a list of problems forms.
3. **Planning care.** As problems are identified, valid care can be planned with the individual and family to solve them. This plan must be based on personal needs and goals, as well as any health problem involved.
4. **Implementing the plan.** Realistic and appropriate actions planned are carried out. In nutritional care and education this will involve decisions and actions about the diet, mode of feeding as needed, and training of the person, staff, and family to carry out the plan.
5. **Evaluating and recording results.** As the plan is carried out, results are monitored carefully to see if the needs are being met, or if revisions in the plan must be made. Records of data, plans, procedures, and progress guide actions and instructions for continuing self-care.

Nutritional assessment
Process of determining individual or group nutritional status as a basis for identifying needs and goals and planning personal health care or community programs to meet these identified goals.

Clinical care process
Interactive process of planning personal health care through five phases of assessment and data collection, analysis of findings, planning care according to a written individual care plan, implementing the plan, and evaluating and recording results.

Community-Centered Public Health

Changing population patterns and health goals. As the 1990 census reports, the United States population continues to increase, reflecting rapid change not only in total numbers but also in greater ethnic diversity, especially in border states such as California and Texas, and in increasing age. In community nutrition, assessment of population groups helps public health officials determine health goals and allocation of resources according to priority of need. Often the focus of this nutrition and health assessment is on groups of people bearing higher health risks: pregnant women, infants and children, adolescents, and elderly adults, especially those under the added stress of poverty, malnutrition, and illness.

Community care process
Program planning to meet defined community health needs through assessment procedures, objectives, program plan, and evaluation.

Phases of the community care process. At whatever level of community nutrition work—national, state, or local—nutrition is an integral component of health and health care. The program-planning process to identify and meet these needs involves four basic areas of activity:

1. **Assessment.** The twofold process of assessment includes: (1) data collection about the population of concern, and (2) analysis of the information to identify nutrition needs and problems.
2. **Objectives.** In relation to the identified needs or problems, both general goals and specific contributory objectives are determined to meet these needs. These goals involve staff and agency decisions about what actions are to be accomplished and a projected timeline for doing the work.
3. **Program plan.** To reach the established objectives, a specific plan of action is developed and carried out as projected. The program plan must consider such items as staff, tools and documents required, sources of funding, and budget for cost control.
4. **Evaluation.** Assessment of program activities and results continues throughout the nutrition project for health promotion or disease prevention. On the basis of this monitoring information, revisions may be made for study purposes or for conversion to a regular, ongoing program status.

Community groups with special life-cycle needs. Several higher-risk groups in the general population will require special nutritional attention, especially if their normal growth and development needs are compounded by such basic problems as poverty.

1. **Pregnant women.** During a woman's pregnancy, she must meet increased nutrient and energy needs to support this period of rapid fetal growth and bring the pregnancy to a successful outcome. At best this period is one of physiologic stress. In poor circumstances this normal stress is compounded by inadequate nutrition, bringing increased stress to both mother and baby. Ongoing nutrition assessment can identify specific needs, help prevent problems and complications, and promote a healthy pregnancy for both mother and baby.
2. **Infants and children.** The highest nutrient requirements per kilogram of body weight during the entire life cycle occur during infancy, when rates of growth and metabolism are at their highest point. Because of this direct relation between growth and nutritional status, close nutrition assessment is required to monitor progress. Over the following period of young childhood, the growth pattern slows and becomes erratic with alternating small growth spurts and plateaus. Continued assessment of progress is essential to promote health.
3. **Adolescents.** With puberty comes the second large growth spurt for the child. In both sexes intensive growth and hormonal changes profoundly affect nutritional needs. Continued monitoring of growth, changing body composition, and nutritional status helps ensure foundations for a healthy adulthood.
4. **Adults and the elderly.** With our increasing lifespan, the gradual aging process

through adulthood requires a sound nutritional base to maintain health and prevent or control chronic diseases, which account for 75% of all deaths in the United States. Nutritional risk factors are associated with most all of these chronic diseases of aging.

Methods of Assessment: Clinical and Population

Whether the assessment is being done in a clinical or community setting, four basic methods are used—anthropometric, biochemical, clinical, and dietary. Community assessment centers mainly on dietary intake surveys and nutrient analyses, but comparative data from biochemical tests, body measurements, and various clinical observations are also used to evaluate individual nutritional status as well as provide practical information about response to nutrition intervention programs. Clinical assessment may include a broader focus on related disease processes with more extensive biochemical and clinical assessment. Whatever the situation, all four methods together provide essential information to identify needs and plan health care. To review assessment basics here, a few of the commonly used measures in each method category are briefly outlined.

Anthropometry. Anthropometry is the process of measuring various dimensions of the human body. Several of these body measures provide valid estimates of muscle and fat components of body composition. They have the advantage of being inexpensive and simple to obtain. Skill gained through careful practice will minimize the margin of error. Selection and maintenance of proper procedures and equipment, as well as attention to careful technique, will help secure accurate data.

Anthropometry
(Gr *anthropos*, man, human; *metron*, measure) The process of measuring various dimensions of the human body to help determine basic body composition and needs.

1. **Weight.** For accuracy, use regular clinic beam balance scales with nondetachable weights, with an additional weight attachment for use with very obese persons. Metric scales with readings to the nearest 20 g provide specific data, but the standard clinic scale is satisfactory. Read and record the person's weight, then obtain information about usual body weight and check standard weight-height tables for comparison. However, approach these tables with caution in applying them to individuals as specific ideals, remembering that wide *normal* variations occur in healthy bodies. Keeping this in mind, interpret personal weight in terms of percentage of the person's usual body weight, with general reference to standard tables. Check for any significant weight loss.

2. **Height.** Use a true vertical bar, such as a flat wall-attached measuring stick or the movable measuring rod on the platform clinical scales. Have the person put his back to the measuring rod, stand as straight as possible, without shoes or hat, heels together, looking straight ahead. The heels, buttocks, shoulders, and head should be touching the vertical measuring surface. Read and record the measure. Compare it with previous recordings to detect possible errors, and to note growth of children or diminishing height of older adults.

3. **Body mass index (BMI).** The weight and height measures can be used to calculate the person's body mass index, a value often used in clinical assessment: weight (kg) divided by height (meters) squared. This ratio is commonly used in evaluating obesity states in relation to risk factors.

Body mass index (BMI)
A calculated assessment of body mass based on weight and height: BMI = [weight (kg) ÷ height (m)]².

4. **Mid–upper arm circumference (MAC).** On the nondominant arm, unless it is affected by edema, use a nonstretchable centimeter tape to locate the midpoint of the upper arm. Measure the circumference at this midpoint. Read this measure accurately to the nearest tenth of a centimeter and record. Compare this result with previous measurements to note possible changes and with standard reference tables.

5. **Triceps skinfold thickness (TSF).** With thumb and forefinger, grasp a vertical pinch of the skin and subcutaneous fat at this previously marked upper-arm midpoint and gently pull away from the underlying muscle. Using a standard millimeter

skinfold caliper and avoiding excessive pressure, measure the skinfold thickness quickly, within 2 or 3 seconds, to the nearest full or fraction of a millimeter. For increased accuracy take three measures and use the mean for calculations. Record results and compare with standard reference tables. This measure provides a good estimate of the subcutaneous fat reserves.

Mid–upper arm muscle circumference (MAMC)
Indirect measure of body's skeletal muscle mass based on mid–arm muscle circumference (MAMC) and triceps skinfold (TSF): MAMC (cm) = MAC (cm) − [π × TSF (mm)].

6. **Mid–upper arm muscle circumference (MAMC).** Using the two previous measures, calculate this value to provide a good indirect measure of the body's skeletal muscle mass: MAMC (cm) = MAC (cm) − [3.14 × TSF (cm)]. If desired, the TSF can be left in millimeters as measured and the value of the mathematical factor pi in the formula changed to 0.314: MAMC (cm) = [0.314 × TSF (mm)].

Standard reference tables for all of these body measures are given in the Appendix.

Biochemical tests. Numerous biochemical tests are available for assessing nutritional status. The most commonly used ones are listed here. Further description, formulas, and reference standards are given in the Appendix.

1. **Plasma protein.** Basic measures of plasma protein include serum albumin, hemoglobin, and hematocrit. Additional ones may include serum transferrin or total iron-binding capacity (TIBC) and ferritin.

2. **Protein metabolism.** Basic 24-hour urine tests are used to measure urinary creatinine and urea nitrogen levels. These materials are products of protein metabolism. The 24-hour excretion of creatinine is interpreted in terms of ideal creatinine excretion for height, the creatinine-height index (CHI). The 24-hour urea nitrogen excretion is used with the calculated dietary nitrogen intake (6.25 g protein = 1 g nitrogen) over the same 24-hour period to calculate nitrogen balance:

$$\text{Nitrogen balance} = \frac{\text{Protein intake}}{6.25} - (\text{Urinary urea nitrogen} + 4)$$

3. **Immune system integrity.** Any diminished capacity of the immune system *(anergy)* is reflected in basic measures such as lymphocyte count, and by additional skin-testing, observing for any delayed sensitivity to common recall antigens such as mumps or purified protein derivative of tuberculin (PPD).

Clinical observations. Careful observations of physical signs of nutritional status provide an important added dimension to the overall assessment of individuals. Using a general examination guide for such physical signs, such as given in Table 2-12, check for any possible evidence of malnutrition. Also, other physical data may include such vital signs as pulse rate, respiration, temperature, and blood pressure. A study of the common procedures of a normal physical examination will provide useful background orientation.[23]

Dietary evaluation. Information about food intake of different groups of people or individuals is usually obtained by use of several basic tools. Choices among these procedures are guided by purposes of the assessment and available staff and funds. More than one tool may be used for crosschecking or expanding the data received. For example, an initial nutrition history to learn basic food patterns may be followed by specific food records to provide some examples of actual food choices, quantities, and meal/snack schedule. A brief review of commonly used diet evaluation methods is outlined here.

1. **Diet history.** Depending on the assessment needs, information about food habits may be obtained by a comprehensive nutrition interview or a tested questionnaire filled out by the individual or parent and followed up by a brief personal review as needed by the nutritionist. Whatever its form, a careful nutrition history including related living situation and other personal, psychosocial, and economic problems, as well as any drugs being used, is a fundamental base of nutrition assessment.

2. **Twenty-four–hour recall.** Individuals are asked to recall the specific food items they ate during the previous day, describing the nature and amount of each. This

TABLE 2-12   Clinical Signs of Nutritional Status

	Good	Poor
General appearance	Alert, responsive	Listless, apathetic; cachexia
Hair	Shiny, lustrous; healthy scalp	Stringy, dull, brittle, dry, depigmented
Neck glands	No enlargement	Thyroid enlarged
Skin, face, and neck	Smooth, slightly moist; good color, reddish pink mucous membranes	Greasy, discolored, scaly
Eyes	Bright, clear; no fatigue circles	Dryness, signs of infection, increased vascularity, glassiness, thickened conjunctiva
Lips	Good color, moist	Dry, scaly, swollen; angular lesions (stomatitis)
Tongue	Good pink color, surface papillae present, no lesions	Papillary atrophy, smooth appearance; swollen, red, beefy (glossitis)
Gums	Good pink color; no swelling or bleeding; firm	Marginal redness or swelling; receding, spongy
Teeth	Straight, no crowding; well-shaped jaw; clean, no discoloration	Unfilled cavities, absent teeth, worn surfaces, mottled, malpositioned
Skin, general	Smooth, slightly moist, good color	Rough, dry, scaly, pale, pigmented, irritated; petechiae, bruises
Abdomen	Flat	Swollen
Legs, feet	No tenderness, weakness, or swelling; good color	Edema, tender calf; tingling, weakness
Skeleton	No malformations	Bowlegs, knock-knees, chest deformity at diaphragm, beaded ribs, prominent scapulae
Weight	Normal for height, age, body build	Overweight or underweight
Posture	Erect, arms and legs straight, abdomen in, chest out	Sagging shoulders, sunken chest, humpback
Muscles	Well developed, firm	Flaccid, poor tone; undeveloped, tender
Nervous control	Good attention span for age; does not cry easily; not irritable or restless	Inattentive, irritable
Gastrointestinal function	Good appetite and digestion; normal, regular elimination	Anorexia, indigestion, constipation, diarrhea
General vitality	Good endurance; energetic, vigorous; sleeps well at night	Easily fatigued, no energy, falls asleep in school, looks tired, apathetic

method is simpler and less costly than a longer diet history, but its usefulness is limited in some groups, such as elderly persons whose memory may be limited. Also, there are measurement problems in determining portion sizes.

3. **Food records.** At times a full dietary analysis of all nutrient and energy values is needed and a 3 to 7 day food record supplies the detailed information. Individuals

are asked to record their food intake for a brief period, or on certain days periodically. Each person is taught how to describe food items used singly and in combination, and how to measure amounts eaten. A 3-day record is usually sufficient to provide accurate information for nutrition analysis. Currently, computer analysis is common.

4. **Food frequency questionnaire.** This assessment tool provides information about an individual's food intake over an extended period of time, useful data when studying a group's disease risk and incidence. It has two basic parts: (1) a list of foods, and (2) a scale for checking frequency of use over a given period of time.

Assessment Evaluation Criteria

Well-nourished persons. Throughout the life cycle, nutritional status monitoring, guided by reference growth standards for each age group and general signs of food nutrition, as outlined in Table 2-12, helps to assure sound nutrition and healthy development. The rapid growth and development of the early years of life and the stress of later adult years of aging carry risks and require special attention.

Pregnancy. During a woman's pregnancy, she must meet increased nutrient and energy needs to support this period of rapid fetal growth and bring the pregnancy to a successful conclusion. Sufficient weight gain to meet maternal-fetal-placental demands during the pregnancy must be assured.[24] Recent criteria for this weight gain, which reflects a positive nutritional status, have been established by the National Academy of Sciences' Institute of Medicine and can serve as a general guide. Optimal nutrient and energy intake to meet both pregnancy and lactation needs can be monitored in general terms by the Recommended Dietary Allowances (see inside book covers) and guidelines discussed in Chapters 4 and 5. At best pregnancy is a period of physiologic stress, and in poor circumstances this normal stress is compounded by inadequate nutrition, bringing increased stress to both mother and baby. Ongoing nutrition assessment can identify specific needs, help prevent problems and complications, and promote a healthy pregnancy for both mother and baby.

Early growth and childhood. The highest nutrient requirements per kilogram body weight during the entire life cycle occur during infancy, when rates of growth and metabolism are at their highest point. Because of this direct relation between growth and nutritional status, close nutrition assessment is required to monitor progress. Over the following period of young childhood, the growth pattern slows and becomes erratic as the child grows in spurts and plateaus. Continued assessment of progress is essential to promote health. Commonly used monitoring tools are the age-specific growth charts from birth through adolescence, such as the National Center for Health Statistics percentile charts included in Appendix A. Age-specific RDA nutrient and energy levels can serve as general criteria, with reference to Chapters 6 and 7 for interpretations and guidance.

Adolescence. With puberty comes the second large growth spurt for the child. In both sexes intensive growth, under control of hormonal changes, profoundly affects nutritional needs. Continued monitoring of growth, changing body composition, and nutritional status helps ensure foundations for a healthy adulthood. In addition to the growth charts through age 18, extensive height-weight tables for the adolescent years are included in Appendix B. The RDA reference standard provides general evaluation criteria for monitoring nutrient and energy needs. Refer to Chapter 8 for specific monitoring guidelines.

Aging and the aged. With our increasing life span, the gradual aging process through adulthood requires a sound nutritional base to maintain health and prevent or control chronic diseases, which account for 75% of all deaths in the United States. Nutritional risk factors are associated with most all of these chronic diseases of aging. The age-adjusted weight-height table developed by Andres (see Appendix C) serves as better evaluation criteria for older adults than the regular standard tables. Also, alternate measures of height and weight for stooped or nonambulatory older adults are included in Appendix C. The RDA provides general nutrient-energy standards, although more specific individual analysis of needs may be required for elderly persons. These needs are discussed in detail in Chapter 9.

Malnourished persons. Poorly nourished persons may be found at both extremes of the nutrient-energy intake range. On one hand, gross deficits are obvious in children suffering from protein-energy malnutrition, while at the other extreme nutrient deficits may be masked by obesity from excess caloric intake.

Protein-energy malnutrition. The high risk of malnutrition in low-income families caught in a cycle of poverty, as well as among the "new poor," is well known and documented. There is also a growing awareness of the extent of various degrees of malnutrition among persons in hospitals, rehabilitation centers, and other long-term care facilities, especially among elderly patients or residents. Assessment procedures in public health services and medical/nursing facilities are designed to identify persons at risk for malnutrition. This assessment can provide the base for planning community intervention programs or individual care plans for needed nutrition support and family food assistance programs, especially for pregnant women, infants, and young children to meet crucial growth needs.

Obesity. In real terms, obesity, especially extreme forms, is a dangerous form of malnutrition because it carries increased risk of chronic disease, such as hypertension, heart disease, and diabetes. Weight assessment and early monitoring, especially of children in high-risk families for obesity and chronic disease, is an important health promotion and disease prevention practice.

Importance of Nutrition Assessment to Health Care and Public Policy

Nutritional care management. In both preventive health care and clinical care of disease, nutrition assessment is the essential first step in identifying individual nutritional needs and planning valid care to meet these needs. Careful assessment in health care can detect underlying risk factors early, so that programs for reducing these risks and thus helping to prevent related disease can be initiated. In clinical care, assessment of nutrition needs can identify and help change lifestyle factors and food habits that contribute to the disease process and thus control its progress. A number of these health promotion and disease prevention or management approaches are discussed in Chapters 3 and 10.

Public nutrition intervention programs. In a similar manner, public health intervention programs must include careful assessment of community need and resources, identifying those persons with problems that hinder care, and the higher cost in the long run of unmet needs. For example, the community cost of simple supportive prenatal care for poor pregnant women is far more cost-effective public policy than is the high long-term cost of neonatal medical technology for salvaging tiny low-birth-weight babies, premature and with multiple medical problems, who then die in infancy or require continuous disability care. Similar situations exist in care of young children and older adults. Poor childhood nutrition, especially during important early growth and development years, contributes to learning disabilities and educational problems. Unmet older adult nutritional needs contribute to progressive chronic disease and long-term costly care.

Summary

Human life and health depends on an appropriate supply of basic nutrients for body energy and tissue building. Of the macronutrients, carbohydrate is the primary fuel to produce energy, with fat as an additional concentrated fuel. Protein provides the amino acids necessary for building tissue. The micronutrients vitamins and minerals serve as control agents for biochemical reactions of body metabolism and structural material for certain tissues. The most basic nutrient, water, provides the life-sustaining solvent base for all the body's metabolic work. Nutrient needs change through the life cycle according to requirements for growth and maintaining body composition, and are supplied by a balanced diet based on variety and moderation.

Nutrition is an integral component of health and health care. Thus, nutrition assessment, both community and clinical, is basic to meeting these nutritional needs. This assessment process includes a variety of methods, including anthropometric, biochemical, clinical, and dietary procedures, and is important to both health care and public policy.

Review Questions

1. Compare the roles of each of the macronutrients in meeting energy needs of the body. How is this energy measured?
2. What are the amino acids? Describe their role in tissue growth and maintenance.
3. What are the two major types of metabolic tasks that the micronutrients perform? Give several examples of each type of task.
4. Describe the basic functions of water, the fundamental nutrient, in maintaining the human body.
5. Describe each of the two major forms of growth and development during the human life cycle. Give examples of how each relates to nutrition and changing nutrient needs.
6. Describe each of the four compartments of body composition based on metabolic activity. What part is most active metabolically? Why?
7. Describe the basic U.S. nutrient standard in terms of its structure and intended use. How is it frequently misused? What is its basic value in nutrition and health throughout the life cycle?
8. Compare the basic food groups, the food exchange groups, and the dietary guidelines for Americans as to purpose and use of each in planning healthy diets.
9. What basic role does assessment play in meeting nutritional needs? Compare this role in both clinical and community nutrition.
10. Identify the four basic methods of nutrition assessment and give examples of each.
11. Describe the importance of this basic assessment to nutritional health care and public policy.

References

1. National Research Council, Food and Nutrition Board: Diet and health: implications for reducing chronic disease risk, Washington, DC, 1989, National Academy Press.
2. Slavin JL: Dietary fiber: mechanisms or magic on disease prevention? Nutr Today 25(6):6, 1990.
3. US Department of Agriculture and US Department of Health and Human Services: Nutrition and your health: dietary guidelines for Americans, ed 3, Home and Garden Bull No 232, Nov 1990.
4. Cho ES et al: Long-term effects of low histidine intake on men, J Nutr 114:369, 1984.

5. National Research Council, Food and Nutrition Board: Recommended dietary allowances, ed 10, Washington, DC, 1989, National Academy Press.
6. Rossouw JE: Kwashiorkor in North America, Am J Clin Nutr 49:588, 1989.
7. Vitamin D: New perspectives, Lancet 1:1122, 1987.
8. DeLuca HF: The vitamin D story: a collaborative effort of basic science and clinical medicine, FASEB (Federation of American Societies for Experimental Biology) 2:224, 1988.
9. Usui Y et al: Vitamin K concentrations in the plasma and liver of surgical patients, Am J Clin Nutr 51:846, 1990.
10. Mertz W: The essential trace elements, Science 213:1332, 1981.
11. Grande F and Keys A: Body weight, body composition, and calorie status. In Goodhart RS and Shils ME, eds: Modern nutrition in health and disease, ed 6, Philadelphia, 1980, Lea & Febiger.
12. Andres R: Mortality and obesity: The rationale for age-specific height-weight tables. In Andres R et al, eds: Principles of geriatric medicine, New York, 1985, McGraw-Hill.
13. Guthrie HA: Recommended dietary allowances 1989: changes, consensus and challenges, Nutr Today 25(1):43, 1990.
14. Houghton B et al: An historical study of the underlying assumptions for United States food guides from 1917 through the Basic Four Food Groups Guide, J Nutr Ed 19(4):169, 1987.
15. Franz MJ et al: Exchange lists: revised 1986, J Am Diet Assoc 87(1):28, 1987.
16. American Dietetic Association: Exchange lists for weight management (1990), Chicago, 1990, ADA.
17. American Dietetic Association: Exchange lists for meal planning, Chicago, 1986, ADA.
18. Report: Dietary guidelines for Americans released, Nutr Today 25(6):44, 1990.
19. Peterkin BB: Dietary guidelines for Americans, 1990 edition, J Am Diet Assoc 90(12):1725, 1990.
20. US Department of Health and Human Services, Public Health Services: The Surgeon General's report on nutrition and health, PHS Pub No 88-50210, Washington, DC, 1988, US Government Printing Office.
21. Shields JE and Young E: Fat in fast food—evolving changes, Nutr Today 25(2):32, 1990.
22. Marens CL et al: Fast-food fare, N Engl J Med 322:557, 1990.
23. Rosenfeld I: The complete medical exam, New York, 1978, Simon & Schuster.
24. Institute of Medicine, Food and Nutrition Board, National Academy of Science: Nutrition during pregnancy, Washington, DC, 1990, National Academy Press.

Further Reading

Executive summary: National Nutrition Monitoring System: nutrition monitoring in the United States: an update report on nutrition monitoring, Nutr Today 25(1):33, 1990.

Just how well are we doing nutritionally as a nation? This report of assessment surveys conducted by the U.S. Departments of Agriculture and Health and Human Services provides some answers. It evaluates the dietary and nutritional status of the U.S. population, as well as the factors that determine status. Overall, it suggests that some changes are occurring in the eating patterns consistent with recommended dietary guidelines for Americans to avoid too much fat, saturated fat, and cholesterol, and to consume adequate amounts of starch and dietary fiber.

McNutt K: Are we pickin' on the kids? Nutr Today 26(3):42, 1991.

This interesting article written in journalistic style provides a good example of national health policy documents used as a basis for a comparative assessment of the nutritional status and food patterns of American adults and children. The author, both a nutritionist and an attorney, makes a generally positive case for the children, but also points out three areas of concern: obesity, iron-deficiency anemia, and dental caries.

3

Nutrition and the Adult: Planning for a Healthy Lifestyle

Sue Rodwell Williams
Eleanor D. Schlenker

Basic Concepts

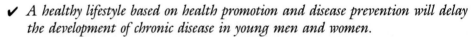

✔ *A healthy lifestyle based on health promotion and disease prevention will delay the development of chronic disease in young men and women.*

✔ *Varied national and community health promotion programs assist individual efforts toward positive health maintenance and disease prevention.*

✔ *The human life cycle begins with the good nutrition and healthy lifestyle that young adults, especially young women, bring to reproduction and the start of a new life.*

✔ *Although genetic factors influence adult health and longevity, personal lifestyle choices determine 50% of an adult's health status.*

Establishing lifestyle patterns that promote personal health and reproductive capacity and a state of well-being and fitness for a lifetime should be a priority for the young adult. Following the tumultuous teen years, when physical growth and development have reached their adult goal, nutrition education and patterns of living focus on food and exercise behaviors that will maintain optimal physical and mental health. Health promotion for adults is often directed toward particular physical problems. Rising medical costs associated with long-term treatment of chronic disorders such as heart disease and diabetes have led to our current emphasis on health education for disease prevention. Our goals are to help individuals identify and adopt those practices that will support optimum health and wellness throughout their adult years.

This chapter looks at some of the ways we can meet these health goals during the adult years. We focus on the nutritional needs of adults, particularly reproductive health of young women and women's health issues, and appropriate health promotion strategies for planning a healthy lifestyle. If signs of chronic disease do become apparent, nutrition intervention can arrest their development and help individuals maintain the highest possible level of personal well-being.

ADULT HEALTH, WELLNESS, AND LIFESTYLE
The Concept of Wellness

Health and *wellness* are words that cannot be used interchangeably. In its simplest form health is defined as the absence of disease, although the World Health Organization (WHO) has expanded this definition to include complete physical, mental, and social well-being, and not merely the absence of disease or dysfunction. The concept of wellness carries this state one step further. It seeks to develop the maximum potential of individuals within their own environments. This implies a balance between activities and goals: work versus leisure, personal needs versus the expectations and goals of others, or lifestyle choices versus health risks. Wellness indicates a positive dynamic state as a person strives toward a higher level of function.

Wellness represents a continuum from high-level wellness and optimum health to low-level wellness, illness, and death. Various body functions will differ in their level of wellness from time to time. As one system or function is improving, another may be deteriorating. However, a strength in one area may compensate for a weakness or stress in another. For example, excellent physical health may help an individual cope with severe emotional stress that occurs with the loss of a family member, job loss, dissatisfaction with a job, or the disapproval of one's peer group.

Approaches to Health and Well-Being

Every day individuals are bombarded with messages that encourage actions to improve their health. However, people approach personal health decisions in many different ways and these approaches may differ at different stages in the life cycle. A healthy child may see little need for appropriate health behavior whereas an overweight man with above-normal serum lipid levels may be concerned about his risk of heart disease and may consider changing his lifestyle to modify predisposing factors. In general, persons use one of three approaches to health care: traditional, preventive, or wellness approach.

Traditional approach. The traditional approach to health leads to change only when the symptoms of illness or disease already exist, and the individual seeks out a physician to diagnose and cure the condition. Because major chronic problems such as heart disease or cancer develop over a period of years, long before overt signs become apparent, this approach is of little value for lifelong positive health.

Preventive approach. The preventive approach to health focuses on identifying risk factors that increase a person's chances of developing a particular health problem, and making behavior choices that will prevent or minimize such risks. Preventive measures may include screening programs to detect the development of a problem while it is still asymptomatic and, thus, allow early intervention. Health fairs, for example, emphasize blood pressure screening and intervention to reduce risk of stroke. The disadvantage of this approach is that it tends to be negative in style, emphasizing disease risk and "do not" rules of care.

Preventive approach
Approach to health that seeks to identify and reduce risk factors for disease.

Wellness approach. The wellness approach focuses on positive lifestyle choices that will enhance physical and mental well-being. On this basis persons may choose to consume more vegetables and whole-grain cereals, rather than a large number of foods high in fat, salt, or sugar. The wellness approach begun early in life allows the development of full personal potential while retarding the onset of degenerative changes and chronic disease.

Wellness approach
Approach to health that promotes positive planning of a healthy lifestyle for physical and mental well-being.

Determinants of Health Status

Good or poor health is determined by five factors: heredity, environment, health outlook, health care, and lifestyle. The first of these factors, heredity, is beyond the individual's control. But the remaining four factors can, at least to some extent, be modified if the person wishes to achieve better health.

Environment. Our environment has two dimensions: the physical environment and the social environment. The *physical environment* encompasses both the near environment and the extended surrounding area. Families living in poor housing with ineffective plumbing and no refrigerator are highly susceptible to infection and disease. Polluted air and water or contaminated food influences health status. The *social environment* can be friendly or hostile. A person may have family or friends for emotional support or be essentially alone. A person may be in a fast-paced environment with high expectations for performance or be in a setting that has low expectations and few demands.

Health outlook. Health outlook relates to personal perception of one's own health and well-being, although perception and reality may not necessarily agree. Individuals who rate their health as excellent or good have a longer life expectancy than those who rate their health as fair or poor.[1] In fact, self-rating of health is a stronger predictor of life expectancy than actual physical status based on a medical examination. Positive feelings about one's health usually reflect a similar attitude toward life in general that supports positive adjustment and adaptation.

Health care. In differing life circumstances health care may or may not be under an individual's control. People in lower socioeconomic groups do not always have access to the same level or quality of medical care as those in higher income groups. Poor reading skills, limited education, or a language barrier may hinder an individual who is attempting to carry out instructions from a health professional about health care or treatment of disease. Health care also includes wise self-care such as seeking medical care when symptoms so indicate, following directions when using medications (including over-the-counter drugs), or exercising regularly.

Lifestyle
A person's unique pattern of living, which depending on its form can be negative or positive in its health results.

Lifestyle. The term **lifestyle** refers to a person's unique pattern of living. These patterns reflect our values and beliefs. They involve what, how much, and when an individual chooses to eat, whether or not an individual exercises regularly, or whether an individual uses drugs. Use of time is a lifestyle choice. An individual may spend leisure time watching television and consuming large amounts of alcohol and snack foods high in sodium and fat. Another person of similar age may spend leisure time practicing tennis or chooses to walk, rather than drive, to a nearby store. A young adult may relieve stress in harmful ways by overeating, smoking, or abusing alcohol. For another, appropriate outlets involving exercise, counseling, or relaxation techniques may be the choice.

Health and wellness throughout adulthood are to a great extent the result of lifestyle choices. When we consider what determines health status, we find that over 50% of this influence is under one's personal control. Diet, exercise, smoking habits, use of alcohol, and stress management all contribute to this total. For those exhibiting early signs of chronic disease, or those at risk because of genetic background, adoption of positive health behaviors can slow or interrupt the degenerative disease process.

Health Promotion

Definitions. Public attention began to focus on health promotion in 1979 with the publication of *Healthy People: The Surgeon General's Report on Health Promotion and Disease Prevention.*[2] The goal was to help people maintain and enhance their well-being by making use of preventive health services and lifestyle modification. While lifestyle changes are a major component of health promotion, some propose that health promotion should also include educational, economic, and environmental adjustments that support behavior conducive to health.[3] An individual with poor reading skills attempting to select a diet lower in saturated fat and cholesterol may be unable to do so if diet counseling or materials written at an appropriate level are not available. Health promotion requires a combination of intervention strategies to bring about behavior change.

Models for behavior change. Health and nutrition educators have examined the social and psychologic factors that influence behavior change. By understanding how people choose to alter their behavior we can best develop programs that will encourage these changes. Several ideas have emerged including the health belief model, the locus of control model, and the idea of self-efficacy.

Health belief model. The health belief model was developed to explain how a person who does not currently have a disease chooses to alter risk factors to prevent future development of this disease.[4] This model suggests that the decision for action is based on three factors: (1) the individual's perception of vulnerability to the disease, (2) the seriousness of the disease, and (3) the difficulty in implementing the lifestyle changes required. A young woman whose mother is confined to a wheel chair as a result of osteoporosis and bone fractures (see p. 81) may begin to exercise regularly and select calcium-rich foods.

Locus of control model. People perceive the world and their ability to control events occurring around them in different ways. Some individuals perceive the day to day events in their lives as being under their (internal) control. They assume responsibility for their life choices and the physiologic and psychologic components of their well-being. Individuals with an internal locus of control tend to be more successful in weight loss as they assume responsibility for their situation.[5] Individuals with an external locus of control consider their situation to be the result of outside forces outside their control. Consequently, they take less responsibility for their lifestyle behaviors. This individual may view his elevated blood pressure as a result of his genetic susceptibility to sodium intake and decide that reducing sodium will not be effective anyway in reducing his risk. Some persons consider all life happenings to be a matter of chance with no particular basis of control. It may be difficult to motivate these individuals to alter lifestyle behavior to improve well-being.

Locus of control
(L *locus,* place, site) A person's perceived control center over his life.

Concept of self-efficacy. The concept of self-efficacy relates to an individual's belief that he or she will be able to make and maintain the health-related changes desired. This feeling of empowerment relates to the facts or skills provided to the individual that support behavior change. Using role play to enable a man at high risk of heart disease to ask diplomatically for juice or a carbonated beverage when offered an alcoholic beverage at a business party will increase his confidence when placed in the situation. As nutritionists/ registered dietitians or other health team members who become involved in health promotion, we must learn to recognize our client's beliefs and attitudes relating to behavior change and develop programs to address these needs.

COMPONENTS OF A PRUDENT HEALTHY LIFESTYLE

Health promotion activities should focus on those lifestyle behaviors known to influence long-term health. These behaviors include dietary patterns, exercise patterns, ability to manage stress, smoking habits, and use of alcohol. This section discusses current recommendations in each of these areas.

Dietary Recommendations

Assessing risks and benefits. Absolute proof of a relationship is especially difficult when evaluating a multifaceted issue such as diet and associated health risks. When developing dietary recommendations policy makers must balance the potential benefits of the dietary pattern recommended against the possible adverse effects of the dietary pattern. Another consideration is the practicality of the diet for implementation by the public. The production of leaner animal products may be as important as public education in lowering dietary fat levels.

An expert panel was recently commissioned by the Food and Nutrition Board of the National Research Council to develop dietary recommendations that would assist persons

ONE STEP FURTHER

Recommendations for Healthy Eating

- Reduce total fat to 30% or less of total kilocalories, saturated fat to less than 10% of total kilocalories, and cholesterol to less than 300 mg per day; polyunsaturated fatty acids should not exceed 10% of total kilocalories.
- Each day eat five or more servings of fruits and vegetables, especially green and yellow vegetables and citrus fruits; eat six or more servings of breads, cereals, or legumes.
- Maintain protein intake at a moderate level, not more than two times the RDA.
- Balance energy intake and physical activity to maintain appropriate weight; avoid diets that are either excessive or severely restricted in kilocalories.
- Limit alcohol consumption to less than one ounce per day (the equivalent of two 12 ounce cans of beer, two 3.5 ounce glasses of wine, or two average cocktails).
- Limit daily intake of salt (sodium chloride) to 6 g or less including salt added in cooking or at the table, and that found in highly processed foods or pickled items.
- Maintain adequate calcium intake with servings of low- and non-fat dairy products and dark green vegetables; use of calcium supplements by healthy people to raise intake above the RDA are not justified.
- Avoid taking dietary supplements that contain above the RDA for any nutrient.
- Maintain an optimal intake of fluoride particularly during the years of tooth formation and growth.

Adapted from Committee on Diet and Health, Food and Nutrition Board: Diet and health: Implications for reducing chronic disease risk, Washington, DC, 1989, National Academy Press.

in reducing their risk of chronic disease.[6] These recommendations for use by nutritionists, government policy makers, and the public are outlined in the box above.

Basis for recommendations. These recommended nutrient and energy guides are based on their relation to established chronic disease risks.

1. **Fats.** Diets high in saturated fat and cholesterol are associated with increased incidence of atherosclerosis and coronary heart disease. Also, high fat diets contribute to the development of obesity and increase cancer risk. Controversy regarding reducing dietary fat centers on the fact that red meat, an important source of iron and zinc, and dairy foods, important sources of calcium and riboflavin, are high in saturated fat and cholesterol. But saturated fat and cholesterol can be limited by using lean meat, poultry without skin, fish, and low- or non-fat dairy products without sacrificing intakes of other important nutrients. Total fat and saturated fat can be reduced further by using polyunsaturated vegetable oils and margarines, and less fried foods.

2. **Complex carbohydrates.** The calories lost by reducing fat intake can be replaced by eating more vegetables, fruits, cereals, and legumes. Plant foods rich in complex carbohydrates and fiber reduce chronic disease risk in several ways. First, a diet high in plant foods is likely to be low or moderate in fat. Also, soluble fiber, found in plant foods, independently lowers blood lipid levels and thereby lowers cardiovascular risk. Fruits and vegetables are good sources of potassium, which seems to play a role in moderating blood pressure levels in some persons and thereby may reduce the risk of stroke. **Carotenoids** present in dark green and deep yellow fruits and vegetables offer some protection against particular forms of cancer. Finally, the fiber component of plant foods assists in maintaining proper function of the large bowel and lower gastrointestinal tract.

Carotenoids
Any of a group of red and yellow pigments chemically similar to and including carotene found in dark green and yellow vegetables and fruits.

3. **Proteins.** Protein intakes among most age groups in the United States are well in excess of the RDA.[6] Protein intakes greater than two times the RDA are associated with increased incidence of certain cancers and coronary heart disease in both animal studies and humans, mainly a result of the high levels of saturated fat and cholesterol usually associated with diets high in animal protein. High protein intakes can also lead to increased urinary loss of calcium and increased risk of osteoporosis.

4. **Energy.** Current trends among young adults include decreased energy intakes, decreased physical activity, and increased body fat as defined by body mass index. Physical activity even at moderate levels will allow an energy intake sufficient to obtain recommended levels of important vitamins and minerals, assist in maintaining normal weight, and improve fitness. Excess body weight increases risk of coronary heart disease, hypertension, non–insulin-dependent diabetes, and gallbladder disease. Weight loss will decrease risk, even if desirable weight is not attained. Excessive alcohol consumption, adding kilocalories that provide few other nutrients, not only undermines energy balance but also increases risk of heart disease, liver disease, high blood pressure, some forms of cancer, and nutrient deficiencies. Pregnant women should totally avoid alcoholic beverages.

5. **Minerals.** It is known that salt (sodium chloride) intakes about 6 g per day (2400 mg of sodium per day) are associated with elevated blood pressure in genetically susceptible individuals. However, it is not possible at this time to identify those particular individuals. The recommended level of intake is likely to prevent the development of high blood pressure in susceptible individuals, and is not deficient for the general population. Foods that are pickled or prepared in brine should be used sparingly. Calcium is receiving increased attention based on the reports associating low calcium intake with elevated blood pressure and increased risk of bone fracture (p. 71 and 81). At the same time there is no strong evidence that calcium intake above the RDA carry any particular benefit.[6]

6. **Supplements.** Protein, vitamin, and mineral supplements in excess of the RDA have not been shown to be beneficial and excess vitamins B_6, A, and D and iron has been shown to be harmful, leading to toxicity or inappropriate interactions with other nutrients. Long-term health risks and benefits related to supplementation have yet to be identified.

Exercise Pattern

Positive effects of exercise. Regular physical exercise contributes to health and fitness in many ways. Some of these benefits include improved energy balance, body composition, cardiac efficiency, and serum lipid levels.

1. **Energy balance.** One of the most obvious health benefits of exercise is its role in energy balance and weight management. Increasing energy expenditure with exercise allows a higher energy intake in food, increasing the likelihood of obtaining adequate amounts of all important nutrients without inappropriate weight gain. An indirect effect of exercise is increased glucose uptake and utilization by muscle cells in the trained versus the untrained individual.

2. **Body composition.** Physical exercise strengthens muscle fibers and helps prevent age-related loss of lean body mass and increase in body fat. Exercise strengthens bone by stimulating bone formation and preventing bone loss. Regular physical stress on the bone through exercise involving the pull of body weight on the bone as occurs in walking, jogging, dancing, or bicycling can prevent or retard the onset of osteoporosis, a common bone disorder among older women.

3. **Cardiovascular efficiency.** Regular exercise increases one's ability to do physical work with increased cardiovascular efficiency and decreased recovery time. Maximal

oxygen consumption is increased while heart rate and blood pressure levels are decreased both during exercise and at rest. Improved condition of the heart as a pump as well as reduced fat deposition in the arterial wall contribute to the maintenance of appropriate blood pressure levels among those exercising regularly. Blood pressure levels increase with age among those with sedentary lifestyles.

4. **Serum lipid levels.** Physical activity retards degenerative changes through its effect on serum lipid levels. Daily exercise increases serum levels of high-density lipoproteins (HDLs) which help protect against coronary artery disease by removing cholesterol molecules from the blood before they can enter the arterial wall. At the same time physical activity assists a low-saturated fat, low-cholesterol diet to significantly lower low-density lipoproteins (LDLs), which carry cholesterol to the cells and increase cardiovascular risk.

Exercise and disease risk. Physically fit persons have a lower risk of death from all causes as compared to their peers. In a study of more than 10,000 men and 3000 women followed for 8 years, mortality rates were four times higher in the least fit persons as compared to the most fit.[7] Survivors and deceased subjects did not differ in age, body mass index, serum cholesterol levels, or blood pressure levels. Those only moderately fit still had less than one half the risk of the least fit. A brisk walk of 30 minutes per day, an exercise level within the physical ability of most persons, can lead to a moderate level of fitness. The duration and resulting energy expenditure of exercise may be more important than the intensity. Daily exercise with an energy cost of 234 kilocalories reduced the incidence of coronary heart disease and death in men with other risk factors including cigarette smoking, elevated serum cholesterol and blood pressure levels, and family history of cardiovascular disease.[8] In fact exercise reduced the risk associated with those factors as compared to sedentary men. Regular exercise may be most critical for those individuals who already suffer from several negative risk factors.

Developing an exercise program. A sedentary individual, regardless of age, should undergo a physical examination before embarking on an exercise program. Also, persons should pay attention to body signals. The appearance of pain suggests that it is time to slow down or stop. To prevent muscular or skeletal injury, or a cardiovascular incident, the progression in both duration and intensity must be gradual. Cardiovascular exercise requires an increase in heart rate to 60% to 85% of maximum (pulse: 220 minus age) continued for at least 20 minutes. However, these levels may need to be achieved over a period of time. For a person with prior cardiovascular problems, heart rate should be carefully monitored.

An individual may be motivated to initiate an exercise program on the basis of health-related beliefs, but long-term adherence is more likely if the activity is enjoyed and family support is provided. Activities of great intensity that are perceived to require great exertion and carry risk of injury are less likely to be continued. Walking can be an ideal activity, leading to energy expenditure and cardiorespiratory fitness, and providing a transition to more vigorous exercise if desired. Characteristics of an exercise program that promote continuing participation include:

- Lack of need for specialized facilities or equipment
- Limited discomfort
- Potential for incorporation in the daily routine
- Opportunity for social interaction

Health professionals need to direct particular attention to the transitions in lifestyle often associated with a decline in physical activity. These include the transition from high school or college to a work situation, a change in residence, or recovery from an illness or injury. Suggestions for exercise activities are given in Table 3-1.

TABLE 3-1   *Energy Cost of Various Physical Activities**

Activity	kcal/kg/hr
Aerobic dancing	8.9
Bicycling (moderate speed)	2.5
Bicycling (racing)	7.6
Golf	3.9
Rowing in race	16.0
Running	7.0
Skating	3.5
Skiing (cross country)	5.9
Swimming (2 mph)	7.9
Tennis	5.3
Walking (3 mph)	2.0
Walking (4 mph)	3.4

* Does not include basal metabolism.

Stress Management

Stress is a specific physiologic or psychologic reaction to a life event. The event may be starting a new job, moving to a different city, getting married, or the death of a family member. The stress response is the same whether initiated by a positive or negative event. Stress can result in adverse physiologic symptoms including (1) gastrointestinal distress, for example, nausea, vomiting, or diarrhea; (2) irregular sleep patterns; (3) increased muscle tension with resulting headache or backache; or (4) cardiovascular responses resulting in constriction of blood vessels and rapid pulse.

Stress
Sum of biologic reactions to adverse stimuli, physical, mental, or emotional, internal or external, that disturbs the state of homeostasis and sense of well-being.

Everyone experiences one or more of these symptoms occasionally, but the danger lies in the long-term consequences resulting from continuing, unalleviated stress. Continued gastric upset and inappropriate secretion of stomach acid can lead to peptic ulcers and associated stomach problems. Heart disease is accelerated by high blood pressure that occurs over time as a stress response. Psychologic distress can have a detrimental effect on food intake resulting in patterns of overeating or binge eating leading to inappropriate weight gain, or at the other extreme, bulimia or anorexia nervosa, now increasing among young adults.

Because poorly managed stress is a threat to both physical and mental health and occupational safety and productivity, cognitive and behavioral approaches have been developed for stress reduction. Group and individual counseling help persons improve understanding and attitude, develop constructive coping mechanisms, and learn positive approaches to problem solving. Behavioral approaches include reduction in use of alcohol, caffeine, or nicotine, along with increased exercise, rest, and relaxation.

Avoidance of Cigarette Smoking

Cigarette smoking is a major risk factor for many chronic conditions and is responsible for more than one of every six deaths in the United States.[9] According to recent statistics smoking accounted for 87% of lung cancer deaths, 21% of coronary heart disease deaths, and 18% of stroke deaths. Use of cigarettes accelerates the development of atherosclerotic lesions, leading to the estimate that more than 40% of deaths from coronary heart disease among men and women less than 65 years of age are attributable to smoking. Smoking exacerbates the risk arising from alcohol use, high blood pressure, and diabetes. Among women who both smoke and use oral contraceptives, coronary risk is 10 times greater than among those who do neither.

Mortality risk for both sexes increases with the number of cigarettes smoked, and is higher for those who began smoking at younger ages. Even at age 30, an individual smoking two packs of cigarettes a day has a life expectancy 8 to 9 years shorter than a nonsmoker of similar age.[9] Until recently, prevalence of lung cancer was lower among women, reflecting their limited use of cigarettes. Lung cancer now has passed breast cancer as the leading cause of cancer death in women. Smokers who quit experience both immediate and long-term benefits. Risk of coronary heart disease is reduced within the first few years. Risk of lung cancer drops substantially in 5 to 9 years, but remains two times that of the lifelong nonsmoker even after 20 years. Although further deterioration of the lung is arrested, smokers with obstructed air passages cannot anticipate major improvement despite cessation of smoking.

A major concern of health professionals should be the prevalence of cigarette smoking among teenagers and young adults. Smoking is now more popular among teenage women than teenage men. Nearly one fourth of all teenage women smoke. Adolescents are beginning to smoke at earlier ages; 15% of those 12 to 17 smoke, with many smoking two packs of cigarettes per day.

A positive result of smoking cessation programs has been the overall decline in adult smokers from 40% to 27% of the population over the last 25 years.[9] Nearly half of all living adults who ever smoked have quit. Smoking cessation programs have focused on behavior modification techniques and coping strategies to assist with the physiologic, psychologic, and social factors related to smoking **addiction.**

Addiction
(L *addictio,* a giving over, surrender) State of being enslaved to some undesirable practice that is physically or psychologically habit-forming to the extent that its cessation causes severe trauma.

Appropriate Use of Alcohol

In the United States alcohol consumption peaks in those aged 20 to 40 with approximately 70% using alcohol to some degree.[6] Alcohol abuse is also most frequent in youth and middle age. Inappropriate use of alcohol has a negative effect on nutritional status and enhances risk of chronic disease. Alcohol has a toxic effect on the gastrointestinal tract and reduces the absorption of many nutrients including vitamins B_6 and B_{12}, folic acid, and zinc. Alcohol further contributes to malnutrition by adding kilocalories to the diet but no protein or important vitamins or minerals. This problem of nutrient density is evident in the diets of some young adults in which alcohol kilocalories replace nonalcohol kilocalories to a level approaching one third of total energy intake. Although this practice avoids weight gain, it further decreases intakes of iron and calcium, nutrients already low in the diets of young adult women.

Alcohol abuse contributes to deteriorating health through its association with elevated serum lipid levels, hypertension, hyperglycemia, and liver disease. Although it was believed that liver damage resulted from a lack of food and nutrients rather than from a direct toxic effect of alcohol itself, studies have found the development of liver abnormalities in well-nourished alcohol abusers. Regular use of alcohol increases risk of stroke and cancer of the oral cavity and esophagus. Depletion of liver stores of vitamin A as a consequence of alcohol abuse may contribute to the association observed between alcohol consumption and cancer of the liver, breast, and pancreas.

HEALTH PROMOTION AND CHRONIC DISEASE

Within this century nutrition research has shifted from the identification of nutrients and deficiency symptoms to the study of the effect of diet and lifestyle on the diseases of civilization such as heart disease and cancer. An abundant food supply along with the decrease in physical activity made possible by modern technology have contributed to widespread incidence of chronic diseases. This has led policy makers and health professionals to examine risk factors associated with these conditions and develop public education approaches that support risk reduction.

Atherosclerotic Heart Disease

Prevalence and impact. The major cause of death in the United States and other Western societies is disease of the heart and blood vessels, accounting for over half of all deaths.[6] Risk is low in early adulthood but increases rapidly with age. Risk is highest for black women and white men. Mortality rates have declined by 28% over the past 2 decades as a result of better medical care following a heart attack, therapeutic intervention such as development of serum lipid–lowering drugs, and changes in diet and exercise patterns.

Development of atherosclerosis. Atherosclerosis, a pathologic series of events occurring in the coronary arteries supplying blood to the heart muscle and the cerebral arteries supplying blood to the brain, actually begins in childhood. Lipid deposits as fatty streaks found in children may regress or progress to form fibrous plaques of accumulated fat and debris. Ulceration or hemorrhage into the plaque causing swelling can occlude the lumen of the artery causing tissue breakdown as blood supply is interrupted. Arterial injury in the coronary arteries results in coronary heart disease, commonly occurring in middle age and carrying risk of myocardial infarction or heart attack. Occlusion or hemorrhage in a cerebral artery usually occurs 10 to 20 years later, resulting in a stroke with paralysis or loss of speech, vision, hearing, or memory. Elevated serum cholesterol or LDL levels and high blood pressure levels increase the severity of atherosclerosis, although high blood pressure is more closely associated with problems in the cerebral arteries.

Risk factors and coronary heart disease. Genetic, dietary, and lifestyle factors as described in Table 3-2 influence the development of atherosclerosis and heart disease. Intervention strategies have been directed toward diet- or drug-induced reductions in LDL levels, smoking cessation, weight loss, limited use of alcohol, and increases in physical activity. High dietary cholesterol and saturated fatty acids lead to increased LDL levels whereas polyunsaturated fatty acids when substituted for saturated fats lower both HDL and LDL cholesterol concentrations. Monounsaturated fatty acids as found in olive oil appear to decrease LDL cholesterol levels without lowering HDL cholesterol levels. Soluble fiber, commonly found in oat bran and starchy vegetables, also appears to lower serum LDL levels. Physical activity increases HDL levels as does moderate use of alcohol. An area of recent investigation has been the omega-3 polyunsaturated fatty acids commonly

TABLE 3-2 *Factors Contributing to Cardiovascular Disease Risk*

Personal Characteristics (No Control)	Lifestyle Behaviors (Intervene and Change)	Background Conditions (Screen and Treat)
Sex	Stress/ability to cope	Hypertension
Age	Smoking cigarettes	Diabetes mellitus
Family history	Abuse of alcohol	Hyperlipidemia (especially
	Sedentary lifestyle	hypercholesterolemia)
	Obesity	
	Food habits	
	Excess saturated fat	
	Excess salt	
	Excess sugar	
	Excess animal protein	

found in fatty (cold water) fish, which seem not only to increase HDL levels but also retard and possibly reverse the formation of atherosclerotic plaques.

Intervention trials for coronary heart disease. Several large-scale diet-heart trials have been conducted with middle-aged hypercholesterolemic men to evaluate strategies for reducing mortality from coronary heart disease. Efforts to reduce serum cholesterol levels included diets low in fat and saturated fat or lipid-lowering drugs. A general finding was that reduction in coronary risk was directly proportional to the decrease in serum cholesterol levels. A 1% decrease in serum cholesterol levels resulted in a 2% decrease in coronary risk.[6] However, a recent summary of many studies suggests that experimental groups experiencing decreased numbers of coronary deaths as a result of dietary or drug intervention had increased numbers of deaths from other causes such that mortality rates did not differ despite the intervention.[10]

An ongoing study in San Francisco is evaluating the influence of lifestyle changes without surgical or drug intervention on atherosclerotic damage.[11] After 1 year a measurable decrease in fatty plaques in the coronary arteries was observed in men who exercised regularly, stopped smoking, and followed a vegetarian diet with less than 10% of energy coming from fat. Such a diet could be deficient in essential fatty acids, vitamin B_{12}, zinc, and iron, and should not be followed without close medical supervision. However, this study may provide evidence that lifestyle changes over a long-term period not only retard but may actually reverse coronary artery disease.

Hypertension

Hypertension or sustained elevated arterial blood pressure increases risk of stroke, coronary heart disease, and kidney damage. Obesity is associated with elevated blood pressure levels that decrease during periods of active weight loss. It appears that regular exercise can prevent the usual age-related increase in blood pressure levels and lead to a decrease in elevated levels, but long-term evaluation of this effect is lacking.[6]

Risk reduction and hypertension. Dietary factors associated with hypertension are alcohol and various electrolytes including sodium, potassium, and calcium. Excessive ingestion of alcohol, more than 1 ounce of alcohol each day, is associated with a high prevalence of hypertension. The effect of nutrients on hypertension is less well understood. Epidemiologic data suggest that a habitual intake of more than 6 g of salt or 2400 mg of sodium per day increases the risk of hypertension, although findings are not consistent.[5] Low intakes of potassium or calcium were associated with high blood pressure and stroke in some U.S. surveys. Unfortunately, efforts to lower blood pressure by supplementing with potassium or calcium have had inconsistent results.[12] In an experimental trial evaluating the influence of a diet moderate in sodium or high in potassium, weight reduction, and drug therapy on blood pressure, the greatest improvement in cardiovascular risk status was achieved with a combination of weight loss and drug therapy.[13] Mild sodium restriction may permit a reduction in the amount of drug required to maintain appropriate blood pressure levels.

Individual response. The impact of electrolyte restriction or supplementation on blood pressure levels is a highly individual response. Clinical trials resulting in no significant change in mean blood pressure have produced striking decreases in blood pressure levels in particular individuals.[12] Diets limited in sodium but generous in food sources of potassium and calcium are of general benefit. Potassium supplementation, unless carefully supervised, is not recommended and is especially dangerous for those using potassium-sparing diuretics or those with compromised kidney function.

Overweight and Obesity

Incidence of overweight. In the United States 25% of white and black men and 25% and 40% of white and black women, respectively, are overweight, and the number is increasing.[14] The popularization of the slim figure and the recommendations of health care professionals have led many adults to attempt to lose weight. Unfortunately, the diets chosen are frequently low in protein, vitamins, and minerals, as well as kilocalories, and lead to nutrient depletion. Moreover, extremely low energy diets do not help the dieter develop new eating patterns; consequently, when the diet is discontinued and the usual eating pattern resumed, the weight is likely to be regained. This can establish a cycle of weight gain, weight loss, and weight gain, which over a period of years can be more detrimental to health than the initial overweight. An approach to weight loss that includes an increase in energy expenditure in the form of physical activity along with a reasonable decrease in energy intake is more effective than either strategy alone, as indicated in the box on p. 62.

Obesity and disease risk. Obesity is an independent risk factor for cardiovascular disease, in addition to contributing to the development of elevated blood pressure and serum cholesterol levels, also independent risk factors. Obesity promotes the development of arthritis and degenerative bone-joint disease, reducing flexibility and hindering mobility. Because physical exercise is difficult, the obese individual is more likely to be sedentary, which sustains the obesity and further contributes to degenerative changes. Obesity is a significant factor in the development of maturity-onset diabetes, as enlarged fat cells resist the action of insulin.

The influence of obesity or overweight upon mortality risk is controversial. Life insurance statistics indicate that individuals greatly above or below average weight are more likely to die at younger ages. In early reports underweight persons had an even greater mortality risk than overweight persons. This led to the assertion by some health professionals that being slightly overweight might actually be protective, particularly in the presence of severe illness or disease. A 25-year followup of the Framingham Heart Study revealed that the high mortality among the underweight men was related to cigarette smoking.[15] Eighty percent of the underweight men were cigarette smokers as compared to only 55% of the overweight men.

The age when an individual becomes obese also influences mortality from cardiovascular disease. Regardless of body weight at age 25, weight gain during the adult years increases cardiovascular risk, whereas weight loss among those who are overweight reduces this risk. Men appear to be more sensitive than women to the detrimental effects of weight gain and the positive effects of weight loss. The location of body fat also influences risk (p. 79). Men and women with thick layers of body fat in the abdominal region have higher risk of coronary heart disease and death than those with similar amounts of fat about their hips.

Even mild overweight can be detrimental to the maintenance of good health. For men ages 40 to 49, mortality rates are doubled in those 20% overweight as compared to those 10% overweight.[15] Moreover, a weight loss of only 10 pounds can cause a significant drop in elevated blood pressure.

Cancer

Cancer is the second leading cause of death in the United States. Although the impact of diet upon cancer mortality has not been determined with certainty, a current estimate suggests that one third of all cancer deaths are diet related.[6] Dietary components that have been linked with specific cancers include alcohol, fat, vitamin C and other antioxidants, beta-carotene, and highly smoked and salted foods.

In humans high fat diets are positively related to cancer incidence and mortality. Polyunsaturated vegetable oils promote tumor growth to a greater extent than do saturated fats. Conversely, omega-3 fatty acids from fish oils and monounsaturated fatty acids from olive oil do not promote tumor growth. Fish oils may actually inhibit tumor growth at high levels of intake. The use of olive oil, high in monounsaturated fats, is believed to

ONE STEP FURTHER

Weight Reduction

Is there an easy way to lose weight? Which weight loss methods are medically safe? The significant number of obese Americans who are always seeking *the* answer provide an eager audience for each newly marketed book, program, or diet.

Particular fad diets have gained popularity by promising quick and easy weight loss by restricting particular nutrients or combining certain foods. Diets providing less than 100 g of carbohydrate daily lead to rapid water loss inducing an early but transient weight loss. However, serious side effects include nausea, vomiting, and binge eating patterns as a result of altered neurotransmitter synthesis following carbohydrate restriction. Diets very low in fat (less than 20% of total energy) are usually high in grains, fruits, and vegetables, but may lack high-quality protein and bioavailable forms of calcium, iron, and zinc. Very low-calorie diets, sometimes referred to as protein-sparing modified fasts, provide less than 800 kilocalories per day in the form of food or a formula drink. Very low-calorie diets were developed, however, to be used only under medical supervision in cases of extreme obesity, but are now being sold over the counter. These products can lead to potassium depletion, cardiac arrhythmias, and in some instances sudden death. Anorectic drugs, such as caffeine or phenylpropanolamine, are marketed for weight loss but can cause dizziness, tachycardia, and hypertension. Human chorionic gonadotropin (HCG) is believed to stimulate fat mobilization but has not led to weight loss in clinical trials.

Surgical interventions for weight loss must be evaluated carefully as the risk may exceed the benefit. Gastric stapling will not in itself result in weight loss unless kilocalories are restricted. An alternative to gastric stapling, approved by the Food and Drug Administration for individuals more than 20% above ideal weight, is the gastric balloon, introduced into the stomach and then inflated. Among 12 highly motivated patients, daily energy intake following gastric placement of the balloon was 615 to 1550 kilocalories.* After 2 to 6 months, weight lost ranged from 1 to 25 kg. The amount of weight lost was not related to the length of time the balloon remained in the stomach.

The weight loss regimens with the greatest long-term success provide moderate energy restriction coupled with exercise and behavior modification. Energy deficits created by energy restriction alone lead to loss of lean tissue as well as fat. Formula diets or bizarre combinations of food lead to immediate loss of weight that is quickly regained. Very low-calorie diets cause significant decreases in resting metabolism that make weight loss even more difficult. Moreover, resting metabolism does not always return to normal following the resumption of normal eating, making further weight gain even more likely.

The California Dietetic Association† recommends that a dietary regimen:
- Satisfy all nutrient requirements except energy
- Meet individual tastes and sociocultural food preferences
- Minimize hunger and fatigue
- Be easily obtained and socially acceptable
- Support the development of an improved food pattern
- Support overall improvement of general health

Such a diet will support lifelong changes in dietary habits and the long-term maintenance of weight loss.

---

*Morrow SR and Mona LK: Effect of gastric balloons on nutrient intake and weight loss in obese subjects, J Am Diet Assoc 90:717, 1990.

†Rock CL and Coulston AM: Weight-control approaches: a review by the California Dietetic Association, J Am Diet Assoc 88:44, 1988.

offer some explanation for the relatively low rate of cancer in the Mediterranean region despite high fat intakes.

Although fat acts as a promoter of tumor growth, the mechanism may differ according to the specific site. In the colon fats may increase the concentration of bile acids that enhance tumor growth. The protective effect of fiber against colorectal cancer may relate to its bulk, diluting the bile acids that are present. Fiber also hastens the passage of the food bolus through the digestive tract thereby shortening the time during which ingested carcinogens are in contact with the intestinal wall. In animal studies diets high in fat and polyunsaturated fat lower the ability of the T-cells in the immune system to attack and destroy beginning cancer cells. This may involve alterations in the cell membrane, which changes in fatty acid composition according to the pattern contained in the diet.

Consumption of dark green and deep yellow vegetables high in carotenoids seems to offer some protection against cancer death. Even among those who smoke, lung cancer is less prevalent if consumption of carotenoid-rich vegetables is high. But carotenoid intake does not completely protect smokers from developing lung cancer. Carotenoids may act on tumor development through control of cell differentiation following their conversion to retinol. Beta-carotene is also an effective antioxidant and can neutralize free radicals, thus, preventing their degenerative action. Finally, substances with vitamin A-like activity enhance T-cell activity, and may in this way inhibit tumor growth.

Diabetes Mellitus

Diabetes mellitus is a metabolic disorder characterized by high blood glucose levels and abnormal carbohydrate utilization caused by inappropriate levels of insulin. Insulin-dependent diabetes mellitus results from destruction of the beta cells of the pancreas. Because no insulin is secreted by the pancreas, insulin must be supplied by injection, or death will result. Destruction of the beta cells is believed to occur through an autoimmune reaction. Age of onset is usually in childhood.

Noninsulin-dependent diabetes mellitus (NIDDM), formerly referred to as adult-onset diabetes, usually occurs after age 40 and is generally associated with obesity. It is more likely caused by secretion of an inappropriate form of insulin or resistance of oversize adipose cells to the action of insulin, rather than a deficiency of insulin. Treatment usually involves weight reduction and diets high in complex carbohydrates (50% to 60% of kilocalories) and low in fat (less than or equal to 30% of kilocalories), although ongoing studies indicate that a moderating of this nutrient ratio may be useful in controlling serum glucose and lipid levels in NIDDM (p. 80). Regular exercise is important, and, if necessary, oral hypoglycemic drugs are prescribed. Atherosclerotic coronary disease is a frequent complication of this disorder; thus, diets high in soluble fiber and low in cholesterol and saturated fat are advisable (p. 59). Maintenance of appropriate weight for height and limiting alcohol intake are important preventive measures for lowering individual risk.

NUTRITION AND HEALTH PROMOTION PROGRAMS
National Health Promotion Programs

National Cholesterol Education Program. The National Cholesterol Education Program (NCEP) sponsored by the National Heart, Lung, and Blood Institute was begun in 1985 in response to the published findings from large scale intervention studies that reducing elevated blood cholesterol levels reduces the rate of heart attacks and associated mortality. The NCEP encourages a team approach including physicians, dietitians, nurses, and pharmacologists in developing intervention strategies and materials to educate professionals, patients, and the public. The guidelines for intervention shown in Table 3-3 and

TABLE 3-3   Classification of Blood Cholesterol Levels and Recommended Follow-Up

Total Blood Cholesterol	Classification	Recommended Follow-up
<200 mg/dl	Desirable	Repeat within 5 years
200-239 mg/dl	Borderline-high	Provide dietary information and recheck blood level annually
≥240 mg/dl	High	Without definite coronary heart disease or two other risk factors* provide dietary information and recheck blood level annually
		With definite coronary heart disease or two other risk factors* do lipoprotein analysis with diet and/or drug treatment depending on LDL cholesterol level

*Risk factors include male sex, family history of premature coronary heart disease, cigarette smoking, hypertension, low HDL cholesterol, diabetes mellitus, definite cerebrovascular or peripheral vascular disease, or severe obesity.
From National Cholesterol Education Program: Report of the expert panel on detection, evaluation, and treatment of high blood cholesterol in adults, NIH Publication No. 88-2925, Washington, DC, 1988, US Government Printing Office.

procedures for dietary and drug treatment present a rational approach applicable to persons of different ages and health status. Since diagnosis of high blood cholesterol depends on the accuracy of a blood test, standardized procedures for cholesterol testing have been established. The NCEP recently defined intervention strategies for children and adolescents whose blood cholesterol levels or family history places them at risk.

Diet and drug intervention requiring professional supervision usually takes place in a physician's office or health care facility. But public education to promote preventive dietary changes and encourage screening of those at high risk must target the community. The Pawtucket (Rhode Island) Heart Health Program provided practical dietary information "wherever people eat." Major supermarkets distributed heart healthy recipes, provided shelf markers noting the cholesterol and sodium contents of important foods, and served as sites for blood cholesterol screening. Restaurants offered menu items carrying a heart healthy logo. School and work-site cafeterias sponsored contests featuring menu items low in cholesterol and saturated fat. Support from community businesses, local health care agencies, and volunteers made the program possible. Such programs encourage participation in screening and follow up counseling.

National health promotion and disease prevention objectives. The U.S. Public Health Service since its beginning has had responsibility for disease prevention and directed programs for the eradication of nutritional deficiency diseases such as pellagra and the control of infectious diseases. In the late 1970s this agency was directed by Congress to establish national goals for health promotion and disease prevention. These goals were publicized nationwide as the 1990 Health Objectives for the Nation. Goals included improved health status, improved health services, improved public awareness of personal health strategies, and improved health and nutrition monitoring. By 1985 there was significant progress toward meeting many of the 1990 objectives with major reductions in illness and death among specific groups of infants, children, and adults.

Based upon this success regional hearings were organized to allow professional organizations, community health groups, and state and local governments to provide input toward the development of new national health objectives for the 1990s targeted for the year 2000.[16] With the findings of these regional hearings, the U.S. Department of Health and Human Services, Public Health Services issued the new goals in 1990: *Healthy People 2000: National Health Promotion and Disease Prevention Objectives.*[17] The target areas are listed below:

- **Health promotion** includes behavioral lifestyle factors that influence health and well-being including use of tobacco, alcohol, and drugs, nutrition, physical fitness, and mental health.
- **Health protection** includes health problems related to the physical and social environment including violence and abusive behavior, air quality, waste disposal, and occupational safety and health.
- **Preventive health services** includes preventive services directed toward specific health problems such as sexually transmitted diseases, adolescent pregnancy, heart disease and other chronic conditions, maternal and infant health problems, and human immunodeficiency virus (HIV).

The Year 2000 Objectives will continue to provide a framework for cooperative activities among state, local, and federal government agencies, health care providers, and community groups through this decade.

Community Sites for Health Promotion

The popular emphasis on health and wellness has led community groups in schools, hospitals, and local government agencies to become involved in health promotion. In the private sector health maintenance organizations (HMOs), businesses, and health clubs are providing health education and screening programs for their members and employees.

Hospital-Based Community Programs

The increasing number of hospitals becoming involved in health promotion is reflective of their changing role from institutions providing care for the sick to those providing a continuum of care, including education for disease prevention, monitoring, and followup care when the patient returns home. Hospital programs include community screening programs to identify those at major risk for chronic disease and educational programs describing lifestyle patterns to reduce risk. Programs may involve blood pressure and cholesterol screening and education, nutrition assessment and counseling, and weight management with support groups for long-term weight loss.

Some hospitals are marketing health promotion services to local employers including employee assistance programs offering counseling and treatment for specific problems such as alcohol and drug dependency, occupational health services for monitoring the safety of the work environment or treating work-related illness or injury, and wellness programs emphasizing improvement of lifestyle habits.

Health Maintenance Organizations

General organization. Health maintenance organizations (HMOs) based on a concept first developed in the early 1900s, operate currently under federal law regulating their practice enacted in the 1960s. They present the option of prepaid medical care, usually by group medical practices. Subscribers pay a set fee per individual or family and in turn are guaranteed all health services required, including visits to physicians and other health-care professionals, hospital care, and related services. HMOs negotiate fees with hospitals, pharmacies, or specialty practice consultants.

As providers of health-care services HMOs have both advantages and disadvantages. From the consumer's point of view HMOs provide an opportunity to control one's own health-care costs as all services required will be provided for the set fee. Such a system effectively insulates an individual or family against the financial devastation that can result from a catastrophic illness or injury. Also, HMOs have a financial incentive to encourage preventive health care. The traditional fee-for-service system rewards providers for treating illness. One disadvantage of the HMO is that individuals may not be able to choose their care provider, but rather must accept the provider under contract to the HMO. Also, any arrangement that does not provide a fee per unit of service may result in a provider limiting services in an effort to control costs.

Health promotion activities. HMOs have taken a leadership role in health promotion activities, often in response to member requests. Seminars and on-going classes are offered on such topics as diet and weight control, smoking cessation, stress management, and physical fitness. Some provide health education libraries, professional counselors including nutritionists or registered dietitians, extensive printed material from public sources, handouts authored in-house, lists of recommended books, or newsletters. Many HMO members consider health education to be an important component of their membership services.

Work-Site Wellness Programs

Goals. Companies with more than 750 employees are most likely to sponsor health promotion programs. But companies of this size employ less than 25% of employed persons in the United States.[18] The incentive for establishing such programs has come at least in part from escalating medical care and insurance costs and efforts to identify causes of this rise. Strategies for health promotion programs usually include four steps:

1. Educate employees as to common health risks.
2. Help employees identify their personal health risks.
3. Assist employees in selecting lifestyle patterns to reduce their health risks.
4. Assist employees in self-monitoring to reinforce the lifestyle changes made.

Health screening programs evaluating blood pressure and serum cholesterol, or promoting smoking cessation, nutrition and weight management, physical fitness, and stress management are the most commonly offered.

Evaluation. Results from many programs indicate that not only do employees lose excess weight, stop smoking, or lower their blood pressure or serum cholesterol levels, but also that this reduction in risk continues after the formal program has been completed. In one work-site program for treatment and monitoring of elevated blood pressure levels over half of those referred for treatment and followup had blood pressure levels below 140/90 mm Hg after 3 years.[19] Among those referred for treatment outside the work-site with no followup program, only one fifth had blood pressure readings of those levels. The success of the work-site program was attributed to the systematic monitoring that provided employees with information about their condition and offered on-going support.

Employer-assisted alterations in the environment that support health promotion are also important to the success of a program. Establishing no-smoking areas or eliminating cigarette machines, or ensuring nutritious food options in the employee cafeteria or vending machines should also be considered when developing a strategy for program evaluation.

Cost effectiveness. Decreasing health risk factors does reduce illness and subsequent costs, although not immediately. In fact, health care costs may rise during the first 6 months following health risk screening when medical intervention needs become apparent. After this initial rise, however, costs decline and this trend continues. In a comparison of health screening participants and nonparticipants from the same company, health care costs over a 4-year period were 24% lower in those receiving health screening.[18] Work-site programs appear to offer vast potential for education and intervention in all aspects of health risk.

Health Clubs

Increasing media attention to physical fitness and weight control have fostered the rapid expansion of for-profit health clubs that offer a variety of services for a comprehensive membership fee. Aerobic exercise and use of physical conditioning equipment are the most common activities, although fitness evaluations and development of personal exercise programs may also be provided. Facilities may include a swimming pool, tennis court, or racquetball courts. Nutrition and diet counseling is often available. Unfortunately, however, in some situations individuals providing dietary evaluations or instruction are not always professional nutritionists or dietitians.

Health Fairs

Over two million people visit health fairs each year. These health fairs are sponsored by service organizations, hospitals, home health agencies, or professional health-related associations. They take place in shopping malls, parking lots, community centers, or parks. They feature displays, posters, hand-out materials, and screening tests for common disorders. Staffed by both professional and lay volunteers, health fairs have as their major purpose health education and sponsors make an effort to attract both the general population and targeted groups.

Because health fairs are unregulated, little is known about the numbers of persons reached or screening procedures attempted. An organization that offers assistance to health-fair sponsors estimates that over 1.5 million measurements of height and weight and over 20 million blood chemistry tests are performed each year at health fairs. Screening tests to detect health problems may be offered as an incentive to attract participants.

The criteria for those tests and the degree of followup within such screening programs concern health professionals. One program initiated telephone followup only when serum cholesterol levels were 360 mg/dl or above, a value considerably above that recommended by the NECP (see Table 3-3, p. 64). False alarms for the well participants as well as false reassurance for the person at risk are an issue in situations where test conditions and the sheer number of tests performed contribute to error. Nevertheless, health fairs serve an important role in drawing attention to healthy lifestyle choices and emphasizing personal responsibility for one's own health.

ADULT STAGE OF THE LIFE CYCLE

We start our application of nutrition to the human life cycle with young adults because they are the biologic *progenitors,* the parents, who must initiate and nourish each new generation. A healthy beginning for each child depends on the degree that these young adults, especially women, nourish their own state of healthy maturity. This healthy adult maturity has both physiologic and psychosocial components born of a healthy lifestyle.

Adult Homeostasis

After the turbulent physical growth and sexual development of adolescence under control of growth and sex hormones, the human body's growth pattern levels off into a state of adult **homeostasis.** The word was first used by Boston physiologist Walter Cannon (1871-1945) in his now classic book to describe what he called the "wisdom of the body."[20] In a state of gene regulation and feedback, the "body's wisdom" maintains an internal dynamic equilibrium and stability within the ebb and flow of its parts through a balancing system of "homeostatic" mechanisms. Physically, then, the adult body has grown up, attained its full genetic size and strength, and now leveled off in a stable state of tissue maintenance and function.

Homeostasis
(Gr *homoios,* same, unchanging; *stasis,* stability) State of the body's internal physiologic balance through constant feedback and adjustment, the operation of homeostatic mechanisms that maintain a dynamic equilibrium within the body in relation to its external environment.

This dynamic balance between body parts and functions is life sustaining. All body constituents are in a constant state of flux, although some tissues are more actively engaged than others. This concept of dynamic equilibrium can be seen in carbohydrate and fat metabolism, but it is especially striking in protein metabolism. The adult body's state of metabolic stability or homeostasis results from a balance between the rates of tissue protein breakdown and resynthesis. In earlier growth years, the tissue protein synthesis rate is higher so that the necessary new tissues can be formed. In later adult years, as in the aging process in the elderly, the rate of tissue protein breakdown gradually exceeds that of synthesis, and the older adult body slowly declines.

Body Composition

Adult body composition is maintained within a rather wide range of individual variance according to sex, weight, and age (see Chapter 2). The most metabolically active tissue is the lean body mass compartment. It requires the greatest amount of energy and is larger in men than in women, accounting for 30% to 65% of the total body weight. The lean body mass will be larger in adults who are physically active and consume a low fat diet. The fat compartment is larger in women than in men and may vary in average weight adults from about 14% to 30% of the total body weight. In overweight persons, too prevalent a situation among Americans due to a relatively sedentary lifestyle and a rich diet, the fat compartment is larger. It is smaller in persons who exercise regularly and eat less fat. In general, as adults grow older and become less physically active, the lean body mass decreases and the relative fat tissue increases. The water compartment in adults of average weight accounts for about 20% of the total body weight. It is larger in thin or less fat persons and smaller in fat persons. The mineral compartment, the smallest part of adult body composition, accounts for only about 5% to 6% of the body weight, most of it in the skeleton.

Physiologic Maturity

The young adult reaches physiologic maturity when full genetic body size is attained and tissue growth continues only on a healthy maintenance basis. There is full development of body functions, including sexual **maturation** and reproductive capacity. During middle and older adulthood, however, there is a gradual cell loss and reduced cell metabolism, with a gradual reduction in the performance capacity of most organ systems.[21] Individuals vary widely in the rate and order at which these changes occur. In general, the age-related decline in lean body mass accelerates in later life.

Maturation

(L *maturus*, mature) Process or stage of attaining one's full physical, psychosocial, and mental development. Individual genetic potential guides physical and mental development, which in turn bears the imprint of environmental, psychosocial, and cultural influences.

Psychosocial Maturity

Psychosocial development continues in individual and changing patterns throughout adulthood with its unique potentials and fulfillments. Throughout the human life cycle, food not only serves to meet nutritional requirements for physical growth and tissue maintenance but also relates intimately to personal psychosocial development. Over the past 30 years, Erikson's structuring of human development in relation to society and culture has greatly influenced our view of the human life cycle.[22] In this pattern, the three adult stages—young, middle, and older—of the human life cycle complete the whole and give meaning to human development.

Young adulthood—ages 18-40. In the years of young adulthood every person, now launched as an individual, must resolve the core problem of intimacy versus isolation (Fig. 3-1). If positive development is achieved, the person is able to build intimate relationships leading to self-fulfillment, either in marriage or in other personal relationships. Persons who have failed to develop psychosocial strengths in previous years of growing up,

FIG. 3-1   The years of early adulthood center on the core psychosocial problem of intimacy versus isolation.
Robert Maust.

however, may become increasingly isolated from others. These are the years of career beginnings, of establishing one's own home, of parenthood, of starting young children on their way through the same life stages, and of early struggles to make one's way in the world.

Middle adulthood—ages 40-60. In the years of middle adulthood the psychosocial problem persons face is **generativity** versus self-absorption. The children have now grown and gone to make their own lives. For some, these are the years of the "empty nest." For others, these years are an opportunity for expanding personal growth—"it's my turn now." There is a coming to terms with what life is all about but a great opportunity of finding expression for stored learning in passing on life's teachings. It is a regeneration of one life in the lives of young persons following the same way. To the degree that these inner struggles are not won, there is increasing self-absorption, a turning-in on oneself, and a withering rather than a regenerating spirit of life.

Older adulthood—ages 60-80+. In the last stage of life the final core psychosocial problem is resolved between integrity and despair. Depending on a person's resources at this point, there is either a predominant sense of wholeness and completeness or a sense of distaste and bitterness and of wondering what life was all about. If the outcome of life's basic experiences and problems has been positive, the individual arrives at old age a person rich in wisdom. Building on each previous level of development, psychosocial growth has reached its individual, positive human resolution. Some elderly persons, however, will not have resolved core psychosocial conflicts and will struggle with conflicts with which they have wrestled in previous stages of life. They arrive at middle and later years poorly equipped to deal with the adjustments and health problems that may face them. Alternatively, many others will have been enriched by life's experiences in their maturing process, and in turn they will bring enrichment to the lives of those around them. The resulting generational relationship is mutually rewarding.

Generativity
(L *generatio,* generation) The dynamic psychosocial process of renewing a society's values from one generation to the next.

BASIC NUTRIENT NEEDS
Physiologic Differences

Beginning with adolescent growth and development, significant body changes occur between the sexes (see Chapter 8). This profound period of physiologic change brings sexual maturity and biologic reproductive capacity to initiate new life. Distinct differences in growth patterns emerge between the sexes and are strengthened in their young adult bodies.

Males. In the male physical growth is manifested more in an increased muscle mass and in long-bone growth. His rate of growth is slower than that of the female body, but he soon passes her in weight and height and becomes the larger of the two young adult forms.

Females. In the female there is an increasing amount of subcutaneous fat deposit, particularly in the abdominal area. The hip breadth increases and the bony pelvis widens in preparation for reproduction. A pelvic girdle of subcutaneous fat results, often a source of anxiety to many figure-conscious young women.

With such profound physical body changes and individual differences, largely revolving around sexual development and preparation for adult roles in a complex society, it is small wonder that many psychosocial tensions result.

Dietary Recommendations

The physiologic differences between the sexes account for differing energy and nutrient recommendations for adult men and women in the three age groups—young-, middle-, and older-age adults.

Adult RDAs. Table 3-4 compares the Recommended Dietary Allowances for males and females during the three age groups.

Energy (kilocalories). The larger male body size and muscle mass accounts for the greater need for energy, especially since the lean body mass is the most metabolically active tissue in the body composition. In adults, the resting energy expenditure (REE) per unit of total body weight, a measure of metabolic rate, differs by approximately 10% between the sexes.[23] The remainder of energy need is for physical activities, which is much smaller than that for metabolic needs. In the past, due to occupational differences, men and women often had markedly different energy expenditures, but their occupational activity requirements now are quite similar. Note that these RDA height-weight reference figures are actual **medians** for the U.S. population of the designated age, as reported by the National Health and Nutrition Examination Survey II (NHANES II), and are not

Median

The middle figure in a rank order listing of an individual group of figures; not an average value of all the figures.

TABLE 3-4   Age and Sex Comparisons of Recommended Dietary Allowances (1989) for Adults

Age (yrs) or cond.	Sex	Weight* kg	Weight* lb	Height* cm	Height* in	Energy† kcal	Pro g	Major Minerals Calcium mg	Major Minerals Phosphorus mg	Major Minerals Magnesium mg
Young adults										
19-24	F	58	128	164	65	2,200	46	1200	1200	300
	M	72	160	177	70	2,900	58	1200	1200	350
Middle adults										
25-50	F	63	138	163	64	2,200	50	800	800	280
	M	79	174	176	70	2,900	63	800	800	350
Older adults										
51+	F	65	143	160	63	1,900	50	800	800	280
	M	77	170	173	68	2,300	63	800	800	350
Pregnancy							+300	60	1200	1200	320
Lactation							+500	65	1200	1200	355
							+500	62	1200	1200	340

RE, retinol equivalents (see full RDAs); α-TE, alpha-tocopherol equivalents (see full RDAs); NE, niacin equivalent (see full RDAs).

*Medians of US population survey figures (NHANES II); does not imply ideal height-weight ratios.

†Light to moderate activity

meant to imply ideal height-to-weight ratios. Additional kilocalories are required to support pregnancy and lactation (see Chapters 4 and 5).

Protein. The adult protein allowances are based on a daily protein intake of approximately 0.75 to 0.8 g/kg of body weight for both sexes and all three age groups.[23] Because of the difference in older adult body composition with a gradually decreasing lean body mass, this continuing basic protein allowance is higher per unit of lean body mass for older adults and should allow for some decrease in utilization efficiency. An additional allowance of 10 g/day of protein throughout pregnancy and 15 g/day during lactation is required (see Chapters 4 and 5).

Minerals. Adult allowances are sufficient if provided on a continuing basis by a well-balanced diet. Two minerals need emphasis: calcium and iron. The RDA for calcium has been increased from 800 to 1200 mg/day for young adults to ensure peak skeletal bone mass, which is attained roughly by age 35.[23,24] For middle and older adults the allowance remains at 800 mg/day, although there is some evidence that older adults, especially postmenopausal women, should have an increased intake to prevent calcium loss from bone and the development of **osteoporosis** (p. 81).[24,25] Poor adult diets may also be deficient in iron, which is needed to prevent iron-deficiency anemia. During the reproductive years, women require more iron intake to prevent deficiency due to menstrual blood loss, so their iron allowance is 15 mg/day; for men it is 10 mg/day. Iron requirements during pregnancy are 30 mg/day, which is difficult to attain by diet so a supplement is usually needed.[24] No increase is needed during lactation.

Vitamins. Intake of the adult vitamin allowances is usually met by ordinary well-balanced diets. The problem in some individual cases may stem from inadequate normal intake rather than from an increased need. A well-selected, mixed diet usually supplies all the vitamins in normally needed quantities. There may be increased therapeutic needs in illness, which should be evaluated on an individual basis.

Osteoporosis
(Gr *osteon,* bone; *poros,* passage) Abnormal thinning of bone, producing a lattice-like formation of enlarged spaces in bone, which increases the risk of fracture.

TABLE 3-4   *Age and Sex Comparisons of Recommended Dietary Allowances (1989) for Adults—cont'd*

Trace Elements				Fat-Soluble Vitamins				Water-Soluble Vitamins						
Iron	Zinc	Iodine	Selenium	A	D	E	K	C	Thiamin	Ribo-flavin	Niacin	B$_6$	Folate	B$_{12}$
mg	mg	μg	μg	μg RE	μg	mg α-TE	μg	mg	mg	mg	mg NE	mg	μg	μg
15	12	150	50	800	10	8	60	60	1.1	1.3	15	1.5	180	2.0
10	15	150	70	1000	10	10	70	60	1.5	1.7	19	2.0	200	2.0
15	12	150	55	800	5	8	65	60	1.1	1.3	15	1.6	180	2.0
10	15	150	70	1000	5	10	80	60	1.5	1.7	19	2.0	200	2.0
10	12	150	55	800	5	8	65	60	1.0	1.2	13	1.6	180	2.0
10	15	150	70	1000	5	10	80	60	1.2	1.4	15	2.0	200	2.0
30	15	175	65	800	10	10	65	70	1.5	1.6	17	2.2	400	2.2
15	19	200	75	1300	10	12	65	95	1.6	1.8	20	2.1	280	2.6
15	16	200	75	1200	10	11	65	90	1.6	1.7	20	2.1	260	2.6

Dietary pattern. The publication *Nutrition and Your Health: Dietary Guidelines for Americans,* issued in its third edition by the U.S. Departments of Agriculture and Health and Human Services, provides a good basic guide for choosing a diet to promote health[26] and is discussed in the box on p. 40. Other general food guides including the basic food groups and the food exchange lists are discussed in Chapter 2. A special daily food guide for women during their reproductive years is discussed below.

WOMEN'S NUTRITION AND REPRODUCTIVE FUNCTION

During the reproductive years of the human life cycle, women conceive, nourish, and bear the new life that begins in turn the new life cycle. Thus health promotion and nutritional support over the life cycle begin in preparation for female reproduction. We therefore focus first on the reproductive function of older adolescent young women and young adult women on whose healthy bodies the foundation for life's continuing cycle depends. We then look briefly at women's special health issues and how they relate to nutritional care and planning a healthy lifestyle.

The Preparation Years

During early childhood in any culture, care of young children involves early psychosocial initiation, consciously or unconsciously, of girls and boys into the cultural pattern of their respective sex roles. Current American cultural diversity allows women an expanded and diverse social role in the world of work and the home, choosing when and if they will have children. Nonetheless, at the same time, physiologic growth and development of young girls during childhood and early adolescence uniquely prepare their bodies and set the biologic time clock for potential reproduction. Both nutritional status and nutrition education play basic roles in this development (see Chapters 6-8).

Nutrition and the Female Hormones

Development of ova. Adult female reproduction begins with the development of ova. The primary form of ova began their development many years before during fetal life, when **primordial ova** differentiate from the germinal **epithelium** covering the outside of the fetal ovary and migrate into the ovary's cortex, carrying with them a layer of the epithelioid **granulosa cells.** An ovum surrounded by this single layer of special granulosa cells is called a **primordial follicle.** By the thirtieth week of gestation the peak number of ova produced reaches about seven million, but most soon degenerate so that less than two million remain in the two ovaries at birth, and only 300,000 at puberty. During the reproductive years of the female only about 450 of these follicles develop sufficiently to expel their ova; the rest degenerate. Finally, at the end of reproductive capability, the **menopause,** only a few primordial follicles remain in the ovaries, and these last few follicles shortly degenerate.[27]

Female hormonal system. A hierarchy of hormones from three sources comprise the cyclic female hormone system. First, initiating the cycle, the **hypothalamus** secretes a releasing hormone called luteinizing hormone-releasing hormone (LHRH), which is a decapeptide chain of 10 amino acids, targeted for the anterior pituitary gland. Second, in response, the anterior pituitary secretes two specific hormones, named by their ovary-stimulating functions: luteinizing hormone (LH) and follicle-stimulating hormone (FSH), both of which are small glycoproteins. Third, in final sequence response, the ovaries secrete **estrogen** and **progesterone,** steroids synthesized from cholesterol and acetyl coenzyme A and transported in the blood loosely bound with the plasma albumin or specific

Primordial ova
(L *primordia,* the beginning; *ovum,* egg) Primitive ovum cells produced in large life supply number in the female fetal uterus before birth.

Epithelium
(Gr *epi-,* on, upon, over; *thele,* nipple) The covering tissue of internal and external surfaces of the body, including linings of vessels and other small cavities.

Primordial follicle
(L *follis,* a leather bag) Primitive ovarian follicle formed during fetal life; a sac- or pouch-like cavity; a small secretory sac or gland. A mature ovarian follicle is an ovum surrounded by specialized epithelial cells.

Hypothalamus
(Gr *hypo-,* under; *thalamus,* inner chamber) A small gland adjacent to the pituitary in the basal mid-brain area. Serves as a collection and dispatching center for information about the internal well-being of the body, using much of this neuroendocrine information to stimulate and control many widespread important pituitary hormones.

binding globulins. The cyclic ovarian changes depend entirely on this systematic sequence of female hormones, which in turn depends on nutritional metabolic support.

Estrogen functions. Of the six different natural estrogens only three are present in significant quantities: beta-estradiol, estrone, and their oxidative product, estriol. Beta-estradiol is by far the most potent, thus the major estrogen. During childhood, only small quantities of estrogens are secreted, but with the beginning of puberty estrogen secretion increases twenty-fold or more, stimulated by the pituitary gonadotropic hormones. Although the principle function of the estrogens is the growth and development of the sexual organs and other tissues related to reproduction, they have other important effects related to mineral metabolism and bone growth.

Sexual organs. With the onset of puberty and the surge of estrogen secretion, the female sexual organs change from those of a child to those of an adult. The uterine size increases two- to threefold and important changes occur in its lining, the endometrium. Estrogens cause marked proliferation of the endometrial tissue and development of the glands that will later be used to nourish the implanting ovum. A similar effect occurs on the mucosal lining of the fallopian tubes, enhancing the activity of the epithelial cilia that sweep toward the uterus to help propel the fertilized ovum.

Breasts. The estrogens cause fat deposits in the breasts and initiate growth and development of milk-producing apparatus, resulting in the appearance of the mature female breast. But estrogens do not convert the breasts into milk-producing organs. This task is not initiated until pregnancy, when lactation is stimulated by the hormone prolactin (see Chapters 4 and 5).

Skeleton. Estrogens cause increased osteoblastic activity and bone growth. Thus at puberty when a girl enters her reproductive years, her growth rate becomes rapid for several years and she is often taller than boys of the same age. However, estrogens have another effect on skeletal growth. They cause early uniting of the epiphyses with shafts of the long bones, causing female growth in height to cease several years earlier than that of the male. Estrogens affect overall bone growth by promoting increased deposits of bone matrix with the subsequent retention of both calcium and phosphorus.

Metabolism and fat deposits. Estrogens increase the metabolic rate in young girls after puberty but not as much as the male sex hormone *testosterone* does in young boys. Estrogen also causes increased deposits of subcutaneous fat in the female body, especially in the buttocks and thighs, causing a broadening of the hips.

Progesterone. The most important function of the second ovarian hormone, *progesterone,* is to promote important secretory changes in the **endometrium** lining the uterus, preparing it for implantation of the fertilized ovum. These secretions also occur in the mucosal lining of the fallopian tubes and provide necessary nutrition for the fertilized, dividing ovum as it moves through the tube to the uterus. Progesterone also helps promote breast development of milk-producing structures, but actual milk production is stimulated only after pregnancy by prolactin from the anterior pituitary. During pregnancy the mild catabolic effect of progesterone helps mobilize proteins for use by the fetus.

Endometrium
(Gr *endon*, within; *metra*, uterus) Inner mucous membrane of the uterus.

The Female Sexual Cycle

The normal female reproductive years, between puberty at age 11 to 15 and the menopause at age 45 to 55, are marked by monthly rhythmic changes in rates of secretion of female hormones and corresponding changes in the ovaries and sexual organs. This rhythmic pattern is correctly called the *female sexual cycle,* or less accurately, the *menstrual cycle.* **Menstruation** is only the visible end phase of the cycle when conception does not occur and all the tissue preparations and blood supply for this target event are expelled by the uterus. The overall cycle averages 28 days in length. Normally it can be as short as 20 days or as long as 45 days. The purpose of the cycle is twofold: (1) to develop and release a mature ovum from the ovaries each month, and (2) to prepare the uterus lining, the endometrium, to receive and nourish the ovum. The entire cycle requires nutritional

Menstruation
(L *mensis*, month) Monthly discharge of blood and mucosal tissues from the non-pregnant uterus. Final phase of the female sexual cycle.

Amenorrhea
(*a-*,negative; Gr *men*, month; *rhoia*, flow) Absence of menses. Nutritional anemorrhea results from extreme weight loss and malnutrition, as in eating disorders such as anorexia nervosa.

Menses
Monthly menstrual period

Follicle
(L *follis*, leather bag) Sac-like secretory cavity encasing an ovum and nourishing its growth.

Ovulation
Monthly process in female sexual cycle of secreting a mature ovum for transport through the fallopian tubes to the uterus.

Corpus luteum
(L *corpus*, body; *uteum*, yellow) Mass of estrogen and progesterone secretory cells. Produced monthly from the ovarian follicle in the postovulation phase of the female sexual cycle.

support to function. **Amenorrhea,** absence of **menses,** is a common and distinct sign of malnutrition in women. The normal monthly functioning of the female sexual cycle in well-nourished women is accomplished through five specific phases: preovulation, follicular growth, ovulation, postovulation, and menstruation.

Preovulation phase. The ovarian changes that produce a mature ovum depend entirely on initial secretion of the stimulating hormones FSH and LH from the anterior pituitary gland. Unstimulated ovaries remain completely inactive. This is the state during childhood until the young girl is about 8 years old, when these hormones gradually awaken and progressively secrete these essential hormones, initiating monthly sexual cycles between the ages of 11 and 15. This culmination is called puberty.

Follicular growth phase. At puberty when secretions of the pituitary gland hormones FSH and LH increase, the entire ovaries and their primordial follicles within begin to grow. Each follicle, dormant since initial development in fetal life, is a sac- or pouch-like cavity lined with secretory cells that encases an ovum and nourishes its growth. The ovum surrounded by these specialized epithelial cells is called an ovarian follicle. Increased surges of FSH and LH at the beginning of each monthly cycle cause one of the follicles to outgrow the others after 1 or 2 weeks and nourish its ovum to maturity while hormonal signals stop the growth of the remainder, which involute, awaiting stimulation at another monthly cycle.

Ovulation phase. About midway, day 14 of a normal 28-day cycle, ovulation occurs, stimulated primarily by a large increase in secretion rate of the anterior pituitary hormone LH assisted by a moderate increase of FSH. This secretion rate peaks about 18 hours before ovulation, causing rapid swelling of the follicle and degeneration of its capsule, allowing final expulsion of the ovum for its transport through the fallopian tubes into the uterus.

Postovulation phase. During the first few hours after ovulation occurs, the remaining secretory cells of the follicle undergo rapid physical and chemical change into a mass of cells called a **corpus luteum**. These lutein cells enlarge and deposit fatty material that gives them a distinctive yellow color and hence their name. The corpus luteum then secretes large quantities of the female hormones estrogen and progesterone, and after another 2 weeks disintegrates. The following decrease in ovarian estrogen and progesterone causes menstruation to follow.

Menstruation phase. Throughout the cycle, marked changes have occurred in the endometrium of the uterus. During the first 11 days of the cycle, estrogen has stimulated a proliferation of tissue, and during the next 12 days progesterone has greatly increased the secretory function. These changes have occurred for the whole purpose of storing large amounts of nutrients to support rapid growth of a fertilized ovum, should it arrive and implant itself. Without such a need, levels of the two hormones decrease sharply, the engorged endometrial tissue detaches along with its blood supply, and contractions of the uterus expel its contents over the final 5 days of the cycle. During normal menstruation about 35 ml of blood and another 35 ml of serous fluid are lost and only the thin initial layer of basic endothelial tissue remains, ready to grow and develop repeatedly in the same sequence during following cycles, supported by the woman's positive nutritional status.[27]

Female Fertility and Contraception

Fertile period. The period of female fertility during each sexual cycle is very short. The ovum remains viable for only about 24 hours, so sexual intercourse and deposit of sufficient viable sperm must occur some time between 1 day before ovulation and 1 day afterward, if fertilization is to take place. The use of some means of contraception helps maintain a mother's health through family planning, thus preventing a high **parity,** that is, frequent pregnancies that drain maternal nutritional resources with no replenishing between.

Rhythm method. The rhythm method of contraception, avoiding intercourse over the period of ovulation, is sometimes practiced but is more often than not unsuccessful. It is usually stated that avoidance of intercourse for 4 days prior to ovulation and 3 days afterward prevents conception. The problem lies in the fact that it is impossible to predict precisely the day of ovulation.

Oral contraceptive agents—the "Pill." This commonly used method of contraception is based on hormonal suppression of fertility by preventing ovulation but allowing menstruation to occur. Most of these oral contraceptive agents (OCAs) contain a combination of synthetic estrogen and synthetic progestins. Because these substances are synthetic they cannot be destroyed by the liver after they are absorbed, as are natural hormones, so they can be taken orally. The pills are usually begun in the early part of the female sexual cycle, continued beyond time of ovulation, and stopped toward end of the cycle to allow menstruation and a new cycle start. Other low-dose combinations of these synthetic hormones may occasionally allow ovulation but prevent conception by other means, such as (1) delaying fallopian tube transport of the ovum (normal time is 3 days), (2) inadequately developing the endometrium, (3) developing abnormal cervical mucus that blocks sperm entry, or (4) abnormal contractions of fallopian tubes and uterus expelling ovum. One prior concern has been the effect of different OCA hormone combinations on lipid and carbohydrate metabolism, elevating serum levels of triglycerides, LDLs, cholesterol, and insulin. Current study and modification of the type and dose of progestin in OCAs, even use of progestin alone, diminishes all of these serum lipid changes.[28]

Barrier methods. An alternate, though sometimes unreliable, method of contraception is use of a **condom** as a sheath or cover for the penis during intercourse to prevent deposit of sperm. With the epidemic incidence of deadly acquired immunodeficiency syndrome (AIDS), however, the condom has an additional function in helping prevent sexually transmitted disease (STD). Also, in the current upsurge of other STDs such as gonorrhea, a condom not only prevents easy entry of the AIDS virus into open gonorrheal lesions on genital tissue, but also spread of the secondary STD. Another barrier device is the diaphragm, vaginally inserted before intercourse as a cover over the cervix entry to the uterus. When used with a spermicidal jelly, the diaphragm may be a helpful but not always reliable method of contraception.

Nutrition and Fertility

Since normal functioning of the female sexual cycle depends on optimal nutritional support, malnutrition greatly reduces fertility. This malnutrition effect may affect whole communities or larger areas in cases of famine from natural disasters such as long-term drought, or from man-made political events such as war and seige. It may also be caused by self-induced starvation, as in eating disorders such as anorexia nervosa or bulimia, occurring in adolescents and young women (see Chapter 8). Whatever the cause, such situations of starvation produce amenorrhea with no conception or poor pregnancy outcomes and high infant mortality.

Menopause

There is a progressive decline in estrogen secretion toward the end of a woman's reproductive life. When she is approximately 50 years of age, her sexual cycles become irregular and ovulation fails to occur during many of them. This period during which the cycles cease altogether and the female sex hormones diminish rapidly to extremely low

Parity
(L *parere*, to bring forth, produce) Number of pregnancies a woman has had with viable offspring.

Condom
(L *condus*, receptacle) A penile sheath serving not only as a barrier method of contraception but also as a means of preventing the spread of sexually transmitted diseases.

TABLE 3-5   *Daily Food Guide for Women*

Food Group	One Serving Equals	Recommended Minimum Servings		
		Nonpregnant		Pregnant/Lactating
		11-24 yr	25+ yr	
Protein foods Provide protein, iron, zinc, and B-vitamins for growth of muscles, bone, blood, and nerves. Vegetable protein provides fiber to prevent constipation.	*Animal Protein:* 1 oz. cooked chicken or turkey; 1 oz. cooked lean beef, lamb, or pork; 1 oz. or ¼ cup fish or other seafood; 1 egg; 2 fish sticks or hot dogs; 2 slices luncheon meat. *Vegetable Protein:* ½ cup cooked dry beans, lentils, or split peas; 3 oz. tofu; 1 oz. or ¼ cup peanuts, pumpkin, or sunflower seeds; 1½ oz. or ⅓ cup other nuts; 2 tbsp. peanut butter	5 A half serving of vegetable protein daily	5	7 One serving of vegetable protein daily
Milk products Provide protein and calcium to build strong bones, teeth, healthy nerves and muscles, and to promote normal blood clotting.	8 oz. milk; 8 oz. yogurt; 1 cup milk shake; 1½ cups cream soup (made with milk); 1½ oz. or ⅓ cup grated cheese (like cheddar, monterey, mozzarella, or swiss); 1½-2 slices presliced American cheese; 4 tbsp. parmesan cheese; 2 cups cottage cheese; 1 cup pudding; 1 cup custard or flan; 1½ cups ice milk, ice cream, or frozen yogurt	3	2	3
Breads, cereals, grains Provide carbohydrates and B-vitamins for energy and healthy nerves. Also provide iron for healthy blood. Whole grains provide fiber to prevent constipation.	1 slice bread; 1 dinner roll; ½ bun or bagel; ½ English muffin or pita; 1 small tortilla; ¾ cup dry cereal; ½ cup granola; ½ cup cooked cereal; ½ cup rice; ½ cup noodles or spaghetti; ¼ cup wheat germ; 1 4-inch pancake or waffle; 1 small muffin; 8 medium crackers; 4 graham cracker squares; 3 cups popcorn	7 Four servings of whole-grain products daily	6	7

Food group	Serving equivalents			
Vitamin C–rich fruits and vegetables Provide vitamin C to prevent infection and to promote healing and iron absorption. Also provide fiber to prevent constipation.	6 oz. orange, grapefruit, or fruit juice enriched with vitamin C 6 oz. tomato juice or vegetable juice cocktail 1 orange, kiwi, mango ½ grapefruit, cantaloupe ½ cup papaya 2 tangerines	½ cup strawberries ½ cup cooked or 1 cup raw cabbage ½ cup broccoli, Brussels sprouts, or cauliflower ½ cup snow peas, sweet peppers, or tomato puree 2 tomatoes	1	1	1
Vitamin A–rich fruits and vegetables Provide beta-carotene and vitamin A to prevent infection and to promote wound healing and night vision. Also provide fiber to prevent constipation.	6 oz. apricot nectar or vegetable juice cocktail 3 raw or ¼ cup dried apricots ¼ cantaloupe or mango 1 small or ½ cup sliced carrots 2 tomatoes	½ cup cooked or 1 cup raw spinach ½ cup cooked greens (beet, chard, collards, dandelion, kale, mustard) ½ cup pumpkin, sweet potato, winter squash, or yams	1	1	1
Other fruits and vegetables Provide carbohydrates for energy and fiber to prevent constipation.	6 oz. fruit juice (if not listed above) 1 medium or ½ cup sliced fruit (apple, banana, peach, pear) ½ cup berries (other than strawberries) ½ cup cherries or grapes ½ cup pineapple ½ cup watermelon	¼ cup dried fruit ½ cup sliced vegetable (asparagus, beets, green beans, celery, corn, eggplant, mushrooms, onion, peas, potato, summer squash, zucchini) ½ artichoke 1 cup lettuce	3	3	3
Unsaturated fats Provide vitamin E to protect tissue.	⅛ med. avocado 1 tsp. margarine 1 tsp. mayonnaise 1 tsp. vegetable oil	2 tsp. salad dressing (mayonnaise-based) 1 tbsp. salad dressing (oil-based)	3	3	3

NOTE: The Daily Food Guide for Women may not provide all the calories you require. The best way to increase your intake is to include more than the minimum servings recommended.

Adapted from California Department of Health Services, Maternal and Child Health: Nutrition during pregnancy and postpartum period: A manual for health care professionals, Sacramento, 1990, CDHS.

Dyspnea
(Gr *dysnia,* difficult breathing) Difficult or labored breathing.

levels is called the menopause. The cause of the menopause is the "burning out" of the ovaries; few primordial follicles remain and production of estrogen by the ovaries decreases as the number of primary follicles approaches zero and the final ones involute and disappear. For most women, this menopausal period is a normal physiologic process with no marked physical or psychologic symptoms. Approximately 15% of women, however, experience a variety of symptoms such as "hot flashes" with extreme flushing of the skin, sensations of **dyspnea,** irritability, fatigue, anxiety, and in a few cases occasional psychotic states.[27] In such cases, estrogen therapy may be indicated.

Nutrition and Pregnancy Planning

Ideally every pregnancy should be a planned pregnancy. However, for many reasons this is not always the case. Certainly for women with preexisting disease such as insulin-dependent diabetes mellitus (IDDM) or maternal **phenylketonuria (PKU),** it is mandatory to achieve the best control status possible to help ensure a successful outcome. Nonetheless, in any case, planning a healthy lifestyle, including both positive nutritional support and physical fitness as described in this chapter, should definitely begin in the early reproductive years of all women. A helpful daily food guide for women that covers the reproductive years, developed by the California Department of Health Services is given in Table 3-5. (See source listing at end of chapter under Further Reading.)

Phenylketonuria (PKU)
Genetic disease that, if untreated, results in severe mental retardation. It is caused by a lack of a key enzyme, phenylalanine hydroxylase, controlling the metabolic conversion of the amino acid phenylalanine to tyrosine. Currently newborn screening and special low phenylalanine diets allows girls with PKU to reach adulthood and have families of their own.

Active pregnancy planning health promotion should be based on nutritional assessment and counseling, with correction of any nutrient or weight deficits and elimination of such lifestyle health hazards as alcohol abuse, smoking, and drug-related problems. These nutrition assessment procedures are reviewed in Chapter 2 and the factors involved in planning a successful pregnancy outcome are discussed in Chapter 4. Of particular concern are drugs that can cause birth defects initiated in early cell differentiation of embryonic life weeks before a woman even knows she is pregnant. Serious effects have been shown, for example, among women who conceive while taking pharmacologic megadoses of vitamin A or vitamin A–related retinoid drugs.[29,30] One such retinoid-drug, *isotretinoin* (13-cis retinoic acid), trade name Accutane, as well as its related compound etretinate, has been used for treating severe cystic acne.[31,32] Since Accutane has been shown to produce spontaneous abortions of malformed fetuses or those with congenital defects started in early embryonic life, it must carry a warning label against its use by sexually active women who do not use a reliable form of contraception. In addition, physicians prescribing this drug for their adolescent or young adult women patients usually order pregnancy testing before starting the drug and monthly during its use.

WOMEN'S NUTRITION AND HEALTH ISSUES
Women and Weight

The health problem of obesity, defined as an excessive accumulation of body fat, has been regarded traditionally as the result of overeating. However, recent studies of twins have indicated that there is a strong genetic component to body fat accumulation and its distribution.[33,34] Men and women differ genetically in their respective sex chromosomes. Men carry an XY combination pair of X (female) and Y (male) chromosomes, whereas women carry a complete XX combination. Cell division of the male XY chromosomes produces the final mature sperm cells, half male (Y) sperm and half female (X) sperm. The sex of the offspring depends on which of these two types of sperm fertilizes the ovum. Thus, it should not be surprising that women may well differ from men in the prevalence of obesity, its time of onset, and their responses to treatment. This genetic factor in obesity helps to explain the "yo-yo" pattern of dieting that compounds the weight problem for many women, as a successful diet will reduce body weight and fat stores but cannot change individual genetic makeup.

FIG. 3-2 Regular physical activity is an important part of planning a healthy lifestyle and reducing chronic disease risks.

From The Image Bank; photographer: John P. Kelly.

Once a person has expressed this genetic predisposition to gain weight, and for women this occurs most often in the early adult years, the obesity is likely to recur again and again unless major changes that promote health and fitness and a healthy lifestyle are made in lifetime habits and environmental factors.[35] Thus, some form of regular exercise and physical activity needs to be a part of that healthy lifestyle. Although effects of exercise on weight loss may be minimal in the short term, long-term followup studies in both men and women show that those who make regular exercise a part of their long-term lifestyle (Fig. 3-2) have dramatically better success at keeping weight off following weight loss dieting.[36,37]

These study results should encourage adolescent and young adult women who face in their early development the twofold gender disadvantage not only of a physiologic propensity for a larger body fat composition but also the social pressure of a society obsessed with thinness as the ideal female form. These results should also encourage middle-age and older adult women whose health concerns include regional body fat distribution, especially abdominal body fat with its association with potential development of chronic disease risks for cardiovascular problems, hypertension, and diabetes.[38] In women, body fat is usually localized in the hips and thighs (*gynoid* or lower body fat distribution). In men, body fat is usually localized in the abdominal region (*android* or upper body fat distribution). However, this sex-related distribution pattern can vary among individual men and women. In both sexes abdominal body fat tends to increase with age, but with the reduction of the female sex hormones at menopause, postmenopausal women experience an acceleration of this upper body fat accumulation.[39]

Coronary Heart Disease

Gender differences. Through earlier adult years, a large gender gap exists between men and women in the incidence of cardiovascular disease, with men at much greater risk, developing the view of heart disease as a "man's disease." However, the gap closes rapidly with menopause and heart disease becomes the leading cause of death for American women aged 50 years and older, accounting for a large number of the nearly 500,000 deaths of men and women annually.[40] Very few women develop cardiovascular disease before menopause due to the protective effect of the female sex hormone estrogen. Thus, women develop coronary heart disease at the same rate as men, but approximately 6 to 10 years later.

Risk factors. Postmenopausal women face the same risk factors for cardiovascular disease as do men (see Table 3-5). They are just as vulnerable to the blood lipid factors, especially elevated cholesterol and the LDLs carrying cholesterol to the cells, that are now recognized as major risk factors in the development of coronary heart disease (p. 59). A high level of LDL is an independent risk factor in both men and women, but a high serum triglyceride level is an independent risk factor only in women.[40,41] Women with diabetes and those who are overweight and hypertensive are at higher risk, and those who smoke compound it further. The devastating effects of smoking leading to peripheral vascular disease and coronary heart disease are now experienced by women as well as men.[40] Thus the coronary heart disease risk profile of a woman can be assessed by a few simple indicators: serum cholesterol, blood pressure, serum glucose, weight, and smoking status.[40] The positive approach of planning a healthy lifestyle, as described earlier, will reduce these risk factors and increase general fitness and well-being.

Noninsulin-Dependent Diabetes Mellitus

Gender differences. NIDDM, the onset of which occurs in adulthood, is closely related in predisposing risk factors for women described above for cardiovascular disease. It occurs mainly in postmenopausal women aged 45 to 60 and has a greater impact on women, sometimes requiring insulin during the initial treatment period to counteract its degree of impaired glucose tolerance. The reasons for this differing gender impact are not entirely clear. It would seem from current studies that obesity (especially an upper body or abdominal pattern of distribution) and elevated serum lipids (especially triglycerides), combined with a low HDL value and the postmenopausal woman's lack of estrogen, help set the stage for impaired glucose tolerance in women.[43,44]

Dietary recommendations. The current standard of dietary guidelines for management of diabetes of the American Diabetes Association and the American Dietetic Association, which generally follow guidelines of the American Heart Association's "prudent" diet, provide the present basis for individual care of diabetes (Table 3-6). Some interesting initial data from recent NIDDM studies, however, document plasma glucose and lipid response to diets that vary from these current standards in the relative amount and type of dietary carbohydrate and fat. One group of investigators found a persistent elevation

TABLE 3-6 Comparison of AHA and ADA Diet Recommendations

	AHA Step 1 (% total kcal)	AHA Step 2 (% total kcal)	ADA/ADA (% total kcal)
Total fat	30	30	30
Monounsaturated	10-15	10-15	12-14
Saturated	10	7	10
Polyunsaturated	<10	<10	6-8
Carbohydrate	50-60	50-60	55-60
Protein	15-20	15-20	0.8 g/kg
Cholesterol	300 mg/day	200 mg/day	300 mg/day

AHA, American Heart Association; ADA/ADA, American Diabetes Association/American Dietetic Association.
From Williams SR: Nutrition and diet therapy, ed 6, St Louis, 1989, Times Mirror/Mosby College Publishing.

of serum triglycerides, an independent heart disease risk factor for women, with the usual high-carbohydrate/low-fat ratio of the standard diet guides.[45,46] Another group found improvement in serum lipid levels with moderation of dietary fat to include more use of monounsaturated fat.[47] For treatment of adults with NIDDM, it would appear that an adjustment of the nutrient ratios may achieve better control of serum glucose and lipids: (1) carbohydrate lowered from a high of 60% to 45% to 50% of total kilocalories, mostly complex in form with little, if any, sucrose; (2) fat moderated from 30% to 35% to 40% of total kilocalories, with the small increase in monounsaturated fat; and (3) protein kilocalories remaining the same at 15% to 20%. Researchers and practitioners agree, however, that any general population guideline must always be applied with reasonable common sense to individuals.

Breast Cancer

Breast cancer is a significant health issue for women. At some time during their lives, one out of 10 American women will develop breast cancer, a rate that has not changed despite current advances in treatment. Diagnosis of breast cancers at earlier stages is achieved through widespread screening. However, researchers agree that only prevention efforts will decrease cancer incidence and prolong survival, because most women with breast cancer do not have a family history or any of the other known risk factors, which include fibrocystic disease, **nulliparity,** or first pregnancy after age 30.[48] Thus, prevention strategies need to be applied to all women. There is an increasing consensus that obesity and the high-fat American diet are primary risk factors, and that weight reduction and maintenance on a low-fat, high fiber diet provide a valuable and practical strategy for breast cancer prevention. Such long-term maintenance goals require planning for a lifetime of healthy lifestyle.

For some years, a vast body of **epidemiologic** evidence has supported this association of increased dietary fat and subsequent increase in incidence of breast cancer in populations migrating to the United States, but controlled studies to rule out other confounding factors from the analysis are needed. Current studies are examining nutritional, hormonal, and physiologic data in conjunction with dietary and lifestyle change that will clarify these effects for breast cancer prevention.[48]

Osteoporosis

Bone growth and maintenance. The health problem of **osteoporosis** in women's later adult years has its roots in earlier growth, development, and maintenance of skeletal bone mass. Thus it provides an excellent example of the importance of the life cycle preventive approach of planning for a healthy lifestyle. Skeletal life cycle homeostasis is a sophisticated response to the alternating pattern of the three basic factors involved in building and maintaining bone mass: nutritional state, physical activity, and hormonal status.[24] There is also a strong genetic role in the development of bone mass in women by the age of about 25, independent of calcium and other nutrients, but dietary factors, physical activity, and hormonal factors constantly modulate the genetically predetermined quantity, size, and shape of bone.[49]

Life cycle bone development. Childhood bone growth is gradual in concert with the child's overall body growth and development, but with puberty a rapid growth period begins. During the healthy adolescent growth spurt of young girls after **menarche,** under the added stimulus of estrogen secretion of the developing ovaries, large quantities of calcium, between 150 and 350 mg/day, are retained by the skeleton.[24] Calcium absorption efficiency is high during this 3 to 5 year period, but dietary calcium must also be sufficient to sustain this high retention rate. Peak adult bone mass is reached by about 35 years of

Nulliparity
(L *nullus,* none; *parere,* to bring forth, produce) Reproductive status of a woman who has never given birth to a viable child.

Epidemiology
(Gr *epidemios,* prevalent; *-ology,* study) Study of factors determining the frequency and distribution of diseases in population groups.

Trabecular

(L *trabes,* a little beam) Small bones in the ends of long bones at joints such as wrist, vertebrae, and hips.

age, although **cortical** bone tissue, the hard outer layer, may reach its full mass during the early adult decade of the 20s. The smaller **trabecular** bone tissue completes its development later, at 35 or afterward. These trabecular bones, which are found in the ends of the long arm bones at the wrists, the vertebrae, and the proximal femurs at the hips, are most susceptible to fractures, beginning at the woman's menopause. Men may sustain fractures at these same sites, but their fracture rates are very much lower than female rates, largely due to the man's greater bone mass and shorter life span.[24] During the decade before menopause, which now occurs in most North American women in the United States and Canada in their early 50s, bone mass begins to decrease at a very low rate, and level of calcium intake appears to have no major effect on the status of this bone mass.[50] At the menopause, the rate of estrogen secretion drops sharply and gradually ceases, a physiologic event that has major impact on the turnover of bone in nearly all women, making them more vulnerable to osteoporosis. If such signs do develop, estrogen replacement therapy may be needed. Continuing an appropriate level of regular exercise during older adult years also helps to maintain the bone mass attained in the premenopause years.[51]

Dietary recommendations. Since the current RDA for calcium for young adults aged 19 through 24 has been raised to 1200 mg/day, matching the already established allowance for adolescent girls, the increased demand for calcium to meet rapid bone growth during this period should be ample for skeletal bone mass needs. The calcium allowance for women from 25 to 50 is set at 800 mg/day, which is sufficient for active women. After the menopause, however, rather than the continued 800 mg/day, the calcium intake probably needs to be increased to 1000 mg/day.[24] Additional calcium supplementation cannot overcome the negative calcium balance that follows the loss of ovarian estrogens.[52] Studies of premenopausal and postmenopausal women suggest that a threshold of calcium intake must be met at the different life cycle stages in order to enhance absorption and retention of calcium, independent of other factors.[51] In short, women who practice good nutrition as a healthy lifetime habit, including not only adequate amounts of calcium but also other bone-building nutrients such as protein, phosphorus, and vitamin D, can develop optimal bone mass during adolescence and young adult years, and maintain that bone mass at a higher level during their postmenopausal years. Planning for a healthy lifestyle is the young adult woman's health promotion, disease prevention approach to osteoporosis, as well as the other health issues of women discussed.

Summary

Adult health and wellness for both men and women depend upon a healthy lifestyle throughout young, middle, and older adulthood. Although genetic factors play a role in determining level of health, lifestyle choices are the major determinant of well-being and the onset and severity of chronic diseases that begin to appear in middle age. Components of a healthy lifestyle include a sound diet with attention to risk factors associated with excess fat, cholesterol, sodium, and body weight; regular physical exercise; stress management; smoking cessation; and avoidance of alcohol and drugs. Widespread chronic diseases of the cardiovascular system, hypertension, diabetes mellitus, and cancer have all been related to one or more of these lifestyle behaviors. A number of health programs have been developed at the national and community levels to heighten public awareness and encourage appropriate behavior change. These public and professional activities include hospital-based community programs, health maintenance organization (HMO) programs, work-site wellness programs, health clubs, community screening programs, and health fairs.

Comparison of nutrient energy needs of men and women reflect their gender differences in body composition and size, as well as in physiologic function. The female sexual cycle, uniquely designed to develop and nourish a healthy new life for the beginning of a life cycle, creates nutrient losses and requires nutritional support for all of its functions to maintain a state of health and well-being. Health promotion through pregnancy planning helps to ensure healthy mothers and babies. Women also encounter special gender-based health issues in their adult years, including weight concerns and health problems such as heart disease, diabetes, breast cancer, and osteoporosis.

Review Questions

1. Describe various approaches to health promotion. Which do you think has the greatest application to current health issues? Why?
2. List and discuss the five components of a healthy lifestyle. How does each influence risk of the major chronic diseases? Develop a healthy 1-day food plan for an adult of your choice, indicating daily activities that would influence the meal pattern or food selection.
3. Describe two national health promotion programs for well-being and disease prevention. List five community agencies or sites that might implemnt these programs at the local level and give strategies for bringing about behavior change in each location.
4. How do women's nutritional needs differ from those of men? Account for each gender difference.
5. Describe the five phases of the female sexual cycle in relation to nutritional needs. Why is amenorrhea a sign of malnutrition?
6. Relate women's nutrition to their gender difference in response to health issues such as obesity, heart disease, diabetes, and breast cancer.
7. Describe the gender differences in bone mass growth and development over the life cycle that create a greater risk for women of developing osteoporosis.

References

1. Mossey JM and Shapiro E: Self-rated health: A predictor of mortality among the elderly, Am J Public Health 72:800, 1982.
2. US Department of Health and Human Services: Healthy people: the Surgeon General's report on health promotion and disease prevention, Washington, DC, 1979, US Government Printing Office.
3. Saunders RP: What is health promotion, Health Educ 19:14, 1988.
4. Holli BB and Calabrese RJ: Communication and education skills. The dietitians guide, ed 2, Philadelphia, 1991, Lea and Febiger.
5. Contento I and Murphy BM: Psycho-social factors differentiating people who reported making desirable changes in their diets from those who did not, J Nutr Educ 22:6, 1990.
6. Committee on Diet and Health, Food and Nutrition Board: Diet and health: implications for reducing chronic disease risk, Washington, DC, 1989, National Academy Press.
7. Blair SN et al: Physical fitness and all-cause mortality. A prospective study of healthy men and women, JAMA 262:2395, 1989.
8. Leon AS et al: Leisure-time physical activity levels and risk of coronary heart disease and death. The Multiple Risk Factor Intervention Trial, JAMA 258:2388, 1987.
9. US Department of Health and Human Services: Reducing the health consequences of smoking, 25 years of progress: A report of the Surgeon General, DHHS Publication No (CDC) 89-8411, Washington, DC, 1989, US Government Printing Office.
10. Muldoon MF, Manuck SB, and Matthews KA: Lowering cholesterol concentrations and mortality: a quantitative review of primary prevention trials, Br Med J 301:309, 1990.
11. Monsen E: Reversing heart disease through diet, exercise, and stress management: an interview with Dean Ornish, J Am Diet Assoc 91:162, 1991.

12. Luft FC: Dietary sodium, potassium, and chloride intake and arterial hypertension, Nutr Today 24:9, 1989.

13. Oberman A et al: Pharmacologic and nutritional treatment of mild hypertension: changes in cardiovascular risk status, Ann Intern Med 112:89, 1990.

14. US Department of Health and Human Services: Nutrition monitoring in the United States. An update on nutrition monitoring, DHHS Publication No (PHS) 89-1255, Washington, DC, 1989, US Government Printing Office.

15. Simopoulos AP and Van Itallie TB: Body weight, health, and longevity, Ann Intern Med 100:285, 1984.

16. Institute of Medicine, National Academy of Sciences: Healthy people 2000. Citizens chart the course, Washington, DC, 1990, National Academy Press.

17. US Department of Health and Human Services, Public Health Services: Healthy People 2000: National Health Promotion and Disease Prevention Objectives, PHS Pub No 91-50212, Washington, DC, 1990, US Government Printing Office.

18. Cohen A and Murphy L: Indicators of health promotion behaviors in the workplace. In: Kar SB, editor: Health promotion indicators and actions, New York, 1989, Springer Publishing Co.

19. Blair SN et al: A public health intervention model for work-site health promotion, JAMA 255:921, 1986.

20. Cannon WB: The wisdom of the body, New York, 1932, WW Norton & Co, Inc.

21. Chernoff R: Aging and nutrition, Nutr Today 22(2):4, 1987.

22. Erikson E: Childhood and society, New York, 1963, WW Norton & Co, Inc.

23. Food and Nutrition Board, National Research Council: Recommended dietary allowances, ed 10, Washington, DC, 1989, National Academy Press.

24. Anderson JJB: Dietary calcium and bone mass through the life cycle, Nutr Today 25(2):9, 1990.

25. Allen L: Calcium and age-related bone loss, Nutr Today 21(3):6, 1986.

26. US Department of Agriculture, US Department of Health and Human Services: Nutrition and your health: dietary guidelines for Americans, ed 3, Washington, DC, 1990, US Government Printing Office.

27. Guyton AC: Textbook of medical physiology, ed 8, Philadelphia, 1991, WB Saunders Co.

28. Godsland IF et al: The effects of different formulations of oral contraceptive agents on lipid and carbohydrate metabolism, N Engl J Med 323:1375, 1990.

29. New York State Department of Health: Use of supplements containing high-dose vitamin A, JAMA 257:1292, 1987.

30. Watson RR: Vitamin A and teratogenesis: recommendations for pregnancy, J Am Diet Assoc 88(3):364, 1988.

31. Lammer EJ et al: Retinoic acid and embryopathy, N Engl J Med 313:837, 1985.

32. Ellis CN and Voorhees JJ: Etretinate therapy, J Am Acad Dermatol 16:267, 1987.

33. Stunkard AJ et al: The body mass index of twins who have been reared apart, N Engl J Med 322:1483, 1990.

34. Bouchard C et al: The response to long-term overfeeding in identical twins, N Engl J Med 322:1477, 1990.

35. Williamson DF et al: The 10-year incidence of overweight and major weight gain in U.S. adults, Arch Intern Med 150:665, 1990.

36. Pavlou KN et al: Exercise as an adjunct to weight loss and maintenance in moderately obese subjects, Am J Clin Nutr 49:1115, 1989.

37. Van Dale D et al: Weight maintenance and resting metabolic rate 18-40 months after a diet/exercise treatment, Ind J Obesity 14:347, 1990.

38. Bouchard C et al: Basic and clinical aspects of regional fat distribution, Am J Clin Nutr 52:946, 1990.

39. Shimokata H et al: Studies in the distribution of body fat: I. Effects of age, sex, and obesity, J Gerontol 44:M66, 1989.

40. Castelli WP: Cardiovascular disease in women, Am J Obstet Gynecol 158:1553, 1988.

41. Bush TL et al: Cholesterol, lipoproteins, and coronary heart disease in women, Clin Chem 34:B60, 1988.
42. Willett WC et al: Relative and absolute excess risks of coronary heart disease among women who smoke cigarettes, N Engl J Med 317:1303, 1988.
43. Golay A et al: Effect of central obesity on regulation of carbohydrate metabolism in obese patients with varying degrees of glucose tolerance, J Clin Endocrinol Metab 71:1299, 1990.
44. Haffer SM et al: Cardiovascular risk factors in confirmed prediabetic individuals, JAMA 263:2893, 1990.
45. Coulston AM et al: Deleterious metabolic effects of high-carbohydrate, sucrose-containing diets in patients with noninsulin-dependent diabetes mellitus, Am J Med 82:213, 1987.
46. Coulston AM et al: Persistence of hypertriglyceridemic effect of low-fat high carbohydrate diets in NIDDM patients, Diabetes Care 12:94, 1989.
47. Gorg A et al: Comparison of high-carbohydrate diet with high-monounsaturated fat diet in patients with noninsulin-dependent diabetes mellitus, N Engl J Med 319:829, 1988.
48. Heber D et al: Weight reduction for breast cancer prevention by restriction of dietary fat and calories: mechanisms and interventions, Nutrition 5(3):149, 1989.
49. Pollitzer WS and Anderson JJB: Ethnic and genetic differences in bone mass: a review with an hereditary vs environmental perspective, Am J Clin Nutr 50:1244, 1989.
50. Riggs BL et al: Dietary calcium intake and rates of bone loss in women, J Clin Invest 80:979, 1987.
51. Halioua L and Anderson JJB: Lifetime calcium intake and physical activity habits: independent and combined effects of bone mass in healthy premenopausal caucasian women, Am J Clin Nutr 49:534, 1989.
52. Riis B et al: Does calcium supplementation prevent postmenopausal bone loss? N Engl J Med 316:173, 1987.

Further Reading

Contento IR and Murphy BM: Psycho-social factors differentiating people who reported making desirable changes in their diets from those who did not, J Nutr Educ 22:6, 1990.

This article applies learning theory to practical approaches for assisting individuals in making positive dietary changes.

Ernst ND et al: The National Cholesterol Program: Implications for dietetic practitioners from the Adult Treatment Panel recommendations, J Am Diet Assoc 88:1401, 1988.

This article provides a comprehensive review of the goals, classification standards, and dietary and drug treatments developed for the National Cholesterol Education Program.

Harris SS et al: Physical activity counseling for healthy adults as a primary prevention intervention in the clinical setting. Report for the U.S. Preventive Services Task Force, JAMA 261:3590, 1989.

This task force provides guidelines for counseling clients beginning physical activity programs and practical suggestions for promoting adherence to these activity regimens.

Newman V and Lee D: Developing a daily food guide for women, J Nutr Ed 23(2):76, 1991.

These authors describe their procedures in developing and assessing the new daily food guide for women as part of California's revision of the state Public Health Services manual for health care professionals, *Nutrition during Pregnancy and Postpartum Period*. This food guide is designed to cover needs of adolescent and young adult women during their reproductive years in three sections: nonpregnant ages 11-24 and 25 + years, and during pregnancy and lactation. Copies of the full manual, as well as single photo-ready copies of the food guide in both English and Spanish, are available from Maternal and Child Health Branch, Department of Health Services, 714 "P" Street, Room 760, Sacramento, CA 95814, (916) 327-8176.

Shields JE and Young E: Fat in fast foods—evolving changes, Nutr Today 25:32, 1990.

These authors review the current trends in the fast food industry in using fat replacements to decrease levels of total and saturated fat.

4

Maternal Nutrition: The Course and Outcome of Pregnancy

Bonnie S. Worthington-Roberts

Basic Concepts

✱✱✱

✔ *Data about nutritional influences on fetal growth guide sound maternal nutrition.*

✔ *The physiology of pregnancy determines answers to maternal nutritional issues.*

✔ *Specific nutritional deficiencies and excesses affect fetal development.*

✔ *Prenatal weight gain follows varying individual patterns.*

✔ *Unusual eating behaviors that occur during pregnancy require evaluation.*

✔ *Nonnutrient dietary components affect pregnancy outcome.*

Food is essential to life and growth. Without an adequate supply of food, and the nutrients it contains, an organism cannot grow and develop normally. Eventually it dies.

In spite of these simple and well established facts, the role that nutrition plays in the course and outcome of pregnancy has not always been recognized. In the controlled conditions of the laboratory, researchers have been able to demonstrate harmful effects of deficient diets on pregnant animals and their offspring in a number of species. However, when studies are made on free-living human populations, direct relationships between what a mother eats during the 9 months of gestation and the course and outcome of her pregnancy are not always evident. Consequently, the emphasis that nutrition has received in prenatal care has varied over the years.

Part of the problem is that the changes occurring during pregnancy, their influence on nutritional needs, and the effects of long term nutritional status on reproductive performance are not fully understood. The application of nutrition principles to pregnancy has had to depend on progress in scientific knowledge about reproduction itself, and as in any science, one of the most important advances is simply learning to ask the right questions. The emphasis of research has changed as more has become known about nutrition, reproduction, and human growth. It is therefore easy to understand why different dietary recommendations for pregnant women have been made.

NUTRITION AND PREGNANCY: HISTORICAL DEVELOPMENT
Early Beliefs and Practices

During the nineteenth century much of what was known and recommended about diet during pregnancy was based on casual observation rather than controlled studies. Little information was available on the nutrient composition of foods or their biologic values. Dietary advice was influenced by belief in imitative magic: belief that the mother or child would acquire the attributes of the foods in the mother's diet. For example, pregnant women were sometimes forbidden to eat salty, acidic, or sour foods for fear the infant would be born with a "sour" disposition. The beliefs were often colored by the emotional and mystical aura surrounding the pregnant state. Eggs were sometimes restricted because of their association with the reproductive function. On the other hand, certain foods were encouraged for their presumed beneficial effects. Pregnant women were often advised to eat broths, warm milk, and ripe fruits to soothe the fetus and ease the birth process.

Problems in nineteenth century obstetric practice also influenced dietary recommendation. During the Industrial Revolution children in Europe had poor diets and worked long hours in dark factories. Rickets, which impairs normal bone formation during the growth years, was a common disorder. A contracted pelvis resulting from rickets was a major obstetric risk. Physicians did not have the modern means of delivering infants from these mothers. Death of both mother and child during childbirth was common.

Experience with his own patients in the 1880s led a German physician, Prochownick, to advocate a fluid-restricted, high-protein, low-carbohydrate diet for women with contracted pelvises to be followed for 6 weeks before birth. Women following this diet produced smaller infants and had easier deliveries. The diet may have had some justification in the 1880s, but it later gained in popularity and became a standard recommendation throughout pregnancy, even when the original rationale no longer applied. Remnants of the Prochownick diet, restricting fluid and carbohydrate, persist today.

There is very little specific information available about diet and pregnancy before the 1930s, other than reports on effects of food shortages during and after World War I. After the war there was much effort to relate food shortages to the size of the baby, but most of the evidence presented was inconclusive and even contradictory.

Reevaluation and Redirection

It was not until the mid-1960s that renewed interest in infant mortality and morbidity rates led to a reappraisal of the influence of diet on pregnancy. Once attention was redirected toward this problem, a number of significant steps were taken. The resulting progress has been rapid. First, two important events occurred in rapid succession.

The White House Conference. The White House Conference on Food, Nutrition, and Health was held in Washington in December 1969. The immediate stimulus was the nationwide shock at the disclosures of widespread hunger and malnutrition in the United States. The determination to do something about it produced the Conference as the first organizational step. Many experts there, involved in the Panel on Pregnancy and Very Young Infants, were also involved with the soon-to-be-published National Research Council (NRC) report on maternal nutrition and the course of pregnancy. They saw the Conference as a priceless opportunity to address the applied issues of diet and pregnancy within the context of their needed health services.

Benchmark NRC Report. The NRC report, *Maternal Nutrition and the Course of Pregnancy,*[1] was issued in 1970. It remains today the major source of research information on the role of nutrition in human reproduction. One of the principal findings of that report was the limited and fragmentary nature of studies on diet and pregnancy. The report singled out the need for long-term longitudinal studies on women and their families, a need which still remains.

FOLLOW-UP GUIDELINES AND PROGRAMS
Initial Guidelines for Practice

In 1973, two sets of guidelines appeared as a direct outgrowth of the stimulus given to nutrition services at the White House Conference: (1) the American Public Health Association[2] guidelines and standards issued primarily for public health workers as an aid to assessments and program planning; and (2) the NRC[3] guidelines for uses and limitations of supplementary food provided during pregnancy. Technical issues, practical problems, and political realities were explored, along with the inherent difficulties involved in multidisciplinary and multifactorial studies.

WIC Program

In 1978, the now well-known WIC program—Special Supplementary Food Program for Women, Infants, and Children[4]—was initiated under court order. The purpose of the WIC program was to provide food as an adjunct to health care during critical times of growth and development. Table 4-1 summarizes the main features of this important program. The WIC program has grown from a pilot program costing $40 million in 1973 to one costing over $1 billion in 1991. Many of the same problems addressed in the 1969 White House Conference are still being encountered in the WIC program today, leading to questions of what the program is accomplishing.

ACOG-ADA Guidelines

In 1981, the American College of Obstetricians and Gynecologists (ACOG) and the American Dietetic Association (ADA) issued a joint publication, *Guidelines for Assessment of Maternal Nutrition.*[5] This was indeed a milestone. The report produced the first national consensus on the relevant risk factors before and during pregnancy. This original listing has been updated by the more recent material in the NRC perinatal guide.

NRC Perinatal Guide

In 1981, the NRC produced the highly useful guide *Nutrition Services in Perinatal Care.*[6] This report was particularly timely because it was designed for use with the rapidly growing regional networks for maternal and perinatal services. It is most helpful because it addresses the nutritional issues of infant feeding and the increasingly important concerns about substance abuse—cigarettes, drugs, and alcohol.

TABLE 4-1   *The Special Supplemental Food Program for Women, Infants, and Children (WIC)*

1. Sponsored by the Food and Nutrition Service of the U.S. Department of Agriculture
2. Originally authorized in 1972
3. Target population: pregnant and postpartum women up to 6 months after delivery if not breastfeeding and up to 12 months if breastfeeding; infants; children up to 5 years of age
4. Eligibility criteria: nutritionally at risk and members of low-income families
5. Program administered by state health departments
6. Regulations require that WIC agencies offer nutrition education and that appropriate health services be available directly or by referral.

The Most Recent Landmark Document

The increasing visibility of maternal services in the United States motivated the National Academy of Sciences to appoint an expert committee with a mandate to evaluate data related to prenatal weight gain and nutrient supplements. The committee's final report entitled *Nutrition during Pregnancy: Weight Gain and Nutrient Supplements* was issued in July 1990.[7] Recommendations made in this report are cited throughout this chapter.

Continued Needs

There is increasing realization of the seamless web of variables that together influence the outcome of pregnancy. Within the constellation of income, health, education, family, and fertility, food and nutrition are just one part, but an important and modifiable one. As one observer stated, "Special efforts to improve prenatal, child, and maternal health showed clear evidence that the services did make a difference. . . . No one has yet teased out the relative effects of different variables."[8] This is the clearest statement of the nature of the problems that need to be addressed in the years ahead.

PHYSIOLOGY OF PREGNANCY

Normal pregnancy is accompanied by anatomic and physiologic changes that affect almost every function in the body. Many of these changes are apparent in the very early weeks. This indicates that they are not merely a response to the physiologic stress imposed by the fetus but are an integral part of the maternal-fetal system, which creates the most favorable environment possible for the developing child. The changes are necessary to regulate maternal metabolism, promote fetal growth, and prepare the mother for labor, birth, and lactation.

The changes that occur in pregnancy are too complex to be given full treatment here, but a look at some changes that have effects on general metabolism will lay the foundation for interpreting nutritional requirements and dietary allowances.

Blood Volume and Composition

Plasma is the fluid component of blood, whereas serum is the part of plasma that remains after its coagulation factors have been removed. Total plasma volume in a nonpregnant woman averages 2600 ml. Near the end of the first trimester of pregnancy, plasma volume begins to increase, and by 34 weeks it is about 50% greater than it was at conception.

There is considerable variation from these averages. Women who have small volumes to begin with usually have a greater increase, as do **multigravidae** and mothers with multiple births.

Researchers have shown that the increase in plasma volume is correlated with obstetric performance. They found that women who have a small increase when compared with the average are more likely to have stillbirths, abortions, and **low-birth-weight** babies. Clearly the restriction of a normal expansion of plasma volume is undesirable in pregnancy.

If the availability of nutrients or the synthesis of normal blood constituents does not keep pace with the expansion of plasma volume, their concentrations per 100 ml of blood will decrease, even though the total amount may rise. This is apparently what happens with red blood cells, serum proteins, minerals, and water-soluble vitamins.

Red cell production is stimulated during pregnancy so that their numbers gradually rise, but the increase is not as large as the expansion of plasma volume (Fig. 4-1). The **hematocrit,** which is normally around 35% in women, may be as low as 29% to 31% during pregnancy. The amount of hemoglobin in each red blood cell does not change,

Multigravida
(L *multus,* many; *gravida,* pregnant) A woman who has had two or more pregnancies.

Low birth weight
Birth weight less than 2500 g (5.4 lb). Very low birth weight: birth weight less than 1500 g (3.3 lb).

Hematocrit (HCT)
(Gr *haima,* blood; *krinein,* to separate) The volume percentage of red blood cells (RBCs) in whole blood; normally about 35% in women. Shows the ratio of RBC volume to total blood volume.

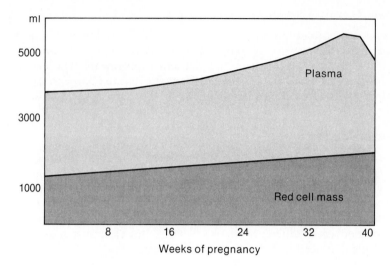

FIG. 4-1 Increase in plasma volume and red cell mass during the course of human pregnancy.

From Worthington-Roberts BS and Williams SR: Nutrition in pregnancy and lactation, ed 4, St Louis, 1989, Times Mirror/Mosby College Publishing.

TABLE 4-2 **Serum Nutrient Levels in Pregnant and Nonpregnant Women**

Nutrient	Normal Nonpregnancy Range	Values in Pregnancy
Total protein	6.5-8.5 g/100 ml	6.0-8.0
Albumin	3.5-5.0 g/100 ml	3.0-4.5
Glucose	<110 mg/100 ml	<120
Cholesterol	120-190 mg/100 ml	200-325
Vitamin A	20-60 µg/100 ml	20-60
Carotene	50-300 µg/100 ml	80-325
Ascorbic acid	0.2-2.0 mg/100 ml	0.2-1.5
Folic acid	5-21 ng/100 ml	3.15
Calcium	4.6-5.5 mEq/L	4.2-5.2
Iron/iron-binding capacity	>50/250-400 µg/100 ml	>40/300-450

Modified from Aubry RH, Roberts A, and Cuenca V, Clin Perinatol 2:207, 1975.

Hemoglobin
(Gr *haima*, blood; L *globus*, a ball) Oxygen-carrying pigment in red blood cells; a conjugated protein containing four heme groups combined with iron and four long globin polypeptide chains; formed by the developing RBC in bone marrow.

Normochromic
Normal red blood cell color.

Normocytic
Normal red blood cell size.

Gestation
(L *gestare*, to bear) Intrauterine fetal growth period (40 weeks) from conception to birth.

but because there are fewer red blood cells per 100 ml of blood, hemodilution occurs. Nonpregnant **hemoglobin** values of 13 to 14 g per 100 ml can drop as low as 10 or 11 g/100 ml in the early months. In a nonpregnant woman this level of hemoglobin would indicate anemia, but in pregnancy the red blood cells are **normochromic** and **normocytic.**

Serum levels of the major nutrients typical for pregnant and nonpregnant women are compared in Table 4-2. The values for pregnant women must be interpreted with caution. Investigators have obtained different values depending on the laboratory methods used. Moreover, levels of certain nutrients can be influenced by a number of maternal factors such as age, parity, smoking, and the use of various medications before or during pregnancy. Even the sex of the fetus can influence the mother's blood levels of some nutrients. The levels will also fluctuate at different times during **gestation.**

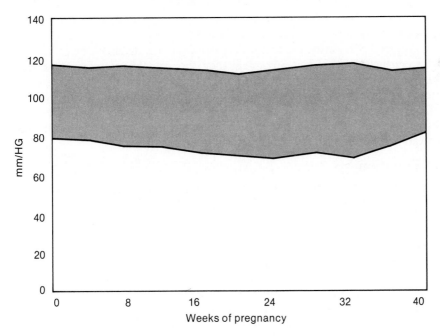

FIG. 4-2 Change in blood pressure during the course of human pregnancy.

From Worthington-Roberts BS and Williams SR: Nutrition in pregnancy and lactation, ed 4, St Louis, 1989, Times Mirror/Mosby College Publishing.

The Cardiovascular System

Extensive anatomic and physiologic changes occur in the cardiovascular system during the course of pregnancy. These adaptations serve to protect the woman's normal physiologic functioning to meet the metabolic demands pregnancy imposes on her body, and to provide for fetal development and growth needs.

The slight cardiac **hypertrophy** or dilation is probably secondary to the increased blood volume and cardiac output. As the diaphragm is displaced upward, the heart is elevated upward and to the left. The degree of shift depends on the duration of pregnancy and the size and position of the uterus.

During the first half of pregnancy, there is a decrease in both systolic and diastolic pressure of 5 to 10 mm Hg. The decrease in blood pressure is probably the result of peripheral **vasodilation** from the hormonal changes during pregnancy. During the third trimester, maternal blood pressure should return to the values obtained during the first trimester (Fig. 4-2).

Cardiac output increases from 30% to 50% by week 32 of pregnancy; it declines to about a 20% increase at week 40. The elevated cardiac output is largely a result of increased stroke volume and is in response to increased tissue demands for oxygen (normal value is 5 to 5.5 L/min). The cardiac output decreases with the woman in the supine position and increases with any exertion such as labor and delivery. The circulation time decreases slightly by week 32. It returns to near normal near term.

Respiration

Respiratory adaptations occur during pregnancy to provide for both maternal and fetal needs. Maternal oxygen requirements increase in response to the acceleration in

Hypertrophy
(Gr *hyper*, above; *trophe*, nutrition) Enlargement of an organ or part due to the process of increasing cell size.

Vasodilation
(L *vas*, vessel; *dilatare*, to spread out) Expansion or stretching of a blood vessel.

metabolic rate and the need to add to the tissue mass in the uterus and breasts. The fetus requires oxygen and a way to eliminate carbon dioxide.

As mentioned previously, the level of the diaphragm is displaced by as much as 4 cm during pregnancy. With advancing pregnancy thoracic breathing replaces abdominal breathing and descent of the diaphragm with respiration becomes less possible.

The pregnant woman breathes deeper (greater **tidal volume,** the amount of gases exchanged with each breath) but increases her respiratory rate only slightly (about two breaths per minute). There is a more efficient exchange of lung gases in the **alveoli;** the oxygen-carrying capacity of the blood is increased accordingly.

Renal Function

In normal pregnancy, renal function is altered considerably. The woman's kidneys must manage the increased metabolic and circulatory demands of the maternal body as well as excretion of fetal waste products. Changes in renal function are caused by pregnancy hormones, an increase in blood volume, the woman's posture, and nutritional intake.

To facilitate the clearance of creatinine, urea, and other waste products of fetal and maternal metabolism, blood flow through the kidneys and the glomerular filtration rate are increased during pregnancy. The change in glomerular filtration rate is partially caused by the lower osmotic pressure, which results from the fall in serum albumin. This is one adaptation that appears to be purely mechanical, since no effects of hormones on this aspect of kidney function have been shown. However, there are consequences for nutrition.

Normally most of the glucose, amino acids, and water-soluble vitamins that are filtered by the nephrons are reabsorbed in the tubules to preserve the body's balance. However, in pregnancy substantial quantities of these nutrients appear in the urine. The most satisfactory explanation at present is that the higher glomerular filtration rate offers the tubules greater quantities of nutrients than they can feasibly reabsorb. Because the change in filtration rate is largely mechanical, there may not be an accompanying mechanism by which the tubules can readjust.

Gastrointestinal Function

The functioning of the gastrointestinal system undergoes a number of interesting changes during the course of pregnancy. The appetite increases, nausea and vomiting may occur, motility is diminished, intestinal secretion is reduced, sense of taste is altered, and absorption of nutrients is enhanced.

Increased progesterone production causes decreased tone and motility of the smooth muscles of the gastrointestinal tract. This leads to esophageal regurgitation, decreased emptying of the stomach, and reverse **peristalsis.** As a result, the pregnant woman may experience heartburn. The decreased smooth muscle tone also results in an increase in water absorption from the colon, and constipation may result. In addition, constipation is secondary to hypoperistalsis, unusual food choices, lack of fluids, abdominal pressure by the pregnant uterus, and displacement of intestines with some compression. **Hemorrhoids** may be everted or may bleed during straining at stool.

Decreased emptying time of the gallbladder is typical. This feature, together with slight hypercholesterolemia from increased progesterone levels, may account for the frequent development of gallstones during pregnancy.

Intraabdominal alterations that can cause discomfort include pelvic heaviness or pressure, **flatulence,** distention and bowel cramping, and uterine contractions. In addition to displacement of intestines, pressure from the expanding uterus increases venous pressure in the pelvic organs. Although most abdominal discomfort is a consequence of normal maternal alterations, occasional bowel obstruction or an inflammatory process may be present.

Tidal volume
  The amount of gases passing into and out of the lungs in each respiratory cycle.

Alveoli
  (L *alveus,* hollow) Small sac-like formations; thin-walled chambers in the lungs surrounded by networks of capillaries through whose walls exchange of carbon dioxide and oxygen takes place.

Peristalsis
  (Gr *peri,* around; stalsis, contraction) A wave-like progression of alternate contraction and relaxation of the muscle fibers of the gastrointestinal tract.

Hemorrhoids
  (Gr *haima,* blood; *rhoia,* to flow) Enlarged veins in the mucous membranes inside or outside of the rectum; causes pain, itching, discomfort, and bleeding.

Flatulence
  (L *flatus,* a blowing) Excessive formation and expulsion of gases in the gastrointestinal tract.

Insofar as taste is concerned, a recent study[9] examined the ability of the pregnant woman to discriminate among different concentrations of salt and sucrose solutions. Results of tests with salt solutions showed that pregnant women were significantly less able to identify concentration differences correctly and preferred significantly stronger salt solutions than did nonpregnant women. The researchers suggest that these observations may reflect a physiologic mechanism for increasing salt intake during pregnancy.

Hormones

The pregnant woman secretes more than 30 different hormones throughout gestation. Some, like those just mentioned, are only present in pregnancy, whereas others that are normally present have altered rates of secretion that are modified by the pregnant state.

Most hormones are proteins or steroids that are synthesized from precursors such as amino acids and cholesterol in endocrine glands throughout the body. Their production is influenced by the mother's general health and nutritional status. Under normal circumstances they are controlling factors in a complex feedback system that maintains homeostasis between cellular and extracellular constituents and metabolism. During pregnancy many of these homeostatic mechanisms are "reset" so that changes occur in the retention, utilization, and excretion of nutrients. Some of the hormones that exert important effects on nutrient metabolism are summarized in Table 4-3. Only those that have more general implications for nutritional management are singled out for discussion here.

Progesterone and estrogen are two hormones that have major effects on maternal physiology during pregnancy. The chief action of progesterone is to cause a relaxation of the smooth muscles of the uterus so that it can expand as the fetus grows, but it also has a relaxing effect on other smooth muscles in the body. Relaxation of the muscles of the gastrointestinal tract reduces motility in the gut, allowing more time for the nutrients to be absorbed. The slower movement is also a cause of the constipation commonly experienced by pregnant women. General metabolic effects of progesterone are to induce maternal fat deposition, reduce alveolar and arterial PCO_2 (partial pressure or tension of the gas carbon dioxide, facilitating exchange of lung gases in respiration and ensuring buffer capacity), and increase renal sodium excretion.

The secretion of estrogen is lower than that of progesterone during the early months of pregnancy, but it rises sharply near term. Its role is to promote the growth and control the function of the uterus, but it too has generalized effects on nutrition. One effect that has caused some difficulties for clinicians is the alteration of the structure of mucopolysaccharides in connective tissue. This alteration is beneficial because it makes the tissue more flexible and therefore assists in dilating the uterus at birth, but it also increases the affinity of connective tissue to water. This **hydroscopic** effect of estrogen and the sodium-losing effect of progesterone produce a confusing clinical picture of the pregnant woman's fluid and electrolyte balance. Because of estrogen, many pregnant women complain of excess fluid retention in the skin. Their faces and fingers become puffy, and there are other indications of generalized **edema.** In addition, changes in cardiovascular dynamics cause extracellular fluid to accumulate in the feet and legs.

Since excess fluid retention is one of the hallmarks of **preeclampsia,** some clinicians view these changes with alarm, and may initiate rather rigorous treatment with diuretics and a sodium-restricted diet to promote water loss. The evidence, however, weighs strongly against this practice. It is now apparent that while the incidence of generalized and peripheral ankle edema is high, it is not associated with an increase in perinatal mortality when the two other symptoms of preeclampsia—hypertension and proteinuria—are absent. In fact, women with mild edema have slightly larger babies and a lower rate of premature births.

The propensity of women to lose sodium from the action of progesterone is compensated for by an increased secretion of aldosterone from the adrenal glands and renin

Hydroscopic
(Gr *hydro*, water; *skopein*, to measure or examine) Possessing tendency to take up and hold water readily.

Edema
(Gr *oidema*, swelling) Accumulation of fluid in the intercellular tissue spaces of the body.

Preeclampsia
(L *prae*, before; *eklampein*, to shine forth) Condition in late pregnancy in which hypertension and edema occur, with or without proteinuria.

TABLE 4-3 *Hormonal Effects on Nutrient Metabolism in Pregnancy*

Hormone	Primary Source of Secretion	Principal Effects
Progesterone	Placenta	Reduces gastric motility; favors maternal fat deposition; increases sodium excretion; reduces alveolar and arterial P_{CO_2}; interferes with folic acid metabolism
Estrogen	Placenta	Reduces serum proteins; increases hydroscopic properties of connective tissue; affects thyroid function; interferes with folic acid metabolism
Human placental lactogen (HPL)	Placenta	Elevates blood glucose from breakdown of glycogen
Human chorionic thyrotropin (HCT)	Placenta	Stimulates production of thyroid hormones
Human growth hormone (HGH)	Anterior pituitary	Elevates blood glucose; stimulates growth of long bones; promotes nitrogen retention
Thyroid-stimulating hormone (TSH)	Anterior pituitary	Stimulates secretion of thyroxine; increases uptake of iodine by thyroid gland
Thyroxine	Thyroid	Regulates rate of cellular oxidation (basal metabolism)
Parathyroid hormone (PTH)	Parathyroid	Promotes calcium resorption from bone; increases calcium absorption; promotes urinary excretion of phosphate
Calcitonin (CT)	Thyroid	Inhibits calcium resorption from bone
Insulin	Beta cells of pancreas	Reduces blood glucose levels to promote energy production and synthesis of fat
Glucagon	Alpha cells of pancreas	Elevates blood glucose levels from glycogen breakdown
Aldosterone	Adrenal cortex	Promotes sodium retention and potassium excretion
Cortisone	Adrenal cortex	Elevates blood glucose from protein breakdown
Renin-angiotensin	Kidneys	Stimulates aldosterone secretion; promotes sodium and water retention; increases thirst

From Worthington-Roberts BS and Williams SR: Nutrition in pregnancy and lactation, ed 4, St Louis, 1989, Times Mirror/Mosby College Publishing.

Juxtaglomerular apparatus

(L *juxta*, near; *glomus*, ball) Complex of special cells located near or adjoining a nephron at the head of a glomerulus of the kidney, responsible for sensing the level of sodium in the blood.

from the **juxtaglomerular apparatus** of the kidneys. If sodium restriction is imposed, this renin-aldosterone system must work harder to maintain normal sodium concentrations in the body. Pushed beyond the stress naturally induced by pregnancy, the system could become exhausted so that, in the long run, less aldosterone and renin are produced. The sodium and water depletion that would result is more dangerous than the mild degree of edema that the treatment is supposed to prevent. This effect has been demonstrated in pregnant rats that are placed on sodium-restricted diets that would be equivalent to 1 g/day of sodium or "no added salt" diet in humans.

Although hormonal effects on fluid and electrolyte balance need more research, the mechanisms that are understood to date suggest that a mild degree of edema is physiologic in pregnancy and that the measures commonly used to prevent it impose an unnecessary risk.

Metabolic Adjustments

The basal metabolic rate (BMR) usually rises by the fourth month of gestation, although small increments may occur before that time. It is normally increased by 15% to 20% by term. The BMR returns to nonpregnant levels by 5 or 6 days postpartum. The elevation in BMR reflects increased oxygen demands of the uterine-placental fetal unit as well as oxygen consumption from increased maternal cardiac work. Peripheral vasodilation assists in the release of the excess heat production, though some women may continue to experience heat intolerance. Lassitude and fatigability after only slight exertion are described by many women in early pregnancy. These feelings may persist along with a greater need for sleep.

A complex series of adjustments in carbohydrate, protein, and fat metabolism occur during gestation to ensure that the fetus receives a continuous supply of fuel when the needs are maximal in late pregnancy. These adjustments are induced by changes in the endocrine milieu and by development of new endocrine tissue, the placenta.

Approximately 50% to 70% of the kilocalories required daily by the fetus in the third trimester (43 kcal/kg/day) is derived from glucose; about 20% of the kilocalories are derived from amino acids, and the remainder from fat. When maternal blood glucose levels fall, the rate of glucose transfer to the fetus declines and fatty acids may become a more dominant fuel source. The net effect of maternal fuel adaptations is to increase the use of fat as a fuel source by the mother to conserve glucose for the fetus. During the second trimester, the mother prepares for the anticipated fetal glucose demand by storing fat. Then in the third trimester, when the fetal glucose demand causes maternal plasma glucose levels to fall, **lipolysis** increases in the maternal compartment.

During a brief fast, such as overnight, maternal plasma glucose concentrations in pregnant women fall significantly below that of nonpregnant women because of continual placental uptake of glucose and impaired hepatic gluconeogenesis. The reduced capacity for gluconeogenesis is related in part to the reduced availability of alanine; the latter is the result of increased placental alanine uptake and restrained maternal muscle breakdown. Lipolysis is enhanced and mild ketosis may occur. In the postprandial period, maternal glucose uptake is lower than in nonpregnant women, despite increased plasma insulin concentrations. More of the glucose removed by the liver is converted to triglycerides; these are stored in maternal adipose tissue to be available for later fasting periods.

Overall, the major adjustment in energy utilization during pregnancy is a shift in the fuel sources. Fat becomes the major maternal fuel whereas glucose is the major fetal fuel. Since the size of the maternal tissue is considerably greater than the size of the fetal mass, lipolysis dominates, causing the respiratory quotient to fall in fasting women. Pregnant women gain weight readily without appreciable changes in energy intake, because water normally comprises about 65% of the weight gain, not because energy is utilized more efficiently. However, there is still some question about the efficiency of energy utilization, especially in the pregnant woman exposed to severe food deprivation.

Role of the Placenta

The **placenta** is not a passive barrier between the mother and the fetus. Rather, it plays an active role in reproduction. The placenta is the principal site of production for several important hormones that regulate maternal growth and development. For the fetus it is the only way that nutrients, oxygen, and waste products can be exchanged.

Lipolysis
(Gr *lipus*, fat; *lysis*, dissolution) The breakdown of fat.

Placenta
(L *placentas*, a flat cake) Characteristic organ of mammals during pregnancy joining mother and offspring, providing supportive nourishment and endocrine secretions for embryonic-fetal development and growth.

Structure and development. Evolving from a tiny mass of cells in the first weeks of pregnancy, the placenta becomes a complex network of tissue and blood vessels weighing about 1.4 lb (650 g) at term. The vital role it plays as a link between mother and child is represented by the two principal parts of the placenta—one uterine and the other fetal.

On the maternal side the placenta is part of the uterine mucosa. When the tiny **blastocyst** implants itself in the uterus 6 to 7 days after fertilization of the **ovum,** the uterine tissue and blood vessels break down to form small spaces called **lacunae** that fill with maternal blood. These spaces are eventually bounded on the maternal side by the decidua or basal plate. Blood begins to circulate in the spaces at about 12 days gestation.

Meanwhile the **trophoblast** grows and sends out rootlike villi into the pools of maternal blood. The villi contain capillaries, which will exchange nutrients and metabolic waste products between the mother and the fetus. In the early weeks of pregnancy the villi are thick columns of cells, but as they subdivide throughout gestation the villi become thinner and produce numerous branches. Some branches become anchored in the maternal tissue, and others remain free or floating in the intravillous spaces. The multiple villus branches provide a large surface membrane area for efficient exchange of nutrients and metabolic waste products between mother and fetus (Fig. 4-3). Even though uterine and embryonic tissues are intermingled, the blood of the mother and the embryo never mix because they are always separated by the placental membrane (Fig. 4-4).

Mechanisms of nutrient transfer. The efficiency of placental nutrient transfer is a determinant of fetal well-being. Reduced surface area of the villi, insufficient vascularization, or changes in the hydrostatic pressure in the intervillous space can limit the supply of nutrients available to the fetus and inhibit normal growth.

Blastocyst

(Gr *blastos*, germ; *kystis*, sac, bladder) A stage in the development of the embryo in which the cells are arranged in a single layer to form a hollow sphere.

Ovum

(L *ovum*, egg) The female reproductive cell (egg) that develops into a new organism.

Lacunae

(L *lacuna*, small pit or hollow cavity) Blood spaces of the placenta in which the fetal villi are found.

Trophoblast

(Gr *trophe*, nutrition; *blastos*, germ) Extraembryonic ectodermal tissue on the surface of the cleaving, fertilized ovum, which is responsible for contact with the maternal circulation and supply of nutrients to the embryo.

FIG. 4-3 Diagrammatic representation of a section through a mature placenta showing the relationship of the fetal placenta (villous chorion) to the maternal placenta (decidua basalis), fetal placental circulation, and maternal placental circulation. Maternal blood is forced into the intervillous space, and exchanges occur with the fetal blood as the maternal blood flows around the villi. Incoming arterial blood pushes venous blood into the endometrial veins, which are scattered over the surface of the maternal placenta. Umbilical arteries carry deoxygenated fetal blood to the placenta, and the umbilical vein carries oxygenated blood to the fetus.

Nutrient transfer in the placenta is a complex process. It employs all the mechanisms used for the absorption of nutrients from the gastrointestinal tract: simple diffusion, facilitated diffusion, active transport, and **pinocytosis** (Table 4-4). The difference, however, is that in the placenta two completely separate blood supplies are maintained. The maternal circulation remains in the intervillous space. The fetal capillaries are separated from the maternal blood by two layers of cells. Their thickness is approximately 5.5 μm (Fig. 4-4).

Pinocytosis
(Gr *pinein*, to drink; *kytos*, cell) Uptake of fluid nutrient material by a living cell by means of incupping and invagination of the cell membrane, which closes off, forming free cell vacuoles.

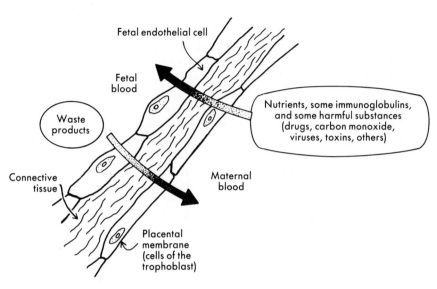

FIG. 4-4 Nutrients, waste products, and other transportable compounds must cross two layers of cells in the process of movement through the placenta.

TABLE 4-4 **Placental Transport Mechanisms and Materials Transported by Each Mechanism**

Transport Mechanism	Substance Transported
Passive diffusion	Oxygen
	Carbon dioxide
	Fatty acids
	Steroids
	Nucleosides
	Electrolytes
	Fat-soluble vitamins
Facilitated diffusion	Most monosaccharides
Active transport	Amino acids
	Some cations (calcium, iron)
	Iodine
	Phosphate
	Water-soluble vitamins*
Solvent drag†	Electrolytes

*At very high concentrations vitamin C has been shown to cross the placenta via diffusion.
†Movement of ions with water as it flows back and forth across the membrane.

Although the same nutrient may be simultaneously transferred by more than one mechanism, the major means of transport can be estimated by comparing nutrient concentrations in maternal and cord blood. If the concentrations are equal, the transfer has most likely occurred by simple or facilitated diffusion. Simple diffusion is a passive process in which nutrients move from high concentrations in the maternal blood to lower concentrations in fetal capillaries until equilibrium is reached. Facilitated diffusion differs from simple diffusion in that the rate of transfer is faster than would be expected. The mechanism of facilitated diffusion is not established, but it is thought that a carrier in the membrane is employed. Active transport requires both a carrier protein and metabolic energy to move a nutrient against an electrochemical gradient.

Most proteins do not cross the placenta since their molecular size is too big to allow penetration through the cells of the villi. This protects the fetus from acquiring harmful agents of high molecular weight, but it also means that the fetus must synthesize its own proteins from its supply of amino acids. An exception is the maternal immunoglobulin IgG. It is not known why this particular protein crosses the placenta, but it appears that the selectivity is related to the structure and not to the size of the molecule. IgG is probably transported by pinocytosis. The benefit to the fetus is that it has the same resistance to infectious diseases as the mother.

Respiratory and excretory exchange. Besides serving as a lifeline for nutrients, the placenta functions in the exchange of respiratory gases and waste products between the mother and fetus.

The delivery of oxygen to the fetus is just as important to proper metabolism as an adequate supply of nutrients. The mother makes adjustments in her breathing to meet fetal oxygen needs, but the amount ultimately depends on the blood flow through the uterus to the placental villi. Near term the rate of flow through the intervillous space is 375 to 560 ml/min. Exchange is made between maternal red cells, which characteristically have a lower affinity for oxygen during pregnancy, and fetal red cells, which have a high affinity.

Maternal nutrition can influence oxygen exchange through the production of hemoglobin. Each gram of hemoglobin carries 1.34 ml of oxygen. In normal concentrations it can deliver up to 16 ml of oxygen per 100 ml of blood to the placenta. If maternal hemoglobin levels are depressed from iron deficiency, the supply of oxygen per 100 ml of blood is reduced. Since the fetus can tolerate little variation in the rate at which oxygen is supplied, the mother must compensate by increasing her cardiac output.

Hyperventilation

(Gr *hyper,* over; L *ventilatio,* ventilation) Increased respiration with larger consequent air intake and oxygen-carbon dioxide exchange in the lungs above the normal amount.

Another function of the placenta is to rid the fetus of metabolic wastes. The placenta is freely permeable to carbon dioxide, water, urea, creatinine, and uric acid. **Hyperventilation** by the mother reduces her Pco_2 (see p. 93) so that carbon dioxide exchange from the fetus is accomplished by simple diffusion. Urea, creatinine, and uric acid, which are the wastes of fetal amino acid metabolism, move through the placenta by diffusion and active transport.

Placental hormones. The production of hormones to regulate the activities of pregnancy is one of the most interesting special functions of the placenta. From the earliest days of pregnancy the cells of the trophoblast and their successors in the placenta manufacture a large variety of hormones. The first to be manufactured in appreciable amounts is the protein hormone *human chorionic gonadotropin (HCG).* Early in the differentiation of the trophoblast this hormone is found coating the trophoblasts's outer cell surfaces, where it is believed to act as an immunologically protective layer, preventing the rejection of the blastocyst and thereby facilitating implantation. HCG also stimulates the synthesis of *estrogen* in the placenta. Synthesis of estrogen actually begins in the free-floating blastocyst where it acts to facilitate implantation. The fact that the cells of the small, primitive blastocyst are already equipped to conduct complex steroid manipulation is a measure of the importance of these hormones at this early stage.

As pregnancy proceeds, large amounts of progesterone are synthesized in the placenta, principally from maternal cholesterol. In addition to sustaining pregnancy, this hormone serves as a raw material for the production of estrogens, mainly estrone, estradiol, and estriol, which in turn act on many organs and tissues of both the mother and fetus. Interestingly, the human placenta lacks the enzymes needed for converting the large amounts of progesterone it makes into certain essential estrogens and other steroids. Consequently, these synthetic events are carried out in the *fetal zone* cells, which are clusters of transient cells found in the developing adrenal glands of the fetus. These cells lack the enzymes necessary to manufacture progesterone but possess the requisite ones for its conversion. In this way the fetal and placental tissues complement each other. When the fetus' endocrine glands become sufficiently mature to take over the manufacture of steroid hormones, the fetal zone cells gradually diminish and eventually disappear. Presumably this sophisticated collaboration is organized and timed by precise genetic instructions and is regulated by equally precise releasing hormones.

Because a great variety of regulatory hormones are synthesized in the placenta, including HCG, human placental lactogen (HPL), chorionic somatomammotropin, and human chorionic thyrotropin (HCT), the placental control during pregnancy must be as comprehensive as that maintained by the pituitary gland throughout life. By means of these hormones the placenta not only carries out the functions of the fetus' pituitary until the organ is ready to perform on its own, but also conducts the entire "endocrine orchestra of pregnancy," which performs largely in the placenta itself.

Immunologic Protection

During pregnancy it is absolutely vital that the embryo be protected from immunologic rejection by maternal tissue. One of the mechanisms that seems to play a part in this task is the nonspecific suppression of lymphocytes, the cells that normally mediate the rejection of a graft. Experiments have shown that lymphocytes can be suppressed by HCG, HPL, prolactin, cortisone, progesterone, the estrogens, and a variety of proteins and glycoproteins.

It is also likely that the embryo is protected by the large tightly packed cells that enclose it soon after the implantation of the blastocyst. This protective barrier prevents the drainage of lymphocytes to maternal tissues. In addition, the maternal blood vessels do not invade the trophoblast of the placenta, so this potential means of graft rejection is blocked. In the early days of the development of the trophoblast further protection is provided by the absence of the expression of antigens. So even though the embryonic tissue is "foreign," it manages to conceal the fact, at least for a while.

Effects of Maternal Malnutrition

Maternal malnutrition has also been found to interfere with normal placental growth and function (Fig. 4-5). This is reflected by lower placental weight, smaller placental size, and reduced deoxyribonucleic acid (DNA) content. Affected placentas also have a reduced peripheral villous mass and villous surface.

STAGES OF HUMAN FETAL GROWTH

After the ovum is released from the mature follicle in the ovary, it enters the fallopian tube. It moves slowly through the tube toward the uterus, encountering potential fertilizing sperm along the way. The stages of human embryonic-fetal growth are illustrated

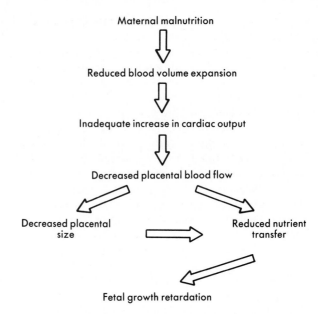

Maternal malnutrition

Reduced blood volume expansion

Inadequate increase in cardiac output

Decreased placental blood flow

Decreased placental size

Reduced nutrient transfer

Fetal growth retardation

FIG. 4-5 Postulated mechanisms responsible for placental and fetal growth retardation as seen with maternal malnutrition in animal models and in human subjects.

Modified from Rosso P: Fed Proc 39:250, 1980.

Morula
(L *morus,* mulberry) Solid mass of cells resembling a mulberry, formed by cleavage of a fertilized ovum.

Ectoderm
(Gr *ektos,* outside; *derma,* skin) Outermost of the three primitive cell layers of the embryo.

Mesoderm
(Gr *mesos,* middle; *derma,* skin) Intermediate layer of embryonic cells developing between the ectoderm and endoderm.

Endoderm
(Gr *endon,* within; *derma,* skin) Innermost of the three primitive embryonic cell layers.

in Fig. 4-6. Fertilization usually occurs in the fallopian tube within 48 hours, after which cell division rapidly proceeds. The resulting solid ball of cells, the **morula,** enters the uterus where it undergoes reorganization into a hollow ball, the *blastocyst.* The blastocyst ultimately buries itself in the endometrial lining of the uterus (5 to 7 days postovulation). Here the precursor cells of the placenta begin to arrange themselves into a functioning placental unit. Nutritional support for the embryo at this time comes from the endometrial lining of the uterus. After its initial development, the placenta grows rapidly throughout gestation. By 34 to 36 weeks the fetus has completed cell division. From that time until term, growth continues only by increase in size of existing cells.

Embryologic studies indicate three stages of fetal growth:

1. **Blastogenesis stage.** The fertilized egg divides into cells that fold in on one another. An inner cell mass evolves, giving rise to the embryo and an outer coat, the *trophoblast,* which becomes the placenta. This process is complete about 2 weeks after fertilization.

2. **Embryonic stage.** This is the critical time when cells differentiate into three germinal layers. The **ectoderm,** outer layer, gives rise to the brain, nervous system, hair, and skin. The **mesoderm,** middle layer, produces all of the voluntary muscles, bones, and components of the cardiovascular and excretory systems. The **endoderm,** inner layer, forms the disgestive and respiratory systems, and glandular organs. By 60 days' gestation all of the major features of the human infant are achieved.

3. **Fetal stage.** This is the period of most rapid growth. From the third month until term, fetal weight increases nearly 500-fold from 6 g (0.2 oz) to 3000-3500 g (6.5 to 7.5 lb) at birth. The average weight curve from 10 weeks to term is shown in Fig. 4-7.

Measurements of DNA and protein in embryonic and fetal tissues show that embryonic growth occurs only by increase in number of cells, **hyperplasia.** Fetal growth continues in cell number, but now also involves increase in cell size, hypertrophy. The stages of cell growth involving hyperplasia and hypertrophy are illustrated in Fig. 4-8.

Hyperplasia
(Gr *hyper,* above; *plasis,* formation) Enlargement of tissue due to a process of rapidly increasing cell number.

Growth-Retarded Infants

From the sequence described, it is possible to estimate the effects of malnutrition on growth at different stages of gestation. In the early months of pregnancy a severe limit on supply or transport of nutrients would have to occur to cause retarded growth because the quantitative requirements of the embryo are extremely small. Nevertheless, a restriction of materials and energy needed for cell synthesis and cell differentiation could produce malformations or cause the embryo to die. Malnutrition after the third month of gestation would not have teratogenic effects, but it could interfere with fetal growth. Nutrient requirements are greatest in the last trimester of pregnancy, when cells are increasing rapidly in both number and size. Even a relatively mild restriction could have serious effects at this time.

Characteristics of SGA Infants

The effects of fetal malnutrition are reflected in the characteristics of small-for-gestational-age (SGA) infants, who though full term are poorly developed. Their conditions are variable, suggesting the multiple causes and importance of timing shown in animal studies. Among those SGA infants that do not have birth anomalies, there are two patterns of growth retardation. One type affects weight more than length; the other affects weight and length equally:

Gestational age
Stage of fetal growth and development at birth, varying from a premature delivery to full term.

1. **Type I: growth retardation primarily affecting weight.** Head size (circumference) and skeletal growth are about normal, but the infants have poorly developed muscles and almost no subcutaneous fat. The resemblance of these infants to the large head and small body features of animals malnourished during the last weeks of gestation, either by maternal dietary restrictions or uterine ligation, is remarkable.
2. **Type II: growth reduction in both weight and height.** Size of all parts of the body, including head circumference and skeleton, is reduced proportionally. The physical characteristics of these infants are similar to those of rat pups whose mothers had deficient diets throughout all of gestation.

NUTRITIONAL INFLUENCES ON FETAL GROWTH

It is not possible, for obvious reasons, to examine maternal-fetal relationships directly at the cellular and molecular levels in humans. Consequently, work toward understanding how maternal nutrition influences growth and development in utero must be done on animals. The technique has usually been to manipulate the diets of pregnant animals and study the effects on cellular morphology and physiology in the offspring at various stages of gestation. Over the past few years much information has accumulated from studies of this type.

Experiments in Animals

Energy and nutrient restriction. Two types of dietary restrictions have been imposed on laboratory animals to study the effects of maternal nutrition on fetal growth and development. One restriction is simply not giving the animals enough food so that the diet is low in kilocalories. The other restriction holds kilocalories at an adequate level but reduces or completely eliminates one or more essential nutrients. The effects of deficiencies

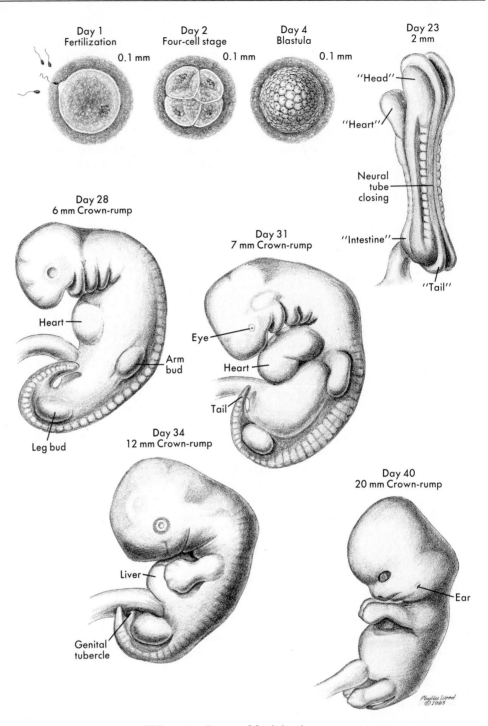

FIG. 4-6 Stages of fetal development.

Day 45
25 mm Crown-rump

Tail

Week 9
44 mm Crown-rump

External
genitalia
(undifferentiated)

Week 12
82 mm Crown-rump

Week 20
185 mm Crown-rump

Week 26
250 mm Crown-rump

Week 38 full term
360 mm Crown-rump

FIG. 4-6, cont'd See opposite page for legend.

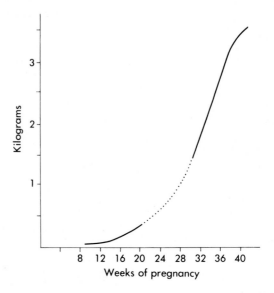

FIG. 4-7   Average curve of fetal growth.

From Hytten FE and Leitch I: The physiology of human pregnancy, ed 2, Oxford, 1971, Blackwell Scientific Publications; reprinted from Thompson AM et al: J Obstet Gynaec Brit Commonw 75:903, 1965.

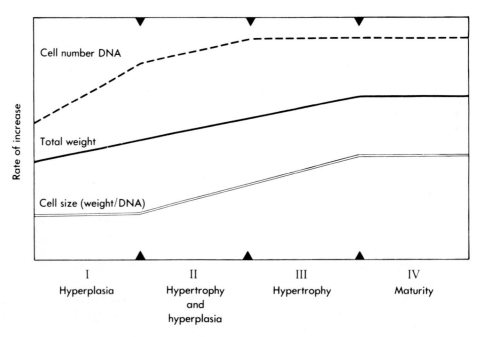

FIG. 4-8   Stages of cell growth.

Modified from Winick M: Nutr Rev 26:195, 1968.

of almost all of the known nutrients have been studied this way, but restrictions of protein and kilocalories have more relevance to humans than restrictions of vitamins or minerals. All animals need energy and use protein in essentially the same way, but the need for vitamins and minerals and their specific functions differ from species to species.

A number of investigators have demonstrated what can happen to fetuses when pregnant animals are fed kilocalorie- or protein-restricted diets. Maternal malnutrition can interfere with the ability of the mother to conceive, it can produce death and resorption or abortion of the fetuses, and it can produce malformations or retarded growth. Of course, the more severe the dietary restrictions are the more serious the effects will be. A reduction of as little as 25% of the total kilocalories without an imbalance in the quality of the maternal diet in rats can reduce both the number of pups born and their ability to survive.

Biochemical studies show why this occurs. One effect of protein-kilocalorie malnutrition is an impairment of cell energy metabolism by interfering with the enzymes involved in glycolysis and the citric acid cycle. Without adequate supplies of amino acids and energy, cell functions break down, and normal processes of growth cannot occur. The effects would be most damaging when cells are normally undergoing rapid division. This implies that the timing of the dietary deficiency, as well as its severity, is important.

Types of growth failure. It is now clear that a number of things can produce growth failure in utero. The cause can be either "intrinsic" or "extrinsic." In differential diagnosis the condition of the placentas of animals born small for gestational age is considered. In intrinsic intrauterine growth failure placentas are usually of normal size. This implies that fetal growth retardation was not caused by inadequate maternal-fetal transport but was the result of other factors. Some examples include chromosomal abnormalities and maternal infections. Extrinsic intrauterine growth failure is usually manifested by placentas that are reduced in size. This indicates that they were incapable of supplying the fetus with adequate nutrition.

The principle feature of intrinsic growth failure is the presence of multiple malformations in the fetuses. These are absent in growth failure produced experimentally by ligation of blood vessels supplying the placenta. They are variable in maternal malnutrition, depending on the timing of the restriction. In both vascular and nutritional failure, placentas are reduced in proportion to fetal weight. In the ligated animals and in late maternal malnutrition, the reduction is caused by a decrease in the average size of the cells. Maternal protein restriction maintained throughout most of the gestation, however, decreases both the number and size of placental cells.

The fetuses themselves also show different patterns of growth retardation. Those subjected to vascular insufficiency show an asymmetric retardation. The fetuses have relatively normal brain sizes and head circumferences, but their livers are greatly reduced, by as much as 50%, and glycogen reserves are completely absent. Proportionally these animals have bigger brains and heads compared to the rest of their bodies. They are extremely hypoglycemic at birth.

When maternal protein restriction is limited to the last few days of gestation, the fetuses show a pattern of growth retardation similar to that produced by vascular insufficiency—proportionally big heads and small bodies. However, when the restriction is imposed throughout most of the gestation period, the pattern of fetal growth retardation becomes more symmetric. There is a 15% to 20% decrease in cell number in all organs including the brain. Head circumference is also reduced. The reduced cell number is greatest in those regions of the brain that are undergoing the most rapid rates of cell division.

Consequences of growth failure. These findings make it obvious that fetuses are *not* perfect parasites that can survive intrauterine insults without adverse effects. Data suggest that inadequate maternal nutrition can affect the fetus in ways that coincide with the stages of cell growth, and that the body reserves of the mother cannot always insulate the fetus from dietary deficiencies. What happens to animals whose mothers were nutritionally deprived during pregnancy depends to a great extent on how they are fed after birth.

Perhaps the finding of most concern is the effect of continued deprivation on the growth of brain cells. If prenatally malnourished pups are restricted after birth by feeding them in litters of 18 pups per dam, they demonstrate a 60% reduction in brain cell number by the time they are weaned. This contrasts with the 20% to 25% reduction associated with prenatal or postnatal malnutrition alone. Thus it seems that continued malnutrition throughout the entire time the brain cells are dividing produces greater deficits than would be expected if the separate effects were simply added together. Experiments have shown that nutritional rehabilitation will not enable these animals to recover their normal size once the period of cell proliferation has passed. They will continue to be small no matter how well fed they are after weaning. Other data suggest that maternal malnutrition may even have intergenerational effect; brain cell numbers were reduced in rats whose mothers were prenatally malnourished, even though these mothers had adequate diets during gestation and after weaning.

These studies would not be so disturbing if size were not related to function. The fact is, however, that alterations in normal biochemical and developmental processes accompany fetal and neonatal malnutrition in several species of animals. Changes in the usual constituents of cells are observed, as well as the delayed appearance of specific enzyme systems. Depending on the timing of the dietary deficiency, degeneration of the cerebral cortex, the medulla, and the spinal cord occurs. Muscular development is also impaired because of a reduced number of muscle cells and fibers.

What has been learned from animal research. Much can still be learned from experiments with animals about the processes of fetal growth and development and the consequences of maternal malnutrition. However the work to date has produced important results, as summarized below:

1. **Growth failure.** Although a number of prenatal influences affect fetal growth, maternal malnutrition can be one cause of growth failure that results in low birth weight.
2. **Nature of tissue effects.** Animals malnourished from restrictions of their mothers' diets throughout most of gestation are characterized by: (1) reduced number and size of cells in the placenta, (2) reduced brain cell number and head size, (3) proportional reductions in the size of other organs, and (4) alterations in normal cell constituents and biochemical processes.
3. **Influencing factors.** The fetal consequences of malnutrition depend on the timing, severity, and duration of the maternal dietary restriction. These consequences may be reversible if the restriction primarily affects growth in cell size. But a reduction in the number of cells may be permanent if the restriction is maintained throughout the entire period of hyperplastic growth.

Human Experience in Fetal Growth

Low birth weight. In view of the risks of early death or permanent disability associated with low birth weight, it is apparent that the animal research on intrauterine failure may have great implications for human problems. Of the annual incidence of low birth weight infants, it is estimated that 10% to 20% is a result of intrauterine growth failure. This means that 80,000 to 120,000 infants who have experienced malnutrition in utero are born each year in the United States. An important thing to understand when interpreting these statistics is that there is no one cause—a number of factors can retard fetal growth.

When the term *fetal malnutrition* is applied to human infants, it simply means that there was a reduction in the maternal supply or placental transport of nutrients so that fetal growth is retarded significantly below genetic potential. It does not necessarily mean that the mother's nutrition was at fault. At present there is no way to judge how many growth-retarded infants are the result of maternal malnutrition.

Relation of animal studies. Although the animal experiments are highly suggestive, caution should be taken in making direct applications to humans. A primary reason for doing animal research is to find out what can possibly happen when certain conditions are imposed. The findings do not guarantee that these things actually happen in the course of human events. There are a number of reasons why the dramatic results of maternal malnutrition demonstrated in animals may not occur as readily in human beings. In effect the consequences of maternal malnutrition on fetal growth and development are all magnified in the animal studies. This is because (1) relative rates of growth and development are much slower in humans compared with laboratory animals, (2) the timing of maximum growth also differs, (3) the number and size of fetuses a mother must nourish in utero compared with her own body size and nutritional reserves are much smaller in humans than in laboratory animals, and (4) the magnitude of dietary deprivation used for experimentation is rarely encountered in human populations under ordinary circumstances.

EFFECTS OF MATERNAL MALNUTRITION

Observations described above provide fertile grounds for speculation, but what is the evidence in human populations that maternal malnutrition causes fetal malnutrition? Of necessity much of the information is incidental. Nonetheless, there have been three kinds of studies that have addressed this question with highly significant results: (1) natural experiments in which birth statistics before, during, and after periods of acute famine are studied and compared; (2) measurements of organ size and cell numbers in stillbirths and neonatal deaths in which all causes not related to maternal malnutrition have been ruled out; and (3) epidemiologic studies of the nutritional correlates of birth weights.

Natural Experiments

The hardships of war afford researchers an opportunity to study the effects of severe dietary restrictions during pregnancy under conditions that fortunately are seldom duplicated. Throughout most of Europe at various times during World War II, food shortages were common. Reports were made on the effects of these shortages during the 1940s, but they are being considered with renewed interest today in light of the findings from animal research. Experiences in Russia and Holland provide examples of these effects:

1. **Russia.** During the seige of Leningrad in 1942 and its immediate aftermath, there was an 18-month period of severe starvation. Comparison of statistics for infants born before, during, and after the seige revealed an expected toll in the course and outcome of pregnancy under such desperate conditions. During the famine period there was a twofold increase in fetal mortality, as well as an increase in the number of infants weighing less than 2500 g (5.4 lb) at birth.

2. **Holland.** Similar findings were reported from Holland. Here the results are more insightful because the famine began suddenly and was limited to about 6 months during the winter of 1944 to 1945. It was not accompanied by other deprivations as severe as those experienced during the seige of Leningrad, and the women of Holland had fairly good diets before the food shortage. During the famine period dietary intake dropped to less than 1000 kcal per day, and protein was limited to 30 to 40 g. Since the famine lasted only 6 months, babies conceived before and during that period were exposed for varying lengths of time, but none was exposed

for the entire course of gestation. On the average, birth weights of infants exposed to the famine were reduced by 200 g (7 oz). Weights were lowest for babies exposed to the famine during the entire last half of pregnancy. Added exposure before that time did not reduce birth weights further. In fact, babies exposed to the famine during the first 27 weeks of gestation, but finishing their terms after the famine ended, had higher average birth weights than those who were only exposed during the last 3 weeks of gestation. The data for stillbirths and congenital malformations followed a different pattern. The rates were lowest for infants conceived before the famine and highest for those conceived during it.

The findings are in line with what is anticipated from knowledge of the stages of human growth. Poor nutrition in the latter part of pregnancy affects fetal growth, whereas poor nutrition in the early months affects development of the embryo and its capacity to survive.

3. **Great Britain.** It is interesting to note that, in contrast with the experiences in Russia and Holland, the prenatal mortality rate in Great Britain, which had been fairly constant before the war, actually declined between 1940 and 1945 despite the poor environmental conditions and no discernible improvements in prenatal care. One possible explanation is that pregnant and lactating women were given priority status for food in Britain as a matter of national policy.

Organ Studies

Studies that attempt to relate the size of organs in human infants to maternal nutrition must control for other conditions known to affect fetal growth. One group of researchers looked at the organs of 252 American stillborn infants and infants who died in the first 48 hours of life, excluding all multiple births, maternal complications, and congenital defects. The infants were grouped as coming from poor or nonpoor families according to income. Comparisons of organs between the two groups showed that the mass of adipose tissue and the size of individual fat cells were smaller in the poor infants. These infants also had smaller livers, adrenal glands, thymuses, and spleens. Heart, kidney, and skeleton were also reduced, but the differences were not as great. The ranking in organ size is consistent with reductions noted in animals who have been prenatally malnourished and in humans who have experienced uterine or placental disorders. Since the last two conditions were ruled out of the study, the investigators concluded that undernutrition could be responsible for prenatal growth retardation in infants from low income families.

The organs in infants who survive intrauterine malnutrition cannot be studied to see if cells are reduced in number or size, but one organ is available. This is the placenta. One scientist reported that the size of placentas and the number of placental cells are 15% and 20% below normal when infants experience growth failure.[10] By comparing placentas from different sources, he has shown that those from indigent populations in developing countries have reductions in cell numbers similar to the reductions noted in placentas from American infants with intrauterine growth failure. In one interesting case in the United States, a mother who was severely undernourished from anorexia nervosa during pregnancy gave birth to an infant weighing less than 2500 g (5.4 lb). When the placenta was examined, it was found to have only 50% of the normal number of cells.

Nutritional Correlates of Birth Weight

Studies of the relationship between maternal nutrition and the birth weight of the infant have tended to focus directly on the nutrient composition of the diet during pregnancy. Because of variations in the nutritional requirements of individuals, these studies have produced conflicting results. However, there are two indicators of long term and immediate nutritional status that have shown consistent associations with birth weight.

These are (1) *maternal body size,* height and prepregnancy weight of the mother; and (2) *maternal weight gain,* the amount of weight gained by the mother during the pregnancy itself.

Maternal body size. It should not be surprising that big mothers have big babies. What is less often appreciated is that the size of the infant at birth largely depends on the size of the mother and is not influenced to a great degree by the size of the father. This was shown years ago in a classic experiment in which Shire stallions were bred with Shetland mares and Shetland stallions with Shire mares. The newborn foals were always an appropriate size to the mothers' breeds. No intermediate sizes were ever produced. The same effects have been demonstrated in a number of animals, and there is indirect evidence for the same phenomenon in humans.

It has been further demonstrated in humans that height and prepregnancy weight of the mother have independent and additive effects on the birth weight of a child. In an analysis of 4095 mothers in Aberdeen, Scotland,[11] it was found that, on average, the tallest and heaviest mothers had babies who weighed 500 g (1 lb) more at birth than babies of the shortest and lightest mothers. It is postulated that maternal size is a conditioning factor on the ultimate size of the placenta and thus controls the blood supply of nutrients available to the fetus.

This idea has support in findings from the Collaborative Perinatal Project of the National Institutes of Health. In this project, Naeye[12] analyzed data from nearly 60,000 pregnancies to discover causes of fetal and **neonatal mortality** among different racial groups. He found that Puerto Ricans experience a higher rate of placental growth retardation than whites. However, this difference disappears when women with prepregnancy weights of 45 kg (101 lb) or less are excluded from the analysis. Naeye concludes that the high rate of placental growth retardation in Puerto Ricans is a result of the greater proportion of women who enter pregnancy with low body weights. Further data from Naeye's study show that, regardless of race or ethnic origin, mothers with low prepregnancy weights have much lighter placentas than heavier mothers.

Maternal underweight. Infants of underweight women show several kinds of morbidity. Edwards and colleagues[13] compared outcomes for women who entered pregnancy at 10% or more below standard weight for height with outcomes for women who entered pregnancy at normal weight (Table 4-5). The women were matched for age, race, parity, and socioeconomic status. The incidence of both low birth weight and prematurity were significantly higher among the underweight mothers. Infants of underweight women also scored lower on the **Apgar scale.** This scale measures the general condition of the neonate as evidenced by heart rate, respiration, muscle tone, reflex irritability, and color at delivery. Differences in Apgar scores were even greater when only those infants of women who were excessive cigarette smokers were compared. Underweight women who smoked more

Neonatal mortality
Number of newborn deaths during the neonatal period (birth to 1 month postpartum) per 1000 live births.

Apgar score
Number defining an infant's condition at 1 minute after birth by scoring the heart rate, respiratory effort, muscle tone, reflex irritability, and color; named for its developer, American anesthesiologist Virginia Apgar (1909-1974).

TABLE 4-5 *Infant Morbidity in Underweight Women and Normal Weight Controls*

Infant Morbidity	Low Prepregnancy Weight (% of births)	Normal Weight Controls (% of births)
Low birth weight	15.3	7.6
Prematurity	23.0	14.0
Low Apgar score	19.0	12.0

From Edwards LE et al: Pregnancy in the underweight woman: Course, outcome and growth patterns of the infant, Am J Obstet Gynecol 135:297, 1979.

than one pack of cigarettes a day during pregnancy had three times the number of infants with low Apgar scores compared with their normal weight controls.

Underweight women were also subject to different rates of pregnancy complications.[13] Anemia occurred more frequently in the underweight group, and those who were both underweight and anemic had an incidence of low birth weight of 17.4%, compared to 3.6% among women who were anemic but of normal weight. The investigators point out that both underweight status and iron deficiency anemia reflect long term suboptimum nutritional intake. They suggest this as a possible explanation for the apparent influence of anemic underweight mothers on the incidence of low birth weight.

Maternal Weight Gain

The weight gained in a normal pregnancy is the result of physiologic processes designed to foster fetal and maternal growth. Much of the weight gain can be accounted for by the products of gestation.

Primigravida
(L *prima*, first; *gravida*, pregnant) A woman pregnant for the first time.

The total number of pounds gained in pregnancy will vary among individual women. Young mothers and **primigravidae** usually gain more than older mothers and multigravidae. A normal gain for most healthy women is about 11 to 15 kg (25 to 35 lb), but current guidelines from the National Academy of Sciences specify appropriate ranges for weight gain related to maternal prepregnancy weight-for-height, height, age, and race (Table 4-6). A chart incorporating these recommendations for underweight, normal weight, and overweight women is provided in Fig. 4-9.

The normal pattern of weight gain is illustrated in Fig. 4-10. Less than half the total weight gain resides in the fetus, placenta, and amniotic fluid. The remainder is found in maternal reproductive tissues, fluid, blood, and "stores." The weight component labeled "maternal stores" is largely composed of body fat, although some increase in the lean body mass, other than reproductive tissue, may also occur. The action of progesterone in the pregnant woman dictates that a fat pad be produced to serve as a caloric reserve for both pregnancy and lactation. Fatfold measurements from 10 to 30 weeks' gestation have shown gradual increases in subcutaneous fat at the abdomen, back, and upper thigh. The pregnant woman who attempts to restrict weight gain to avoid development of the fat pad will simultaneously affect to some degree normal development of the other products of pregnancy (Fig. 4-10).

TABLE 4-6   *Recommended Total Weight Gain Ranges for Pregnant Women,* by Prepregnancy Body Mass Index (weight/height²)†*

Weight-for-Height Category	Recommended Total Gain	
	kg	lb
Low (BMI <19.8)	12.5-18	28-40
Normal (BMI of 19.8-26.0)	11.5-16	25-35
High‡ (BMI >26.0 to 29.0)	7-11.5	15-25

*Young adolescents and black women should strive for gains at the upper end of the recommended range. Short women (<157 cm or 62 inches) should strive for gains at the lower end of the range.
†Body mass index (BMI) is calculated using metric units.
‡The recommended target weight gain for obese women (BMI >29.0) is at least 7.0 kg (15 lb).
From Institute of Medicine: Nutrition during pregnancy: weight gain and nutrient supplements, Washington, DC, 1990, National Academy Press.

FIG. 4-9 A "modern" weight gain chart for pregnant women. Adapted from the National Academy of Science's Nutrition during Pregnancy, 1990.

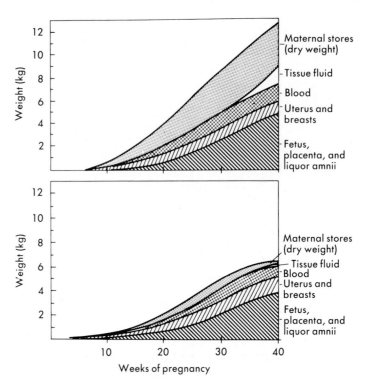

FIG. 4-10   Estimated composition of weight gain during pregnancy for a normal, healthy, Northern European woman *(top)* and a poor, underfed woman from India *(bottom)*.

Modified from Hurley LS: Developmental nutrition, Englewood Cliffs, NJ, 1980, Prentice-Hall, Inc.

A sudden weight gain that greatly exceeds this rate is likely to be caused by excess fluid retention. As stated repeatedly in this chapter, mild generalized edema and some accumulation of fluid in the lower limbs is not unphysiologic. Women with edema can gain as much as 9 L of fluid and still have clinically normal pregnancies. However, it should be emphasized that this accumulation is gradual. A large shift in water balance reflected by a sudden increase in weight is usually an indication of preeclampsia, particularly if it occurs after the twentieth week.

The more liberal attitude about weight gain during pregnancy that prevails today should not detract from the logic of avoidance of excessive weight gain. While large weight gain may have little or no adverse impact on the developing fetus, it may be detrimental to the mother during pregnancy and afterward.[14] Women who gain excessively large amounts of weight during pregnancy are at greater risk for the development of hypertension and are more likely to require cesarean delivery. Evidence also suggests, not surprisingly, that excessive weight gain during pregnancy may increase risk of long-term problems in controlling weight gain later in life.

Supplementation/Intervention Trials

It is now well recognized that the provision of extra food, with or without education, will improve pregnancy outcome in groups of high-risk, low-income pregnant women. The value of supplemental food varies from woman to woman but obviously the severity of the original deficit is predictive of the value of the added food resources. A series of supplementation studies in developing countries have proved the positive impact on birthweight that such interventions can have. Even in developed countries, however, the benefits of nutrition intervention programs for high-risk women have been demonstrated.

The experiences at the Montreal Diet Dispensary in Canada show that the benefits of extra kilocalories and special dietary management during pregnancy are not confined to chronically malnourished women in developing countries.[15,16] They can also improve the pregnancy performance of high-risk mothers in more affluent nations. Knowing the risk of reproductive problems associated with low income, Higgins and colleagues selected the hospital handling the highest percentage of poor patients in Montreal. All patients from two of the hospital's public maternity clinics were enrolled for a total of 1544 women between 1963 and 1970. A unique feature was that dietary needs for kilocalories and protein were individually calculated for each woman based on her body weight for height with adjustments for protein deficiency, underweight, and other stress conditions. Women whose family incomes fell below specified levels (70% of all women in the study) were given supplies of milk, eggs, and oranges every 2 weeks. All of the women received counseling on food selection to meet their individual needs every time they visited the clinic, and nutritionists visited them at home at least once during their pregnancies.

Such intensive nutritional care enabled the women to average 93% of their total kilocalorie needs and 96% of their total protein requirements throughout gestation. Since the majority started out with large average daily deficits, they all showed significant improvements in the quality of their diets. Birth statistics indicate how the mothers and their infants benefited from these measures. The incidence of low birth weight in this high-risk study group decreased to the point that it equaled the all-Canada rate and was lower than the rate for Quebec province. Stillbirths, neonatal mortality, and **perinatal mortality** were also lower than the rates prevailing in Canada and Quebec.

Perinatal mortality
(Gr *peri*, around; L *natus*, born) Infant deaths in the perinatal period (before and after birth, from approximately week 20-28 of gestation to 1-4 weeks postpartum) per 1000 live births.

It is impossible to know how much of the improvements in pregnancy performance and outcome demonstrated in this study can be attributed to the diets of the women, the food supplements, or the special attention they received. What is important about the study is that it shows how high-risk mothers, against all odds, can experience successful pregnancies when superior nutritional guidance is a part of their prenatal care.

Other clinicians have made aggressive efforts to improve pregnancy outcome through nutrition intervention for underweight pregnant women and women demonstrating poor weight gain during pregnancy. Between 1984 and 1988, approximately 2000 women receiving prenatal services in Virginia Health Department clinics were provided individualized nutrition interventions based on techniques developed at the Montreal Diet Dispensary. Those responding to the food intake and weight gain guidelines showed a marked reduction in low-birth-weight deliveries (Fig. 4-11).[17]

Similarly, in a large urban clinic, a group of 52 underweight pregnant women who received no counseling were compared with a similar group of 57 underweight and failure-to-gain pregnant women who received extensive nutrition counseling during the course of pregnancy. Women in the counseled group gained significantly more weight during their pregnancies than did the controls. They also delivered babies that averaged 300 g heavier than those born to women in the control group, a difference not related to ethnic background, income status, age, or smoking habit. The percentage of women having low-birth-weight babies was 8% in the counseled group compared with 17% among controls.[18]

Orstead and colleagues took the process one step further by estimating the cost effectiveness of individualized nutrition counseling for a group of high-risk women in Chicago. The nutrition services for the counseled group cost about $44,500 more than the usual program, but the cost of caring for the extra low-birth-weight babies in the control group was approximately $230,700. The benefit-to-cost ratio was therefore close to five to one.[19]

FIG. 4-11 Low birth weight rates of underweight pregnant women enrolled in the Virginia Nutrition Intervention Project, 1984 to 1988, who were ≤90% of expected weight at the initial visit and either >90% *(open bars)* or ≤90% *(solid bars)* of expected weight at the last visit.

From Clements DF: The Nutrition Intervention Project for underweight women, Clin Nutr 7:205, 1988. Reprinted with permission from Churchill Livingston Medical Journals.

Finally, numerous efforts have been made over the years to evaluate the massive Special Supplement Food Program for Women, Infants, and Children (WIC). In 1986, the U.S. Department of Agriculture published a five volume report based on a nationally representative low-income population.[20] The researchers concluded after 5 years of study that WIC had a significant beneficial effect on the duration of pregnancy, birthweight, head growth, fetal mortality, and neonatal mortality. The program's effects were most clearly seen in high-risk pregnant women.

Not all nutrition intervention programs provided to high-risk pregnant women have demonstrated the degree of positive impact that was shown in the studies cited above. This varied response should certainly be expected, given the different populations served, the different supplements employed, the various methods of supplement administration, and a variety of other differing variables. Overall, however, the findings appear to suggest that *the poorer the nutritional condition of the mother entering pregnancy, the more valuable the prenatal diet and nutritional supplement will be in improving her pregnancy course and outcome.*

NUTRIENT FUNCTIONS AND NEEDS

The nutrients enter into all of the major metabolic processes involving the production of energy, synthesis of cells, maintenance of their structure and function, and the regulation of body processes. First we examine the basis for the Recommended Dietary Allowances

(RDA) nutrient and energy standards for pregnancy. Then, in considering each of these nutrient functions, emphasis is given to those nutrients that have major roles in pregnancy and why their requirements during pregnancy increase.

Recommended Dietary Allowances

The Food and Nutrition Board of the National Research Council is well aware of the problems of determining nutrient requirements during pregnancy and considers them when setting dietary allowances and making recommendations about the need for supplementation. Recommended Dietary Allowances are based on the best available evidence from metabolic balance studies and from indirect estimates.[21]

The current 1989 edition of the RDA standards for pregnant and nonpregnant adult women is presented in Table 4-7. The figures in the table indicate the needs of a "reference" woman who is 25 to 50 years of age, 160 cm (64 in) tall, and weighs 63 kg (138 lb) when she conceives. Women may need more or less of the amounts listed for kilocalories and protein depending on body size, activity, and health status. The allowances for vitamins and minerals provide sufficient room for individual variation, an important consideration, so that they can be applied to all healthy women. They may not be adequate for women who enter pregnancy in poor nutritional status or who suffer from chronic disease or other complicating conditions. They may not be appropriate for the young pregnant adolescent or the woman who is very overweight.

TABLE 4-7 *Recommended Dietary Allowances for Women of Reproductive Age (1989)*

	Age				
Nutrient	11-14	15-18	19-24	25-50	Pregnancy
Energy (kcal)	2200	2200	2200	2200	+300*
Protein (g)	46	48	46	50	60
Vitamin A (µg RE)	800	800	800	800	800
Vitamin D (µg)	10	10	10	5	10
Vitamin E (mg α-TE)	8	8	8	8	10
Vitamin C (mg)	50	60	60	60	70
Folate acid (µg)	150	180	180	180	400
Niacin (mg NE)	15	15	15	15	17
Riboflavin (mg)	1.3	1.3	1.3	1.3	1.6
Thiamin (mg)	1.1	1.1	1.1	1.1	1.5
Vitamin B_6 (mg)	1.4	1.5	1.6	1.6	2.2
Vitamin B_{12} (µg)	2.0	2.0	2.0	2.0	2.2
Calcium (mg)	1200	1200	1200	800	1200
Phosphorus (mg)	1200	1200	1200	800	1200
Iodine (µg)	150	150	150	150	175
Iron (mg)	15	15	15	15	30
Magnesium (mg)	280	300	280	280	320
Zinc (mg)	12	12	12	12	15
Selenium (µg)	45	50	55	55	65

*Second and third trimesters.

From Food and Nutrition Board, National Council, National Academy of Sciences: Recommended Dietary Allowances, ed 10, Washington, DC, 1989, National Academy Press.

Energy

Pregnancy requirements. During pregnancy, two factors determine energy requirements: (1) changes in the mother's usual physical activity, and (2) increase in her basal metabolism to support the work required for growth of the fetus and the accessory tissues. The cumulative energy cost of pregnancy has been estimated at 40,000 to 70,000 kilocalories.[22,23] This amount is derived from the kilocalorie equivalents of protein and fat stored in the products of conception and from increased oxygen consumption of the mother. The total 40,000 to 70,000 kilocalories break down to an addition of only 200 to 300 extra kilocalories during the second and third trimesters of pregnancy to the daily allowance of the nonpregnant reference woman. A portion of the energy increment may be offset by the tendency of pregnant women to reduce their physical activity in the last trimester.

Protein

Pregnancy requirements. Requirements for protein during pregnancy are based on the needs of the nonpregnant reference woman plus the extra amounts needed for growth. The easiest way to determine how much extra protein is needed daily to support the synthesis of new tissue is to divide the amounts contained in the products of conception and maternal body by the average length of gestation. About 925 g of protein are deposited in a normal weight fetus and in the maternal accessory tissues.[22] When this is divided by the 280 days of pregnancy, the average is 3.3 g of protein that must be added to normal daily requirements. The rate at which new tissue is synthesized, however, is not constant throughout gestation. Maternal and fetal growth does not accelerate until the second month, and the rate progressively increases until just before term. The need for protein follows this growth rate. Only about an extra 0.6 g of protein is used each day for new tissue synthesis in the first month of pregnancy, but by 30 weeks gestation protein is being used at the rate of 6.1 g per day. If this is added to the normal maintenance needs of the reference woman, 18.6 to 24 g of protein per day are required.

Protein utilization. These calculations of protein need would equal dietary allowances if 100% of the protein eaten could be used in the body. Actually, however, the efficiency of protein utilization depends on its digestibility and amino acid composition. Proteins that do not contain all of the essential amino acids in amounts proportional to human requirements are utilized less efficiently. Even a high quality protein, such as that in eggs, is utilized much less than 100%. Protein utilization from a mixed diet is about 70% and from a totally vegetarian diet it is even less efficient. Protein utilization also depends on kilocalorie intake. It has been shown that an extra 100 kcal during pregnancy will have the same effect on nitrogen retention as an additional 0.28 g of nitrogen itself. This means that kilocalories from nonprotein sources, that is, carbohydrates and fats, have a protein-sparing effect. If these kilocalories are inadequate, protein requirements would increase. Finally, the trials that measure nitrogen loss are conducted on a limited number of subjects. There is a great deal of variation from the averages obtained. Since a dietary allowance must cover the needs of all healthy women, room for individual differences must be built in.

RDA standard. Because of these considerations, RDAs for protein are set much higher than calculated requirements of 18.6 to 24 g per day.[21] The National Research Council allows 50 g of protein a day for the nonpregnant reference woman with an extra 10 g per day starting in the second month of pregnancy. If individual allowances are calculated on the basis of body weight, daily need would be about 1.3 g/kg of pregnant body weight or about 0.6 g/lb. The RDA standard is based on a mixed diet in which at least one third of the protein comes from high-quality animal foods. Thus vegetarian diets that exclude all animal products can only be made adequate when more total protein is consumed, or when foods are selected so that those low in a particular amino acid are complemented by foods in which that amino acid is high.

Protein deficiency. Adverse consequences of protein deficiency during pregnancy are difficult to separate from the effects of kilocalorie deficiency in real life situations. Almost all cases of limited protein intake are accompanied by limitation in availability of kilocalories. Under such circumstances decreased birth weight has been reported. As indicated in a Guatemalan study,[24] provision of supplemental kilocalories alone to pregnant women with deficient levels of protein intake was just as effective as provision of both protein and kilocalories in influencing birth weight of babies.

Protein excess. Adverse effects of excessive protein during pregnancy are poorly understood at the present time. The New York supplementation study[25] has provoked much discussion of this issue, since use of the high protein supplement was associated with an increased number of very prematurely born infants and excessive neonatal deaths. In light of these findings other data have been reviewed. Analysis of a number of past supplementation studies in human populations[26] has suggested that providing a supplement with more than 20% of the kilocalories from protein is associated with retarded fetal growth, whereas supplements providing less than 20% of the kilocalories from protein yield increments in birth weight of offspring. Although these data suggest that too much protein, presented in an unbalanced nutritional package, may have negative effects on pregnancy course and outcome, data are limited and the debate continues about the relevance of the observations.

Micronutrients: General

It is well recognized that food is the optimal vehicle for delivering nutrients. It therefore follows that nutrient supplementation is an intervention that requires justification. This viewpoint was stated in no uncertain terms by the expert committee appointed by the National Academy of Sciences.[7] In essence, there is limited evidence that multivitamin-mineral supplementation significantly improves fertility or pregnancy outcome in most women. There are situations, however, that justify individualized supplement prescription (Table 4-8). These circumstances are defined throughout this section of the chapter.

Folate

The B-complex vitamin folate is required for cell division to proceed. If this vitamin is lacking, detrimental effects are especially great in body tissues that have high turnover rates. One of the first signs of folate deficiency is megaloblastic anemia, caused by the production of abnormal red blood cells. These cells are arrested in their development, so bone marrow contains a large number of immature megaloblasts and hemoglobin levels are reduced. Hemoglobin levels below 11 g/dl during the first and third trimesters or below 10.5 g/dl during the second trimester are criteria for diagnosis of anemia (Table 4-9). Anemia is associated with increased risk of adverse pregnancy course and outcome.

The treatment of anemia with appropriate dietary changes and nutrient supplement is not an issue subject to much debate. There is, however, controversy about the need for folate supplementation by pregnant women who are not anemic. Much of this controversy stems from our limited knowledge base about the impact of folate deficiency on pregnancy outcome. Maternal folate deficiency in experimental animals is associated with increased incidence of problems related to pregnancy and increased delivery of abnormal offspring.[27] Fetal malformations have been reported in offspring of women using drugs that are folate antagonists.[28] Some evidence in humans suggests that deficiency of this vitamin may be associated with abruptio placentae, spontaneous abortion, preeclampsia, fetal malformations, and subnormal infant development. Such reports, however, are not direct proof of association.

TABLE 4-8   Current Supplementation Recommendations: National Academy of Sciences (1990)

Nutrient	Candidates for Supplementation	Level of Nutrient Supplementation
Iron	All pregnant women (2nd and 3rd trimesters)	30 mg ferrous iron daily
Folic acid	Pregnant women with suspected dietary inadequacy of folate	300 µg/day
Vitamin D	Complete vegetarians and others with low intake of vitamin D-fortified milk	10 µg/day
Calcium	Women under age 25 whose daily dietary calcium intake is less than 600 mg	600 mg/day
Vitamin B_{12}	Complete vegetarians	2 µg/day
Zinc/copper	Women under treatment with iron for iron deficiency anemia	15 mg Zn/day 2 mg Cu/day
Multivitamin-mineral supplements	Pregnant women with poor diets and for those who are considered high risk: multiple gestation, heavy smokers, alcohol/drug abusers, other	Preparation containing: iron—30 mg zinc—15 mg copper—2 mg calcium—250 mg vitamin B_6—2 mg folate—300 µg vitamin C—50 mg vitamin D—5 µg

From Institute of Medicine: Nutrition during pregnancy: weight gain and nutrient supplements, Washington, DC, 1990, National Academy Press.

TABLE 4-9   Current Definition of Anemia

Trimester	Hemoglobin (g/dl)
First	<11.0
Second	<10.5
Third	<11.0

Data from National Academy of Sciences: Nutrition during pregnancy: weight gain and nutrient supplements. Washington, DC, 1990, National Academy Press.

The biggest controversy relates to the role of folate deficiency in the etiology of neural tube defects. The work of Smithells[29-32] and Laurence[33] in northern Europe suggests that multivitamin or folate supplementation of women with previous neural tube defect offspring is associated with significant reduction in second occurrence of the problem. Since methodologic details of these projects have been heavily criticized, the merit of these reports has been questioned. A carefully controlled trial is currently underway in northern Europe to examine the possible preventive value of periconceptional vitamin supplementation.[34] If this trial is completed successfully, it will be possible to develop scientifically based recommendations about vitamin supplementation before and during pregnancy.

In the meantime, several research groups have attempted to address the question indirectly. Three surveys have been conducted in the United States to assess periconceptional vitamin supplementation practices of women delivering and having a diagnosed offspring with neural tube defects and selected "control" women.[35-37] The results have been mixed. In two of the three studies, use of vitamin supplements around the time of conception was associated with a reduced risk of neural tube defect in the offspring. In the third study with a similar protocol, the periconceptional vitamin use was not different between mothers of neural tube defect babies and mothers of other infants. It is obvious that the last word is not yet in. For the time being, the expert panel from the National Academy of Sciences states: "Pending further research, the subcommittee considers it prudent to supplement the diet with low amounts of folate (300 μg per day) if there is any question of the adequacy of intake of this vitamin."[7]

Vitamin B_{12}

Vitamin B_{12}, or cobalamine, like folate, is also an important contributor to the process of cell division. Deficiency of this vitamin can therefore lead to the development of megaloblastic anemia with consequences described above. Fortunately, deficiency of vitamin B_{12} is rare; high-risk women include those who choose a strict vegetarian diet. Such women need vitamin B_{12} supplements of 2 μg per day.[7]

Vitamin B_6

Vitamin B_6, or pyridoxine, is concerned with amino acid metabolism and protein synthesis. In its active form of pyridoxal phosphate the vitamin is a cofactor in reactions involving a group of enzymes known as transaminases. Vitamin B_6 requirements increase in pregnancy not only because of the greater need for nonessential amino acids in growth but also because the body is making more niacin from tryptophan.

Fetal needs. Urinary excretion of vitamin B_6 metabolites during pregnancy is 10 to 15 times higher than in nonpregnant women, but blood values are typically reduced. Investigators are not sure of the clinical significance of this. There is evidence that the placenta concentrates vitamin B_6 and that levels in cord blood are much higher than in the maternal circulation. This could mean that the reduced maternal blood levels are simply the result of physiologic adjustments. On the other hand, there is also evidence that the fetus takes up more vitamin B_6 and that maternal levels increase when oral supplements are used.[38] Limited animal data suggest adverse pregnancy outcome in the presence of vitamin B_6 deficiency.[39] In addition, European researchers[40] observed that the depth of pregnancy depression correlated negatively with serum vitamin B_6 concentration. Roepke and Kirksey[41] and Schuster's group[42] observed significantly lower Apgar scores in newborns of mothers with evidence of vitamin B_6 deficiency when compared with offspring of controls. The meaning of these observations remains to be determined.

Maternal nausea and vomiting. While the precise etiology of nausea and vomiting during pregnancy remains unknown, interest continues in the possibility that vitamin B_6 status may be important. Vitamin B_6 is known to catalyze a number of reactions involving neurotransmitter production and in that capacity could conceivably affect an assortment of physiologic states. However, a clear connection between vitamin B_6 and pregnancy nausea remains to be observed.[43,44] In one small study[45] relief of symptoms of pregnancy sickness appeared to be superior in women using Bendectin (an anti-nausea drug now off the market) with added vitamin B_6, as compared with women using Bendectin alone. Additional controlled double-blind studies are required to draw any firm conclusions about the value of vitamin B_6 supplements in the management of nausea during pregnancy.

Vitamin C

Vitamin C deficiency has not been shown to affect the course or outcome of pregnancy in humans. But questions have arisen about the possible association of vitamin C with several specific conditions made known through isolated clinical observations. For example, low plasma levels of vitamin C have been reported in association with premature rupture of the membranes[46] and preeclampsia.[47] An extra 10 mg of vitamin C a day is recommended for the pregnant woman. This total recommendation of 70 mg a day is easily met by the U.S. diet. Large intakes of vitamin C supplements may adversely influence fetal metabolism. Metabolic dependency on high doses may develop in the fetus, causing possible scurvy in the neonatal period.[48,49]

Thiamin, Riboflavin, and Niacin

Since thiamin, riboflavin, and niacin are all part of the reactions that produce energy in the body, requirements are related to caloric intake. Since kilocalorie allowances increase during pregnancy, the allowances for thiamin, riboflavin, and niacin automatically increase also. In addition, evidence from urinary excretion studies indicates that pregnant women have higher requirements for thiamin and riboflavin than nonpregnant women. The RDA for these two nutrients therefore include additional adjustments.

In animals, severe deficiencies of thiamin, riboflavin, or niacin during pregnancy have resulted in fetal death, reduced growth, and congenital malformation. The skeleton and organs that arise from the ectoderm appear to be especially susceptible to riboflavin deficiency. Lack of riboflavin in the mother's diet was once thought to be a cause of prematurity in humans, but recent studies have failed to find a correlation.

Researchers have evaluated the thiamin status of pregnant women at various stages of gestation and have found that 25% to 30% have values that would be considered deficient by nonpregnant standards. Although there have been some reported cases of congenital beriberi from maternal thiamin deficiency, there is no evidence of impairment at the levels consumed by women in developed countries. The niacin status of pregnant women has been inadequately investigated. However, there are no cases indicating that niacin deficiency in humans produces the malformations noted in experimental animals.

Vitamin D

Vitamin D has long been appreciated for its positive effects on calcium balance during pregnancy. Evidence suggests that vitamin D may be involved in neonatal calcium homeostasis. Observations in Great Britain indicate that the peak season for neonatal hypocalcemia coincides with the time of least sunlight.[50] In addition, serum vitamin D levels are often low in such infants, suggesting that some cases of neonatal hypocalcemia and enamel hypoplasia may relate to maternal vitamin D deficiency and subsequent limitation in placental transport of vitamin D to the fetus.[51,52] A study of pregnant Asian women showed that vitamin D supplementation during the third trimester was associated with an improved rate of maternal weight gain, higher maternal and newborn serum 25 (OH)D levels at term, a reduced incidence of symptomatic hypocalcemia in newborns, and a lower percentage of small-for-gestational-age infants.[53] However excessive amounts of vitamin D may be harmful during gestation. Severe infantile hypercalcemia and associated problems have been reported in newborn animals and in human infants.

Vitamin A

Both vitamin A and carotene cross the placenta, and fetal storage of vitamin A accounts in part for the recommendation that pregnant women consume an extra 1000 IU of this vitamin daily. An intake of this level can readily be provided by dietary sources, and there appears to be no need for routine supplementation. Although vitamin A deficiency is teratogenic in lower animals, confirmatory evidence in humans is lacking. Excessive use and the toxic effects have posed problems.

Megadose toxicity. Excessive vitamin A consumption is believed to be teratogenic in humans, but most scientific evidence describes developmental anomalies in animals. However, one report has described a human infant with congenital renal anomalies associated with maternal ingestion of large doses of vitamin A, about 10 times the RDA, during pregnancy.[54] Another report[55] from Scandinavia indicated that a **microcephalic** child with multiple malformations of the central nervous system was born to a mother who consumed 150,000 IU of vitamin A daily during gestation days 19 to 40.

Vitamin A analog. The adverse effects of excessive vitamin A intake in early pregnancy have been dramatically illustrated by the recent introduction of isotretinoin (Accutane) into the marketplace.[56-58] This drug, used for the treatment of cystic acne, is an analog of vitamin A (see p. 78). Since its first appearance on pharmacy shelves in the early 1980s, cases of birth defects and spontaneous abortion have been associated with its use. This toxicity syndrome has been called the *isotretinoin teratogen syndrome* and was described by Benke.[56] Major features include prominent **frontal bossing, hydrocephalus, microphthalmia,** and small, malformed, low-set, undifferentiated ears (Fig. 4-12). More cautionary labeling has now been provided with the product and physicians are warned about the possible dangers of prenatal exposure.[58]

Vitamin E

Requirements for vitamin E are believed to increase somewhat during pregnancy, but deficiency in humans rarely occurs and has not been linked with either reproductive causality or reduced fertility. Since vitamin E deficiency in experimental animals has long been associated with spontaneous abortion, interest in the use of vitamin E for prevention of abortion has been a popular idea. In general, however, studies in humans have not supported this preventive measure. Several studies have shown, however, that the fetal vitamin E level is one third to one fourth the maternal concentration in both premature and term infants. Maternal levels of vitamin E rise during pregnancy such that by the third trimester these levels become 60% greater than in the nonpregnant controls. It has been found, however, that the maternal level must be from 150% to 500% of the value of the nonpregnant controls if the cord blood values are to reach the low normal adult vitamin E concentrations.

Microcephaly
(Gr *mikros,* small; *kephale,* head) Small size of the head in relation to the rest of the body.

Frontal bossing
(ME *boce,* lump, growth) A rounded protuberance of the forehead. In general, a boss is a knob-like rounded protuberance on the body or some body organ.

Hydrocephalus
(Gr *hydro,* water; *kephale,* head) Condition characterized by enlargement of the cranium caused by abnormal accumulation of fluid.

Microphthalmia
(Gr *mikros,* small; *ophthalmos,* eye) Abnormal smallness of one or both eyes.

FIG. 4-12   Front and lateral view of a child affected prenatally by isotretinoin.
From Benke PJ: JAMA 251:3267, 1984.

Although the vitamin E level in the infant at birth is significantly less than in the mother, the infant's level has been shown to correlate directly with the maternal concentration.[59] Attempts to raise the fetal level by supplementing the mother with vitamin E during the last trimester confirmed the direct correlation of fetal and maternal vitamin E concentrations. It has been concluded, however, that parenteral vitamin E administration to the mother before delivery is not enough to prevent an infant from having the hemolytic anemia of vitamin E deficiency. Since this problem develops within 6 weeks after birth, it can best be prevented by oral supplementation of the infant during the postnatal interval.

Vitamin K

Data are insufficient for the RDA committee of experts to establish a standard for vitamin K during pregnancy. Additional increments to usual intakes are not recommended because consumption of this vitamin by adult women exceeds the RDA. Efforts to determine if vitamin K supplementation of pregnant women can improve the vitamin K status of their preterm offspring have yielded conflicting results.[60,61]

Other Vitamins

Little is known about the dietary requirements for biotin and pantothenic acid. Safe and adequate dietary intakes for these vitamins were suggested in the 1989 edition of the RDA (Table 4-10).

Iron

During pregnancy, iron is needed for the manufacture of hemoglobin in both maternal and fetal red blood cells. The fetus accumulates most of its iron during the last trimester. At term a normal weight infant has about 246 mg of iron in blood and body stores. An additional 134 mg are stored in the placenta. About 290 mg are used to expand the volume of the mother's blood.

Erythropoiesis
(Gr *erythros*, red; *poiesis*, making) Production of erythrocytes, red blood cells.

Maintenance of **erythropoiesis** is one of the few instances during pregnancy when the fetus acts as a true parasite. It assures its own production of hemoglobin by drawing iron from the mother. Maternal iron deficiency, therefore, does not usually result in an infant who is anemic at birth. The most common cause of iron deficiency anemia in the infant is prematurity. The infant who has a short gestation simply does not have time to accumulate sufficient iron during the last trimester.[62]

TABLE 4-10   *Estimated Safe and Adequate Daily Dietary Intakes of Additional Selected Vitamins and Minerals for Adolescents and Adults*

| | Age Group | |
	Adolescents	Adults
Age	11+	
Vitamins		
Biotin (μg)	30-100	30-100
Pantothenic acid (mg)	4-7	4-7
Trace elements (mg)		
Copper	1.5-2.5	1.5-3.0
Manganese	2.0-5.0	2.0-5.0
Fluoride	1.5-2.5	1.5-4.0
Chromium	0.05-0.2	0.05-0.2
Molybdenum	0.075-0.250	0.075-0.250

Modified from Food and Nutrition Board, National Research Council, National Academy of Sciences: Recommended dietary allowances, Washington, DC, 1989, US Government Printing Office.

Iron deficiency in the mother may have adverse effects on her obstetric performance.[63] A reduction in hemoglobin concentration means that the mother must increase her cardiac output to maintain adequate oxygen use by placental and fetal cells. This extra work fatigues the mother and makes her more susceptible to other sources of physiologic stress. A very low maternal hemoglobin places the mother at risk of cardiac arrest and leads to a poor prognosis for survival should she hemorrhage on delivery.

Setting requirements for iron during pregnancy is complicated by changes in the erythropoiesis system. Even when women have adequate iron status at conception, the plasma volume increases faster than the number of red blood cells so that hemodilution occurs. However, erythropoiesis is stimulated in the last half of pregnancy, and the rate of red blood cell production goes up. If sufficient iron is available, hemoglobin levels should rise to at least 11 mg/100 ml by term.

Generally, the initial drop in hemoglobin is a normal physiologic phenomenon, but there is concern that the usual iron intakes of pregnant women may not support increased erythropoiesis and fetal demands in the last half of pregnancy.[64] Iron absorption increases during pregnancy (to as much as 30%) compared with the usual 10% absorption from the diet. Also working in the mother's favor is the 120 mg or so that she saves over the course of gestation because she is not menstruating. However, even when these adjustments are taken into account, the pregnant woman still may need to consume about 30 mg of iron each day to maintain iron reserves. This amount could be supplied if large servings of iron-rich foods were eaten, but unfortunately, such foods are limited to organ meats, oysters, clams, and prune juice. These are not foods that people typically consume. From an average mixed diet, about 6 mg of iron are obtained from each 1000 kcal of food. At this rate a pregnant woman would have to eat 3000 to 5000 kcal of food per day to meet her iron needs. Furthermore, studies have shown that most women enter pregnancy with low iron stores so they have little to draw on to maintain normal hemoglobin.

For this reason, the expert panel from the National Academy of Sciences[7] concluded: "Iron is the only nutrient for which requirements cannot be met reasonably by diet alone. To meet the increased need for iron during the second and third trimesters of pregnancy, the average woman needs to absorb approximately 3 mg of iron per day in addition to the amount of iron usually absorbed from food. Evidence from iron supplementation studies indicates that low-dose supplements (e.g., 30 mg of ferrous iron daily during the second and third trimesters) can provide this amount of extra iron." The committee went on to say that since low doses of iron pose no known dangers to the mother or fetus, the potential benefits of iron supplementation outweigh the risks.

Calcium

The fetus acquires most of its calcium in the last trimester when skeletal growth is maximum and teeth are being formed. Widdowson[65] has calculated that the fetus draws 13 mg per hour of calcium from the maternal blood supply, or 250 to 300 mg per day. At birth the infant has accumulated approximately 25 g. Additional calcium is stored in the maternal skeleton as a reserve for lactation.

Extensive adjustments in calcium metabolism are routinely observed in the pregnant woman.[66] Hormonal factors are largely responsible.

1. **Human chorionic somatomammotropin** (from placenta). Progressively enhances the rate of bone turnover throughout pregnancy.
2. **Estrogen** (largely from placenta). Inhibits bone resorption and thus provokes a compensatory release of parathyroid hormone (PTH), which maintains the serum calcium level while enhancing intestinal calcium absorption and decreasing its urinary excretion.

The net effect of this hormonal action is the promotion of progressive calcium retention. The prenatal changes begin well ahead of the time when fetal mineralization starts.

It thus appears that anticipatory adjustments prepare the maternal organism for the increased calcium demands later on. Mineralization of the fetal skeleton is ultimately stimulated, largely through active placental calcium transport, leading to fetal hypercalcemia and subsequent endocrine adjustments. Vitamin D and its metabolites also cross the placenta and appear in fetal blood in the same concentration found in maternal circulation.

The current RDA standard for calcium during pregnancy is 1200 mg daily, a level 400 mg higher than recommended for the nonpregnant woman. Some argue that this allowance is set too high, since apparently successful pregnancies occur in many other cultures with calcium intakes substantially below those recommended. The explanation likely relates to the large calcium reservoir in the maternal skeleton, of which the total requirements of pregnancy amounts to about 2.5%. Also, in many other cultures diets contain less protein and this factor might serve to reduce the degree of calcium loss in the urine. Researchers[67] have reported data from balance studies suggesting that if maternal intake of calcium is low, stores of calcium will be depleted to meet fetal needs. If this is the case, frequent pregnancies and consistently low calcium intakes throughout the childbearing years could contribute to suboptimal bone density in later life. Clinical osteomalacia in **multiparous** women has been observed.[68]

Whether or not calcium status is etiologically related to the development of pregnancy-induced hypertension is currently the subject of much debate. Several studies have been conducted to determine if calcium supplementation reduces the incidence of this problem.[69-72] Results to date are highly suggestive of beneficial effects from calcium supplementation. A large, multicenter trial is scheduled in the United States to further explore the role that calcium might play in this mysterious prenatal condition.

Multiparous
(L *multus*, many; *parere*, to bring forth) Referring to women who have had two or more pregnancies resulting in live births.

Phosphorus

The RDA standard for phosphorus is the same as that for calcium, 800 mg with an extra 400 mg during pregnancy. It is so widely available in foods that a dietary deficiency is rare. In fact, it is possible that many problems may be caused by too much phosphorus rather than too little. Most adults can tolerate relatively wide variation in dietary calcium-phosphorus ratios when vitamin D is adequate.

Calcium-phosphorus balance relates to maintenance of normal neuromuscular action. Twenty years ago it was suggested that sudden clonic or tonic contractions of the *gastrocnemius muscle* (posterior "calf" muscle that flexes knee and ankle joints), occurring often at night, was caused by a decline in serum calcium. Prevention or relief was proclaimed to come from reduction of milk intake, a high phosphorus and calcium beverage. Supplementation with nonphosphate calcium salts was also recommended, along with regular use of aluminum hydroxide to form insoluble aluminum phosphate salts in the gut. While anecdotal reports have suggested benefit of these measures, controlled and double blind studies have failed to show any correlation between leg cramps and either intake of dairy products or the type of calcium supplement used.

Magnesium

Magnesium is much like calcium and phosphorus in that most of it is stored in the bones. The amounts that are biochemically active are concentrated in nerve and muscle cells. Deficiencies of magnesium produce neuromuscular dysfunction characterized by tremors and convulsions. Magnesium-deficient pregnant rats show impaired abdominal contractions during parturition. Not a great deal is known about the need for magnesium during pregnancy. The RDA standard is based on estimates of the amounts accumulated by the mother and the fetus.

Zinc

Zinc has an active role in metabolism for several reasons: (1) it is a component of insulin, (2) it is part of the carbonic anhydrase enzyme system that helps maintain acid-base balance in the tissues, and (3) it acts in the synthesis of DNA and RNA, which gives it a very important role in reproduction.

Much recent interest has centered on the significance of zinc deficiency in adversely affecting pregnancy course and outcome.[73-76] Zinc is a known constituent of a number of important metalloenzymes and a necessary cofactor for other enzymes. Zinc deficiency in rats leads to development of congenital malformations.[77] Nonhuman primates also are affected. Abnormal brain development and behavior have been described in offspring of zinc-deficient monkeys.[78] Evidence from human populations suggests that the malformation rate and other poor pregnancy outcomes may be higher in populations where zinc deficiency has been recognized.[79-81] For example, Jameson[82] observed in Scandinavia that women with low serum levels of zinc had higher incidence of abnormal deliveries, including congenital malformations. However, since conflicting reports also appear in the literature[83-85] and questions remain about satisfactory measures of zinc status, the true role of zinc deficiency in adverse course and outcome of human pregnancy remains unknown. The potential hazard of prenatal zinc supplements has not been determined in human populations. Haphazard use of such supplements, however, has no role in wise prenatal care.

Iodine

For many years it has been understood that maternal iodine deficiency leads to cretinism in offspring. It is still seen in some parts of the world today. Recent data also suggest that suboptimum iodine nutrition of the mother may compromise development of her fetus, even when cretinism does not occur. Several research groups[86] have evaluated the performance of children born to mothers living in iodine-deficient regions of New Guinea and India. Children born to mothers given adequate iodine were significantly faster and more accurate in tests of mental and manual function than children of control mothers. These findings indicate that iodine deficiency may lead to a spectrum of subclinical deficits that place children at a developmental disadvantage.

Fluoride

The role of fluoride in prenatal development is poorly understood at present. Some questions have existed over the past 50 years about the degree of fluoride transport across the placenta. Should it cross the placenta, questions still remain about its value in the development of caries-resistant permanent teeth.

Development of the primary dentition begins at 10 to 12 weeks of pregnancy. From the sixth to ninth months of pregnancy, the first four permanent molars and eight of the permanent incisors begin to form. Thus 32 of the ultimate teeth are forming and developing during human pregnancy. Since there is no indication that color of the teeth is adversely affected and some evidence that caries resistance and morphologic characteristics are improved, prenatal fluoride supplementation may be justified. *It should be recognized, however, that this issue is highly controversial and to date formal support for routine prenatal fluoride supplementation has not been voiced by any established medical or dental organization.*

Sodium

The metabolism of sodium is altered during pregnancy under the stimulus of a modified hormonal milieu. Glomerular filtration increases markedly over time to "clean up" the increased maternal blood volume. An additional filtered sodium load of 5000 to 10,000 mEq daily is typically seen during pregnancy. Compensatory mechanisms come into play to maintain fluid and electrolyte balance.

Restriction of dietary sodium has been common in the past among pregnant women with edema, but moderate edema is normal during pregnancy and should not be combated with diuretics and low-sodium diets. The increased fluid retained normally during pregnancy actually somewhat increases the body's demand for sodium. Rigorous sodium restriction in pregnant animals stresses the renin-angiotensin-aldosterone system to the point of breakdown. Such animals show reduced weight gain and altered fluid consumption patterns.[87] They also tend to develop water intoxication along with renal and adrenal tissue degeneration.[88] Neonatal hyponatremia (low blood sodium) has been observed in offspring of women who unduly restricted sodium intake before delivery.[89] The damage potential to the maternal renin-angiotensin-aldosterone system also exists. Although moderation in the American habit of excessive salt use is appropriate for all people, aggressive restriction is unwarranted during pregnancy. No less than 2 to 3 g of sodium should be consumed daily.

Other Minerals

One of the more recent advances in nutrition research is the discovery that many other trace elements are necessary for human growth, general health, and reproduction. Chromium, manganese, copper, selenium, molybdenum, vanadium, tin, nickel, and silicon have all been shown to be needed by the body. Like iodine, calcium, and phosphorus, these elements (and likely others as well) participate in reactions that control body processes. Studies in animals have revealed that deficiencies produce widespread and serious metabolic defects. Limited knowledge of requirements in humans makes it impossible to establish RDA standard for the majority of these minerals. The current RDA does, however, list estimated safe and adequate daily dietary intakes for copper, manganese, fluoride, chromium, and molybdenum (see Table 4-10). No figures are available for pregnant women. Since toxic levels for many of the trace elements may be much higher than usual intakes, pregnant women should not take supplements that would greatly exceed the upper limits recommended.

FOOD BELIEFS, CRAVINGS, AVOIDANCES, AND AVERSIONS

Most women change their diets during the course of pregnancy. Some changes are based on medical advice, others on folk medical beliefs, and others on changes in preference and appetite that may be idiosyncratic or culturally patterned. Since those changes that are culturally sanctioned will affect a woman's willingness to follow prescribed dietary regimens, the health care provider should be sensitized to their existence.

Food Beliefs and Food Behaviors

Many beliefs have been recorded about prenatal diet, such as the idea that the mother can mark her child before birth by eating specific foods. Overuse of a craved food during pregnancy is thought to explain physical or behavioral peculiarities of the infant. More often, unsatiated cravings are thought to explain birthmarks that mimic the shape of the desired food (such as strawberry- or drumstick-shaped marks). Behavioral markings have also been thought to derive from the prenatal diet; that is, the mother's consumption of many foods has been said to cause the child to like such foods after birth.

Another important group of beliefs concerns dietary means by which the mother can ensure an easier delivery. Most important, from the biomedical viewpoint, are beliefs that lead a woman to avoid animal protein foods or to avoid "excessive" weight gain. Most lay people know very well that a smaller weight gain during pregnancy produces a smaller infant. Thus, since a smaller baby may be "easier to deliver," low weight gain has been proposed as desirable, especially since it is commonly believed that the baby can "catch up" after birth.

Food avoidances are those foods that the mother consciously chooses not to consume during her pregnancy, usually for a reason she can articulate and that seems reasonable to her. The four most commonly avoided foods are sources of animal protein: milk, lean meats, pork, and liver. Cravings and aversions are powerful urges toward or away from foods, including foods about which women experience no unusual attitudes outside of pregnancy. The most commonly reported craved foods are sweets and dairy products. The most common aversions are reported to be alcohol, caffeinated drinks, and meats. However, cravings and aversions are not limited to any particular food or food groups.

The nutritional significance of these food-related behaviors is difficult to evaluate. Available information has often been collected in an anecdotal or one-sided manner. Thus there is limited detailed information on dietary alterations that appear to be detrimental and little knowledge of total subcultural prenatal dietary intakes. As a result, it is difficult to quantify the nutritional effect of restrictive beliefs, avoidances, cravings, or aversions. The nutritional importance of such practices cannot be assessed without reference to the rest of the woman's diet. Overall, however, most cravings result in increased intakes of calcium and energy, whereas aversions often result in decreased intake of animal protein. Such cravings and aversions are not necessarily deleterious.

Pica

One type of compulsive food behavior or craving during pregnancy, however, does carry potential danger.[90-92] This practice is termed *pica* (from the Latin word for magpie, with reference to the bird's **omnivorous** appetite). Human pica refers to the compulsion for persistent ingestion of unsuitable substances having little or no nutritional value. Pica of pregnancy most often involves consumption of dirt or clay (geophagia) or starch (amylophagia). However, compulsive ingestion of a variety of nonfood substances such as ice, burnt matches, hair, stone or gravel, charcoal, soot, cigarette ashes, mothballs, antacid tablets, milk of magnesia, baking soda, coffee grounds, and tire inner tubes has been noted. The practice of pica is not new nor is it limited to any one geographic area, race, creed, culture, sex, or status within a culture.

Omnivorous (L *omnis*, all; *vorare*, to eat) Eating all kinds of foods, both animal and plant.

The medical implications of pica are not well understood, although several speculations have been made. The displacement effect of pica substances could result in reduced intake of nutritious foods, leading to inadequate dietary intakes of essential nutrients. Alternatively, substances that provide kilocalories, for example, starch, could lead to obesity if ingested in large amounts above the usual dietary intakes. Some pica substances may contain toxic compounds or quantities of nutrients not tolerated in disease states. Some pica substances interfere with the absorption of certain mineral elements, such as iron. Other less commonly reported complications of pica include:

1. **Lead poisoning.** Congenital lead poisoning secondary to maternal pica for wall plaster.
2. **Irritable uterus.** Tender, irritable uterus with dystocia associated with fecal impaction from clay ingestion.
3. **Anemia.** Fetal hemolytic anemia caused by maternal ingestion of mothballs and toilet air fresheners.
4. **Obstruction.** Parotid enlargement and gastric and small bowel obstruction from ingestion of excessive laundry starch.
5. **Infection.** Parasitic infection from ingestion of contaminated soil or clay.

The etiology of pica is poorly understood, although several proposals have been made. One theory suggests that the ingestion of nonfood substances relieves nausea and vomiting. Another theory suggests that the deficiency of an essential nutrient such as calcium or iron results in the eating of nonfood substances that contain these nutrients. When pregnant women were questioned about the practice of pica, they gave a variety of answers:

- A taste for clay existed.
- Clay kept the baby from being marked at birth.
- Nervous tension was relieved.
- Starch made the newborn lighter in color.
- Starch helped the baby "slide out" more easily during delivery.

CASE STUDY

Pica Cases

Case 1. In England a 21-year-old woman was hospitalized at 38 weeks gestation because of severe anemia. She was generally tired, occasionally dizzy, and had edema of the ankles and mild anorexia. After 3 weeks of concentrated treatment with iron and folic acid she showed no improvement. Through further questioning it was found that throughout her pregnancy she had been eating toilet air freshener blocks at the rate of one to two per week. Cessation of this practice led to immediate improvement.

Case 2. A 31-year-old black woman was admitted to a rural emergency room with extreme weakness, severe nausea and vomiting, and fever. The patient reported no bowel movements during the preceding 2 weeks. On examination she was lethargic and appeared critically ill. Within 10 minutes of arrival she experienced a grand mal seizure followed by cardiorespiratory arrest. Efforts at resuscitation were unsuccessful and the woman died. Autopsy findings included 3 L of pus within the peritoneal cavity and a 4 cm perforation of the sigmoid colon. Free within the cavity were stones measuring 2.5 cm in diameter and a clay ball measuring 5 cm in diameter. Near the site of perforation, the colon was impacted with hardened claylike material. Subsequent inquiry of the family revealed that clay ingestion in the rural area was commonplace, and the husband noted that three of the patient's four children occasionally ate clay from the same bank their mother had used.

- Clay quieted hunger pains.
- Clay and starch were pleasant to chew.
- Pica carries social approval.

Many of these reasons given are based on superstition, customs and traditions, or practices passed from mother to daughter over generations. Two examples of pica, one of which caused maternal death, are described in the box above.

EFFECTS OF POTENTIALLY HARMFUL FOOD COMPONENTS

A number of food components have shown harmful effects on the course and outcome of pregnancy. Several of these agents and their effects are described here, including alcohol, caffeine, food additives, and food contaminants.

Alcohol

Fetal alcohol syndrome (FAS). During the past 15 years health researchers have become aware of the adverse effect of excessive consumption of alcohol on fetal development. In 1973 pediatricians in Seattle, Washington, described a unique set of characteristics of infants born to women who were chronic alcoholics. These infants exhibited specific anomalies of the eyes, nose, heart, and central nervous system that were accompanied by growth retardation, small head circumference, and mental retardation. The investigators named the condition *fetal alcohol syndrome* (Table 4-11). The condition does not necessarily lead to death but is associated with permanent disabilities (Fig. 4-13).

There is a high rate of prenatal mortality among infants with FAS. Infants who survive are generally irritable and hyperactive after birth. These symptoms are attributed to alcohol withdrawal. Physical and mental development is impaired. FAS infants exhibit poor rates of weight gain and failure to thrive despite concerted efforts at nutritional rehabilitation. The box on p. 130 illustrates the occurrence of FAS due to maternal ingestion of alcohol, in this instance in the unusual form of large amounts of cough syrup.

TABLE 4-11   *Facial Characteristics in Fetal Alcohol Syndrome*

	Features Necessary to Characteristic Face	Associated Features
Eyes	Short palpebral fissures	
Nose	Short and upturned in early childhood, hypoplastic philtrum	Flat nasal bridge; epicanthal folds
Maxilla	Flattened	
Mouth	Thinned upper vermilion	Prominent lateral palatine ridges, cleft lip with or without cleft palate; small teeth
Mandible		Retrognathia in infancy; micrognathia or relative prognathia in adolescents
Ears		Posterior rotation, abnormal concha

From Clarren and Smith, N Engl J Med 298:1063-67, 1978. Reprinted with permission from The New England Journal of Medicine.

FIG. 4-13   Child with FAS at day 1 and 8 years of age. This child was diagnosed at birth and has spent all his life in a foster home where the quality of care has been excellent. His IQ has remained stable at 40 to 45. Although he is more seriously retarded than most children with FAS, he demonstrates the resistance of the disability to environmental intervention.

Courtesy of Dr. Ann P. Streissguth, University of Washington, Seattle.

CASE STUDY

Fetal Alcohol Syndrome

An infant with typical features of FAS, including a head circumference below the tenth percentile on the National Center for Health Statistics growth chart, was born at term to a 24-year-old mother who reported consumption of 480 to 840 ml per day of a nonprescription cough syrup. The alcohol content of the syrup was 9.5%, or 36.5 to 63.8 g per day, equivalent to the alcohol content of 1 to 2 L of 4% beer or 0.5 to 1.0 L of wine.

Intensive prenatal care had been instituted with entry into an addiction treatment program at an undefined point in pregnancy. No evidence of distortion of truth was found with urinary test for substance abuse. Whether pregnancy outcome was related to alcohol, to other drugs, or to their interactive effects is not clear. The case emphasizes the need for awareness of the full content of over-the-counter drugs used in pregnancy.

Fetal alcohol effects. The impact of more moderate levels of alcohol consumption on fetal development has been the focus of much research during the past decade. It is now well recognized that moderate drinkers may produce offspring with "fetal alcohol effects" showing more subtle features of FAS. Such women also demonstrate a higher rate of spontaneous abortion, abruptio placentae, and low-birth-weight delivery.

General actions of alcohol. At present, the mechanisms by which alcohol produces such widespread effects on the fetus are not completely understood. Since alcohol can cross the placenta, the current hypothesis is that high alcohol levels build up in the fetus and produce direct toxic effects that are most severe in the early phases of pregnancy during blastogenesis and cell differentiation. Another theory is that some of the effects of alcohol may be caused by maternal malnutrition. We may not think of alcohol as a food, but it yields 7 kcal/g. Alcohol is considered an "empty kilocalorie" food because most alcoholic beverages supply little or no nutrients. Women who derive a substantial portion of their daily caloric needs from alcohol may not have an appetite for more nutritious foods. Deficiencies of folic acid, magnesium, and zinc have been shown to be highly teratogenic in animals, so it is reasonable to suspect that deficiencies of these nutrients could play a role in FAS.

Alcohol use by pregnant women. Although the adverse effects of maternal alcohol consumption on fetal development have been known for over a decade, a significant number of women still choose to drink alcohol while they are pregnant. One research team[93] reported that among women delivering in a large urban hospital in Massachusetts, 82% had consumed alcohol during pregnancy: 3% consumed alcoholic beverages more than 20 times per month, and 3% consumed more than 20 oz (600 ml) per month. Streissguth and coworkers[94] reported patterns of alcohol use among pregnant women in a large urban area who had been exposed to a heavy media campaign aimed at preventing fetal alcohol effects. Looking at precampaign and postcampaign data (1974 to 1975 and 1980 to 1981), the number of women who reported any alcohol use around the time of the first prenatal visit dropped from 81% to 42%, but among drinkers, there was no decrease in the proportion of women who reported heavier drinking. As these authors suggest, the relative constancy in the proportion of "heavier" drinkers and binge drinkers, particularly around the time of conception, indicates the need for more attention to this important period of gestation in advice to women who are planning a pregnancy.

Prenatal care for alcoholic mothers. According to Rosett and colleagues,[95,96] pregnancy course and outcome can be significantly improved if problem drinkers agree to change their habits after conception has occurred. These workers reported that infants born to women who reduced their heavy drinking did not differ in growth from offspring of rare and moderate drinkers. They did, however, show a higher frequency of abnormalities. This group urges that facilities providing routine prenatal care integrate therapy for heavy drinking into their counseling sessions. Since the desire to have a healthy baby is a powerful motivating force, therapeutic success can be achieved with some of the heaviest drinkers.

Caffeine

Animal studies. The danger of caffeine to the developing fetus has been studied in several animal models. Massive doses appear to be teratogenic in mice, but the effects of smaller quantities have not been satisfactorily examined. One research group[97] did observe that offspring of rats fed coffee during pregnancy had reduced body, liver, and brain weight at birth. By 39 days, these animals had recovered in size but demonstrated increased locomotion, decreased grooming time, and decreased time spent with a novel object. Another research team[98] reported that when caffeine was introduced into the diet of rats throughout pregnancy and lactation, offspring of successive pregnancies showed growth reductions, although teratogenic effects were not seen with this moderate level of caffeine exposure.

A 1980 report from the Food and Drug Administration (FDA) suggested that rather modest amounts of caffeine provided to pregnant rats may increase the incidence of defects in development of the digits.[99] Pregnant rats provided an amount of caffeine (per unit size) equivalent to about 12 to 40 cups of coffee per day for humans produced offspring with an increased incidence of partial or complete absence of the digits of the paws. A Virginia woman subsequently claimed that her 15-year-old child with no fingers or toes was damaged in utero by her daily consumption of 10 to 12 cups of coffee. Although data were limited in relation to human use of caffeine in pregnancy, a general warning was voiced to the public in 1981 to avoid unnecessary caffeine consumption during pregnancy.

Conclusions. Since this warning was released in the early 1980s, three systematic observations of large groups of pregnant women have not provided cause for alarm.[100-102] However, another recent report suggested that a rather low level of daily caffeine consumption (about 150 mg) is associated with greater risk of late first and second trimester spontaneous abortion.[103] Since available data from observations of human populations are inconclusive, common sense suggests that caution should be exercised and pregnant women should be advised to use caffeine in moderation, if at all.

Food Additives

The teratogenicity of common food additives is largely unknown in human situations. Metabolism of cyclamate and red dye no. 2 reportedly damage developing rat embryos,[104] but both of these additives have now been banned for use in the U.S. food supply. Saccharin, mannitol, xylitol, aspartame, and other artificial sugar substitutes have come under careful scrutiny in the last several decades. Kline and co-workers[105] have reported, however, that incidence of spontaneous abortion in a human population was not associated with ingestion of any sugar substitute.

Saccharin. Because saccharin has been shown to be weakly carcinogenic in rats, moderation in its use seems appropriate. This is especially true for women of reproductive age, since studies in rats indicate that saccharin can most effectively initiate bladder cancer when the mother is exposed to high doses before pregnancy and the offspring are exposed in utero and throughout their lives. Saccharin can also markedly promote or enhance the potential of other carcinogens in rats, providing another reason for moderation in use.[106]

Aspartame. The increasing use of aspartame in the American food supply has been associated with outcries from a minority of scientists who propose that one or more of the breakdown products of aspartame may interfere with normal fetal development. Chemically, aspartame is L-aspartyl-L-phenylalanine methyl ester. The dipeptide ester is metabolized into three moieties in the small intestine, so that studies of the safety of aspartame are essentially studies of aspartic acid, phenylalanine, and methanol.

Human studies with pregnant women. Human subjects have been fed up to six times the 99th percentile of the projected daily intake (6 × 34 = 200 mg/kg). No evidence of risk to the fetus has been observed. Aspartate does not readily cross the placenta. Small elevations of blood methanol following the above abuse doses of aspartame have not led to measurable increases in blood formic acid, which is the product responsible for the acidosis and ocular toxicity of methanol poisoning. Phenylalanine is concentrated on the fetal side of the placenta.

Phenylalanine and PKU. The phenylalanine component of aspartame has raised the most concern due to the unknown damaging impact of phenylalanine on brain tissue of children with phenylketonuria (PKU). Individuals with this genetic disease lack the liver enzyme that converts phenylalanine to tyrosine. Thus, blood levels of phenylalanine rise to high levels and mental retardation is the ultimate result. Aspartame in abuse doses up to 200 mg/kg in normal subjects, or to 100 mg/kg in PKU **heterozygotes** (carriers of the gene for PKU), have not been found to raise blood phenylalanine levels to the range generally accepted to be associated with mental retardation in offspring.

Conclusions. One might conclude that, under foreseeable conditions of use, aspartame poses no risk for use in pregnancy. However, since limited data are available to date on pregnancy course and outcome in heavy aspartame users, it may be wise to recommend moderation in aspartame use during pregnancy, especially in women known to be PKU heterozygotes.

Food Contaminants

General toxicity. A number of "contaminants" are found in food. Some of these may adversely affect pregnancy course and outcome if consumed in sufficient amounts. Most heavy metals are embryotoxic but only mercury, lead, cadmium, and possibly nickel and selenium have been implicated in this regard. Lead toxicity has long been known to be associated with abortion and menstrual disorders. Evidence as to whether lead is teratogenic is conflicting. Some authors report a correlation between atmospheric lead levels and congenital malformations, whereas others deny these associations. In sheep, prenatal lead exposure has also been shown to affect the offspring's learning ability.

Mercury poisoning. Probably the earliest instance of massive, unplanned exposure of a local population to an environmental toxicant occurred in 1953 in and around Minamata, a town located on a bay in southern Japan. Unusual neurologic problems (for example, mental confusion, convulsions, and coma) began afflicting villagers. Over one third of the affected individuals died, and many infants and children suffered permanent brain damage from prenatal and neonatal exposure. Mercury was transported across the placenta and also appeared in breast milk of mothers consuming contaminated fish. Eventually the source of the mercury was traced to the effluent discharged from a local plastics factory into Minamata Bay. A similar incident occurred in Niigata, Japan in 1964.

Another massive methylmercury disaster occurred in Iraq during the winter of 1971

Heterozygote

(Gr *hetero*, other; *zygotos*, yoked together) Individual possessing different *alleles* (gene forms occupying corresponding chromosome sites) in regard to a given trait.

to 1972. In this case barley and wheat grain treated with methylmercury as a fungicide had been purchased from Mexico. The grain sacks carried a written warning—but only in Spanish. Thirty one pregnant women who ate the grain were hospitalized with methylmercury poisoning. Almost half of them died. Infants born to surviving mothers showed evidence of cerebral palsy, blindness, and severe brain damage. Similar outbreaks have occurred in Russia, Sweden, and elsewhere.[107]

Other heavy metals. Several other heavy metals probably affect the fetus and infant. Cadmium (which is derived accidentally from tobacco smoke, the electroplating industry, and deterioration of rubber tires) is a known cause of developmental malformations in rodents. Low doses of nickel causes embryotoxicity and eye malformations in the progeny of rats. Selenium is also a suspect teratogen.

Pesticides. A number of pesticides have been a major concern among public health professionals for quite some time. The Environmental Protection Agency reports that about one third of the 1500 active ingredients in registered pesticides are toxic, and one quarter are mutagenic and carcinogenic. Although the agency has established limits on the amounts of pesticide residues that are allowed in foods, it has restricted the use of only five: heptaclor, chlordane, DDT, Mirex, and DBCP. Once deposited in the food chain, they are almost impossible to eliminate. The effects of exposure to low concentrations of these toxins is not only unknown but also difficult to investigate because of the problem of finding pesticide-free control populations.

PCBs. Polychlorinated biphenyls (PCBs), used as plasticizers and heat exchange fluids, comprise another group of chemicals that endanger health. In Kyushu, Japan in 1968, a number of pregnant and lactating women ingested cooking oil contaminated with PCBs. As a result, they had small-for-gestational-age infants with dark skin, eye defects, and other abnormalities. Although prenatal exposure was probably significant, evidence indicated that transfer of PCBs through breast milk was the most significant route of exposure. Polybromated biphenyl (PBB), produced commercially as a fire retardant, also provoked attention after its accidental entry into cattle feed in Michigan in 1973 to 1974. Over 30,000 cattle and many sheep, swine, and poultry died or were slaughtered. Contaminated meat, milk, and eggs were identified in local food supplies, and stillbirths among affected cattle increased. Adverse effects in human pregnancy have not been reported, but considerable concern still exists.

EFFECTS OF RIGOROUS PHYSICAL ACTIVITY

For many years questions have been raised about the effect of heavy maternal physical activity during pregnancy on fetal growth. Some insight may be gained from studies related to heavy physical labor, modern fitness programs, and athletic training.

Heavy Physical Labor

In a study conducted in Ethiopia, trained nutritionists visited pregnant women in their homes for a period of 3 consecutive days. During this time dietary surveys were conducted. Two groups of women who had similar energy and protein intakes during pregnancy were then compared. One group of mothers was forced by circumstances beyond their control to engage in hard physical work throughout pregnancy. The second group of mothers had servants to do such physical labor. Mothers in both groups ate on the mean about 1550 kcal a day.

When the two groups of Ethiopian women were compared, the women who engaged in hard physical labor had significantly lower pregnancy weight gains and smaller babies than did mothers who did not have to engage in such work. Kilocalorie deficiency was likely involved in the etiology of fetal growth retardation that was seen. In addition, however, the oxygen debt incurred by moderate exercise is increased in human pregnancies, and this may lead to fetal hypoxia. This response is also evident in animal studies where uterine blood flow decreases during maternal exercise.

Fitness Programs

The circumstances of mandatory physical labor described above, further imposed on an underlying state of moderate undernutrition, may seem far removed from today's modern fitness-conscious woman who opts to engage in a rigorous exercise program during pregnancy. But some useful comparisons can be made.

The fitness-conscious pregnant woman often gets conflicting advice from her physician and other health professionals. The obstetric textbooks rarely offer more than a single paragraph concerning physical activities during pregnancy. Obstetricians tend to form their own philosophies about various physical activities or athletic participation during pregnancy, and their recommendations often are based on their own (or their wives') experiences. Traditional advice to women from the obstetric community has been to decrease activity and increase periods of rest during pregnancy, particularly in the third trimester.

Over the past 15 years, a number of studies have been conducted to examine the true relationship between physical activity programs and pregnancy course and outcome. A variety of fitness and training regimens have been evaluated.[108] Most studies have reported no difference in pregnancy outcome related to physical activity. However, most pregnant women followed by these investigators decreased frequency, duration, or intensity of exercise in the latter part of pregnancy. One research group at the University of Vermont was able to compare a group of women who maintained frequent vigorous endurance exercise routines throughout the third trimester with other less active pregnant women.[109] While the incidence of antenatal and neonatal complications was similar in all groups, those exercising vigorously in the third trimester had babies with a mean birth weight of 2633 g (5.5 lb); mean birth weights of offspring from both control groups exceeded 3000 g (6.25 lb).

More recently, this group from Vermont[110-112] examined pregnancy course and outcome in women who continued a regular running or aerobics program during pregnancy at or above 50% of preconceptional levels; active control women were also observed. As can be seen in Table 4-12, the vigorously exercising women has somewhat fewer spontaneous abortions, superior labor and delivery characteristics, better fetal condition at birth, and no greater level of preterm delivery or premature rupture of membranes. However, babies of the vigorously exercising women demonstrated growth restriction; they were clearly born with reduced levels of body fat (Table 4-13). While the authors speculate that this difference in fat mass at birth may have long term beneficial effects on health of the offspring, one might also wonder if this smaller kilocaloric reserve increases the risk of an infant not successfully combatting a major nutritional or medical insult during infancy. Until additional data are available, it seems prudent to advise women not to engage in very rigorous conditioning exercise during the third trimester.

Some high-risk women, such as those with diabetes, heart disease, or history of spontaneous abortion, may be well advised to be particularly cautious about the selection of exercise programs. The American College of Obstetricians and Gynecologists provides exercise guidelines for all pregnant women that go well beyond discouraging endurance training in the third trimester (Table 4-14).[113] While these guidelines may be overly restrictive for many pregnant women, they provide a common sense base from which to start.

TABLE 4-12 **Features of Pregnancy Course and Outcome in Runners and Aerobic Dancers versus Active Control Women**

Characteristic	Controls (%)	Exercisers (%)
Spontaneous abortion	25	17 (runners)
		18 (aerobic dancers)
Onset of labor		
Preterm (263 days)	9	8
Premature rupture of membranes	29	30
Induction of labor	13	13
Labor management		
Artificial rupture of membranes	50	23
Stimulation for abnormal labor pattern	20	13
Second stage arrest	14	2
Method of delivery		
Spontaneous	50	88
Forceps	20	6
Cesarean section	30	6
Fetal condition and outcome		
Meconium in fluid	25	14
Abnormal heart rate	25	14
1 min Apgar score less than 7	25	14

From Clapp JF: The effects of maternal exercise on early pregnancy outcome, Am J Obstet Gynecol 161:1453, 1989; and Clapp JF: The course of labor after endurance exercise during pregnancy, Am J Obstet Gynecol 163:1799, 1990.

TABLE 4-13 **Characteristics of Infants Born to Runners and Aerobic Dancers versus Active Control Women**

Characteristics	Controls	Exercisers	Significant Difference
Birth weight (g)	3691	3381	Yes
Birth weight percentile	65th	45th	Yes
Length (cm)	51.3	51.4	No
Head circumference (cm)	35.2	35.0	No
Placental weight (g)	456	449	No
Indices of soft tissue growth restriction			
Skinfolds (sum of triceps and subscapular) (mm)	11.8	9.3	Yes
Skinfold percentile	58	28	Yes
Calculated body fat (%)	16.2	11.2	Yes
Calculated fat mass (g)	603	382	Yes

From Clapp JF and Capeless EL: Neonatal morphometrics after endurance exercise during pregnancy, Am J Obstet Gynecol 163:1805, 1990.

TABLE 4-14 *American College of Obstetricians and Gynecologists' Guidelines for Exercise during Pregnancy and Postpartum*

1. Regular exercise (at least three times per week) is preferable to intermittent activity. Competitive activities should be discouraged.
2. Vigorous exercise should not be performed in hot, humid weather or during a period of febrile illness.
3. Ballistic movements (jerky, bouncy motions) should be avoided. Exercise should be done on a wooden floor or a tightly carpeted surface to reduce shock and provide a sure footing.
4. Deep flexion or extension of joints should be avoided because of connective tissue laxity. Activities that require jumping, jarring motions, or rapid changes in direction should be avoided because of joint instability.
5. Vigorous exercise should be preceded by a five-minute period of muscle warm-up. This can be accomplished by slow walking or stationary cycling with low resistance.
6. Vigorous exercise should be followed by a period of gradually declining activity that includes gentle stationary stretching. Because connective tissue laxity increases the risk of joint injury, stretches should not be taken to the point of maximum resistance.
7. Heart rate should be measured at times of peak activity. Target heart rates and limits established in consultation with the physician should not be exceeded.
8. Care should be taken to gradually rise from the floor to avoid orthostatic hypotension. Some form of activity involving the legs should be continued for a brief period.
9. Liquids should be taken liberally before and after exercise to prevent dehydration. If necessary, activity should be interrupted to replenish fluids.
10. Women who have led sedentary life-styles should begin with physical activity of very low intensity and advance activity levels very gradually.
11. Activity should be stopped and the physician consulted if any unusual symptoms appear.

Pregnancy only
1. Maternal heart rate should not exceed 140 beats/minute.
2. Strenuous activities should not exceed 15 minutes in duration.
3. No exercise should be performed in the supine position after the fourth month of gestation is completed.
4. Exercises that employ the Valsalva maneuver should be avoided.
5. Caloric intake should be adequate to meet not only the extra energy needs for pregnancy, but also of the exercise performed.
6. Maternal core temperature should not exceed 38° C.

Reprinted with permission from the American College of Obstetricians and Gynecologists: Exercise during pregnancy and the postnatal period (ACOG Home Exercise Programs). Washington, DC, 1985, American College of Obstetricians and Gynecologists.

EFFECTS OF CIGARETTE SMOKING

Fetal growth retardation is often seen in offspring of cigarette smokers, as shown in Fig. 4-14. It has been postulated that this condition is due to the reduced food intake of the mother. Observations have shown that this is not true. Women who smoke often consume more kilocalories per day than women who do not smoke.[114]

The growth retarding impact of smoking relates to the effects of carbon monoxide, nicotine, and possibly other compounds on placental perfusion and oxygen transport to the fetus. It is also likely that efficiency of kilocalorie utilization is reduced in women who smoke. Whether or not encouraging greater weight gain among smoking mothers will increase the infant's size is as yet an unanswered question. However, several reports have suggested that greater maternal weight is directly related to greater infant birth weight

FIG. 4-14   Maternal cigarette use and infant birth weight.

Modified from Niswander KR and Gordon M: The women and their pregnancies, Philadelphia, 1972, WB Saunders Co. In Martin J: Neurobehav Toxicol Teratol 4:421, 1982.

in this population.[114,115] In any event, the wisest counsel to mothers who smoke is to stop—at least during the pregnancy.

COMMON COMPLAINTS WITH DIETARY IMPLICATIONS

General nutritional guidance may also be needed during pregnancy for common functional gastrointestinal difficulties encountered. These complaints are highly individual in form and extent. They will, therefore, require individual counseling and assurances for control. Usually these difficulties are relatively minor. But if they persist or become extreme, they will need medical care. In most cases general investigation of food practices will reveal some areas where diet counseling may help relieve gastrointestinal problems. Some of the more common difficulties include nausea, constipation, hemorrhoids, or heartburn.

Nausea and Vomiting

Difficulty with nausea and vomiting is usually mild and limited to early pregnancy. It is commonly called "morning sickness" because it tends to occur early in the day, but it can come at any time of day. Usually it lasts only a brief period at the beginning of the pregnancy, but in some women it may persist longer.

A number of factors may contribute to the usual mild condition. Some are physiologic, based on normal hormonal changes that occur early in pregnancy. Other factors may be psychologic, such as various tensions and anxieties concerning the pregnancy itself. Simple treatment generally improves food toleration. Small frequent meals, fairly dry and consisting chiefly of easily digested energy foods such as carbohydrates, are more readily tolerated. Cooking odors should be avoided as much as possible. Liquids are best taken between meals instead of with food. If the condition persists and develops into hyper-emesis—severe, prolonged, persistent vomiting—medical attention is required to prevent complications and dehydration. However, such an increase in symptoms is rare. Most conditions pass early in the pregnancy and respond to the simple dietary remedies given here. Women should be reassured that mild short-term nausea is common in early pregnancy and will not harm the fetus.

Constipation

The condition of constipation is seldom more than minor. Hormonal changes in pregnancy tend to increase relaxation of the gastrointestinal muscles. Also, the pressure of the enlarging uterus on the lower portion of the intestine, especially during the latter part of the pregnancy, may make elimination somewhat difficult at times. Increased fluid intake, use of naturally laxative foods and fiber, such as whole grains with added bran, fibrous fruits and vegetables, dried fruits (especially prunes and figs), and other fruits and juices generally induce regularity. Laxatives should be avoided. They should only be used in special situations under medical supervision.

Hemorrhoids

A fairly common complaint during the latter part of pregnancy is that of hemorrhoids. These are enlarged veins in the anus, often protruding through the anal sphincter. This vein enlargement is usually caused by the increased weight of the fetus and the downward pressure it produces. The hemorrhoids may cause considerable discomfort, burning, and itching. Occasionally they may rupture and bleed under the pressure of a bowel movement, therefore causing more anxiety. The difficulty is usually remedied by the dietary suggestions given above to control constipation. Also, observing general hygiene recommendations concerning sufficient rest during the latter part of the day may help to relieve the pressure of the uterus on the lower intestine.

Heartburn or Full Feeling

The related complaints of "heartburn" or "full feeling" are sometimes voiced by pregnant women. These discomforts may occur especially after meals, usually caused by the pressure of the enlarging uterus crowding the adjacent digestive organ, the stomach, thereby causing some difficulty after eating. Food mixtures may sometimes be pushed back into the lower part of the esophagus, causing a "burning" sensation from the gastric acid mixed with the food mass. This burning sensation is commonly called heartburn simply because of the proximity of the lower esophagus to the heart. Obviously, however, it has nothing to do with the heart and its action. A full feeling comes from general gastric pressure, caused by a lack of normal space in the area, and is accentuated by a large meal or gas formation. These complaints are generally remedied by dividing the day's food intake into a number of small meals during the day. Attention may also be given to relaxation, adequate chewing, eating slowly, and avoiding tensions during meals. Comfort is also improved by wearing loosefitting clothing.

SELECTED EXAMPLES OF HIGH-RISK PREGNANCY
General Comments

A number of risk factors may contribute to a poor pregnancy outcome. In a joint report, the American College of Obstetricians and Gynecologists and the American Dietetic Association have issued a set of risk factors to identify women with special nutritional and health-care needs during pregnancy.[116] These factors, summarized in Table 4-15,

TABLE 4-15   Risk Factors in Pregnancy-Induced Hypertension

Before Pregnancy	During Pregnancy
Nulligravida	Primigravida
Diabetes mellitus	Large fetus
Preexisting condition (hypertension, renal or vascular disease)	Glomerulonephritis
Family history of hypertension or vascular disease	Fetal hydrops
Diagnosis of pregnancy-induced hypertension in a previous pregnancy	Hydramnios
Dietary deficiencies	Multiple gestation
Age extremes	Hydatidiform mole
20 years or younger	
35 years or older	

GUIDELINES FOR POSITIVE TEACHING TO CORRECT NUTRIENT DEFICIENCIES

- **General counseling approach**
  Reinforce good habits
  Encourage needed changes in food practices
- **Basic counseling actions**
  Identify unmet needs
  Clarify reasons for increased nutrient needs
  Identify reasons for dietary deficiencies
  1. Low income
  2. Food aversions or intolerances
  3. Cultural food pattern
  4. Vegetarian food patterns
  Evaluate need for nutrient supplements
  1. Kilocalories/protein
  2. Vitamins
  3. Minerals

---

relate to nutritional status, habits, needs, and problems. The nutritional factors identified in this report are based on clinical evidence of inadequate nutrition. A better approach, suggested by King,[117] provides useful criteria for predicting nutritional risk, instead of waiting for clinical signs of poor nutrition to appear. Three types of dietary patterns, she summarizes, would not support optimal maternal and fetal nutrition: (1) insufficient food intake, (2) poor food selection, and (3) poor food distribution through the day. These patterns, added to the list of risk factors in Table 4-15, would be much more sensitive for nutritional risk. On this basis, practitioners can plan personal care and provide for special counseling needs (see box above).

Pregnancy-Induced Hypertension (PIH)

Formerly labeled *toxemia*, PIH is a risk factor related to nutrition and treated according to its symptoms:

1. **Clinical symptoms.** PIH is generally defined according to its manifestations, which usually occur in the third trimester toward term. Among these symptoms are hypertension, abnormal and excessive edema, albumuria, and in severe cases, convulsions or coma—*eclampsia*.
2. **Treatment.** Specific treatment varies according to the patient's symptoms and needs. In any case, optimal nutrition is a fundamental aspect of therapy. Adequate dietary protein is essential. Correction of plasma protein deficits stimulates normal operation of the capillary fluid shift mechanism and restores circulation of tissue fluid, inducing subsequent correction of the **hypovolemia.** In addition, adequate salt and sources of vitamins and minerals are needed for correction and maintenance of metabolic balances.

Hypovolemia
(Gr *hypo*, under; ME *volu(me)*, volume; Gr *haima*, blood) Low blood volume.

Preexisting Disease

Preexisting clinical conditions complicate pregnancy and increase risks. They are managed according to the general principles of care related to pregnancy and to the particular disease involved. Examples of these preexisting conditions include hypertension, diabetes mellitus, and phenylketonuria (PKU).

Hypertension. Preventive screening and monitoring of blood pressure are essential. The hypertensive disease process begins long before any signs and symptoms appear and later symptoms are inconsistent.[118] Risk factors for hypertension before and during pregnancy are given in Table 4-16. Nutritional care centers on prevention of weight extremes, either underweight or obesity, and correction of any dietary deficiencies by maintaining optimal nutrition. Sodium intake can be moderate but should never be unduly restricted because of its relation to fluid and electrolyte balances during pregnancies.

Diabetes mellitus. The management of diabetes in pregnancy presents special problems. Routine screening is therefore necessary to detect gestational diabetes, and team man-

TABLE 4-16   Nutritional Risk Factors in Pregnancy

Risk Factors Present at the Onset of Pregnancy	Risk Factors Occurring during Pregnancy

Age
  15 years or younger
  35 years or older
	Low hemoglobin or hematocrit
	  Hemoglobin less than 12.0 g
	  Hematocrit less than 35.0 mg/dl

Frequent pregnancies: three or more during a 2-year period	Inadequate weight gain Any weight loss
Poor obstetric history or poor fetal performance	Weight gain of less than 2 lb per month after the first trimester
Poverty	Excessive weight gain: greater than 1 kg (2.2 lb) per week after the first trimester
Bizarre or faddist food habits	
Abuse of nicotine, alcohol, or drugs	
Therapeutic diet required for a chronic disorder	

Inadequate weight
  Less than 85% of standard weight
  More than 120% of standard weight	

agement is required for control of pre-existing insulin-dependent diabetes mellitus (IDDM).[119,120]

Screening. Most prenatal clinics do routine screening for diabetes and provide careful followup for every patient who shows glycosuria. Risk factors detected in initial history include (1) family history of diabetes, (2) previous unexplained stillbirths, (3) large babies weighing 4 kg (9 lb) or more, (4) recurrent miscarriage, (5) births of babies with multiple congenital anomalies, and (6) excessive obesity.

Gestational diabetes. During pregnancy glycosuria is not uncommon because of the increased circulating blood volume and its load of metabolites. However, only 20% to 30% of women showing glycosuria or somewhat abnormal glucose tolerance subsequently develop diabetes. Nonetheless, identification of women with this condition and their close followup observation are important because of the higher risk of fetal damage during this period. Most of these women revert to normal glucose tolerance after delivery.

Preexisting IDDM. Because of the course of diabetes during pregnancy, as well as the altered course of pregnancy in the presence of diabetes, a team of specialists is necessary for sound management and prevention of problems to reduce risk of fetal death and increase the probability of a successful outcome. Close personalized nutritional care by the team nutritionist is mandatory throughout. The insulin requirement increases during pregnancy and drops dramatically upon delivery.

Maternal phenylketonuria (MPKU). Mandatory screening of all newborns for the genetic disease PKU and low phenylalanine diet have supported normal growth in PKU children. Now a generation of young women with childhood PKU are having children of their own. Maternal PKU presents potential fetal hazards associated with increased abortions and stillbirths, congenital anomalies often causing death, and intrauterine and postnatal growth and development retardation in surviving infants. A planned pregnancy, with careful management of the mother's diet *before* conception, and close followup care *throughout* the pregnancy itself, can improve the outcome of these high-risk pregnancies. A strict diet low in phenylalanine and a special formula of other amino acids is required.

 ## CASE STUDY

Preconceptional Counseling

A professional woman 35 years of age visits her health care provider for advice. She and her husband are planning a pregnancy and she wishes to approach this project systematically. An interview and physical examination reveals that she:

- Has been using oral contraceptives for 10 years
- Smokes
- Is 10 pounds underweight
- Enjoys wine with her meals
- Has a family history of diabetes
- Has a typical 60-hour work week
- Intends to continue her career during and after pregnancy

Analysis
1. Outline appropriate recommendations for the preconception period.
2. Define those issues that require discussion about the pregnancy period itself.
3. Summarize appropriate anticipatory guidance for the postpartum period.

Summary

The relative importance of nutrition in prenatal development has been studied and debated for a number of years. Available evidence strongly supports a key role for maternal nutrition in significantly affecting the fate of both mother and child. Animal data convince, and human observations clearly suggest, that maternal prepregnancy weight and weight gain during pregnancy positively correlate with birth weight of the offspring.

Supplementation programs for pregnant women are successful when they are properly administered and focused on needy populations. The benefit of such programs may also be substantial even when health care workers or food program administrators are unable to measure that benefit with available tools. With limited time and resources in prenatal settings, priority should be given to those women with greatest need. Dietary recommendations must be tailored to meet the specific needs of each woman served.

Review Questions

1. Describe significant historic observations about the relationship between maternal diet and pregnancy outcome.
2. Discuss current dietary recommendations during pregnancy and justify each of them.
3. Define appropriate weight gain guidelines for pregnancy.
4. Define known effects of specific nutrient deficiencies and excesses in human pregnancy.
5. Summarize current information about the impact of alcohol, caffeine, and other food substances on pregnancy course and outcome.
6. Outline appropriate management recommendations for the common gastrointestinal complaints of pregnancy.

References

1. Committee on Maternal Nutrition, Food and Nutrition Board, National Research Council: Maternal nutrition and the course of pregnancy, Washington, DC, 1973, National Academy of Sciences.
2. Christakis G, ed: Maternal nutrition assessment, Am J Public Health 63(Suppl):1, 1973.
3. Committee on Maternal Nutrition, Food and Nutrition Board, National Research Council: Nutritional supplementation and the outcome of pregnancy, Washington, DC, 1973, National Academy of Sciences.
4. Select Panel for the Promotion of Child Health, US Department of Health and Human Services: Better health for our children: a national strategy, vols 1-3, Pub No (PHS) 79-55071, Washington, DC, 1981, US Government Printing Office.
5. Task Force on Nutrition: Assessment of maternal nutrition, Chicago, 1978, American College of Obstetricians and Gynecologists.
6. Committee on Nutrition of the Mother and Preschool Child: Nutrition services in perinatal care, Washington, DC, 1981, National Academy Press.
7. Institute of Medicine, National Academy of Sciences: Nutrition during pregnancy: weight gain and nutrient supplements, Washington, DC, National Academy Press.
8. Starr P: The social transformation of American medicine, New York, 1982, Basic Books.
9. Brown JE and Toma RB: Taste changes during pregnancy, Am J Clin Nutr 43:414,1986.
10. Winick M: Fetal malnutrition, Clin Obstet Gynecol 13:526, 1970.
11. Thomson AM et al: The assessment of fetal growth, J Obstet Gynaecol Br Commonw 75:903, 1968.
12. Naeye PL: Causes of fetal and neonatal mortality by race in a selected U.S. population, Am J Public Health 69:857, 1979.

13. Edwards LE et al: Pregnancy in the underweight woman: course, outcome, and growth patterns of the infant, Am J Obstet Gynecol 135:297, 1979.
14. Shepard MJ et al: Proportional weight gain and complications of pregnancy, labor, and delivery in healthy women of normal prepregnant status, Am J Obstet Gynecol 155:947, 1986.
15. Primrose T and Higgins A: A study of human antepartum nutrition, J Reprod Med 7:257, 1971.
16. Higgins AC et al: Impact of the Higgins Nutrition Intervention Program on birth weight: a within mother analysis, J Am Diet Assoc 89:1097, 1989.
17. Clements DE: The nutrition intervention project for underweight pregnant women, Clin Nutr 7:205, 1988.
18. Bruce L and Tsabo J: Nutrition intervention program in a prenatal clinic, Obstet Gynecol 74:310, 1989.
19. Orstead C et al: Efficacy of prenatal nutrition counseling: weight gain, infant birthweight, and cost effectiveness, J Am Diet Assoc 85:40, 1985.
20. Rush D: The National WIC Evaluation: an evaluation of the Special Supplemental Food Program for Women, Infants, and Children, vols I and II, Research Triangle Park, NC, 1986, Research Triangle Institute and New York State Research Foundation for Mental Hygiene.
21. Food and Nutrition Board, National Research Council, National Academy of Sciences: Recommended dietary allowances, ed 10, Washington, DC, 1989, National Academy Press.
22. Hytten FE and Leitch I: The physiology of human pregnancy, ed 2, Oxford, 1971, Blackwell Scientific Publications, Inc.
23. Durnin JVGA: Energy requirements of pregnancy: an integration of the longitudinal data from the five-country study, Lancet 2:1131, 1987.
24. Lechtig A et al: Effect of food supplementation during pregnancy on birth weight, Pediatrics 56:508, 1975.
25. Rush D et al: A randomized controlled trial of prenatal supplementation in New York City, Pediatrics 65:683, 1980.
26. Rush D et al: Controlled trial of prenatal nutrition supplementation defended, Pediatrics 66:656, 1980.
27. Giroud A: Nutritional requirements of the embryo, World Rev Nutr Diet 18:195, 1973.
28. Dansky LV: Anticonvulsants, folate levels and pregnancy outcome: a prospective study, Ann Neurol 21:176, 1987.
29. Smithells RW et al: Vitamin deficiencies and neural tube defects, Arch Dis Child 51:944, 1976.
30. Smithells RW et al: Possible prevention of neural tube defects by periconceptional vitamin supplementation, Lancet 1:339, 1980.
31. Smithells RW et al: Apparent prevention of neural tube defects by periconceptional vitamin supplementation, Arch Dis Child 56:911, 1981.
32. Smithells RW et al: Further experience of vitamin supplementation for prevention of neural tube defect recurrences, Lancet 1:1027, 1983.
33. Laurence KM et al: Double-blind randomized controlled trial of folate treatment before conception to prevent recurrence of neural tube defects, Br Med J 282:1509, 1981.
34. Wald NJ: Neural tube defects and vitamins: the need for a randomized clinical trial, Br J Obstet Gynaecol 91:516, 1984.
35. Mulinara J et al: Periconceptional use of multivitamins and the occurrence of neural tube defects, JAMA 260:3141, 1988.
36. Milunsky A et al: Multivitamin/folic acid supplementation in early pregnancy reduces the prevalence of neural tube defects, JAMA 262:2847, 1989.
37. Mills JL et al: The absence of a relation between periconceptional use of vitamins and neural tube defects, N Engl J Med 321:430, 1989.
38. Ejderjamm J and Hamfelt A: Pyridoxal phosphate concentration in blood in newborn infants and their mothers compared with the amount of extra pyridoxal taken during pregnancy and breast-feeding, Acta Paediatr Scand 69:327, 1980.

39. Worthington-Roberts BS, Vermeersch J, and Williams SR: Nutrition in pregnancy and lactation, ed 4, St Louis, 1989, Times Mirror/Mosby College Publishing.
40. Pulkkinen MO et al: Serum vitamin B_6 in pure pregnancy depression, Acta Obstet Gynecol Scand 57:471, 1978.
41. Roepke B and Kirksey A: Vitamin B_6 nurtriture during pregnancy and lactation, I. Vitamin B_6 intake, levels of the vitamin in biological fluids, and conditions of the infant at birth, Am J Clin Nutr 32:2249, 1979.
42. Schuster K et al: Vitamin B_6 status of the low-income adolescent and adult pregnant women and the condition of their infants at birth, Am J Clin Nutr 34:1731, 1981.
43. Schuster K et al: Effect of maternal pyridoxine HCl supplementation on the vitamin B_6 status of mother and infant and on pregnancy outcome, J Nutr 114:977, 1984.
44. Schuster K et al: Morning sickness and vitamin B_6 status of pregnant women, Hum Nutr Clin Nutr 39C:75, 1984.
45. Wheatley D: Treatment of pregnancy sickness, Br J Obstet Gynaecol 84:444, 1977.
46. Wideman CL et al: Ascorbic acid deficiency and premature rupture of fetal membranes, Am J Obstet Gynecol 88:592, 1964.
47. Clemetson CAB and Anderson L: Ascorbic acid metabolism in pre-eclampsia, Obstet Gynecol 24:774, 1964.
48. Cochrane WA: Overnutrition in prenatal and neonatal life: a problem? Can Med Assoc J 93:893, 1965.
49. Norkus EP and Rosso P: Effects of maternal intake of ascorbic acid on the postnatal metabolism of this vitamin in the guinea pig, J Nutr 111:624, 1981.
50. Roberts RA et al: Antenatal factors in neonatal hypocalcemic convulsions, Lancet 2:809, 1973.
51. Purvis RJ et al: Enamel hypoplasia of the teeth associated with neonatal tetany: a manifestation of maternal vitamin D deficiency, Lancet 2:811, 1973.
52. Delvin EE et al: Vitamin D supplementation during pregnancy: effect on neonatal calcium homeostasis, J Pediatr 109:328, 1986.
53. Brooke OG et al: Vitamin D supplements in pregnant Asian women: effects on calcium status and fetal growth, Br Med J 1:751, 1980.
54. Bernhardt JR and Dorsey DJ: Hypervitaminosis A and congenital renal anomalies in a human infant, Obstet Gynecol 43:750, 1974.
55. Strange L et al: Hypervitaminosis A in early human pregnancy and malformations of the central nervous system, Acta Obstet Scand 57:289, 1978.
56. Benke PI: The isotretinoin syndrome, JAMA 25:3267, 1984.
57. Lammar EJ et al: Retinoic acid embryopathy, N Engl J Med 313:837, 1985.
58. Marwick C: More cautionary labeling appears on isotretinoin, JAMA 251:3208, 1984.
59. Haga P et al: Plasma tocopherol levels and vitamin B-lipoprotein relationships during pregnancy and in cord blood, Am J Clin Nutr 36:1200, 1982.
60. Kazzi NJ et al: Placental transfer of vitamin K1 in preterm pregnancy, Obstet Gynecol 75:334, 1990.
61. Morales WJ et al: The use of antenatal vitamin K in the prevention of early neonatal intraventricular hemorrhage, Am J Obstet Gynecol 159:774, 1988.
62. Sisson TRC and Lund CJ: The influence of maternal iron deficiency on the newborn, Am J Clin Nutr 6:376, 1958.
63. McFee JG: Anemia: a high-risk complication of pregnancy, Clin Obstet Gynecol 16:153, 1973.
64. Romslo I et al: Iron requirement in normal pregnancy assessed by serum ferritin, serum transferrin saturation and erythrocyte protoporphyrin determinations, Br J Obstet Gynaecol 90:101, 1983.
65. Widdowson EM: Growth and composition of the fetus and newborn. In Assali NE, ed: Biology of gestation, vol 2, New York, 1968, Academic Press.
66. Villar J and Belizan JM: Calcium during pregnancy, Clin Nutr 5:55, 1986.

67. Duggin GG et al: Calcium balance in pregnancy, Lancet 2:926, 1974.

68. Felton DJC and Stone WD: Osteomalacia in Asian immigrants during pregnancy, Br Med J 1:1521, 1966.

69. Villar J and Repke JT: Calcium supplementation during pregnancy may reduce preterm delivery in high-risk populations, Am J Obstet Gynecol 163:1124, 1990.

70. Lopez-Jaramillo P: Calcium supplementation reduces the risk of pregnancy-induced hypertension in an Andes population, Br J Obstet Gynaecol 96:648, 1989.

71. Belizan JM: The relationship between calcium intake and pregnancy-induced hypertension: up-to-date evidence, Am J Obstet Gynecol 153:898, 1988.

72. Villar J: Calcium supplementation reduces blood pressure during pregnancy: results of a randomized controlled clinical trial, Obstet Gynecol 70:317, 1987.

73. Allen LH: Trace elements and outcome of human pregnancy, Clin Nutr 5:72, 1986.

74. Apgar J: Zinc and reproduction, Annu Rev Nutr 5:43, 1985.

75. Solomans NH et al: Zinc needs during pregnancy, Clin Nutr 5:63, 1986.

76. Soltan MH and Jenkins MH: Maternal and fetal plasma zinc concentration and fetal abnormality, Br J Obstet Gynaecol 89:56, 1982.

77. Hurley LS: Trace metals in mammalian development, Johns Hopkins Med J 148:1, 1981.

78. Sandstead HH et al: Zinc deficiency in pregnant rhesus monkeys: effects on behavior of infants, Am J Clin Nutr 31:844, 1978.

79. Bergmann KE et al: Abnormalities of hair zinc concentration in mothers of newborn infants with spina bifida, Am J Clin Nutr 33:2145, 1980.

80. Cherry FF et al: Plasma zinc hypertension-toxemia and other reproductive variables in adolescent pregnancy, Am J Clin Nutr 34:2367, 1981.

81. Meadows NJ et al: Zinc and small babies, Lancet 2:1135, 1981.

82. Jameson S: Effects of zinc deficiency in human reproduction, Acta Med Scand 593(suppl): 1976.

83. Ghosh A et al: Zinc deficiency is not a cause for abortion, congenital abnormality, and small-for-gestational-age infant in Chinese women, Br J Obstet Gynaecol 92:886, 1985.

84. Hunt IF et al: Zinc supplementation during pregnancy: effects on selected blood constituents and on progress and outcome of pregnancy in low-income women of Mexican descent, Am J Clin Nutr 40:508, 1984.

85. Mukherjee MD et al: Maternal zinc, iron, folic acid, and protein nutriture and outcome of human pregnancy, Am J Clin Nutr 40:496, 1984.

86. Connolly KJ et al: Fetal iodine deficiency and motor performance during childhood, Lancet 2:1149, 1979.

87. Bursel RG and Watson ML: The effect of sodium restriction during gestation on offspring brain development in rats, Am J Clin Nutr 37:43, 1983.

88. Pike RL et al: Juxtaglomerular degranulation and zona glomerulosa exhaustion in pregnant rats induced by low-sodium intakes and reversed by sodium load, Am J Obstet Gynecol 95:604, 1966.

89. Lelong-Tissier MC et al: Hyponatremie maternofetale carentielle par regime desode, Arch Fr Pediatr 34:64, 1977.

90. Horner RD et al: Pica practices of pregnant women, J Am Diet Assoc 91:34, 1991.

91. National Research Council, Food and Nutrition Board: Alternative dietary practices and nutritional abuses in pregnancy, Washington, DC, 1982, National Academy of Sciences.

92. Lackey CJ: Pica—pregnancy etiological mystery. In National Academy of Sciences: Alternative dietary practices and nutritional abuses in pregnancy, Washington, DC, 1982, National Academy of Sciences.

93. Lillien LJ et al: Diet and ethanol intake during pregnancy, J Am Diet Assoc 81:252, 1982.

94. Streissguth AP et al: Comparison of drinking and smoking patterns during pregnancy over a six-year interval, Am J Obstet Gynecol 145:716, 1983.

95. Rosett HL et al: Patterns of alcohol consumption and fetal development, Obstet Gynecol 61:539, 1983.

96. Rosett HL et al: Treatment experience with pregnant problem drinkers, JAMA 249:2029, 1983.
97. Groisser DS et al: Coffee consumption during pregnancy: subsequent behavioral abnormalities of the offspring, J Nutr 112:829, 1982.
98. Dunlop M and Court JM: Effects of maternal caffeine ingestion on neonatal growth in rats, Biol Neonate 39:178, 1981.
99. Collins TFX et al: A study of the teratogenetic potential of caffeine ingestion in drinking water, Food Chem Toxicol 21:763, 1983.
100. Kurppa K et al: Coffee consumption during pregnancy, N Engl J Med 306:1548, 1982.
101. Linn S et al: No association between coffee consumption and adverse outcomes of pregnancy, N Engl J Med 306:141, 1982.
102. Rosenberg L et al: Selected birth defects in relation to caffeine-containing beverages, JAMA 247:1429, 1982.
103. Furuhashi N: Effects of caffeine consumption during pregnancy, Gynecol Obstet Invest 19:187, 1985.
104. Streitfeld PP: Congenital malformation: teratogenic foods and additives, Birth Fam J 5:7, 1978.
105. Kline J et al: Spontaneous abortion and the use of sugar substitutes, Am J Obstet Gynecol 130:708, 1978.
106. Hoover R: Saccharin—bitter aftertaste? N Engl J Med 302:573, 1980.
107. Koos BJ and Longo LD: Mercury toxicity in the pregnant woman, fetus, and newborn infant: a review, Am J Obstet Gynecol 126:390, 1976.
108. Culpepper L: Exercise during pregnancy. In Merkatz IR et al, eds: New perspectives in prenatal care, New York, 1990, Elsevier, pp 193-210.
109. Clapp JF and Dickstein S: Endurance exercise and pregnancy outcome, Med Sci Sports Exer 16:556, 1984.
110. Clapp JF and Capeless EL: Neonatal morphometrics after endurance exercise during pregnancy, Am J Obstet Gynecol 163:1805, 1990.
111. Clapp JF: The effects of maternal exercise on early pregnancy outcome, Am J Obstet Gynecol 161:1453, 1989.
112. Clapp JF: The course of labor after endurance exercise during pregnancy, Am J Obstet Gynecol 163:1790, 1990.
113. American College of Obstetricians and Gynecologists: Exercise during pregnancy and the postnatal period (ACOG Home Exercise Programs). In ACOG Technical Bulletin: Women and exercise, no 87, Washington, DC, 1985, ACOG.
114. Picone TA et al: Pregnancy outcome in North American women, I. Effects of diet, cigarette smoking, and psychological stress on maternal weight gain, Am J Clin Nutr 36:1205, 1982.
115. Papoz L et al: Maternal smoking and birth weight in relation to dietary habits, Am J Obstet Gynecol 142:870, 1982.
116. Task Force on Nutrition: American College of Obstetrics and Gynecology and American Dietetic Association, Chicago, 1978.
117. King JC: Dietary risk patterns during pregnancy. In Weinger J and Briggs G, eds: Nutrition update 1:206, 1983.
118. National High Blood Pressure Education Program Working Group Report on High Blood Pressure in Pregnancy, Am J Obstet Gynecol 163:1691, 1990.
119. Summary of Recommendations of the Second International Workshop Conferences on Gestational Diabetes Mellitus, Diabetes 34(suppl 2), 1985.
120. Nuwayhid BS, Brinkman CR, and Leib SM, eds: Management of the diabetic pregnancy, New York, 1987, Elsevier.

Further Reading

Brown JE: Nutrition for your pregnancy, Minneapolis, 1983, University of Minnesota Press.

This well written popular book on diet and nutrition during pregnancy continues to provide an excellent resource for the general public.

Hess MA and Hunt AE: Pickles and ice cream, New York, 1982, McGraw-Hill.

This award-winning book on diet and pregnancy designed to help mothers through their pregnancies continues to be an excellent practical resource.

Institute of Medicine, National Academy of Sciences: Nutrition during pregnancy: weight gain and nutrient supplements, Washington, DC, 1990, National Academy Press.

This new report provides detailed background for current recommendations for maternity care in the two areas of concern for both mothers and their care providers, weight gain and nutrient supplements.

Worthington-Roberts BS and Williams SR: Nutrition in pregnancy and lactation, ed 4, St. Louis, 1989, Times Mirror/Mosby College Publishing.

This manual provides detailed background on issues related to nutrition during pregnancy and lactation.

5

Lactation and Human Milk

Bonnie S. Worthington-Roberts

Basic Concepts

❖❖

- ✔ *Specific female anatomy and physiology provide the required structures and functions for normal postpartum lactation.*
- ✔ *Human milk is designed to meet human infant needs.*
- ✔ *Successful lactation requires nutritional support.*
- ✔ *Breastfeeding provides the primary means of supporting growth and development of young infants.*
- ✔ *Physiologic knowledge and personal skills underlie sensitive counseling for the breastfeeding mother.*

*L*actation is a physiologic process accomplished by females since the origin of mammals. Today, as in times past, the process of breastfeeding is successfully initiated by at least 99% of women who try. All that is required of the lactating mother is an intact mammary gland (or preferably two) and the presence and operation of appropriate physiologic mechanisms that allow for adequate milk production and release.

From this basic physiologic view, the establishment and maintenance of human lactation are determined by at least three factors:

1. The anatomic structure of the mammary tissue and the development of milk-producing cells (alveoli), ducts, and nipples to produce and then deliver the milk
2. The initiation and maintenance of milk secretion
3. The ejection or propulsion of milk from the alveoli to the nipple

But the most significant term above is the word "human." This brings an added personal dimension to the physiologic process. Breastfeeding is a very personal process for a mother.

In this chapter, then, we look at lactation, human milk, and breastfeeding in both physiologic and "human" terms. Clear knowledge of the physiologic factors listed above, which includes nutritional needs, is essential for effective lactation management. Furthermore, sensitivity to the personal needs involved is essential for helping mothers have satisfying breastfeeding experiences. Both of these aspects will be explored to provide individual support for today's mother who is largely inexperienced in breastfeeding.

BREAST ANATOMY AND DEVELOPMENT
Anatomy of the Mammary Gland

Basic structure. The **mammary gland** of the human female consists of milk-producing cells (glandular epithelium) and a duct system embedded in connective tissue and fat (Fig. 5-1).[1] The size of the breast is variable, but in most instances it extends from the second through the sixth rib and from the central breast bone (sternum) to the arm pit. The

Mammary glands
(Gr *mamme,* mother's breast) Milk-producing glands in the females of all mammal species, humans and animals, distinguished from all other animal life by bearing live young and producing milk to nourish them.

FIG. 5-1 **A,** General anatomic features of the human breast showing its location on the chest, more specifically, the anterior region of the thorax between the sternum and the anterior axillary line. **B,** Detailed structural features of the human mammary gland showing the terminal glandular (alveolar) tissue of each lobule leading into the duct system, which eventually enlarges into the lactiferous duct and lactiferous sinus. The lactiferous sinuses rest beneath the areola and converge at the nipple pore.

mammary tissue lies directly over the large chest muscle (pectoralis major muscle) and is separated from this muscle by a layer of fat, which is continuous with the fatty tissue of the gland itself.

Areola. The center of the fully developed breast in the adult woman is marked by the **areola,** a circular pigmented skin area from 1.5 to 2.5 cm in diameter. The surface of the areola appears rough because of the presence of large, somewhat modified fluid-producing glands, which are located directly beneath the skin in the thin subcutaneous tissue layer. The fatty secretion of these glands is believed to lubricate the nipple. Bundles of smooth muscle fibers in the areolar tissue serve to stiffen the nipple for a better grasp by the sucking infant.

Nipple and duct system. The nipple is elevated above the breast and contains 15 to 20 **lactiferous ducts** surrounded by modified muscle cell tissues and covered by wrinkled skin. Partly within this compartment of the nipple and partly below its base, these ducts expand to form the short lactiferous sinuses in which milk may be stored. The sinuses are the continuations of the mammary ducts, which extend outward from the nipple toward the chest wall with numerous secondary branches. The duct system ends in masses of milk-producing cells, which form subsections or **lobules** of the breast (Fig. 5-1).

Adolescent-adult development. During adolescence, as indicated in Chapter 3, the female breasts enlarge to their adult size. Frequently, one breast is slightly larger than the other, but this difference is usually unnoticeable. In a nonpregnant woman the mature breast weighs approximately 200 g, the left being somewhat larger than the right. During pregnancy there is some increase in size and weight such that by term the breast may weigh between 400 and 600 g. During lactation this weight increases to between 600 and 800 g.

Variation after childbirth. Wide variation in the structural composition of the human breasts has been observed in women after childbirth. Some breasts contain little secretory tissue; some large breasts contain less glandular tissue than much smaller organs. It is well known, however, that neither size nor structural composition of the breast significantly influences **lactation** success in the average woman. Almost all women who want to breastfeed find that they can.

Breast Development

Infancy and childhood. In the human newborn the mammary glands are developed sufficiently to appear as distinct, round elevations, which feel like movable soft masses. Through the microscope future milk ducts and glandular lobules can be recognized easily. These early glandular structures can produce a milk-like secretion ("witch's milk") 2 or 3 days after birth. All of these **neonatal** phenomena related to the mammary glands probably result from the intensive developmental processes that occur in the last stages of intra-uterine life. Usually they subside in the first few weeks after birth. Some shrinkage or involution in the breast takes place by the time the infant is several weeks old, and this is followed by the "quiescent" period of mammary growth and activity during infancy and childhood.

Adolescence. With the onset of puberty and during adolescence, an increased output of estrogenic hormone accomplishes ovarian maturation and follicular stimulation (p. 73). As a result of this response, the mammary ducts elongate, and their lining cells reduplicate and proliferate. The growth of the ductal cells is accompanied by growth of fibrous and fatty tissue, which is largely responsible for the increasing size and firmness of the adolescent gland. During this period the areola and nipple also grow and become pigmented.

Areola
(L *areola*, area, space) Pigmented area surrounding the nipple of the human breast.

Lactiferous ducts
(L *lac*, milk; *ferre*, to bear; *ducere*, to lead or draw) Vessels producing or conveying milk from producing cells to storage and release areas of the breast; tube or passage for secretions.

Lobule
(L *lobus*, lobe, a well-defined area) Smaller branching vessels that make up a lobe of the mammary gland.

Lactation
(L *lactare*, to suckle) Process of milk production and secretion in the mammary glands.

Neonatal
(Gr *neos*, new; L *natus*, born) Relating to the period surrounding birth, especially the first 4 weeks after birth when the newborn is called a neonate.

Breast Maturation

Hormonal effects. As the developing woman matures and ovulation patterns become established, the regular development of progesterone-producing corpora lutea in the ovaries (p. 74) promotes the second stage of mammary development. Lobules gradually appear, giving the mammary glands the characteristic lobular structure found during the childbearing period. This differentiation into a lobular gland is completed about 12 to 18 months after the first menstrual period, but further development continues in proportion to the intensity of the hormonal stimuli during each menstrual cycle and especially during pregnancies.

Functional mammary tissue. Some young women enter reproductive life with insufficient functional mammary tissue to produce enough milk for their baby's total nourishment. In some cases this relates to underdevelopment of the mammary ductwork associated with periodic cessation of menstruation (amenorrhea) or very late menarche. In addition, there are women who have had surgery to remove cysts, tumors, or other growths; others have undergone surgery for breast reduction or reconstruction. For whatever reason, circumstances exist in which functional mammary tissue is insufficient to fully support a nursing infant. Fortunately these situations are rare.

Preparation during pregnancy. The mammary gland of a nonpregnant woman is inadequately prepared for secretory activity. Only during pregnancy do changes occur that make satisfactory milk production possible. In the first trimester of pregnancy the small ducts sprouting from the mammary ducts proliferate to create a maximum number of surface cells for future alveolar cell formation. In the mid-trimester the reduplicated small ductules group together to form large lobules. Their central cavities begin to dilate. In the last trimester the existent clumps of milk-producing cells progressively dilate in the final preparation for the lactation process.

Role of the placenta. The placenta plays an important role in mammary growth in pregnancy. It secretes ovarian-like hormones in large quantities. A number of these hormones have been identified as contributing to mammary gland growth.

Antepartum preparation. Although mammary growth and development occur rapidly throughout pregnancy, additional proliferation of lining cells takes place in the **antepartum** period shortly before delivery of the baby or at **parturition.** The proliferation of these cells that begins just before parturition in response to increasing levels of the hormone **prolactin** results in new cells with a new complement of enzymes.

THE PHYSIOLOGY OF LACTATION
General Activity

Initial postpartum secretions. Full lactation does not begin as soon as the baby is born. During the first 2 or 3 days **postpartum** a small amount of **colostrum** is secreted. In subsequent days a rapid increase in milk secretion occurs, and in usual cases lactation is reasonably well established by the end of the first week. In first-time mothers (primiparas), however, the establishment of lactation may be delayed until the third week or even later. Generally, therefore, the first 2 or 3 weeks are a period of lactation initiation, and this is followed by the longer period of maintenance of lactation.

Milk production stages. Initiation and maintenance of lactation comprises a complex process involving both nerves and hormones. It involves the sensory nerves in the nipples, the spinal cord, the hypothalamus, and the pituitary gland with its various hormones. The process of milk production occurs in two distinct stages: (1) secretion of milk and (2) propulsion or ejection whereby the milk passes along the duct system. The two events are closely related and often occur simultaneously in the nursing mother.

Antepartum
(L *ante*, before; *partum*, parting, a separate part) Period of gestation before onset of labor and the birth of the infant.

Parturition
(L *parturitio*, to give birth) Act or process of childbirth; labor and delivery.

Prolactin
(Gr *pro-*, before; L *lac*, milk) Hormone of the anterior pituitary gland that stimulates and maintains lactation in postpartum mammals.

Colostrum
(L *colostrum*, bee sting swelling and secretions) Thin, yellowish milky liquid, mother's initial breast secretion before and immediately after birth of her baby; rich in immune factors and nutrition, especially protein and minerals; foremilk.

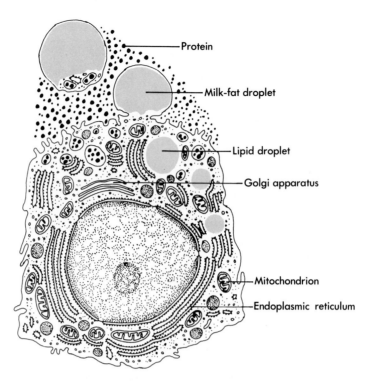

Protein

Milk-fat droplet

Lipid droplet

Golgi apparatus

Mitochondrion

Endoplasmic reticulum

FIG. 5-2   Diagrammatic representation of a mammary gland cell showing the basic square shape with typical wavy surface border and nucleus. Cytoplasmic organization is characteristic of cells undergoing active protein synthesis and secretion. The synthetic apparatus consists of many free ribosomes and an extensive system of rough endoplasmic reticulum. A large Golgi body is located above the nucleus, and associated with it are some vacuoles containing particulate material that condenses into a central core or granule. Toward the top, the granules become progressively larger and contain more dense protein granules. The vacuoles fuse with the surface membrane and liberate their contents intact into the lumen. Fat droplets are found throughout the cell but are largest near the top. They protrude into the lumen and appear to pinch off from the cell proper along with a small bit of cytoplasm. Other cytoplasmic structures include large mitochondria lysosomes, and a small number of smooth membranous tubules and vesicles.

Modified from Lentz TL: Cell fine structure: an atlas of drawings of whole cell-structure, Philadelphia, 1971, WB Saunders Co.

The secretion of milk involves both the synthesis of the milk components and the passage of the formed product into the ducts (Fig. 5-2). These events may be under independent control, since the accumulation of both fat and protein reaches a high level during the latter part of pregnancy. Shortly before delivery the accumulated secretory products begin to pass into the duct system. The secretory process is activated again by the sucking stimulus of the infant.

In general, each milk-producing **alveolar** cell proceeds through a secretory process that is preceded and followed by a resting stage (Fig. 5-3). Milk synthesis is most active during the suckling period but occurs at lower levels at other times. The secretory cells are square but change to a cylindric shape just before milk secretion while cellular water uptake is increased. As secretion commences, the enlarged cell with its thickened surface becomes clublike in shape. The tip pinches off leaving the cell intact. The milk constituents

Alveoli
(L *alveolus,* hollow) Small sac-like outpouching areas in the mammary gland, secretory units that produce and secrete milk.

Resting cell   Beginning milk synthesis   Active milk secretion   Regression to resting state

FIG. 5-3 Diagrammatic representation of the cycle of changes that occur in secretory cells of the alveoli from resting stage through milk production and secretion with eventual return to the resting stage.

are then free in the secreted solution, and the cell retains a cap of membrane. Between periods of active milk secretion, alveolar cells return to their characteristic resting state.

Fat Synthesis and Release

Initial synthesis. Fat synthesis takes place in the **endoplasmic reticulum** from compounds synthesized intracellularly or imported from the maternal circulation. Alveolar cells are able to synthesize short chain fatty acids, which are derived predominantly from available acetate. Long chain fatty acids and triglycerides are derived from maternal plasma; these fatty acids are predominantly used for the synthesis of milk fat. Synthesis of triglyceride from intracellular carbohydrate also plays a predominant role in fat production for human milk.

Final preparation and release. The process of **esterification** of fatty acids takes place in the endoplasmic reticulum. The resultant triglycerides accumulate as small fat droplets in the endoplasmic reticulum but eventually coalesce in the basal region of the cell to form large droplets that migrate toward the top of the cell. Ultimately these droplets bulge into the lumen for eventual discharge. **Apocrine** secretion involves the protrusion of the cell surface into the lumen with eventual pinching off of the protruded unit. This discharged material usually contains fat globules, protein, and a small amount of **cytoplasm,** all of which will appear in human milk.

Protein Synthesis and Discharge

Initial synthesis. The vast majority of proteins present in normal milk are specific to mammary secretions and are not identified in any quantity elsewhere in nature. The formation of milk protein including mammary enzymes is induced by prolactin and further stimulated by other hormones. Studies using sophisticated microscopic techniques have clearly shown that the abundant rough endothelial reticulum is the site of protein synthesis in the secretory cell.

Final preparation and release. Protein granules accumulate within the Golgi complexes before transport through the cell and release into the lumen by apocrine secretion or reverse **pinocytosis.** The proteins in milk are derived from two sources: (1) some are synthesized **de novo** in the mammary gland, and (2) others are derived as such from plasma. Inclusion of plasma-derived proteins in the milk secretion occurs primarily in the

Endoplasmic reticulum
(Gr *endon,* within; *plassein,* to form; L *rete,* net) A protoplasmic network of flattened double-membrane sheets in cells; important metabolic cell organelles, some with rough surfaces bearing ribosomes for protein synthesis and other smooth surfaces synthesizing fatty acids.

Cytoplasm
(Gr *kytos,* hollow vessel; *plasma,* anything formed or molded) Protoplasm of the cell outside the nucleus, a continuous gel-like aqueous solution in which the cell organelles are suspended; site of major cell metabolism.

De novo
(L *anew,* from the beginning) To make afresh from primary components; "from scratch," as in cooking.

early secretory product colostrum. Thereafter the three main proteins in milk—casein, alpha-lactalbumin, and beta-lactalbumin—are synthesized within the gland from amino acid precursors. All of the essential and some of the nonessential amino acids are taken up directly from the plasma, but some of the nonessential amino acids are synthesized by the milk-producing cells of the gland.

Carbohydrate Synthesis and Release

Golgi apparatus
A complex cup-like structure of membranes with associated vesicles first described by Italian Nobel prize-winning histologist Camillo Golgi (1843-1926); synthesis site of numerous carbohydrate metabolic products such as lactose, glyco-proteins, and muco-polysaccharides.

Vesicle
(L *vesica*, bladder) A small bladder or sac containing liquid; se-cretory transport sacs that move out into the cell cytoplasm to aid metabolism.

Lactose synthesis. The predominant carbohydrate in milk is lactose. Its synthesis occurs within the **Golgi apparatus** of the alveolar cell. The synthesis of lactose combines glucose and galactose. Most of the intracellular glucose is derived continually from circulating blood glucose; galactose is synthesized from glucose.

Final preparation and release. Once synthesized within the Golgi complex, lactose is attached to protein and carried to the cell surface in a **vesicle.** It is then released from the surface of the cell by reverse pinocytosis, as occurs with several other milk components.

The Role of Hormones

Milk secretion. The stimulus for milk secretion derives largely from the hormone prolactin (Fig. 5-4). This hormone acts on alveolar cells and promotes continual milk production and release. Maintenance of milk secretion, however, requires other hormonal factors from the anterior pituitary. If sucking is discontinued during the lactation period, pituitary release of these necessary hormones ceases and milk secretion usually stops in the following few days, with accompanying deterioration and sloughing of alveolar cells.

Relation of oral contraceptive agents. Estrogen inhibits milk production, especially in the early stage of lactation. However, studies of the use of combined estrogen-progestin oral contraceptive agents (OTAs) (p. 75) indicate that lactation is not inhibited in women who wish to nurse their infants, as long as the pill is not used in the immediate postpartum

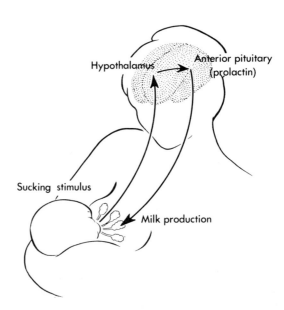

FIG. 5-4 Diagrammatic representation of the basic physiologic features of milk production. The sucking stimulus provided by the baby sends a message to the hypothalamus. The hypothalamus stimulates the anterior pituitary to release prolactin, the hormone that promotes milk production by alveolar cells of the mammary glands.

period. Some dose-related suppression of the quantity of milk produced and the duration of lactation is found with extended use. Even though several reports suggest that measurable composition changes occur in the milk produced by women taking OTAs, results are inconsistent and largely viewed as insignificant.

The "Let-Down" Reflex

Primary stimulus. Once milk production and secretion have been accomplished, the baby may then obtain this milk by promoting its ejection from the ducts. The milk ejection or "let-down" reflex is a mechanism involving both nerves and hormones that is regulated in part by central nervous system factors (Fig. 5-5). The primary stimulus is sucking on the nipple, which triggers the discharge of the hormone **oxytocin** from the posterior pituitary. Oxytocin is carried in the bloodstream to the muscle-like **(myoepithelial) cells** around the alveoli and along the duct system, where it is easily available to the nursing baby.

Psychologic influences. The milk ejection reflex appears to be sensitive to small differences in circulating oxytocin level. Thus even minor emotional and psychologic disturbances can influence the degree to which breast milk is released to the baby. The significance of psychologic influences on the milk ejection reflex in humans has been demonstrated by numerous case histories. These experiences illustrate the fact that milk ejection can be inhibited by embarrassment or stress, or it can be set off by the mere thought of the baby or the sound of his cry. This observation has been confirmed by experimental stimulation (or inhibition) of the milk ejection reflex. Signs of successful let-down of milk are easily recognized by the nursing mother. Common and significant occurrences include: (1) milk dripping from the breasts before the baby starts nursing, (2) milk dripping from the breast opposite to the one being nursed, (3) contractions of

Oxytocin
(Gr *oxys*, sharp, sour; *tokos*, birth) Pituitary hormone causing uterine contraction and milk ejection.

Myoepithelial cells
(Gr *mys*, muscle; *epi-*, on; *thele*, nipple) Tissue composed of contractile epithelial cells surrounding the alveoli and duct system of the lactating breasts.

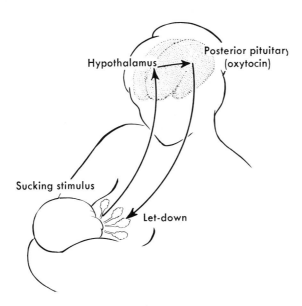

FIG. 5-5 Diagrammatic representation of the basic features of the "let-down reflex." The sucking stimulus arrives at the hypothalamus, which promotes the release of oxytocin from the posterior pituitary. Oxytocin stimulates the contraction of the muscle-like (myoepithelial) cells around the alveoli in the mammary glands. Contraction of these muscle-like cells causes the milk to be propelled through the duct system and into the lactiferous sinuses, where it becomes available to the nursing infant.

the uterus during breastfeeding, often causing slight pain or discomfort, and (4) a tingling sensation in the breast.

Sucking stimulus. Sucking stimulation is widely accepted as the most effective means of maintaining adequate lactation. There is considerable evidence in human subjects that the restriction of sucking significantly inhibits lactation. Artificial sucking stimulation in the form of manual expression or a breast pump has repeatedly been recommended as a means of increasing milk yield or maintaining yield in the absence of the baby. Evidence suggests that feeding on demand optimally stimulates the lactation process.

Duration of lactation. Local and cultural patterns of infant feeding are of great significance in determining the duration of breastfeeding for a given mother. Although successful lactation can continue as long as sucking stimulation is maintained, a gradual fall in the amount of milk produced generally develops after 12 months. This drop in milk output largely relates to reduced demand and loss of recurrent nipple stimulation by the baby.

GENERAL NATURE OF MAMMALIAN MILK
Unique Species Variation

Many investigations during the past decade have defined the biochemical and nutritional properties of different types of mammalian milk. It is clear from these studies that each type of milk is unique and consists of a highly complex mixture of organic and inorganic compounds.

Mother-child relation and nature of milk. It is likely that the characteristics of mammalian milks relate directly to variable mother-child relationships that take place in infancy. Shaul found support for this idea while examining five groups of wild animals[2]:

Marsupial

(L *marsupium*, a pouch) Member of the animal class of mammals who bear undeveloped young, which they carry and nourish in an abdominal pouch until their development is complete; includes such animals as kangaroos and koala bears.

Group 1. Marsupials and animals that bear their young while in hibernation. In these animals the mother is available at all times and the milk is dilute and low in fat.

Group 2. Animals born in a relatively mature state that follow or are carried by their mothers at all times. Here the maternal attentiveness is high and the milk produced is rather low in fat and dilute. The low fat content is often seen in milks of animals that nurse frequently.

Group 3. Animals that leave their young in a secluded place and return to them at widely spaced intervals. The lioness is a good example of this type. This group of animals has very concentrated milk that is high in fat.

Group 4. Animals born in a relatively immature state and that remain for a considerable time in nests or burrows. The mother must leave for several hours at a time and nursing is more "on schedule" rather than "on demand."

Group 5. Animals that spend much time in cold water or when on land are frequently made wet by the mother returning from the water. In all these cases the milk is very concentrated and has an extremely high fat content.

Comparison of human milk. Human milk is dilute and thus resembles the milk of the marsupials and hibernating bears whose offspring feed constantly. It is therefore not surprising that the human baby demands to be fed frequently (Table 5-1). For this reason, in many parts of the world the mother carries the baby where she goes at all times.

The Nature of Human Milk

Variable basic content. Reports during the past 15 years on the biochemical composition of human milk have included over 1000 publications. Large numbers of new components continue to be characterized such that more than a hundred constituents are now recognized. Basically human milk consists of a solution of protein, sugar, and salts

TABLE 5-1   *Nutrient Content of Mature Human Milk*

Constituent (per Liter)	Human Milk	Constituent (per Liter)	Human Milk
Energy (kcal)	680	Minerals	
Protein (g)	10.5	Calcium (mg)	280
Fat (g)	39.0	Phosphorus (mg)	140
Lactose (g)	72.0	Sodium (mg)	180
Vitamins		Potassium (mg)	525
Vitamin A (RE)*	670	Chloride (mg)	420
Vitamin D (μg)	0.55	Magnesium (mg)	35
Vitamin E (mg)	2.3	Iron (mg)	0.3
Vitamin K (μg)	2.1	Iodine (μg)	110
Thiamin (mg)	0.21	Manganese (μg)	6.0
Riboflavin (mg)	0.35	Copper (mg)	0.25
Niacin (mg)	1.5	Zinc (mg)	1.2
Pyridoxine (μg)	93	Selenium (μg)	20
Folic acid (μg)	85	Fluoride (μg)	16
Cobalamine (μg)	0.97	Chromium (μg)	50
Ascorbic acid (mg)	40		

*RE, retinol equivalents.
Data from Institute of Medicine: Nutrition during lactation. Washington, DC, 1991, National Academy Press.

in which a variety of fatty compounds are suspended (Table 5-2). The composition varies from one human to another, from one period of lactation to the next, and even hourly during the day. The composition of a given milk sample is related not only to the amount secreted and the stage of the lactation but also to the timing of the withdrawal and to individual variations among lactating mothers. These latter individual variations may be affected by such variables as maternal age, parity, health, and social class. **Gestational age** of the infant also makes a difference.

Milk volume. Observations of completely breastfed babies who appear to be thriving suggest that daily volume of breast consumption ranges from 340 to over 1000 ml/day. The mean falls between 600 and 900 ml/day, at least for representative North American women.[3] Mothers of twins may show an enhanced capacity for milk production. Hartmann, in Western Australia, compared milk outputs of mothers of single infants with that of mothers of twins.[4] The obvious difference in milk production is demonstrated in Fig. 5-6. Severe food restriction may limit the volume of milk production.[3] A lifestyle involving vigorous exercise, however, does not have a detrimental impact on milk output.[5]

Relation to maternal nutrition. Although many data have been recorded on the differences in samples of human milk, the general picture is the same throughout the world. Except for vitamin and fat content, the composition of human milk appears to be largely independent of the state of the mother's nutrition, at least until malnutrition becomes severe. Even after prolonged lactation for 2 years or more, the quality of the milk produced by Indian and African women appears to be relatively well maintained, although the quantity may be small. Also, it is well known that severely undernourished women during time of famine often manage to feed their babies reasonably well.[3]

Colostrum

In the first few days after birth, the mammary glands secrete a small amount of opaque fluid called colostrum. The volume varies between 2 and 10 ml per feeding per day during

Gestational age
(L *gestare,* to bear) Period of embryonic-fetal growth and development from ovum fertilization to birth; varying with degree of preterm development to full-term mature newborn.

TABLE 5-2   Classes of Constituents in Human Milk

Protein and nonprotein nitrogen compounds

Proteins
Caseins
α-Lactalbumin
Lactoferrin
Secretory IgA and other immunoglobulins
β-Lactoglobulin
Lysozyme
Enzymes
Hormones
Growth factors

Nonprotein nitrogen compounds
Urea
Creatine
Creatinine
Uric acid
Glucosamine
α-Amino nitrogen
Nucleic acids
Nucleotides
Polyamines

Water-soluble vitamins
Thiamin
Riboflavin
Niacin
Pantothenic acid
Biotin
Folate
Vitamin B_6
Vitamin B_{12}
Vitamin C
Inositol
Choline

Cells
Leukocytes
Epithelial cells

Carbohydrates
Lactose
Oligosaccharides
Bifidus factors
Glycopeptides

Lipids
Triglycerides
Fatty acids
Phospholipids
Sterols and hydrocarbons
Fat-soluble vitamins
  A and carotene
  D
  E
  K

Minerals
Macronutrient elements
Calcium
Phosphorus
Magnesium
Potassium
Sodium
Chlorine
Sulfur

Trace elements
Iodine
Iron
Copper
Zinc
Manganese
Selenium
Chromium
Cobalt

Modified from National Academy of Sciences: Nutrition during lactation, Washington, DC, 1991, National Academy Press.

the first 3 days, related in part to the parity of the mother. Women who have had other pregnancies, particularly those who have nursed babies previously, usually demonstrate colostrum output sooner and in greater volume than other women. Colostrum is typically yellow, a feature associated with its relatively high carotene content. Also, it contains more protein and less sugar and fat than milk produced thereafter. As might be expected from these composition differences, it is lower in kilocalories than mature milk—67 versus 75 kcal/100 ml. The ash content of colostrum is high, and concentrations of sodium,

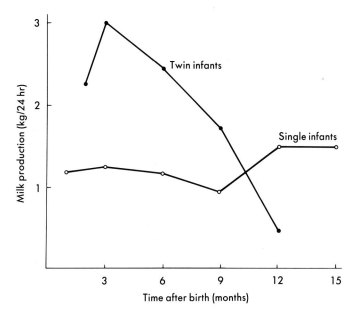

FIG. 5-6 Milk outputs of Western Australian women breastfeeding twins and exclusively breastfeeding single babies.

Based on data from Hartmann PE et al: Birth Fam J 8:215, 1981.

potassium, and chloride are greater than in mature milk. The few composition analyses of human colostrum that have been reported show striking variability during any one day and from day to day. It is likely that these differences partially reflect the unstable secretory patterns that exist in the mammary apparatus as it begins active production, secretion, and ejection of milk.

Transitional Milk

Colostrum changes to transitional milk between the third and sixth day, at which time the protein content is still rather high. By the tenth day the major changes have been completed, and by the end of the first month the protein content reaches a consistent level that does not fall significantly thereafter. As the content of protein falls, the content of lactose progressively rises. This is also the case for fat, which increases to typical levels as lactation becomes more firmly established.

Preterm Milk

With the renewed interest in the feeding of human milk to preterm infants, substantial attention has been focused on the composition of milk produced by mothers who deliver prematurely.[6] Early reports suggested that the protein and nonprotein nitrogen content of **preterm milk** was higher than that of term milk. Additional observations revealed that preterm milk might also be higher in its concentration of calcium, IgA, sodium, potassium, chloride, phosphorus, magnesium, medium chain and polyunsaturated long-chain fatty acids, and total lipids, but lower in its lactose level than term milk. Thus the opinion developed that premature infants who are fed their mother's milk might demonstrate superior growth and development to that observed in premature infants fed banked human milk. In general this suspicion has proved to be true for very low-birth-weight infants as reported by researchers who have completed appropriate comparisons. It appears, how-

Preterm milk
Milk produced by mothers of premature infants.

ever, that commercial infant formulas designed for low-birth-weight infants may also be superior to banked human milk in supporting growth of these babies.

The controversy surrounding the nutritional adequacy of human milk for very low-birth-weight infants still exists. Although recent observations suggest that premature infants can thrive on milk from their own mothers, it is known that protein and sodium concentrations are marginal and calcium and phosphate levels are too low to support optimum development of the skeleton. In the face of immature gastrointestinal and renal function and poor nutrient stores, the very low-birth-weight infant who is provided human milk will often profit from an organized supplementation program.

It is even possible to supplement human milk with a powdered or liquid product designed to improve nutritional adequacy for very low-birth-weight infants.* The powdered fortifier contains protein and carbohydrate and increases the caloric density of breast milk to about 24 kilocalories per ounce. The product is sold in premeasured packets; one packet is designed for addition to 25 ml of human milk. The liquid fortifier is similar in composition and is designed to be mixed with human milk or fed alternately with human milk.

COMPOSITION OF MATURE HUMAN MILK
Protein

Amount and types of protein. It is well known that different animals show different rates of growth. This fact appears to be related to their milk. The slowest rate of growth is found in humans and human milk contains the least protein. The major proteins found in breast milk are caseins and whey proteins. Caseins are phosphorus-containing proteins that occur only in milk. The **whey** proteins, like lactalbumin and lactoferrin, are synthesized in the mammary gland. Other proteins, including protein hormones and serum albumin, are transported to the milk from the plasma. The concentration of protein found in human milk is lower than the previously accepted value of 1.5 g/100 ml that was calculated from analyzed nitrogen content. Since human milk has been found to contain 25% of its nitrogen in nonprotein compounds, the lower protein concentration (0.8 to 0.9 g/100 ml) is now accepted as the true amount.

Initial changes. The protein content of human milk, like that of other mammals, falls rapidly over the first few days of lactation and reflects a relatively higher loss of those proteins important in immune functions. Colostrum averages about 2% protein; transitional and mature milk average 1.5% and 1.0%, respectively.

Relation to maternal diet. Observations of many women in a variety of countries have shown that protein content of human milk is not reduced in mothers consuming a diet low in protein or poor in protein quality. A study in Pakistan supports this idea.[7] Here the protein quality and quantity of milk collected from women of a very low socioeconomic group in Karachi were similar to those of well-nourished women there and in other parts of the world. Of interest, however, was the observation that the concentration of lysine and methionine in the free amino acid content of milk samples from malnourished women was reduced when compared with milk from healthy, well-nourished mothers. The investigators suggest that this finding could imply a reduction in nutritional *quality* of the protein in these samples. It is important to recognize, however, that dietary amino acid deficits may be readily subsidized from maternal tissues as long as reserves are available from which to draw in order to maintain protein homeostasis (p. 67). Temporary fluctuations in free amino acid levels may be apparent, but alterations in

Whey
The thin liquid of milk remaining after the curd, containing the mild protein casein, and the cream have been removed; contains other milk proteins lactalbumin and lactoferrin.

---

*Human Milk Fortifier, Mead Johnson Laboratories (powdered); Similac Natural Care, Ross Laboratories (liquid).

quantity or quality of intact milk proteins are much less likely to occur until maternal protein stores are severely depleted.

Effect of chronic maternal protein deficit. With chronic protein undernutrition, breast milk composition may change. One study was carried out to assess the effects of prolonged lactation on the quantity of protein and patterns of amino acids in breast milk obtained from Thai women at various times during lactation.[8] Protein levels decreased from 1.56% during the first week to a low of about 0.6% from 180 to 270 days and then rose to about 0.7%. Using these data, one can calculate that a 3-month-old infant in the 50th percentile for weight would require about 1250 ml of milk per day to meet protein needs. Since few infants in developing countries would receive this volume of milk daily and since supplemental sources of protein are scarce, the protein status of such infants could be significantly compromised.

Amino acids. The amino acid content of human milk is recognized as ideal for the human infant. It is relatively low in several amino acids that are known to be detrimental if found in the blood at high levels, for example, in the genetic disease phenylalanine; on the other hand it is high in other amino acids that the infant cannot synthesize well, such as cystine and taurine. Some of the positive features of amino acid composition of human milk are summarized in Table 5-3. These characteristics are especially useful to infants whose biochemical capabilities are underdeveloped at birth.

Nonprotein nitrogen. The total amount of nonprotein nitrogen in human milk averages nearly 25% of all nitrogen and is significantly higher than that found in cow's milk (about 5%). The importance of this to infant nutrition and health is unknown. Nonprotein nitrogen sources consist of a variety of organic, and trace amounts of inorganic, compounds shed into the milk supply. Among these compounds are peptides and free amino acids, the latter of which may provide a nutritional advantage to the infant. Nonprotein nitrogen sources also include urea, creatinine, and sugar amines. Scientists have speculated that it is of nutritional significance that each species of mammal seems to carry a characteristic pattern of free amino acids in its nonprotein nitrogen pool.

TABLE 5-3 *Significant Features about the Amino Acid Composition of Human Milk*

Characteristic	Explanation
Lower in methionine and rich in cystine	An enzyme, cystathionase, is late to develop in the fetus; this impairs optimum conversion of methionine to cystine, which is needed for growth and development; methionine may increase in the bloodstream of an infant fed cow's milk but not one fed human milk; hypermethioninemia may damage the central nervous system
Lower in phenylalanine and tyrosine	The enzymes tyrosine aminotransferase and parahydroxyphenyl pyruvate oxidase are late in developing: cow's milk-fed babies may develop hyperphenylalaninemia and hypertyrosinemia, which may adversely affect development of the central nervous system, especially in the premature; breast milk offers much less problem
Rich in taurine	Breast milk provides taurine for bile acid conjugation, and it *may* also be a neurotransmitter or neuromodulator in the brain and retina; humans cannot synthesize taurine well; cow's milk contains little taurine; the requirement for taurine in the developing neonate is uncertain

Eicosapentanoic acid (EPA)
(Gr *eicosa*, twenty; *penta*, five) Long-chain polyunsaturated fatty acid composed of a chain of 20 carbon atoms with 5 double (unsaturated) bonds; one of the omega-3 fatty acids found in fatty fish and fish oils.

Docosahexanoic acid (DHA)
(Gr *docosa*, twenty-two; *hexa*, six) Long-chain polyunsaturated omega-3 fatty acid having a 22 carbon chain with 6 double (unsaturated) bonds; metabolic product of omega-3 EPA, found in fatty fish and fish oils. The body synthesizes both EPA and DHA from the essential fatty acids linoleic and linolenic acids.

Omega-3 fatty acids
Group of long-chain polyunsaturated fatty acids having important precursor roles in producing highly active hormone-like substances, the *eicosanoids*, involved in critical metabolic activities such as vascular muscle tone and blood clotting.

Depot fat
Body fat stored in adipose tissue.

Taurine. Much recent discussion has centered on the amino acid taurine. Since taurine is found in particularly high levels in fetal brain tissue, it has been proposed that it may play a role in the development of the brain. In addition, taurine is associated with bile acid and thus plays an important role in digestion and may function in the management of cholesterol in the body. Since human milk contains much more taurine than does cow's milk, it has been speculated that the breastfed infant might profit significantly from the higher taurine intake. Interestingly, however, observations have shown that breastfed babies maintain plasma taurine levels that are similar to those of formula-fed infants. It would therefore appear that taurine is not an essential amino acid for infants. However, the general consensus is that taurine is a conditionally essential nutrient for human infants and children, especially those born prematurely.[9]

Lipids

Amount. The total lipid content of human milk varies considerably from one woman to another and is even affected by parity and season of the year. Separate observations by different investigators around the world give the following average levels of fat in human milk: 2.02%, 3.1%, 3.2%, 3.27%, 3.95%, 4.5%, and 5.3%. Sampling methods may affect fat content, since the first milk (fore-milk) is low in fat and the last milk (hind-milk) shows about a threefold increase in the fat content.

Types. Nearly 90% of the lipid in human milk is present in the form of triglycerides. But small amounts of phospholipids, cholesterol, diglycerides, monoglycerides, glycolipids, sterol esters, and free fatty acids are also found. The fatty acid composition of human milk differs greatly from that of cow's milk. The content of the essential fatty acid linoleic acid is considerably greater in human milk than in cow's milk. The content of short-chain saturated fatty acids (C4 to C8) is greater in cow's milk. Of equal interest is the observation that human milk contains more cholesterol than cow's milk and much more cholesterol than commercial infant formulas. A beneficial effect of this higher cholesterol level has been suggested on grounds that (1) it is needed by the rapidly growing central nervous system for **myelin** synthesis, and (2) in early life it stimulates the development of enzymes necessary for cholesterol degradation.

Recent research has demonstrated that human milk contains not only linoleic acid and linolenic acid but also **eicosapentanoic acid (EPA)** and **docosahexanoic acid (DHA).** Interestingly, infant formula does not contain the longer-chain forms EPA and DHA. Since animal experiments have provided evidence that these **omega-3 fatty acids** may be essential for the normal prenatal and postnatal development of the brain and retina, the contribution that human milk makes to this developmental process is receiving much attention.[10]

Maternal diet effect on composition. The composition of the fat in human milk varies significantly with the diet of the mother. Lactating women fed a diet rich in polyunsaturated fats, such as corn and cottonseed oils, produce milk with an increased content of polyunsaturated fats. This is best seen by comparing total vegetarians with nonvegetarians, as seen in Table 5-4. Over the years, as dietary unsaturated fat intake has increased in the United States, the fatty acid composition of breast milk samples has reflected this change (Table 5-5).

When maternal energy intake is severely restricted, fatty acid composition of human milk resembles that of **depot fat.** This effect is to be expected; it represents fat mobilization in response to the reduction in energy intake. A substantial increase in the proportion of dietary kilocalories from carbohydrate will result in an increase in milk content of fatty acids with carbon chain lengths less than 16. The significance of this latter observation is unknown.

TABLE 5-4 *Mean Breast Milk Fatty Acid Concentration in Vegetarians (Vegans) and Nonvegetarians (Controls)*

Methyl Esters	Vegans*	Controls*
Lauric ($C_{12:0}$)	39	33
Myristic ($C_{14:0}$)	68	80
Palmitic ($C_{16:0}$)	166	276
Stearic ($C_{18:0}$)	52	108
Palmitoleic ($C_{16:1}$)	12	36
Oleic ($C_{18:1}$)	313	353
Linoleic ($C_{18:2}$)	317	69
Linolenic ($C_{18:3}$)	15	8

*Mean values expressed as milligrams per gram total methyl esters detected for four vegans and four controls (nonvegetarians).
Modified from Sanders TAB et al: Am J Clin Nutr 31:805, 1978.

TABLE 5-5 *Reports of Fatty Acid Composition of Human Milk*

Fatty Acid	Breast Milk Content (Percent of Total Fatty Acid)	
	1953*	1977†
Lauric ($C_{12:0}$)	5.5	3.8
Myristic ($C_{14:0}$)	8.5	5.2
Palmitic ($C_{16:0}$)	23.2	22.5
Palmitoleic ($C_{16:1}$)	3.0	4.1
Stearic ($C_{18:0}$)	6.9	8.7
Oleic ($C_{18:1}$)	36.5	39.5
Linoleic ($C_{18:2}$)	7.8	14.4
Linolenic ($C_{18:3}$)	—	2.0

*Based on data from Macy IG et al.: The composition of milks, Pub No 254, Washington, DC, 1958, National Research Council.
†Based on data from Guthrie HA, Picciano MF and Sheehe D: J Pediatr 90:39, 1977.

As far as cholesterol is concerned, there is no evidence that its concentration in human milk is altered by the maternal diet. In fact, milk cholesterol level stays between 100 and 150 mg/L even in hypercholesterolemic women and increases only in severe cases of pathologic hypercholesterolemia.

Fat-digesting enzymes. Human milk contains several lipases. One is a serum-stimulated lipase (lipoprotein lipase) that may appear in the milk as a result of leakage from the mammary tissue. Another fat-digesting milk enzyme has a similar activity to that of pancreatic lipase, breaking down triglycerides to free fatty acids and glycerol. This enzyme is present in the fat fraction and appears to be inhibited by bile salts. It probably is responsible for **lipolysis** of milk refrigerated or frozen for later use. Additional lipases in

Lipolysis
(Gr *lipos,* fat; *lysis,* dissolution) Fat digestion or break-down.

the skim milk fraction are inactive until they encounter bile. These lipases, the bile salt-stimulated lipases, are believed to be present only in the milk of primates and are thought to serve some useful purpose for this species. Since the bile salt-stimulated lipases have been clearly shown to be stable and active in the intestine of infants, they can contribute significantly to the hydrolysis of milk triglycerides and partly account for the greater ease in fat digestion that is commonly demonstrated by breastfed babies.

Carnitine. Both human milk and cow's milk contain **carnitine,** which plays an important role in the oxidation of long-chain fatty acids by facilitating their transport across the **mitochondrial** membrane. The body's supply of carnitine is derived in part by ingestion of dietary carnitine and in part by endogenous synthesis from the essential amino acids lysine and methionine. Newborns are especially in need of carnitine since fat provides a major source of energy. It has been suggested that carnitine may be an essential nutrient for the newborn since infants may have a limited synthetic capacity, especially those born prematurely.[11] Human milk contains about 50 to 100 **nmol** of carnitine per milliliter; formula products based on milk or beef contain 50 to 656 nmol/ml. Those formulas prepared from soy isolate, and specialized formulations from egg white and casein, carry an amount equal to or less than 4 nmol/ml. For this reason most manufacturers of soy-based infant formulas now add carnitine to their products. Whether or not infants using any of these formulas or provided human milk require additional carnitine has been the subject of much debate. At this point, it appears that supplemental carnitine is unnecessary for the vast majority of **neonates.**

Carbohydrate

Lactose. Lactose, a disaccharide composed of glucose and galactose, is the main carbohydrate in human milk. In all species of mammals studied, milk is isotonic with plasma, which helps keep the cost of milk secretion low. Lactose exerts 60% to 70% of the total osmotic pressure of milk. The concentrations of lactose in human milk are remarkably similar among women and there is no good evidence that they can be influenced by maternal dietary factors.

Lactose is relatively insoluble and is slowly digested and absorbed in the small intestine. The presence of lactose in the gut of the infant stimulates the growth of microorganisms that produce organic acids and synthesize many of the B vitamins. It is believed that the acid milieu that is created helps to check the growth of undesirable bacteria in the infant's gut and to improve the absorption of calcium, phosphorus, magnesium, and other minerals. Since human milk contains much more lactose than cow's milk (7% and 4.8%, respectively), these gut-associated benefits of lactose are more significant in the breastfed than in the bottle-fed infant.

Other carbohydrates. Chromatographic processing of human milk samples has revealed trace amounts of glucose, galactose, and an array of moderate chain length carbohydrates (**oligosaccharides**). Some of these appear to be protective even though they are present in low concentrations. Nitrogen-containing sugars promote the growth of lactobacilli, the dominant acid-producing bacteria in the lower intestinal tract of breastfed infants. Specialized oligosaccharides inhibit the binding of selected bacterial pathogens or their toxins to epithelial cells by acting as "trapping receptors."

Amylase. Although human milk does not contain much complex carbohydrate, it does contain a starch-splitting enzyme, amylase, which is quite stable at pH levels found in the stomach and small bowel.[12] This enzyme may provide an alternative pathway for digestion of glucose **polymers** and starches in early infancy when pancreatic amylase is low or absent in duodenal fluid. The physiologic importance of mammary amylase may be analogous to that of the bile salt-stimulated lipase found in human milk.

Mitochondrion

(Gr *mitos*, thread; *chondrion*, granule) Cell's "powerhouse," small elongated organelle located in the cell cytoplasm; principal site of energy generation (ATP synthesis); contains enzymes of the final energy cycle (citric acid cycle) and cell respiratory chains, as well as ribonucleic acid (RNA) and deoxyribonucleic acid (DNA) for some synthesis of protein.

Nanomole (nmol)

(Gr *nanos*, dwarf; *molekul*, molecule) Metric system unit for measuring extremely small amounts. Prefix *nano-* used in naming units of measurement to indicate one-billionth of the unit with which it is combined. Mole is the chemical term for the molecular weight of a substance expressed in grams—gram molecular weight.

Polymer

(Gr *poly-*, many; *meros*, part) Large compound formed by chains of simpler repeating molecules, e.g., glucose polymer oligosaccharide.

Minerals

Comparison with cow's milk. One of the most striking differences between human and cow's milk lies in the mineral composition. As with protein, it is believed that this difference may be related to the rate of growth of the species for which the milk was intended. According to typical estimates, there is six times more phosphorus, four times more calcium, three times more total ash, and three times more protein in cow's milk than in human milk. The high mineral and protein composition of cow's milk distinctly affects the amount of mineral and protein waste products provided to the kidney. One might speculate that the kidney of the newborn infant is prepared to handle the "waste" derived from breast milk but is stressed unduly by the requirements placed on it when cow's milk, especially nonfat milk, is selected as an alternate.

Major and trace minerals. The major minerals found in mature human milk are potassium, calcium, phosphorus, chlorine, and sodium. Iron, copper, and manganese are found in only trace amounts, and since these elements are required for normal red blood cell synthesis, infants fed too long on milk alone become anemic. Minute amounts of zinc, magnesium, aluminum, iodine, chromium, selenium, and fluoride are also found in breast milk. Infants who are not provided with fluoridated water in addition to breast milk may benefit from a daily oral fluoride supplement of regulated dosage predetermined by the physician or pharmacist. Providing the lactating woman with a fluoride supplement does not significantly alter her milk output of fluoride (Fig. 5-7).

Varying mineral composition. The total mineral content of human milk is fairly constant, but the specific amounts of individual minerals may vary with the status of the mother and the stage of lactation. Observations from a number of laboratories have shown declining concentrations of several minerals over the weeks and months following the onset of lactation (Fig. 5-8). Of substantial interest are other reports in which dietary intake and supplementation habits of mothers have been compared with mineral com-

FIG. 5-7 Plasma *(open symbols)* and breast milk *(closed symbols)* fluoride concentrations in mothers after oral dose of 1.5 mg fluoride as sodium fluoride solution. (Conversion: fluoride— 1 mol/L ≈ 19 ng/ml.)

From Ekstrand J: No evidence of transfer of fluoride from plasma to breast milk, Br Med J 283:761, 1981.

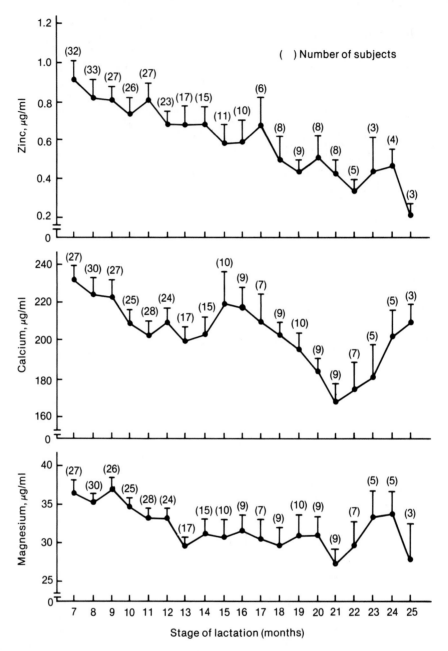

FIG. 5-8 Concentrations of zinc, calcium, and magnesium in milk samples collected at a morning feeding from 7 to 25 months of lactation. *Vertical bars* represent SEM.

Based on data from Karra MV et al: Am J Clin Nutr 43:495, 1986.

position of milk. In most situations little relationship has been found between maternal mineral intake and mineral content of milk. However, since the adequacy of maternal intake of some minerals has been questioned, this may place the mother at risk.

Iron and zinc bioavailability. Some minerals are more easily absorbed from breast milk than from cow's milk or commercial formulas. McMillan and others reported that nearly 50% of the iron in human milk is absorbed, whereas availability of iron from cow's milk and iron-fortified formulas is only 10% and 4%, respectively.[13,14] More recently Garry and associates found that iron absorption from human milk may be much higher than 50% during the first 3 months of life.[15] An explanation for this improved absorption has not been found.

Iron supplementation. Whether or not breastfed infants should receive iron supplements is still the subject of much debate.[15,16] Several studies suggest that infants who are breastfed during the first 6 months of life and receive little or no dietary iron other than that in human milk appear to be iron sufficient at age 6 months. However, based on changes in total body iron determined by body weights and hemoglobin and ferritin concentrations, Owen and others concluded that some nonsupplemented breastfed infants are in negative iron balance between ages 3 and 6 months.[16] One might suggest that human milk alone cannot provide sufficient iron for optimum infant nutrition after 5 or 6 months of life.

Like iron, the **bioavailability** of zinc is substantially better from human milk than from other alternative preparations.[17] In one study the bioavailability of zinc fed to rats in various milk solutions was 59.2% for human milk, 42% for cow's milk, and 26.8% to 39% for commercial formulas. In other work human subjects demonstrated better absorption of zinc from human milk than from cow's milk or selected infant formulas (Fig. 5-9). An explanation for the better absorption of zinc from human milk is still being sought. It has been suggested, however, that the unique distribution and binding of zinc, and some other elements, to high and low molecular weight fractions of milk very likely are related to the differences in bioavailability that have now been demonstrated by a number of investigators.

Bioavailability
Amount of a nutrient ingested in food that is absorbed and thus available to the body for metabolic use.

Fat-Soluble Vitamins

General vitamin content. All the vitamins, both fat- and water-soluble, required for good nutrition and health are supplied in breast milk, but the amounts vary markedly from one person to another. The major factor influencing the vitamin content of human milk is the mother's vitamin status. In general, when maternal intakes of a vitamin are chronically low, the levels of that vitamin in human milk are also low. As maternal intakes of the vitamin increase, levels in milk are also low. As maternal intakes of the vitamin increase, levels in milk also increase. For many vitamins, however, a plateau develops that is not exceeded in the face of further augmentation in vitamin intake through diet or supplement. As a general rule, milk concentrations of water-soluble vitamins are more responsive to maternal dietary intake than are the concentrations of fat-soluble vitamins.

Vitamin D. The amount of biologically active vitamin D in human milk has been found to be low (0.5 to 1.5 μg/L). However, maternal sunshine exposure and dietary intake affect infant vitamin D status through their effects on breast milk vitamin D content. This is supported by the recent finding that a short course of oral vitamin D (60 μg/day) supplementation or exposure to ultraviolet phototherapy quickly raised the levels of **antirachitic** (vitamin D) sterols in the plasma and milk of lactating women.[18] There was a peak effect in 1 week with oral vitamin D supplementation and 2 to 3 days after ultraviolet irradiation. The levels then rapidly returned to baseline. Other reports show a direct relationship between maternal and infant levels of 25-hydroxyvitamin D, implying that maternal vitamin D intake directly affects the vitamin D concentration in breast milk.

Antirachitic
(Gr *anti-*, against; *rachitis*, a spinal disorder) Agent that is therapeutically effective against rickets, a nutritional deficiency disease affecting childhood bone development in which vitamin D is lacking.

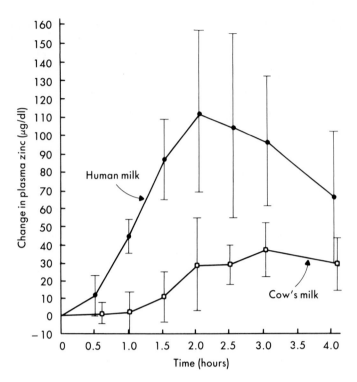

FIG. 5-9   Changes in plasma zinc concentration after ingestion of 25 mg of zinc with human milk (five subjects) and cow's milk (seven subjects). Points represent means ± SD variation from baseline value.

From Casey CE, Walravens PA, and Hambidge KM: Availability of zinc: loading tests with human milk, cow's milk, and infant formulas. Pediatrics 68:394, 1981. Reproduced by permission of Pediatrics.

A question remains regarding the need for vitamin D supplementation in the term infant who is exclusively breastfed. Although some clinicians do not believe it is necessary, the bulk of data support the practice. Greer and associates found low serum 25-hydroxy-vitamin D concentrations and early decreases in bone mineral content in breastfed infants not receiving supplemental vitamin D.[19,20] Ozsoylu and Hasanoglu reported low serum 25-hydroxyvitamin D levels at 1 month of age in breastfed infants not supplemented with vitamin D.[21] In some of the sunniest parts of the world, such as the Middle East, rickets is common in certain breastfed infants because cultural practices keep the babies well clothed and indoors for the first year.[22] Even in the United States, reports of resurgence in rickets among breastfed infants provoke considerable concern.[23,24] Since no harm is associated with vitamin D supplementation at 10 μg/day and since expense and inconvenience are trivial, support of this practice seems justifiable. For light-skinned suburban populations in sunny regions and seasons, one may worry less about compliance with this recommendation.

Vitamin A. Milk is a good source of vitamin A and its precursors. Its concentration in human milk is influenced by the quality and quantity of the dietary elements consumed by the mother. The vitamin A content of breast milk is reportedly much lower in some developing countries than in the West. Maternal serum vitamin A levels in these same regions are also typically low. Vitamin A or carotene intake of some Western mothers is higher in the spring and summer months because of greater supplies of green leafy and yellow vegetables. Modern methods of preservation, however, have extended the length of seasons for many vegetables and fruits so that dietary differences from season to season may be minimal for many women with access to supermarkets, home freezers, and other such luxuries of modern society.

Vitamin E. Levels of vitamin E in human milk are substantially greater than those in cow's milk. As might be expected, serum levels of vitamin E rise quickly in breastfed infants and are maintained at normal levels without much fluctuation. Cow's milk-fed babies demonstrate depressed circulating levels of vitamin E unless supplemented. Fortunately manufacturers of infant formulas have increased their levels of vitamin E fortification to avoid potential deficiency.

Vitamin K. In mature human milk vitamin K is present at a level of 2 µg/L. Cow's milk contains much more than this amount with a typical reported value of 60 µg/L. Vitamin K is produced by the intestinal flora, but it takes several days for the sterile infant gut to establish an effective microbe population. Even then, onset of hemorrhagic disease with bleeding as late as 4 weeks after delivery has been associated with breastfeeding if no vitamin K had been given at birth. It is recommended, therefore, that all newborn infants receive vitamin K.

Water-Soluble Vitamins

Effect of maternal intake. The levels of water-soluble vitamins in human milk are more likely to reflect maternal diet or supplement intake more than most other ingested compounds. Maternal dietary supplements with most of these vitamins have been shown to increase their content in breast milk. This is especially true in women whose dietary patterns or nutritional status are suboptimum. It appears that with some of these vitamins a plateau may be reached where increased intake has no further impact on milk composition. This idea was nicely demonstrated when varying levels of supplemental ascorbic acid were provided to lactating women.[25] With comparable diets, women consuming either 90 mg or 250 mg per day of ascorbic acid produced milk with similar concentration of this vitamin. Women taking 1000 mg of ascorbic acid per day produced milk that was only slightly higher in its ascorbic acid content.

Vitamin B$_6$. Felice and Kirksey have provided evidence that milk concentration of vitamin B$_6$ may be a sensitive indicator of vitamin B$_6$ status of the mother.[26] They further suggest that the majority of lactating women produce milk with a vitamin B$_6$ content that is substantially less than that recommended for good health and growth of infants. These researchers observed that mothers receiving 2.5 mg/day of supplemental vitamin B$_6$ failed to supply their breastfeeding infants with 0.3 mg of vitamin B$_6$ per day, which is the RDA for young infants.[27]

Vitamin B$_{12}$. The vitamin B$_{12}$ content of human milk has been found to range from 0.33 to 3.2 **ng**/ml (mean 0.97 ng/ml), and ingestion of supplemental B$_{12}$ does not significantly affect milk content.[28] Human milk from well-fed mothers was found to contain adequate amounts of B$_{12}$. Its bioavailability, however, depends on the sufficiency of **proteolytic enzymes** to release it from its bound form. Infantile neurologic disorders related to vitamin B$_{12}$ deficiency have been reported in breastfed infants of strict vegetarian women.[29,30]

Resistance Factors

A thorough discussion of the composition of breast milk must include mention of the beneficial components of human milk that are not classified as nutrients (Table 5-6).

Bifidus factor. One of the earliest resistance factors to be described in human milk was

Nanogram (ng)
(Gr *nano-*, dwarf) One billionth gram; also called millimicrogram.

Proteolytic enzymes
(Gr *protos*, first; *lysis*, dissolution) Series of enzymes that progressively split proteins, large molecular compounds, into their respective individual amino acids.

TABLE 5-6   *Antiinfectious Factors in Human Milk*

Factor	Function
Bifidus factor	Stimulates growth of bifidobacteria, which antagonizes the survival of enterobacteria
Secretory IgA (sIgA), IgM, IgE, IgD, and IgG	Act against bacterial invasion of the mucosa and/or colonization of the gut (show bacterial and viral neutralizing capacity; activate alternative complement pathway)
Antistaphylococcus factor	Inhibits systemic staphylococcal infection
Lactoferrin	Binds iron and inhibits bacterial multiplication
Lactoperoxidase	Kills streptococci and enteric bacteria
Complement (C_3, C_1)	Promotes opsonization (the rendering of bacteria and other cells susceptible to phagocytosis)
Interferon	Inhibits intracellular viral replication
Lysozyme	Lyses bacteria through destruction of the cell wall
B_{12}-binding protein	Renders vitamin B_{12} unavailable for bacterial growth
Lymphocytes	Synthesize secretory IgA; may have other roles
Macrophages	Synthesize complement, lactoferrin, lysozyme, and other factors; carry out phagocytosis and probably other functions

Lactobacillus bifidus
(*L. bifidus*) Predominant fermentative lactobacillus in the intestinal flora of breastfed infants.

Candida albicans
(L *candidus*, glowing, white) Most frequent agent of *candidiasis*, a yeast-like fungus infecting moist tissue areas of the body, involving skin, vagina, and oral mucosa.

Lymphocytes
Mature leukocytes, special lymphoid white blood cells, T cells and B cells, forming major components of the body's immune system; also found in human milk.

the bifidus factor, which may be a nitrogen-containing polysaccharide that favors the growth of *Lactobacillus bifidus*. Its uniqueness to human milk has recently been confirmed.[31] *L. bifidus* confers a protective effect against invasive enteropathogenic organisms. **Immunoglobulins.** Various **immunoglobulins** are present in human milk, including IgA, IgG, IgD, and IgE. Although IgG appears to migrate from maternal serum into milk, evidence suggests that IgA, IgD, and IgE are produced locally in mammary tissue. A variety of studies support the idea of migration of **lymphoblasts** from maternal gut-associated lymphoid tissue to the mammary glands followed by local production of immunoglobulins at this site and secretion of them into the milk. This mechanism allows for maternal lymphoblasts to obtain antigenic exposure from distant sites and carry this experience to the mammary tissue where synthesis of appropriate antibodies can occur for protection of the suckling infant.

Secretory IgA (sIgA) is the predominant immunoglobulin in human milk. It is found in large amounts in colostrum and in smaller, but still significant, levels in mature breast milk. Secretory immunoglobulins have been shown to be a major host resistance factor against organisms that infect the gastrointestinal tract, in particular *E. coli* and the enteroviruses. Also, a protective effect against other organisms has been demonstrated. Human milk clearly exhibits a prophylactic effect against septicemia of the newborn.

Other host resistance factors. Some of the other host resistance factors in breast milk are also worthy of mention. **Lysozyme,** an antimicrobial enzyme, occurs in breast milk at 300 times the concentration found in cow's milk. **Lactoferrin** has been described recently as a compound with a "monilia-static" effect against *Candida albicans*. It inhibits the growth of staphylococci and *E. coli* by binding iron, which the bacteria require to proliferate. **Lactoperoxidase,** which has been shown in vitro to act with other substances in combatting streptococci, is also found in human milk. Specific **prostaglandins** have also been defined, and these may protect the integrity of the gastrointestinal tract epithelium against noxious substances.[32]

Lymphocyte-macrophage activities. Of additional interest is the discovery that the **lymphocytes** in human milk produce the antiviral substance interferon. **Macrophages**

are also found in colostrum and mature milk; 21,000/mm^3 reportedly are present in a typical colostrum specimen. Macrophages are motile and phagocytic and have been shown to produce **complement,** lactoferrin, lysozyme, and other factors. The full role of the macrophages is still under investigation, but they undoubtedly have a protective function, both within the mammary lacteals and subsequently within the baby. A number of investigators have studied the activities of lymphocytes in human milk. Milk samples from lactating mothers have been collected at various times postpartum and examined for cell types present and in vitro activities of the various identified cells. The greatest number of cells appear in colostrum with numbers dropping significantly during the following 8 weeks.

Effect of maternal malnutrition. As one might expect, maternal malnutrition adversely affects not only the nutritional composition of human milk but also its content of immunologic substances. Observations of malnourished Colombian women showed that colostrum contained only one third the normal concentration of IgG and less than half the normal level of albumin. Significant reductions in colostrum levels of IgA and the fourth component of complement (C4) were also observed.[33] These differences tended to disappear in mature milk, accompanied by improvement in the nutritional status of the malnourished mothers during the first several weeks postpartum. Therefore, the protective qualities of colostrum and milk may be significantly influenced by maternal nutritional status.

Contaminants

The lactating woman is often exposed to a variety of nonnutritional substances that may be transferred to her milk. Such substances include drugs, environmental pollutants, viruses, caffeine, alcohol, and food allergens. Although moderate amounts of many of these agents are believed to pose no risk to nursing infants, some substances provoke concern because of known or suspected adverse reactions.

Drugs. Much research has focused on the release of drugs into the milk of lactating women. Whether the mother drinks it, eats it, sniffs it, inserts it as an anal or vaginal suppository, or injects it, some level of the active agents in the drug enters the maternal tissues and blood and finally migrates to the breast milk. The difference in method of administration determines the amount of drug that finally enters the blood and the speed with which it reaches the capillaries of the breast. In general the amount of a drug excreted in milk is not more than 1% to 2% of the maternal dose. Although concern exists about the amount of a given drug in the breast milk, of greater concern is the amount that actually reaches the infant's bloodstream. Unfortunately, there is no accurate way to measure this because other factors also affect the level in the infant's bloodstream. The tolerance of the chemical to the pH of the stomach and the enzymatic activity of the intestinal tract is significant. The volume of milk consumed by the infant is a factor as well.

Some drugs appear in human milk in sufficient quantities to be harmful to the infant (Table 5-7).[34] Sedatives used to relieve tension may produce drowsiness in the baby as well as the mother. Lithium and reserpine produce a bluish tint to the skin along with other disorders. Valium residuals in mother's milk induce lethargy in breastfed babies. Lithium carbonate, a drug prescribed for relief of manic depression, may induce lowered body temperature, loss of muscle tone, and bluish skin in the nursing infant. Both cyclophosphamide and methotrexate cause bone marrow depression when ingested by infants. A variety of disorders follow intake by infants of breast milk contaminated with antimicrobial agents of one kind or another. Penicillin in breast milk may produce an allergic reaction in a sensitive infant. Other antibiotics may produce similar reactions, as well as sleepiness, vomiting, and refusal to eat. Radioactive thyroid may damage the thyroid

Complement
Series of enzymatic serum proteins that interact with an antigen-antibody complex to promote phagocyte activity or destroy other cells.

TABLE 5-7   *Abbreviated Guide to Drug Therapy in Nursing Mothers*

Drugs That Are Contraindicated during Breastfeeding	
Drug	**Reported Sign or Symptom in Infant or Effect on Lactation**
Bromocriptine	Suppresses lactation
Cocaine	Cocaine intoxication
Cyclophosphamide	Possible immune suppression; unknown effect on growth or association with carcinogenesis; neutropenia
Cyclosporine	Possible immune suppression; unknown effect on growth or association with carcinogenesis
Doxorubicin	Possible immune suppression; unknown effect on growth or association with carcinogenesis
Ergotamine	Vomiting, diarrhea, convulsions (doses used in migraine medications)
Lithium	⅓ to ½ therapeutic blood concentration in infants
Methotrexate	Possible immune suppression; unknown effect on growth or association with carcinogenesis; neutropenia
Phencyclidine (PCP)	Potent hallucinogen
Phenindione	Anticoagulant; increased prothrombin and partial thromboplastin time in one infant (not used in USA)

Drugs of Abuse That Are Contraindicated during Breastfeeding	
Drug	**Effect**
Amphetamine	Irritability, poor sleep pattern
Cocaine	Cocaine intoxication
Heroin	
Marijuana	Only one report in literature; no effect mentioned
Nicotine (smoking)	Shock, vomiting, diarrhea, rapid heart rate, restlessness; decreased milk production
Phencyclidine	Potent hallucinogen

gland. Bowel problems in infants may result from maternal consumption of some laxatives, such as anthraquinone, aloes, cascara, emodin, and rheum (rhubarb). Safe laxatives include magnesia, castor oil, mineral oil, bisacodyl (Ducolax), senna phenophthalein or nonprescription Ex-Lax, and fecal softeners. Heroin or the painkiller dextropropoxyphene (Darvon) can lead to infant addiction. Treatment of the heroin-addicted mother with methadone is problematic, since one infant death has been reported during maternal methadone therapy.

If a mother needs a specific medication and the hazards to the infant are believed to be minimal, the following important adjustments can be made to minimize the effects:

1. **Action time.** Do not use the long-acting form of the drug because the infant has even more difficulty in excreting the agent, which usually requires detoxification in the liver. Accumulation in the infant is then a genuine concern.
2. **Dose schedule.** Schedule the doses so the least amount of the drug gets into the milk. Given the usual absorption rates and peak blood levels of most drugs, having the mother take the medication immediately after breastfeeding is the safest time for the infant.
3. **Observations.** Watch the infant for any unusual signs or symptoms such as change in feeding pattern or sleeping habits, fussiness, or rash.

CHAPTER 5: *Lactation and Human Milk* **173**

TABLE 5-7 *Abbreviated Guide to Drug Therapy in Nursing Mothers—cont'd*

Radiopharmaceuticals That Require Temporary Cessation of Breatfeeding*

Drug	Recommended Alteration in Breastfeeding Pattern
Gallium-67 (^{67}Ga)	Radioactivity in milk present for 2 wk
Indium-111 (^{111}In)	Small amount present at 20 hr
Iodine-125 (^{125}I)	Risk of thyroid cancer; radioactivity in milk present for 12 days
Iodine-131 (^{131}I)	Radioactivity in milk present 2 to 14 days depending on study
Radioactive sodium	Radioactivity in milk present 96 hr
Technetium-99m (^{99m}Tc), ^{99m}Tc macroaggregates, ^{99m}TcO$_4$	Radioactivity in milk present 15 hr to 3 days

Drugs That Have Caused Significant Effects on Some Nursing Infants and Should Be Given to Nursing Mothers with Caution†

Drug	Effect
Aspirin (salicylates)	Metabolic acidosis (dose related); may affect platelet function; rash
Clemastine	Drowsiness, irritability, refusal to feed, high-pitched cry, neck stiffness (one case)
Phenobarbital	Sedation; infantile spasms after weaning from milk containing phenobarbital, methemoglobinemia (one case)
Primidone	Sedation, feeding problems
Salicylazosulfapyridine (sulfasalazine)	Bloody diarrhea in one infant

*Consult nuclear medicine physician before performing diagnostic study so that a radionuclide with the shortest excretion time in breast milk can be used. Before study, the mother should pump her breast and store enough milk in freezer for feeding the infant; after study, the mother should pump her breast to maintain milk production but discard all milk pumped for the required time that radioactivity is present in milk.
†Measure blood concentration in the infant when possible.
Adapted from American Academy of Pediatrics, Committee on Drugs: Transfer of drugs and other chemicals into human milk, Pediatrics 84:924, 1989. Reproduced by permission of Pediatrics.

4. **Drug amount in milk.** When possible, choose the drug that produces the least amount in the milk.

One of the best sources of information on drugs in relation to human milk and infant health is the family pharmacist. It is also wise to read the product label to evaluate product composition and precautionary statements. Effective December 26, 1979, all drug manufacturers in the United States were required to provide relevant information on the labels of new drugs developed and marketed since that date. Whatever is known about excretion of the drug into milk and whatever is known of the effect on the infant will be indicated on the label. If nothing is known, the label will state that fact. In such a case, and in all use of drugs, the prudent mother will exercise due caution.

Environmental contaminants. The current concern over pesticide residues, industrial wastes, and other environmental contaminants is not without cause. Many of these compounds have accidentally contaminated food and water supplies around the world. In general the chemical contaminants that appear in breast milk have high lipid solubility, resistance to physical degradation or biologic metabolism, wide distribution in the en-

Organohalides
(Gr *organon*, organ; Chem *halides*, compounds of fluorine, chlorine, bromine, or iodine) Chemical compounds used as pesticides or in industrial processes, e.g., DDT and PCBs.

vironment, and slow or absent excretion rates. Of greatest concern among such chemicals are the **organohalides** such as polychlorinated biphenyls (PCBs) and dichlorodiphenyl trichloroethane (DDT).[35] Long-term low-level exposure to the organohalides results in a gradual accumulation of residues in fat, including the fat of breast milk. Lactation is the only way in which large amounts of such residues can be excreted.

Savage and associates conducted a study of environmental contaminants that focused on levels of chlorinated hydrocarbon insecticide residues in nearly 1500 human milk samples around the United States.[36] The majority of samples showed low but detectable levels of most of these insecticides or their metabolites, but significant differences were found among the five geographic regions. The southeastern United States had the highest mean residue levels, whereas the northwest had the lowest levels. Although nursing infants around the United States would generally receive low levels of some of these residues, a small number could be exposed to fairly high amounts.

It is clear that human milk is a variable source of contaminants, but it is difficult to define a "safe" level of exposure to these compounds. However, both the World Health Organization and the U.S. Food and Drug Administration have set "regulatory" or "allowable" levels for daily intake of several organohalides (Table 5-8). These standards provide a large margin of safety, so the fact that a given infant exceeds the level does not mean that such exposure is toxic. Much remains to be learned about the chemical contamination of human milk. Meanwhile, it is heartening to know that very few cases of illness caused by transmission of environmental chemicals through breast milk have appeared.

Heavy metals. Lead and mercury, both heavy metals, are transferred placentally to the fetus and also to the infant via maternal milk. Rat studies have shown that lactation increases lead absorption from the gut, which leads ultimately to an increased level of lead excretion via the milk. The exact mechanism for this phenomenon is not known. However, lactose may play a dominant role, since it is known to facilitate the absorption of calcium, other trace elements, and lead.

Nicotine. Nicotine enters human milk and can cause nicotine "poisoning" of the breastfed infant. Infants 3 to 4 days of age whose mothers smoked 6 to 16 cigarettes a day were reported to refuse to suckle, to become apathetic, vomit, and retain urine and feces. In a chain-smoking mother the nicotine content of milk may reach 75 µg/L. In the case of

TABLE 5-8 *"Typical" Levels, FDA Action Levels, Allowable Daily Intake, and Calculated Daily Intake of Representative Breastfed Infants*

Substance	Typical Levels* (ppb)	FDA Action Levels for Cow's Milk† (ppb)	Allowable Daily Intake (µg/kg)	Daily Intake of Breastfed Infants‡ (µg/kg)
Dieldrin	1-6	7.5	0.1	0.8
Heptachlor epoxide	8-30	7.5	0.5	4
PCBs	40-100	62.5	1	14
DDT (including metabolites)	50-200	50	5	28

*Levels considered typical in whole milk in the United States.
†Assuming 2.5% fat. FDA action levels represent the limit at or above which the FDA will take legal action against a product to remove it from the market.
‡Intake of a 5 kg infant drinking 700 ml of milk per day; levels are based on high values given under typical levels.
Modified from Rogan WJ, Bagniewska A, and Damstra T: N Engl J Med 302:1450, 1980.

mothers who smoke very little it is likely that the amount of nicotine the infant would get from breathing cigarette smoke in the immediate environment would be more significant than that obtained from milk. The long-term impact of such exposure is unknown.

Caffeine. Caffeine passes from the maternal bloodstream into breast milk. Although a small dose of caffeine comparable to that obtained from a cup of coffee is transported at low levels from the mother to her milk (1%), caffeine does reach the infant where it can accumulate over time.[37] Wakeful, hyperactive infants sometimes are victims of caffeine stimulation. A mother who drinks more than six to eight cups of any caffeine-containing beverage in a day's time might expect her infant to demonstrate "coffee nerves." Such an infant does not require hospitalization, and verification of blood caffeine levels is not mandatory, although it might be helpful. An elimination trial should suffice to evaluate the role of maternal caffeine ingestion, and subsequent elimination, on infant behavior.

Alcohol. Beverage alcohol also passes from the mother's bloodstream into her breast milk. **Ethanol** has been shown to reach human milk in a similar concentration to that in maternal blood. Interestingly, however, the major breakdown product of ethanol, acetaldehyde, does not appear in human milk even though significant amounts may have been measured in maternal blood.

The role of the mammary gland in eliminating acetaldehyde may be similar to that of the placenta. If human milk contains large amounts of ethanol, the nursing infant may develop a pseudo-**Cushing's syndrome,** as described by Binkiewicz, Robinson, and Senior.[38] The 4 month-old infant they describe (Fig. 5-10) was breastfed by a mother who consumed at least fifty 12-oz cans of beer weekly, plus generous amounts of other more

Ethanol
Chemical name for beverage alcohol.

Cushing's syndrome
Condition first described by Boston surgeon Harvey Cushing (1869-1939), due to hypersecretion of adrenal corticotropic hormone (ACTH) or excessive intake of glucocorticoids, with rapidly developing fat deposits of face, neck, and trunk, giving a characteristic cushingoid "moon face" appearance.

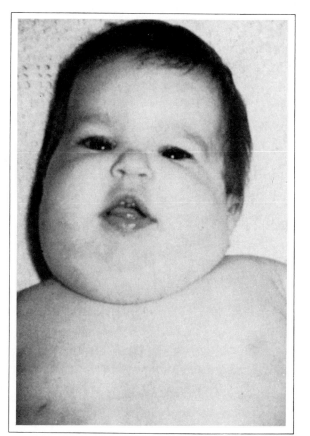

FIG. 5-10 Cushingoid appearance in a 4-month-old infant whose mother consumed at least 50 cans of beer weekly plus generous portions of other, more concentrated alcoholic beverages.

From Binkiewiez A, Robinson MJ, and Senior B: Pseudo-Cushing syndrome caused by alcohol in breast milk. J Pediatr 93:965, 1978.

concentrated alcoholic drinks. When the mother stopped drinking but continued to nurse, the infant's growth rate promptly increased and her appearance gradually returned to normal. The mother also noted that she did not sleep as much as she did before.

Recent observations of lactating women consuming various levels of alcohol suggest that regular consumption of several drinks per day is associated with delayed psychomotor development at 1 year of age.[39] Whether or not this adverse result indicates permanent damage is unknown. Until more information is available, lactating women are well advised to limit consumption of alcoholic beverages.

The AIDS virus. Evidence suggests that the AIDS virus can be transmitted from mother to infant through breast milk. This recent finding has provoked much concern from the standpoint of providing appropriate advice about infant feeding to high-risk women. Should one encourage or discourage breastfeeding for such women? The current thinking in the United States is that breastfeeding should be discouraged when a woman is known to carry this virus. The World Health Organization, however, supports the concept that infants in many developing countries run greater risks of dying of diarrheal disease if they are not breastfed than of developing AIDS from the breast milk exposure. Debate on this issue continues around the world. In the meantime, breast milk banks are taking special precautions to screen out donors who potentially could contribute virus-contaminated specimens. Samples are also pasteurized sufficiently to destroy viruses that might be present.[40-43]

DIET FOR THE NURSING MOTHER
General Recommendations

The Committee on Recommended Dietary Allowances (RDA) of the Food and Nutrition Board considers the optimum diet for the lactating woman to be one that supplies somewhat more of each nutrient than that recommended for the nonpregnant female (Table 5-8).[44] Obviously, the needs of specific women relate directly to the volume of milk produced daily.

Energy

Prenatal storage. During pregnancy most women store approximately 2 to 4 kg of body fat, which can be mobilized to supply a portion of the additional energy for lactation. It is estimated that stored fat will provide 200 to 300 kcal per day during a lactation period of 3 months. This amount of energy represents only part of the energy needed to produce milk. The remainder of the energy needs should derive from the daily diet the first 3 months of lactation. During this time lactation can be successfully supported and readjustment of maternal fat stores can take place. If lactation continues beyond the initial 3 months or if maternal weight falls below the ideal weight for height, the daily extra energy allowance may need to be increased accordingly. If more than one infant is being nursed during the first few months of life, maternal kilocalorie stores will be more quickly used, and daily supplemental energy needs may double when maternal stores are depleted.

Efficiency of milk production. The efficiency of milk production has been estimated by several researchers by the observation of energy intake and energy utilization of breast-feeding and non-breastfeeding mothers. English and Hitchcock compared the energy intake of 16 nursing mothers and 10 nonnursing mothers and found that the energy intake of breastfeeders in the sixth and eighth postpartum week was 2460 kcal/day.[45] The energy intake of nonnursing mothers during the same postpartum period was 1880 kcal/day—a difference of 580 kcal. In a later study lactating women were found to take in

2716 kcal/day and nonnursing mothers 2125 kcal/day—a difference of 590 kcal. By adding the assumed energy equivalents of body weight being lost, total energy available to the two groups was about 2977 and 2364 kcal/day, respectively. If one assumes that the energy requirements for basal metabolism and activity are equivalent for the two groups, the energy needed for daily milk production is close to 560 kcal. The production efficiency of human milk is therefore about 90%.

Energy needs. Recent observations of lactating women have led some researchers to propose that energy needs have been overestimated. Butte and others found that typical women who were producing about 750 ml of milk per day had a mean daily energy intake of 2171 plus 545 kcal per day.[46] Observations of postpartum weight loss patterns and subsequent calculations of energy balance led them to an estimation of 80% efficiency in energy utilization for milk production. When energy available from the diet (2171 kcal/day) was added to the energy derived from tissue mobilization (315 kcal/day) and the caloric equivalent of the milk was subtracted (597 kcal/day), a net balance of 1889 kcal/day was left for maintenance and activity. These findings suggest that successful lactation is compatible with gradual weight reduction and attainable with energy intakes less than current recommendations.

Similarly, Manning-Dalton and Allen evaluated postpartum weight loss patterns, breastfeeding completeness, and daily kilocalorie intakes of well-nourished North American women.[47] In spite of low mean kilocalorie intakes (2178 kcal/day), breastfeeding was successful, and weight loss during the 12 to 90 days postpartum averaged only 2.0 kg for the entire sample and 1.6 kg for the solely breastfeeding women. These authors emphasize that almost every aspect of maternal energy balance in lactation needs further investigation. In the meantime it should be recognized that the U.S. Recommended Dietary Allowance for energy in lactation is probably higher than necessary, especially for the well-nourished woman with a sedentary life style. It is also apparent that the commonly held belief that breastfeeding helps the mother lose weight cannot be substantiated.[48]

Postpartum maternal weight concerns. For many women the usual slow rate of weight loss after childbirth may not satisfy their desires for immediate return to prepregnancy body weight. It is therefore likely that dietary restriction may be self-imposed, even though it is discouraged by health professionals. It is important to recognize, however, that moderate to severe restriction of caloric intake during lactation will compromise the woman's ability to synthesize milk. This is especially significant in the early weeks of lactation initiation before the process is firmly established. As a result of this effect of caloric restriction on milk production, lactating women should be advised to accept a gradual rate of weight loss in the first 6 months after childbirth. Otherwise, lactation success may be limited and the infant may suffer from insufficient milk supply to meet growth needs.

Protein

Along with the recommended energy increment, a 15 to 20 g increase in daily protein intake is advised for lactating women. The extra protein is believed to be necessary to cover the requirement for milk production with an allowance of 70% efficiency of protein utilization.

The increased needs for protein, as well as energy, can be met easily by consumption of about three to four extra cups of milk per day. Although this will provide the needed protein and energy, it will not cover the increased recommendations for other nutrients—ascorbic acid, vitamin E, and folic acid. Thus other foods such as citrus fruits, vegetable oils, and leafy green vegetables will also need to be added to the daily diet to supply these nutrients. The Daily Food Guide for Women, discussed in Chapter 3 (p. 76), provides a helpful food pattern for the reproductive years, including increases needed for pregnancy and lactation.

Vegetarian Diets

Maintenance of lactation while consuming a vegetarian diet can be managed well, providing all the basic principles of sensible vegetarian eating are followed carefully. The nutritional needs of the lactating vegetarian woman are the same as those of the lactating woman with a more traditional diet. Appropriate extra sources of kilocalories and protein must be clearly defined. If dairy products are acceptable in the chosen dietary regimen, extra milk can be used as indicated. If dairy products are not included in the accepted list of foods, extra energy and high quality protein must be obtained from appropriately combined vegetables, legumes, grains, nuts, and other such food sources in larger amounts. Calcium needs can be met by eating large quantities of some green leafy vegetables (for example, kale), calcium-fortified foods, and other significant sources of vegetable calcium. Dietary supplements may be unacceptable. Thus, intelligent daily diet planning is essential for maintenance of successful lactation and health of the vegetarian mother.

The Question of Supplementation

Although lactation increases a woman's requirement for nearly all nutrients, these increased needs can be provided by a well-balanced diet as outlined. For this reason nutritional supplements are generally unnecessary except when there is a deficient intake of one or more nutrients. It is true, for example, if the lactating woman does not tolerate milk, calcium supplementation as well as alternative energy and protein sources are needed to help prevent unnecessary calcium withdrawal from bones.

Although there is no evidence that calcium composition of human milk can be influenced by dietary intake of calcium, it is clear that dietary calcium deficiency promotes mobilization of calcium from bones to maintain milk calcium levels during lactation. Older clinical literature documents cases of **osteomalacia** in mothers who nursed their infants for long periods of time while on inadequate diets. Also, it has been proposed that the relatively high incidence of osteomalacia and **osteoporosis** (p. 71) in the United States is partially related to the waning intake of dairy products by adult women. Whether or not this is the case is still unknown. It stands to reason, however, that prolonged lactation accompanied by poor calcium intake may significantly compromise the calcium status of the skeletal system and increase its susceptibility to fractures and other forms of trauma.

Cost of Nutritional Support for Lactation

The cost of providing adequate nutritional support for the lactating mother depends heavily upon what foods she selects to meet her nutritional needs. Some older studies suggest that human milk costs more than bottle-feeding because of the extra nutrients the mother must consume. It is clear, however, in examining the costs of appropriate extra foods for the lactating mother that human milk is cheaper than proprietary cow's milk formulas if economical food choices are made (Tables 5-9, 5-10, and 5-11). The present difference between the costs of commercially prepared cow's milk formulas and human milk undoubtedly will continue to increase in coming years, since the price of "double cycle" animal food products, including cow's milk, continues to escalate. Beyond the price consideration, however, it is hard to justify "wastage" of human milk and the resultant unnecessary draw on the precious supply of other animal protein available to the world's population. Human milk represents a vital national resource that, if utilized

Osteomalacia

(Gr *osteon*, bone; *malakia*, softness) Condition marked by softening of the bones due to impaired mineralization with excess accumulation of osteoid tissue (immature young bone matrix that has not had mineralization to harden); results from deficiency of vitamin D and calcium.

TABLE 5-9 **Recommended Daily Dietary Allowances for Lactation**

	First 6 Months	Second 6 Months
Energy (kcal)	+500	+500
Protein (g)	65	62
Vitamin A (RE*)	1300	1200
Vitamin D (μg)	10	10
Vitamin E activity (mg αTE)†	12	11
Ascorbic acid (mg)	95	90
Folacin (μg)	280	260
Niacin (mg‡)	20	20
Riboflavin (mg)	1.8	1.7
Thiamin (mg)	1.6	1.6
Vitamin B_6 (mg)	2.1	2.1
Vitamin B_{12} (μg)	2.6	2.6
Calcium (mg)	1200	1200
Phosphorus (mg)	1200	1200
Iodine (μg)	200	200
Iron (mg)	15	15
Magnesium (mg)	355	340
Zinc (mg)	19	16

*RE, Retinol equivalents.

†α-Tocopherol equivalents; 1 mg d-α-tocopherol = 1 αTE.

‡Although allowances are expressed as niacin, it is recognized that on the average, 1 mg of niacin is derived from each 60 mg of dietary tryptophan.

Modified from Food and Nutrition Board, National Research Council, National Academy of Sciences: Recommended dietary allowances, ed 10, Washington, DC, 1989, US Government Printing Office.

to its fullest extent, could markedly improve not only the health and nutritional status of today's children but also the "natural resource base" of many underdeveloped countries.

ADVANTAGES OF BREASTFEEDING
Basic Values

Human milk was designed for human infants. The process of lactation is normal for mammals. It is therefore not surprising that a number of advantages have been defined for mothers and infants who participate in the breastfeeding experience (see box on p. 181). The degree of advantage varies among mother-infant pairs, since availability of alternative foods, environmental conditions, and lifestyle characteristics are markedly different from one setting to another. Reviewing the issue with an open mind, however, leaves no doubt that in the majority of situations breastfeeding provides distinct benefits for both child and family.

Antiinfective Properties

Around the turn of the century there was little knowledge of microbiology or of immunology, and bottle-fed infants suffered from a much higher incidence of diarrhea and acute gastrointestinal tract infection. They also experienced higher mortality rates than breastfed infants. Throughout much of the United States and the industrialized West,

TABLE 5-10 *Nutrients, Amounts, and Estimated Cost of Foods Needed to Meet Additional Nutritional Requirements of a Lactating Woman: Standard (Nonbudget) Plan*

Suggested Foods	Amounts	Cost*	Calories	Protein	A	C	B_1	B_2	B_3	Calcium	Iron
Milk, fresh, 2%	2 cups	.36	290	18	700		0.14	0.82	0.4	576	1.7
Meat (round steak)	2 oz	.87	150	13	35		0.04	0.11	2.8	6	0.6
Vegetable, dark green or yellow (broccoli, cooked)	¾ cup	.25	20	2.5	1990	70	0.07	0.15	0.6	68	
Other vegetable or fruit (grapefruit)	½	.15	45	1	10	44	0.05	0.02	0.2	19	0.5
Citrus fruit (orange juice)	½ cup	.14	60	1	275	60	0.11	0.01	0.5	12	0.1
Enriched (or whole grain)	1 slice	.16	65	3			0.09	0.03	0.8	24	0.8
TOTAL		1.93	630	38.5	3010	174	0.5	1.14	5.3	705	3.7

*Costs of May 1991, Seattle, Wash.

TABLE 5-11 *Nutrients, Amounts, and Estimated Cost of Foods Needed to Meet Additional Nutritional Requirements of a Lactating Woman: Budget Plan*

Suggested Foods	Amounts	Cost*	Calories	Protein	A	C	B_1	B_2	B_3	Calcium	Iron
Nonfat dry milk (prepared for drinking)	2 cups	.26	180	18	20		0.18	0.88	0.40	592	
Peanut butter	2 oz	.32	190	8			0.04	0.04	4.8	18	0.6
Vegetable, dark green or yellow (carrots, cooked)	¾ cup	.20	25	0.5	7610	4.5	0.04	0.03	0.04	24	0.45
Citrus fruit (tomato juice)	½ cup	.15	25	1	970	20	0.06	0.04	0.95	86	1.1
Enriched (or whole grain) bread	2 slices	.16	130	6			0.18	0.06	1.6	48	1.6
TOTAL		1.08	550	33.5	8600	24.5	0.5	1.05	7.79	768	3.75

*Costs of May 1991, Seattle, Wash.

ONE STEP FURTHER

techniques for microbial control of the artificial diet have lessened the differences in mortality between bottle-fed and breastfed infants. However, small differences are still apparent in the number and severity of illnesses contracted by bottle-fed and breastfed infants.

Although the protective effect of breast milk is fully appreciated, not all studies show that breastfed babies demonstrate reduced morbidity. It is also true that the reported morbidity among breastfed infants may have nothing to do with the antiinfectious properties of human milk but might instead relate to different parenting strategies or lifestyle characteristics of mothers who choose to breastfeed instead of bottle-feed. Whatever the case, substantial data suggest that breastfeeding reduces infant morbidity, especially in the early months of life.[49]

Optimum Nutrition

A main advantage of breastfeeding is freedom from "formulogenic disease." The complications of improper dilutions, such as incorrect caloric density and excessive renal solute load, are not concerns for breastfed babies. Colostrum and breast milk contain factors whose functions are unclear, as well as micronutrients whose value to the newborn only become apparent when they are omitted from infant formulas. Human milk appears to have a fat composition and protein content ideally suited to the growth rate of the human infant; it is the standard by which formulas are measured.

Appropriate Growth and Development

Bottle-fed and breastfed infants follow similar growth curves from birth until the third or fourth month of age. From the fourth month on, the bottle-fed infant gains weight at a faster rate, especially beyond the sixth month of life. A sizable number of pediatric specialists feel that the slower rate of growth among older breastfed infants represents the ideal pattern for optimum health. It has even been suggested that the National Center for Health Statistics standards are not appropriate for evaluating the growth performance of breastfed infants and that growth curves based exclusively on breastfed infants should be used for that purpose. Thus far such curves are not available, and agreement about what represents optimum growth in infancy has not yet been reached.

Butte and others have demonstrated recently, however, the efficiency with which human milk is utilized by the young infant for maintenance and growth.[50] Forty-five healthy full-term infants who were exclusively breastfed were observed for the first 4 months of life. The amount of breast milk ingested over a 24-hour period was determined by test weighing using automatic electronic scales. At each feeding over a subsequent 24-hour period, milk samples were expressed from alternate breasts for analysis. Although adequate growth was demonstrated by the infants, this was accomplished with energy and protein intakes substantially less than that currently recommended. In the case of energy the following observations were recorded:

	Energy intake (kcal/day)	Energy intake (kcal/kg/day)
1 month	520 ± 131	110 ± 24
2 months	468 ± 115	83 ± 19
3 months	458 ± 124	74 ± 20
4 months	477 ± 111	71 ± 17

Reduced Risk of Allergy

Development of food allergy has been associated with the penetration into the body of intact proteins or large peptide fragments with antigenic determinants. Under ordinary circumstances, secretory antibodies, efficient intraluminal digestion, and impermeable intestinal epithelial cells and intercellular junctions combine to form a "mucosal barrier" in the healthy intestine. Intestinal absorption of whole protein macromolecules is thought to be maximum in the newborn period and to decrease with age. Formula feeding, as opposed to breastfeeding, has been associated with increased susceptibility to food allergies. Whether this is more directly related to exposure to "foreign" **antigens** in commercial formulas, to differences in intestinal morphology with different food sources, to a protective action of breast milk, or to a combination of these mechanisms has not been determined. Recent studies suggest that breast milk may promote early closure of the mucosal barrier. In other studies **antibodies** directed toward milk components have been found in human milk, and these may be involved in the prevention of allergies by hindering the intestinal absorption of intact immunogenic food proteins by the neonate.

Although arguments against the value of breastfeeding for allergy prevention have been presented in the literature with some vigor, these contributions clearly represent the minority viewpoint. It seems appropriate, therefore, that families with a history of allergy should be counseled about the desirability of breastfeeding combined with an allergen-avoidance diet for the baby during the majority of the first year of life.

Allergy to breast milk is uncommon, and some researchers question whether it exists at all. It has been shown, however, that allergens from foods that a mother consumes may enter her breast milk and occasionally promote an allergic reaction in a sensitive infant.[51] Sometimes alteration of maternal diet may be useful.[52] Gerard proposes that if food allergies are present on both sides of the family, the lactating mother should vary her diet and avoid large intake of any one specific food, particularly of cow's milk and egg products.[53] If the baby later develops symptoms suggestive of allergy, the mother should modify her diet rather than place her baby on a cow's milk or soy formula.

Normal Psychologic Development

Breastfeeding has been referred to as the period of "exterior gestation" because it provides continuity with the intrauterine environment while providing security and nourishment. Some workers have suggested that prolactin, coupled with sensory input from the baby, produces "mothering" responses in most women. Many women who have raised both breastfed and bottle-fed infants state that they feel a special closeness to the breastfed child that persists into adult life. Much attention has been focused on what might be termed *maternal-infant bonding*. Breastfeeding promotes strong emotional ties while meeting the infant's most basic physical need.

Antigens
(*antibody* + Gr *gennan*, to produce) Any disease agents, such as toxins, bacteria, viruses, and other foreign substances, that stimulate the production of *antibodies* to combat and destroy them.

Antibodies
Immune system components, specific immunoglobins, especially secretory IgA in the bowel and upper respiratory mucosa, that destroy invading antigens.

Reduced Risk of Obesity

Attempts have been made to assess the value of breastfeeding as protection against the development of obesity. But present data do not allow for satisfactory assessment of the merits of these statements. Published reports have yielded conflicting findings. For the time being it therefore seems inappropriate to advocate breastfeeding as a means of protection against infantile obesity.

Other Infant Benefits

An array of other advantages for babies have been proposed as being associated with breastfeeding. Many clinicians have suggested that low-birth-weight infants who are provided human milk are less likely to develop **necrotizing enterocolitis**.[54] Several researchers have proposed that breastfeeding protects against the development of clinical symptoms of **celiac disease, Crohn's disease,** and insulin-dependent diabetes mellitus (IDDM).[55-56] Support for these and other hypotheses are limited, but future observations may confirm their validity.

Necrotizing enterocolitis (Gr *nekrosis*, deadness; *enteron*, intestine) Infectious tissue-destroying intestinal disease; acute inflammation of intestinal mucosa.

Maternal Benefits

Involution of uterus. One of the earliest documented maternal benefits of breastfeeding is the effect of oxytocin on the **involution** of the uterus. Early breastfeeding, even on the delivery table, stimulates contractions of the uterus that help to control blood loss.

Suppression of ovulation. The stimulation of the nipples and resultant secretion of prolactin suppress ovulation in many women, particularly when supplements and solids are not offered to the baby. This is believed to be of major significance in promoting short-term child spacing in the developing countries. When solid foods become a major source of nourishment for the child, nipple stimulation and prolactin levels decrease in the lactating mother, and ovulation and menstruation usually begin again.

Ease of feeding. One of the prime benefits expressed by most women who breastfeed is the ease with which feeding is managed, particularly at night. The actual time spent

Involution (L *involutio: in,* into, *volvere,* to roll) Process of rolling or turning inward, shrinking an organ to its normal size, as the uterus after childbirth.

TABLE 5-12   Cost per Day of the Most Commonly Used Prepared Formulas, Basic Equipment, and Fuel*

Formula Products and Other Expenses	Cost per Day with Bottles and Nipples			Cost per Day with Disposable Holders and Liners		
Dry, powdered (52 scoops per can)	$1.87			$1.87		
Double-strength liquid (13 oz. can)		2.10			2.10	
Ready-to-feed liquid (32 oz can)			2.49			2.49
Unbreakable bottles with nipples ($10.68/dozen)	.12	.12	.12			
Extra nipples ($3.32/dozen)	.03	.03	.03			
Electricity (to clean and sterilize water/bottles)	.04	.04	.04			
or						
Disposable holders				.11	.11	.11
Liners (one used per feed)				.30	.30	.30
TOTAL	2.06	2.29	2.68	2.28	2.51	2.90

*Costs of May 1991, Seattle, Wash.

nursing the infant may be greater during the first 2 weeks for the breastfeeding mother, since the infant eats more frequently to build up the mother's milk supply. More total time is spent in "nursing" by the bottle-feeding mother, however, since she must make the formula, clean the bottles, and heat the feedings before serving them.

Economy. Economy can no longer be used as a *major* reason for breastfeeding in the United States, but for some women it may be a relevant factor. Although the "old" evaporated milk formula costs about the same as the additional food required by the lactating woman, **proprietary formulas,** especially ready-to-feed ones (the only type that rivals breastfeeding in convenience), may be more expensive than breastfeeding (Table 5-12). For some people, both in the United States and elsewhere, the expense of a commercial formula is prohibitive.

Proprietary
(L *proprietarius,* owner) Referring to commercial products, such as infant formulas and medicinal items, which are designed, manufactured, and sold only by the owner of the patent, formula, brand name, or trademark associated with the product.

INCIDENCE OF BREASTFEEDING
General Background

In spite of the recognized benefits of breastfeeding for the child and the mother, the number of babies in the United States who were formula-fed climbed to an estimated 82% in the 2 decades before 1970. Comparable statistics were reported from England and France in the period following World War II.

Current Trends

Increased practice. More recent reports indicate that this prior trend reversed in the early 1970s and reached a peak in the early 1980s (Fig. 5-11).[3] More mothers are not only breastfeeding but also continuing to do so for a longer period of time throughout the months of their infants' most rapid growth and high nutritional demands. It is also apparent that the increased incidence of breastfeeding has not been limited to higher income, better-educated mothers. From 1971 to 1981 the incidence at 2 months postpartum more than tripled among mothers in lower income families. The incidence of breastfeeding increased five times among mothers whose education did not extend beyond elementary or high school. Incidence of breastfeeding among mothers on the WIC program has increased. As might be expected, breastfeeding in any 1 year, especially long term, is much more common among mothers who have successfully breastfed a previous child. Even mothers of preterm infants, however, may nurse for long periods of time. Current trends in breastfeeding are summarized in Table 5-13.

Maternal employment. Recent surveys have considered the employment status of the mother as it relates to choices about infant feeding.[57,58] One report involved a large population of women in the Baltimore area.[57] These women were interviewed twice during the first 3 months postpartum. Planning to be employed during the first 6 months of the postpartum period did not affect the choice to initiate breastfeeding. However, actually being employed was significantly associated with cessation of breastfeeding as early as 2 or 3 months postpartum. Less than one half of mothers who were employed were still breastfeeding at the second postpartum interview, whereas two thirds of those who were not employed were still breastfeeding. Among employed mothers, working no more than 20 hours/week appeared to be associated with continued breastfeeding.

Regional differences. Regional differences have been reported in the current incidence of breastfeeding.[3] The highest rates of initiating breastfeeding in the hospital (Fig. 5-12) and at 5 or 6 months postpartum (Fig. 5-13) are found in the Mountain and Pacific regions. Rates in the East South Central region are the lowest. Ethnic differences within census regions are the same as those seen in national data.

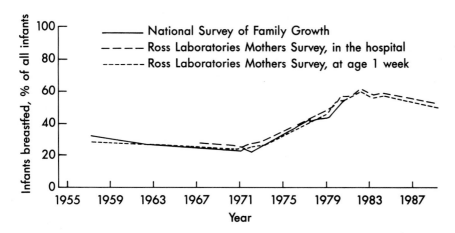

FIG. 5-11 Percentage of infants breastfed, by survey and year.

From Institute of Medicine, National Academy of Sciences: Nutrition during lactation, Washington, DC, 1991, National Academy Press.

Influence of change in medical attitude. One of the greatest influences on the current trend toward breastfeeding is the change in medical attitude. Today the American Academy of Pediatrics (AAP) actively recommends breastfeeding, as indicated by its Committee on Nutrition.

Beginning with its 1978 report, the AAP has recommended that all physicians encourage mothers to breastfeed their infants.[59,60] The AAP Committee on Nutrition declared:

1. Despite technologic advances in infant formulas, breast milk is "the best food for every newborn infant."
2. All physicians need to become "much more knowledgeable" about infant nutrition in general and breastfeeding in particular.
3. Attitudes, practices, and instruction in prenatal clinics and maternity wards should be changed to encourage breastfeeding.
4. In hospitals, mothers and infants should be kept together after birth so babies can be fed on demand.
5. Not only should information about breastfeeding be supplied to all school children, but nursing should also be portrayed as natural on television and other media.
6. To prevent conflict between breastfeeding and employment, legislation should mandate 3 to 4 months postdelivery leaves so that working mothers can breastfeed.

This hearty endorsement was followed in 1982 by a critical evaluation of how and why breastfeeding should be encouraged.[60] The AAP again voiced its support for the promotion of breastfeeding but made note of the maternal characteristics and family circumstances that may need attention when deciding on infant feeding strategies.

To reinforce the needed changes in health care practices, the AAP provided specific guidelines for activities to support breastfeeding. The final recommendations of the AAP include the following practices[60]:

- Education about breastfeeding in school for boys as well as girls since later support by the father helps breastfeeding succeed
- Public education through television, newspapers, magazines, and radio to enhance the acceptability of breastfeeding

TABLE 5-13 *Percentage of Mothers Breastfeeding Newborn Infants in the Hospital and Infants at 5 or 6 Months of Age in the United States in 1989,* by Ethnic Background and Selected Demographic Variables*

Category	Total		White		Black		Hispanic†	
	Newborns	5-6 Month Infants	Newborns	5-6 Month Infants	Newborns	5-6 Month Infants	Newborns	5-6 Month Infants
All mothers	52.2	19.6	58.5	22.7	23.0	7.0	48.4	15.0
Parity								
Primiparous	52.6	16.6	58.3	18.9	23.1	5.9	49.9	13.2
Multiparous	51.7	22.7	58.7	26.8	23.0	7.9	47.2	16.5
Marital status								
Married	59.8	24.0	61.9	25.3	35.8	12.3	55.3	18.8
Unmarried	30.8	7.7	40.3	9.8	17.2	4.6	37.5	8.6
Maternal age								
<20 years	30.2	6.2	36.8	7.2	13.5	3.6	35.3	6.9
20-24 years	45.2	12.7	50.8	14.5	19.4	4.7	46.9	12.6
25-29 years	58.8	22.9	63.1	25.0	29.9	9.4	56.2	19.5
30-34 years	65.5	31.4	70.1	34.8	35.4	13.6	57.6	23.4
≥35 years	66.5	36.2	71.9	40.5	35.6	14.3	53.9	24.4
Maternal education								
No college	42.1	13.4	48.3	15.6	17.6	5.5	42.6	12.2
College‡	70.7	31.1	74.7	34.1	41.1	12.2	66.5	23.4

Family income								
<$7,000	28.8	7.9	36.7	9.4	14.5	4.3	35.3	10.3
$7,000-$14,999	44.0	13.5	49.0	15.2	23.5	7.3	47.2	13.0
$15,000-$24,999	54.7	20.4	57.7	22.3	31.7	8.7	52.6	16.5
≥$25,000	66.3	27.6	67.8	28.7	42.8	14.5	65.4	23.0
Maternal employment								
Full time	50.8	10.2	54.8	10.8	30.6	6.9	50.4	9.5
Part time	59.4	23.0	63.8	25.5	26.0	6.6	59.4	17.7
Not employed	51.0	23.1	58.7	27.5	19.3	7.2	46.0	16.7
U.S. census region								
New England	52.2	20.3	53.2	21.4	35.6	5.0	47.6	14.9
Middle Atlantic	47.4	18.4	52.4	21.8	30.6	9.7	41.4	10.8
East North Central	47.6	18.1	53.2	20.7	21.0	7.2	46.2	12.6
West North Central	55.9	19.9	58.2	20.7	27.7	7.9	50.8	22.8
South Atlantic	43.8	14.8	53.8	18.7	19.6	5.7	48.0	13.8
East South Central	37.9	12.4	45.1	15.0	14.2	3.7	23.5	5.0
West South Central	46.0	14.7	56.2	18.4	14.5	3.8	39.2	11.4
Mountain	70.2	30.4	74.9	33.0	31.5	11.0	53.9	18.2
Pacific	70.3	28.7	76.7	33.4	43.9	15.0	58.5	19.7

*Mothers were surveyed when their infants were 6 months of age. They were asked to recall the method of feeding the infant when in the hospital, at age 1 week, at months 1 through 5, and on the day preceding completion of the survey. Numbers in the columns labeled "5-6 Month Infants" are an average of the 5-month and previous day responses.

†Hispanic is not exclusive of white or black.

‡College includes all women who reported completing at least 1 year of college.

Data from A Ryan, Ross Laboratories, personal communication, 1990, as presented in Institute of Medicine, National Academy of Sciences: Nutrition during lactation, Washington, DC, 1991, National Academy Press.

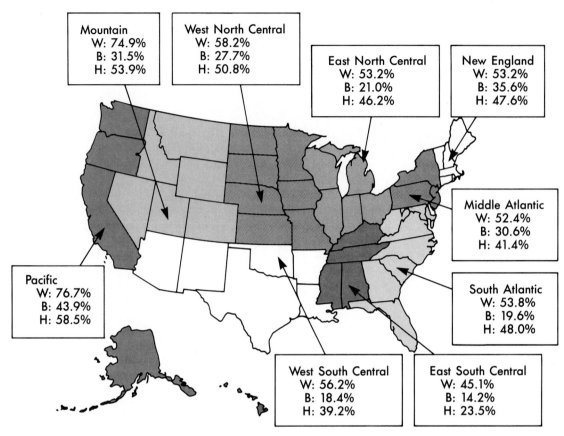

FIG. 5-12 Breastfeeding initiation rates, by census region and ethnic background. *W,* white; *B,* black; *H,* Hispanic.

Data from the 1989 Ross Mothers Survey (A. Ryan, Ross Laboratories, personal communication, 1990). Institute of Medicine, National Academy of Sciences: Nutrition during lactation, Washington, DC, 1991, National Academy Press.

- Improved education about breastfeeding techniques in medical and nursing schools, and residency programs in obstetrics, pediatrics, and family practice
- Factual educational material designed to present advantages of breastfeeding
- Encouragement not to use breastfeeding alternatives for relief, vacation, or night feeding until nursing is well established
- Breastfeeding information provided in prenatal classes and at any prenatal contact
- Decreased sedation of the mother for labor and birth
- Extended contact between mother and infant in the first 25 hours
- Rooming in encouraged except when specifically contraindicated
- Avoidance of routine supplemental feeding
- Lactation suppressants not given unless requested by the mother
- Discharge packs of formula given only at the discretion of the physician or at the request of the mother, not as a routine hospital practice
- Development of day nurseries adjacent to school or work places to encourage and support working and school-aged mothers to breastfeed

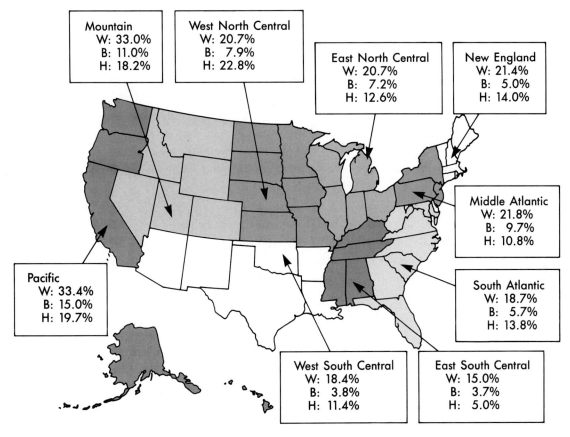

FIG. 5-13   Breastfeeding rates at 5 to 6 months postpartum, by census region and ethnic background. *W,* white; *B,* black; *H,* Hispanic.

Data from the 1989 Ross Mothers Survey (A. Ryan, Ross Laboratories, personal communication, 1990). Institute of Medicine, National Academy of Sciences: Nutrition during lactation, Washington, DC, 1991, National Academy Press.

- Utilization of lay support groups such as La Leche League
- Encouragement of continued breastfeeding of the hospitalized child
- Relactation instruction when necessary

PRENATAL AND POSTPARTUM COUNSELING
The Decision to Breastfeed

The decision to breastfeed is a significant one for the parents and is usually made relatively early in the pregnancy. The factors that influence this decision are complex and interrelated.

Where parents have not yet made a decision or have not been exposed to the advantages of breastfeeding, it is the responsibility of the health care professionals to support lactation as the optimum method of infant feeding. Although health professionals must support the parents' ultimate decision regarding feeding method, they too often fail to take a positive stand in support of lactation early enough in the prenatal period to influence the decision-making process. It has long been recognized that physicians who support lactation have higher percentages of breastfeeding mothers.

When the decision has been made to breastfeed, an individual or small group instruction session is indicated. Simply handing out pamphlets is not very effective. These sessions may be held early in the second trimester. Both parents should be included in the instruction session if possible. Fathers tend to be more supportive if they know what to expect and understand possible difficulties they may encounter. The prenatal visit provides the opportunity to get to know the parents, to find out how much they know about breastfeeding, what fears and apprehensions they may have, and to estimate how much help and support the mother is likely to need in the early weeks of breastfeeding. It is important to remember that there is a typical breastfeeding personality. Women who appear to be "nervous" can learn to breastfeed successfully if they cultivate a relaxed and confident attitude. This is best accomplished by adequate instruction along with professional and family support.

Lactation Education Program

In the beginning of the lactation education program, the health professional should discuss the advantages of breastfeeding as outlined earlier here. She should listen and respond to any concerns that the parents may have. Then the physiology of lactation and the mother's diet should be discussed.

The general physiology of lactation should be covered, explaining briefly the structure of the breast and hormonal controls of the process. A good understanding of mammary gland physiology is a great aid in promoting confidence in the ability to lactate. Women should realize that breast size is not a factor in the success of lactation. They should be informed that the glandular structure is adequately developed in virtually all women during pregnancy and differences in breast size are mainly the result of variation in the content of adipose tissue. Simplified diagrams and explanations such as those provided in this chapter may be useful for breastfeeding education.

A brief discussion of the dietary requirements for lactation should be included in the prenatal visits. It is usually sufficient to stress that additional amounts of the same types of foods that belong in any well-balanced diet, with special attention to good sources of calcium and vitamin C, will adequately provide the additional nutrition. Although fluid is an essential component of breast milk and its consumption should be encouraged, thirst dictates fluid requirements in most women. The body's ability to conserve fluid by concentrating urine allows women to succeed in lactation with wide variations in levels of fluid intake.

Nipple Conditioning

Although several studies suggest that prenatal nipple conditioning does not prevent nipple soreness during early lactation, it may be useful for some women. In societies where the breast is uncovered or where clothing is loosely worn, nipple soreness is much less a problem. The woman who plans to breastfeed should purchase a nursing brassiere that will suffice for the increased size required for the last few months of pregnancy, as well as for lactation. If her breasts are very heavy, or if the woman feels uncomfortable with the weight unsupported, the brassiere can be worn day and night. One of the easiest ways to get the nipples used to tactile stimulation is to leave the flaps on the brassiere open as much as possible during the day and night. This allows the nipples to rub against clothing, gradually desensitizing them.

Lanolin
(L *lana*, wool) Fatty substance extracted from wool, used in ointments and salves.

No special ointments or preparations are generally required for nipple conditioning. Pure **lanolin,** a component of many of the breast creams on the market, appear to be harmless, but products containing alcohol or petroleum-based products are to be avoided,

FIG. 5-14   Breast shield in place.

since they remove natural lubricants from the nipple and areola. Since soap is drying, it is advisable to wash the nipple area with water only.

Inverted Nipples

Inverted nipples occasionally occur. They can be diagnosed by pressing the areola between the thumb and forefinger. A flat or normal nipple will protrude; a truly inverted nipple will retract. Truly inverted nipples are rare. When they do occur, they can usually be treated by massage.

Not only may exercises be helpful in the prenatal period to prepare flat or inverted nipples for lactation, but also use of a nipple shield, or breast shield, may be even more effective (Fig. 5-14). The rubber nipple tip of the shield should be removed and only the plastic base with the hole in the center applied over the areola inside a well-fitting brassiere. The constant even pressure will cause the nipple to evert through the hole. The shield can be worn daily for the last weeks or months of pregnancy.

If inverted nipples are discovered at the first feeding in the hospital, the mother should use the electric pump to pull the nipples out, then place the infant quickly on the breast. If an electric pump is not available, a manual cylinder-type pump can be used. Between feedings, the mother should wear a breast shield and supportive brassiere.

Effect of Anesthetics

Another major consideration to be discussed during prenatal visits is the effect of anesthetics and analgesics given during labor and delivery on early feedings. Research indicates that even the nerve conduction anesthetics affect the newborn's reflexes and may impair ability to suck well. The baby may be lethargic and disinterested in feeding or may take the breast and suck only weakly until the effects of the anesthesia have worn off. This information may be useful to the mother in selecting an anesthetic, if it is to be used. The baby who is uncooperative because of sedation can still breastfeed successfully. Probably it will take just a few days longer to establish a let-down reflex and to produce an adequate milk supply. The baby who is severely affected may not suck well until after the third or fourth day of life. With the current trend toward early hospital discharges, it might be beneficial to keep mother and baby in the hospital for an extra day or to provide good follow-up care at home to ensure that lactation gets off to a good start.

Resources

The mother should be encouraged to jot down questions that arise. Several excellent books on breastfeeding are referenced at the end of this chapter. Most are available in paperback and from public libraries. Some large clinics have established their own lending libraries. Clients will benefit from talking with mothers who are already successfully breastfeeding. If no suitable candidates can be found from office files, local chapters of La Leche League, an international organization of mothers and professionals dedicated to spreading information about breastfeeding, will usually be able to assist the parents.

In-Hospital Postpartum Support

Breastfeeding will often be a new experience for the mother, as well as for the baby. The new mother may be apprehensive and unsure of herself, and need help and guidance in handling the infant. The clinician who is to instruct the mother at the first feeding should try to make her feel as much at ease as possible. The father should be encouraged to be present at feedings and during instruction if the hospital permits it and if the mother is comfortable with his presence. The father's support, knowledge, and understanding will be valuable later on. He may remember techniques and advice the mother has forgotten.

Positions for feeding. There are two basic breastfeeding positions, each of which is subject to a wide variety of individual adaptations. The chief requirements are (1) the comfort of the mother throughout the feeding, and (2) the positioning of the baby so that the process of swallowing is not impaired.

Episiotomy
(Gr *epision*, pubic region; *tome*, a cutting) Surgical incision into the peritoneum and vagina for obstetric purposes.

If the mother has had an **episiotomy** or operative delivery (cesarean section), she may be more comfortable breastfeeding lying down. She should position herself comfortably on her side, using pillows for additional support as required. The baby should be placed on his side with his mouth parallel to the nipple. A roll of receiving blankets makes a good support for the baby's back. This position is illustrated in Fig. 5-15. The baby can then feed comfortably from the lower breast without undue nipple traction or unnecessary distortion of the infant's alimentary tract. Both baby and mother will probably need help in repositioning to feed from the other breast.

FIG. 5-15 Recommended recumbent position for breastfeeding.

The second common position for breastfeeding is that in which the mother sits in a comfortable chair that provides good back support, arm rests, and, if possible, foot and leg support. She cradles the baby in her arm, placing his head over her elbow so that his mouth is adjacent to the nipple. A pillow may be required on her lap to support the baby's body and under her elbow to prevent her arm from becoming too tired while holding the baby's head in the proper position for feeding. This position is illustrated in Fig. 5-16 and must be reversed for feeding on the opposite breast. This position can be modified for use in the hospital bed (Fig. 5-17). If this is to be successful, the head of

FIG. 5-16 Recommended positioning for breastfeeding while sitting in a comfortable chair.

FIG. 5-17 Modified positioning for breastfeeding while sitting in a hospital bed.

FIG. 5-18   Baby is tucked under right arm like a football and is nursing on right breast.

the bed should be raised fully and the foot adjusted to provide leg support. Pillows will be required to support the arm holding the baby's head. An additional blanket roll or pillow under the mother's knees may make the position more comfortable. After feeding has begun, the position should be checked to make sure that nipple traction and distortion of the infant's alimentary tract are at a minimum.

Another popular position, especially with small babies or twins, is the "football hold." The baby's head is held in the palm of the hand while the forearm is used to support the baby's torso (Fig. 5-18). This allows the mother to move the baby easily until the proper position of the baby's mouth relative to the nipple is achieved. The "football hold" can be used while "tailor" sitting in bed with the mother's back supported. It is especially comfortable for mothers who have had cesarean deliveries.

TYPICAL CONCERNS OF THE BREASTFEEDING MOTHER

Even though the prenatal and early postnatal assistance with lactation may have been of high quality, mothers will likely have additional problems and questions during the first few weeks. A variety of concerns often develop and attention to these concerns may well determine the duration of breastfeeding for some distraught mothers.

Anxiety over Quantity and Quality of Milk Supply

Sufficient quantity. Milk is produced to equal demand in almost all women. If the letdown reflex is functioning adequately, insufficient quantity is rarely a problem. The mother's concern may come from a well-meaning friend or relative who has casually remarked, "Mrs. X didn't have enough milk for her baby so she had to bottle-feed." Nurses and other helpers should try to impress on the new breastfeeding mother that in many societies of the world *all* women breastfeed their babies and virtually *all* women in our society who really want to breastfeed can do so, too. If feeding sessions have been frequent and of adequate duration, milk supply is probably ample. Pediatricians suggest careful monitoring of the infant's growth by weighing every week during the first month of life. A gain of about one third to one half pound per week is suggested. This can be reassuring to the mother and can help the clinician detect growth problems early on.

Baby's responses. Mothers may need to be reminded that babies do not always cry from hunger. Sometimes they may need to be "bubbled" or have diapers changed. Often they may merely require companionship and sometimes a baby cries for no apparent reason. If the baby is growing well and has at least six wet diapers a day, assuming he is receiving no additional water or formula, the mother should be comforted by knowing that the milk supply is adequate and that this fussy baby might be even fussier if he were being bottle-fed.

Milk quality. Too many well-meaning "advisors" are quick to volunteer that "your milk obviously doesn't agree with him" or "he's got gas (or colic); it must be something you ate." Such comments immediately give the mother a sense of guilt. Although the protein and fat content of human milk varies slightly according to time of day, stage of lactation, and the individual woman, evidence indicates that maternal nutrient stores "subsidize" the requirements of lactation if occasionally dietary intake is inadequate. Breast milk is therefore seldom "too rich" or "too thin" if the maternal diet is adequate and the let-down reflex functions.

Mother's diet and rest. Adverse reaction to foods in the maternal diet has been known to occur. From 4 to 6 hours are required for components of metabolites of a specific food to appear in breast milk. The food producing a reaction can often be identified and omitted from the mother's diet. Most foods that could be tolerated during pregnancy will be well tolerated by the mother and the infant during lactation. If a food consistently seems to bother mother or child, it can be omitted to see if relief, real or imagined, occurs.

Adequate rest, diet, and fluids are essential, especially if the milk supply needs to be increased. Mothers do not "lose" their milk. However, sometimes a busy schedule and lack of food or rest interfere with milk production. When this happens it is wise to take a day off to "make more milk." With rest, fluids, good diet, and of course more frequent feedings, milk supply usually parallels demand within 24 to 48 hours. Growth spurts, and thus increasing demand, are common at about 6 to 12 weeks of age.

Other general anxieties. Other causes for anxiety are the softening of the breast that occurs once lactation has become established, the presence (or absence) of milk leaking, changes in infant stool patterns, and lack of sleeping through the night. All of these are normal and do not indicate lack of breast milk. Growth failure is the only true indication of inadequate nutrition in the normal breastfed infant. When this occurs it is most frequently observed after the baby is 6 months of age. About this time some women find that their breast milk alone does not provide sufficient nutrition to maintain optimum growth. In fact, however, research has demonstrated that exclusive breastfeeding can be adequate for periods varying from 2 to 15 months and that there is no specific age at which breastfeeding becomes inadequate.

Excess milk flow. Sometimes the mother's concern is actually an oversupply of milk. She should be encouraged to use manual expression to slow the flow of milk before a feeding and to express to a comfort level between feedings. This expressed milk may be frozen for supplements or donated to milk banks for premature or critically ill infants. The mother should continue to offer both breasts at each feeding but decrease time to 5 to 10 minutes per side. The use of a pacifier for increased sucking time may be desirable.

Nipple Soreness

Normal reaction versus true problem. Many women who breastfeed experience varying degrees of general nipple discomfort when feeding. The discomfort associated with the first few seconds of feeding and alleviated by the feeding is normal. It is caused by the stimulation of the breast tissue by oxytocin during let-down. True nipple soreness, which is accompanied by tenderness and redness of the areola, is evidence of tissue breakdown and is better prevented than treated.

Treatment. Some women, particularly those with fair skin, seem more susceptible to this problem. If nipples must be treated, they should be treated promptly rather than allowing the condition to progress to cracked and fissured nipples open to infection. In addition to the techniques already discussed for nipple conditioning and prevention of soreness, the following suggestions may be useful:

1. Check for proper tongue position below nipple and make sure the baby's grasp includes some of the areola. Express milk if necessary to allow proper grasp of nipple.
2. Feed the baby on demand. If he gets too hungry he may suck harder, causing further soreness.
3. Vary the position with each feeding, allowing the baby to suck on slightly different areas of the areola with each feeding.
4. Begin each feeding on the breast that is least tender. Allow the baby to suck until the let-down reflex has occurred, then switch to the tender side and allow the baby to empty the breast. Promptly return to the less tender side to finish the feeding.
5. Promptly terminate feedings when completed. Allowing an infant to suck on an empty breast causes increased tissue damage. From 7 to 10 minutes on each side should be sufficient if nipples are tender. Offer a pacifier if necessary.
6. Let nipples dry well before replacing brassiere flaps, allowing air to circulate on them as freely as possible. Air drying for 10 minutes after a feeding and before using any breast cream is a good precedure.
7. Avoid soaps, alcohol, and especially petroleum-based compounds on the nipple area, as they cause further irritation. Lanolin or a commercial breast cream may be applied after the areola has dried. **Tannic acid** has long been recognized for its role in promoting healing. Thus some mothers have found that a used tea bag, thoroughly cooled and applied to the nipple area two or three times a day, helps to promote healing.

Tannic acid
Compound of certain plants such as tea leaves, giving an astringent taste and having astringent properties that promote local tissue healing; an herbal remedy.

Engorgement

Causes. Engorged breasts are hot, heavy, and hard with milk. Many physicians and nurses see this as basically a hospital-acquired condition caused by infrequent feeding. This is at least partly true, and the consequences may be a hungry frustrated baby and a mother suffering from pain and stress. However, in some women a general increase in circulation to the mammary tissue and edema in the tissues are thought to combine with the newly produced milk to cause mild to extreme discomfort, regardless of feeding frequency. The only component of this situation that can be remedied is the milk. There is no more effective "breast pump" than a hungry baby.

Treatment. During engorgement the baby should be put to breast at least every 3 hours. The mother should compress the areola between two fingers to make it easier for the infant to grasp (Fig. 5-19). If the milk supply greatly exceeds demand, the baby should be allowed to suck only to relieve the sensation of fullness (about 5 minutes) at each breast. Some milk may be manually expressed before offering the breast to the baby if the nipple is difficult for the baby to grasp. If the baby is uncooperative, for example, sleepy, manual expression will have to be used to relieve the pressure of accumulating milk. A firmly fitting brassiere may make engorgement less painful.

Many women find relief from discomfort by the application of moist heat to the breast. This may be done with wet towels, a warm shower or bath, or steam from a sink or basin

FIG. 5-19   When breast is offered to infant, areola is gently compressed between two fingers and breast is supported to ensure that infant is able to grasp areola adequately.

From Lawrence R: Breastfeeding: a guide for the medical profession, St Louis, 1980, Times Mirror/Mosby College Publishing.

of water. For the ambulatory mother suffering from engorgement, face cloths wet with warm water and folded into plastic bags can be held in place by the brassiere. Since much of the discomfort is caused by **edema** resulting from **venous stasis,** moist heat to increase the circulation would seem a more beneficial prescription than ice packs. However, some women have found that ice or cold packs make them feel better, possibly because cold merely dulls the sensation of discomfort. Massage is also useful to help soften the breast and assist the baby in draining the ducts. If the mother is really uncomfortable, a mild analgesic can be recommended. Typical engorgement occurs only on the first full day of milk production and is of short duration, usually about 24 hours.

Leaking

A number of women experience leaking from their breasts during the first few weeks of breastfeeding. Usually it is caused by fullness in the breast or the milk letting down and is part of the normal breastfeeding experience. It may occur during a nursing from the opposite breast, just before a nursing when the breasts are full, or when nursings are missed altogether. Sometimes it is caused by psychologic conditioning. For example, a woman may leak in response to hearing a baby cry, picking up her own baby to nurse, or simply thinking about breastfeeding her baby. Some mothers may be reassured by leaking, since it is a sign of a plentiful milk supply and a functioning let-down. Often the mother and baby only need time to adjust to one another, and leaking will subside as harmony develops between supply and demand.

Supplemental Feedings

Occasional bottle-feeding. Rare is the mother who does not want—indeed, need— to be away from her infant for a brief period that will undoubtedly include a feeding. For this reason it is a good idea to introduce the baby to an occasional bottle at least by

Edema
(Gr *oidema,* swelling) Unusual increase of fluid in the intercellular tissue spaces, local or generalized.

Venous stasis
(L *venosus,* vein; Gr *stasis,* standing still) A stoppage, or decreased flow, of blood draining an organ, causing engorgement of the affected tissue.

the end of the first month and about once a week or so thereafter. Many infants do not accept a bottle from their mothers but will take it from father or a sitter. The breastfeeding infant will often swallow more air with a bottle-feeding and may need to be "bubbled" more frequently, particularly if he seems to take the milk very quickly.

Preparation of single feeding. Powdered formula offers advantages for use as a single feeding supplement when human milk is not available. The proper number of measures of powder can be placed in the bottle and the nipple and cap put in place. Then if the bottle is needed, about half of the required amount of cold water can be added. The bottle should be shaken thoroughly to dissolve the powder, and then the remainder of the liquid should be added as very warm water. With this method, formula dilutions are less likely, the bottle is at serving temperature, and the cost is considerably less than ready-to-feed formula—a real advantage if the baby only takes 1 or 2 oz and the remainder has to be discarded. Any unmixed unneeded bottle can safely be left in the diaper bag for the next time. If refrigerated, a can of formula powder will last at least 6 months.

Expression of Milk

Manual technique. Manual expression of milk is a useful technique for the breastfeeding mother to learn. Although some women may find it a laborious procedure, there is often no substitute. Actually, the procedure is simple. First apply moist heat to the breast and massage gently for 5 to 10 minutes before expression or until a let-down reflex can be obtained. Then place the thumb on top and the forefinger under the areolar margin, gently pushing the finger and thumb back toward the chest wall to grasp behind the milk sinuses (Fig. 5-20). Squeeze gently in a "pumping" motion toward the nipple to remove the milk that has collected in the milk sinuses. Repeat the procedure, rotating the position of the grasp on the nipple occasionally so that all the sinuses are drained. Some women will find that the milk flows freely once a let-down occurs. Others will only be able to express a few drops at a time.

Breast pump. Mothers who need to express milk for a period of a day or weeks, such as in the case of a working mother or the mother of a hospitalized infant, might find it considerably easier and more comfortable to use a breast pump. Some very good manual pumps are now on the market (Fig. 5-21), and several high-quality electric breast pumps (Fig. 5-22) are also available. Each one simulates the nursing experience by providing alternating periods of negative and positive pressure. Many cities have rental sources of breast pumps. La Leche League maintains a rental supply of electric breast pumps in some cities. Manual breast pumps frequently do not work well and can cause considerable discomfort and even nipple damage because of the tremendous uninterrupted negative pressure used to extract the milk.

FIG. 5-20   Manual expression of breast milk. Front view, side view, and two-handed method for efficient women with good aim.

FIG. 5-21 Several popular varieties of manual breast pumps. **A,** Marshal or Kaneson. **B,** Medela. **C,** Lloyd-B. **D,** Egnell hand-operated pump.

From Worthington-Roberts BS and Williams SR: Nutrition in pregnancy and lactation, ed 4, St Louis, 1989, Times Mirror/Mosby College Publishing.

FIG. 5-22 Typical electric breast pump.

From Worthington-Roberts BS and Williams SR: Nutrition in pregnancy and lactation, ed 4, St Louis, 1989, Times Mirror/Mosby College Publishing.

Storage of Milk

If expressed human milk is to be saved for future feeding, care must be taken to assure that it is safe from microbes with minimal loss of its nutritional or protective characteristics. Fresh human milk is bacteriologically safe for up to, but no longer than, 6 hours after expression.[61] Freezing not only protects milk from contamination but also promotes minimal change in milk composition.[62] Membranes of milk cells are destroyed by this process and some hydrolysis of triglycerides occurs.[63] However, immunoglobulin levels, antibody titers, and nutritional properties are virtually unchanged. Heat treatment and **lyophilization** promote additional losses.[64,65] Fat and protein digestibility are reduced and milk cells damaged. Also levels of many of the protective factors are substantially reduced. Recent data suggest, however, that rapid high-temperature treatment allows for retention of nutritional and immunologic qualities.[66]

Several efforts have been made to determine if the type of storage container influences the quality of the milk. Paxson and Cress reported that the placement of human milk into glass containers markedly reduces retrieval of the white cells even though **phagocytosis** is unaffected.[67] These workers recommended that human milk be collected in plastic containers. However, Goldblum and associates reported that the type of container made little difference in the number of identifiable cells after 4 hours of storage.[68] They also found that levels of some of the protective factors declined with storage during the 4-hour period, but no one type of container proved to be superior for the storage of all of the measured immunologic factors. These investigators concluded that because of the profound loss of sIgA antibodies in polyethylene bags, the difficulty in handling the flexible bags, and the potential breakage of the Pyrex glass containers, polypropylene containers were best for future work.

Duration of Breastfeeding

The tradition in most parts of the world is to breastfeed for 2 to 3 years. Weaning is rather natural at this age, since the child can now feed himself and eat a full adult diet. He also has teeth and can walk and talk a little and thus express wishes and disagreements. The mother, too, may again become pregnant at this time so that her attention will need to be directed toward the new infant.

Spontaneous termination. Many young children spontaneously give up breastfeeding at about 1 year of age or soon thereafter, especially if they are receiving adequate supplementary foods. Some mothers feel much relief, and others feel sad or rejected. Some children cling to the breast for years, and again maternal response to this behavior is mixed. There are also a few children who cling to the breast and refuse to eat solid foods. These are usually children a year of age who have had solids introduced too late. It is essential that these children be trained to eat solid food, and the sooner the training takes place, the easier it will be for the parent.

The individual mother-child couple must determine their own ideal duration of breastfeeding. Factors to consider include:

1. Convenience of the mother
2. Needs of the child, both psychologic and physiologic
3. Availability of satisfactory alternative or supplemental feeds
4. Custom in the community

Whether a mother breastfeeds her child for 2 months or 2 years, the main concern of the health care provider is to support the mother in her decision, and to help her avoid cessation of breastfeeding against her wishes.

Lyophilization
(Gr *lyein,* to dissolve; *philein,* to love, having an affinity for a stable solution) Process of rapid freezing and dehydration of the frozen product under high vacuum to stabilize or preserve a biologic substance.

Phagocytosis
(Gr *phagein,* to eat; *cyte,* hollow vessel, anything that contains or covers) Engulfing of microorganisms, other cells, or foreign particles by phagocytes.

SPECIAL PROBLEMS
Maternal and Infant Conditions

Contraindications to lactation. Although each case must be evaluated on its own merit, there are very few conditions that automatically preclude breastfeeding. The genetic disease **galactosemia** is one *absolute* contraindication to breastfeeding. Breast milk is a rich source of lactose, and the very survival of infants with galactosemia depends on their receiving a non-lactose-containing formula. Galactosemia is a rare disorder, occurring in approximately 1 in every 60,000 births. Another genetic disease **phenylketonuria (PKU)** is also often mentioned as a contraindication to breastfeeding. However, breast milk has relatively low levels of phenylalanine. In fact, infants who are exclusively breastfed may receive a phenylalanine intake near the amount recommended for treating PKU. Total or partial nursing can therefore be used, although close monitoring of the infant's blood phenylalanine levels is required.

> **Galactosemia**
> Rare inherited disease in newborns caused by a missing enzyme (galactose-1-phosphate uridyl transferase—G-1-PUT), required for conversion of galactose (from lactose) to glucose. Untreated galactose accumulation in the blood causes extensive tissue damage and potential death. Normal growth and development now follows newborn screening and immediate initiation of a galactose-free diet with a special soy-base formula.

Mothers with a known transmissible viral disease, such as acquired immunodeficiency syndrome (AIDS) should probably not breastfeed. Breastfeeding is also inappropriate in cases of alcoholism, heroin addiction, malaria, or severe chronic disease resulting in maternal malnutrition. Patients with active tuberculosis should not breastfeed. However, if the mother is being treated with an antituberculosis drug and is culture negative, breastfeeding is allowed. In such cases, careful checks of mother and infant are necessary because an accumulation of the antituberculin drug, Isoniazid, can cause liver damage. Women with diagnosed breast cancer are usually advised not to breastfeed so that the needed treatment can be given immediately.

Mothers requiring drug therapy for management of chronic medical conditions may not be able to breastfeed if the only drug of choice is contraindicated during lactation. Recommendations of the American Academy of Pediatrics related to lactation and drug use are periodically updated (Table 5-7).

Cesarean birth. Mothers who have had operative deliveries ("C-sections") usually find that they can breastfeed successfully after the effects of the anesthesia have worn off for both the mother and child. In fact the mother can minimize the effects of pain medication on her baby by taking it 15 to 30 minutes directly before nursing. It may be possible for the mother to avoid some discomfort by requesting that the intravenous line be placed in a position that allows her maximum ability to handle her baby. Use of plenty of pillows will allow her to reduce the discomfort of pressure on her incision. If she can be comfortable in more than one position, she may be able to increase the number of nursing positions and reduce the severity of nipple soreness. Despite the few potential problems, the rate of successful breastfeeding among cesarean mothers is no different from that of mothers who deliver vaginally.

Poor let-down function. Some women seem to have more trouble than others in establishing a satisfactory let-down reflex. The extent to which the mother's emotional state contributes to the problem must be assessed. Anxiety and stress are known separately to decrease milk output since adrenalin inhibits oxytocin release. Anything that encourages relaxation should enhance let-down. A warm bath, moist heat to the breasts, gentle massage, and tactile stimulation, as well as soft lights and soft music, have been known to help. A moderate amount of alcohol seems to be beneficial as a relaxant for the mother and seems to enhance the let-down. Excessive amounts of alcohol and caffeine, however, have both been reported to interfere with the let-down reflex. The mother who habitually smokes to relax should avoid doing so during nursing and use other means, such as mental exercises. Failing that she should at least wait until the infant is sucking vigorously and the ejection is well established, then in the meanwhile continue her efforts to quit smoking entirely. Marijuana contains a psychoactive chemical (9-tetrahydrocannabinol) that acts on the hypothalamus and eventually disrupts pituitary production of prolactin as well as other hormones.

Colds and influenza. The presence of colds or other mild viral infections such as influenza is usually no reason to discontinue lactation as long as the mother feels able to breastfeed. The infant has usually been exposed to the infection by the time the mother realizes that she is affected. There is good evidence that the infant has some immunity through maternal antibodies. If the infant is infected, it is often a very mild form. When the infant has a cold, congestion makes breathing difficult during nursing. Use of a nasal aspirator to remove mucus and aid breathing may be of some help.

Clogged milk ducts. This condition is caused by incomplete emptying of one or more ducts. This sometimes occurs when the infant's feeding position does not allow for equal drawing on all of the milk sinuses, causing stasis. Milk or cast-off cells accumulate within a duct and form a localized plug or blockage. Milk then builds up behind the plug. Tenderness may develop in the area of the plug, and a lump may be felt at the point of blockage. Under these circumstances of simple obstruction, no fever, flulike symptoms, or systematic reactions typically occur. The remedy is (1) more frequent feeding, especially on the affected side; (2) rest; (3) analgesics, if necessary; and (4) application of moist heat. If the mother can lie down and allow the infant to nurse on the affected breast for half an hour or longer, the improvement is often dramatic. If treatment is prompt, recovery should be nearly complete within 24 hours.

It is highly desirable that the plug be removed quickly, since plugged ducts can develop into larger blocked-off areas called a "caked breast." This may be followed by a breast infection and considerable discomfort. If the plug can be released, however, improvement can be rapid. Sometimes plugs dissolve or are reabsorbed by maternal tissues. If the plug is released and comes out with the milk, it may be brownish or greenish and thick and stringy. This is no danger for the baby, but he may temporarily reject the milk.

Mastitis. The symptoms of **mastitis,** breast infection, are similar to those of engorgement. The breast is tender, distended with milk, and may feel hot to touch. Fever may be present. Treatment consists of prompt medical attention, antibiotic therapy, bed rest, and continued breastfeeding. Discontinued feeding causes increased stasis and further pain. Frequently the source of the infection is an untreated infection in the infant. Recurrent breast infections may require culturing of the milk or the baby's mouth to determine which antibiotics to prescribe. Infrequently the cause of the infection may be exposure to bacteria carried by other family members. If all other treatments prove ineffective, cultures should be taken from the rest of the family to determine the source of bacteria and prescribe simultaneous treatment for all involved. In any case, weaning should not be attempted until the infection has cleared up.

Abscess. When breast infections are not successfully treated, they may develop into a serious and painful condition called an abscess, in which there is localized pus and swelling of tissue. An abscess should be viewed as a serious problem requiring immediate medical attention. Diagnosis is made by culturing the secretions from the breast. Usual treatment includes antibiotics along with massage, pumping, and sometimes surgical drainage. It may be necessary to discontinue nursing on the affected side, but usually it can continue on the unaffected breast.

Maternal Disease

Chronic disease. Heart disease, diabetes, hepatitis, nephrosis, and most other chronic medical conditions are not themselves a contraindication to breastfeeding. Usually if the condition can be managed well enough to allow successful maintenance of pregnancy, breastfeeding may be the feeding method of choice because it is less tiring for the mother.

Mastitis
(Gr *mastos*, breast; *itis*, inflammation) Breast infection; inflammation of the mammary gland.

Diabetes. Since management of the diabetic woman in pregnancy has become increasingly more successful, many diabetic mothers are now choosing to breastfeed. In fact some mothers with diabetes enjoy a postpartum remission of their diabetes, which may last through lactation and in some cases several years longer. The remission has been attributed to the hormone interactions that affect the hypothalamus and pituitary gland during pregnancy, labor, delivery, and lactation.

Since persons with diabetes are known to be prone to infection, mastitis may pose a significant threat, and vaginitis may be more common. Infection of the nipples may also occur because of *Candida albicans*. Careful anticipatory care, avoidance of fatigue, and early antibiotic management of developing problems are wise.

Thyroid disease. When hypothyroidism is diagnosed in the mother, it is generally treated with full replacement therapy of desiccated thyroid. Under such circumstances breastfeeding is not contraindicated. If the mother is truly hypothyroid, care should be taken to rule out hypothyroidism in the infant. Diagnosis is made by evaluating blood values and is not a hazard to the nursing infant.

Unlike hypothyroidism, the diagnostic procedures and therapeutic management of the mother with hyperthyroidism present some hazards to the breastfed infant. Treatment includes antithyroid medication, which inhibits the synthesis of thyroid hormones. Compounds in this medication may appear in breast milk and may build up in the infant's circulation. With careful monitoring and thyroid medication, nursing may proceed successfully. However, care must be taken to watch for **bradycardia** and other signs of hypothyroidism, including goiter.

Bradycardia
(Gr *bradys*, slow; *kardia*, heart) A slow heart beat, evidenced by slowing of the pulse rate to less than 60 beats/min.

Cancer. A mother with a diagnosis of breast cancer should not nurse her infant in order to have definitive treatment immediately for herself. However, not all lumps in the lactating breast are cancer, or even benign tumors. The lactating breast is lumpy by nature, and the lumps shift day by day. If a mass is located and the physician thinks it should be biopsied, it can be done under local anesthesia without weaning the infant. Usually such a lump is diagnosed as a benign mass. Immediate surgery to remove the mass may relieve tremendous anxiety without necessarily sacrificing breastfeeding.

Infectious disease. Infectious diseases that require isolation of the mother from other adults, as well as from children, may be a contraindication to breastfeeding.

Family and Social Situations

Multiple births. It is entirely possible to nurse more than one infant and many case reports support this fact. Historical observations of wet nurses indicate that support of six babies simultaneously is within the realm of physiologic capability. The key deterrent to nursing twins or triplets is not usually the milk supply but the time. Nursing two infants at the same time is clearly more efficient. A number of tricks have been proposed to accommodate more than one infant, but as they become larger and more active, it may be a real challenge to keep them simultaneously nursing without assistance from the father or a friend. The nursing mother of more than one infant needs to conscientiously attend to her own rest and nourishment.

Working during lactation. Many women believe that breastfeeding conflicts with working outside the home. This is a myth, since the two can go nicely together. The reduced incidence and severity of illness in the breastfeeding infant may actually reduce the days the mother misses from work. It is desirable for the working mother to have a minimum of 4 to 6 weeks at home with her nursing infant before returning to a full-time job. This time will allow for the successful establishment of lactation and the development of a close mother-child relationship. This strong foundation will provide the mother with substantial motivation to continue breastfeeding as her work commitments increase and her time with the infant decreases. The dedicated working mother will want to learn to express her milk so that she can provide it to her infant and maintain her lactation capacity for the days she has to work.

Pregnancy during lactation. Occasionally a mother may wish to nurse an infant after she becomes pregnant again. This circumstance is physiologically possible, but the nutritional and psychologic demands on the mother are substantial. Some women may even experience uterine contractions while nursing and in some cases may need to consider weaning to avoid the possibility of spontaneous abortion. The child may become discouraged from nursing because of the changing composition and taste of the milk produced as the pregnancy proceeds. The mother's milk supply may also decrease, and this may cause her child to lose interest in nursing.

Nursing siblings—tandem nursing. With sufficient sucking stimulus, most mothers can produce enough milk to successfully nurse a young infant, as well as an older child. It is important, however, to consider the emotional needs of the older sibling and the physical well-being of the mother. If the mother feels that the older child may satisfy his sucking needs and benefit emotionally from the breastfeeding experience, she may decide to continue nursing both children. However, if she feels that this undertaking is too demanding or she resents the older child nursing, she is well advised to wean the older child as soon as possible.

If the mother decides to wean the toddler, she should go about it gradually. It may be rather difficult while she is nursing the young baby, since the older one may want to nurse when he sees the younger sibling at the breast. An obvious solution is to nurse the baby at the times when the older child is not around or is happily occupied with other things. The mother will need to decide on some alternative activities and snacks to take the place of breastfeeding so that the transition from nursing to total weaning will go smoothly.

Relactation. Relactation is the resumption of lactation after it has been stopped some time beyond the immediate postpartum period. This process may be attempted by women who have for various reasons not nursed their infant for a while or by women who change their minds about lactation after weaning has taken place. To reactivate the lactation process requires that appropriate stimuli are provided to the breasts. The baby's sucking or manual stimulation may be accompanied by use of medications or hormones. Success generally depends on the mother's determination and the baby's willingness to suckle at the less than satisfying breast. The longer the interlude between initial lactation and relactation, the more likely the effort is to fail.

A mother needs to decide if she really wishes to attempt relactation. Considerable motivation is required, and initially the effort may be very time consuming. It should be clear to the mother that she may not be able to produce an adequate milk supply to meet all the infant's nutritional requirements. In fact such a goal may be unrealistic and undesirable. The majority of mothers who express great pleasure in their relactation experience indicate that the mother-infant relationship is of far greater short- and long-term importance than the act of the breastfeeding alone. They emphasize that breastfeeding is as much *nurturing at* the breast as it is *nutrition from* the breast. In many instances undue emphasis on a complete milk supply actually hinders the mother's ability to achieve it.

The mother who is attempting relactation needs to build up her milk supply by making sure that she receives satisfactory rest and nutrition along with frequent sucking stimulus. She may encourage the infant to suckle by simply cuddling and stroking, but in addition may apply a sweet-tasting substance to the end of the nipple. She may effectively offer the baby a supplement and avoid nipple confusion between the bottle and the breast by use of a nursing supplementer, the Lact-Aid. The Lact-Aid Nursing Trainer is a plastic bag that can be filled with formula and affixed to the mother's clothing near the breast

FIG. 5-23 Lact-Aid nursing trainer in use.

Courtesy of Lact-Aid International, Inc, PO Box 1066, Athens, TN 80206.

during a feeding. A similar product called the Lactation Supplementer has recently been developed by Medela. While the baby nurses at the mother's breast, he receives formula through a small tube attached to the bag at one end and taped to the mother's nipple at the other (Fig. 5-23). Gradual weaning from the Lact-Aid or the Lactation Supplementer can be provided by putting less and less in the bag, in response to cues indicating an increase in maternal lactation, that is, excess supplement left in bag after nursing, very wet diapers, soft stools, spitting up after feedings, and increased time between feedings.

Nursing the adopted infant. It is extremely time consuming, and sometimes impossible, to induce lactation without having been pregnant. Even when a pregnancy has been carried out in the past, great motivation is required to nurse an adopted infant. Chances increase if the mother has given birth or nursed another baby. If she is currently nursing another baby or has recently weaned one, her chances for success are good. A mother embarking on this nursing experience should have realistic motives and goals. She should not expect to provide all the infant's nutrition through lactation but should look forward to a satisfying emotional experience.

The nipple preparation and relactation techniques described above apply also to the adoptive mother. In addition, it is useful for the mother to pump her breasts to stimulate milk production. She can gradually increase the frequency and duration of this activity until it reaches a level of about 20 minutes every 2 hours when the baby's arrival is near. The mother should realize that it may be quite a while before she sees any results from her pumping and that even a small amount of milk means success. The milk supply will increase rapidly when the baby begins suckling. If the mother is not able to obtain her baby soon after birth, however, her chances of success may decline, since the baby will have been bottle-fed and may suffer from nipple confusion.

The fact that some women have succeeded in nursing their adoptive infants does not mean that all adoptive mothers can nurse or should attempt to do so. This point was well made by a physician whose family had recently adopted a young infant.[69] He pointed out that adoptive parents often have decided to adopt a child after a long period of reproductive failure and a trying experience with an adoptive agency. When the adopted infant finally arrives, the parents have to cope with a considerable role handicap. In view of the substantial time commitment of induced lactation and the stress and frustration that can be associated with it, one must really ask whether the advantages outweigh the disadvantages. Attempting lactation may set the mother up for another failure of physical function and loss of self-esteem, and in addition it requires much time and energy that could be devoted to more significant areas of social adjustment. *No pressure should ever be put on the adoptive mother to breastfeed*. If she wishes to try, she should have support and guidance. However, if she finds that she and her family are frustrated and exhausted, she should immediately reevaluate her intentions and not be encouraged to continue.

Teenage mothers. Most teenage mothers elect to keep their babies even when their home environments are neither supportive nor conducive to successful lactation. The self-image of the teenager may be poor, and she may have much doubt about her self-worth. She frequently feels uncomfortable in her new role as a mother. If the young mother expresses some interest in breastfeeding, effort should be made to determine her motives, and advantages and disadvantages should be discussed. It should be determined whether or not breastfeeding would significantly compromise her ability to continue in school or provide for the infant's other needs. Physiologically, teenagers are entirely capable of breastfeeding, although some will have less functional breast tissue than adult women. Teenage mothers are capable of satisfactory milk production and experience the same difficulties as other women. When problems arise, however, teenagers are less likely to overcome them and continue breastfeeding. They obviously require much support. Those with good support systems often breastfeed for the same amount of time as older mothers.

Failure to Thrive

Causes. Failure of some breastfed infants to thrive has been reported for several decades and in many respects is no less puzzling today than when it was first described. A flow chart summarizing possible maternal and infant causes of the problem is provided in Fig. 5-24. In some cases there may be no history of excessive crying or dissatisfaction. The infant takes the breast well, nurses for a sufficient length of time, and sleeps well. There may be nothing to indicate abnormal nutrition, or whether the infant is getting enough to eat (see box on p. 207), until marked signs of dehydration and even marasmus appear.

Suckling process. According to Frantz and Fleiss, a major cause of failure to thrive in the totally breastfed infant is a weak or ineffective suck.[70] As these clinicians have repeatedly observed, the baby who is gaining weight poorly often has a rapid flutter-type chewing suckle that does not seem to have any drawing pause between the jaw motions, and swallowing occurs only every 3 to 15 suckles. On the other hand, they have noted that the babies who gain weight well also have a chew action to their jaw motions but display a slight pause in their cheeks between each suckle, and they appear to swallow with every suckle. The quality of the suckle often improved when an effort was made to hold the tongue down at the start of the feed and the tongue position was periodically checked. It also helped to have the mother switch breasts frequently, switching when inappropriate suckling began to develop. In some cases the Lact-Aid Nursing Trainer was found to be useful. Since minumum effort is required by infants to fill their mouths with milk, they have to create a chain reaction of suckle, swallow, suckle, and swallow.

Evaluation of growth rate. The breastfed infant should be evaluated regularly to determine if growth is proceeding normally (see box on p. 208). If the infant fails to thrive, even after techniques to enhance let-down and improve milk supply, and then

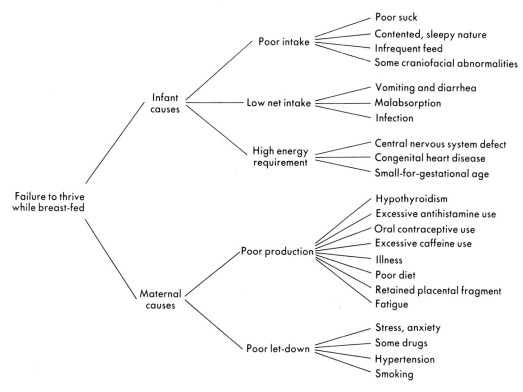

FIG. 5-24 Diagnostic flowchart for failure to thrive.

Modified from Lawrence R: Breast-feeding: a guide for the medical profession, ed 2, St Louis, 1986, Times Mirror/Mosby College Publishing.

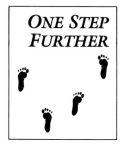

ONE STEP FURTHER

How to Tell If the Infant Is Getting Enough to Eat

1. Urination six or eight times a day. Most breastfed infants will have at least one or two stools a day during the first few weeks and may have as many as one every feeding.
2. Adequate weight gain.
3. Good color and skin tone.
4. Feeding every 1½ to 3 hours, after which baby seems content.

improves when placed on a formula, breastfeeding should either be abandoned or a regular program of supplementary feeding established. The important point is to monitor growth closely enough that a life threatening emergency and panic-weaning to bottle can be avoided. In some cases of failure to thrive at the breast, the mother should receive additional support to allay feelings of guilt and failure that will inevitably arise. Breastfeeding of a subsequent child is not necessarily contraindicated.

CASE STUDY

A Breastfeeding Infant's Early Growth Pattern

A young mother and her 3-month-old infant appear in the clinic for routine well-baby care. The infant appears to be healthy but small. The body measurements reveal that weight falls on the 5th percentile and height plots on the 40th percentile. The mother reports that she is breastfeeding her baby, that things are going well although she is very tired, and that the baby is well behaved and rarely cries.

Questions for analysis
1. Define appropriate questions for the mother.
2. Outline a strategy to determine if the infant is receiving sufficient nutritional support through breast milk.
3. Propose an acceptable monitoring protocol.
4. Suggest solutions to the various problems that might be identified.

COMMON REASONS FOR FAILURE OF LACTATION
Poor Maternal Attitude

Probably the chief reason for failure of breastfeeding is a poor maternal attitude toward lactation in the first place. The mother who does not sincerely want to breastfeed her infant but agrees to do so to placate her family, friends, or nurse will have a very difficult time. Fear, worry, distraction, anger, and other such emotions have a potent effect on the let-down reflex. When this reflex functions poorly, the infant receives only a portion of the milk supply because the bulk of the milk stored in the alveoli is not released. The infant cries from hunger and eventually fails to gain weight. This provides negative feedback to the mother and a vicious cycle begins.

Inadequate Milk Supply

Failure to establish adequate milk supply by frequent feeding on demand is a great deterrent to successful lactation. Before breastfeeding is abandoned, the clinician should check to see if caloric intake has been adequate to support lactation. Are there anxieties and distractions to nursing that can be eliminated? Is the mother getting enough rest? Is she taking oral contraceptives or other medication that suppresses lactation? The problem may be inhibition of the let-down reflex rather than failure of milk production. Is the hospital routine nonsupportive? Other problems can stem from use of supplements too soon and too frequently, and from early introduction of solid foods.

Lack of Information and Support

Another common reason for failure of lactation is lack of information and support for the mother. Many women do not have the support of friends or relatives who have successfully breastfed infants. These women are often poorly informed about the physiology of lactation and about the virtually fool-proof method of meeting the infant's nutritional needs. New breastfeeding mothers may have fears of the milk supply being too low in quality or quantity to support the infant's growth requirements. They may become discouraged when the infant does not feed well because he has been sedated during labor and delivery. They may be discouraged by nipple discomfort or engorgement, common complaints during the first few days of breastfeeding. Often a new mother feels mildly depressed around the fourth or fifth day postpartum, and any initial lactation problems will be magnified out of proportion. This is particularly true if the mother does not see these occurrences as normal. If the parents have had adequate prenatal instruction and good counseling during the hospital stay, the chances of weathering these storms are greatly increased. If the breastfeeding mother has the support of her partner and understanding professionals who can provide kind words to bolster her confidence even when things are going fine, she will feel she has a place to turn for help and advice when things go badly. Under these circumstances problems that cannot be avoided can be more easily overcome.

Summary

From many standpoints evidence supports the suitability of breast milk for the human infant. The important role of the health professional in counseling breastfeeding mothers is now recognized. Effective functioning as a breastfeeding counselor demands a thorough understanding of the process of lactation and a sincere desire to help inexperienced mothers decide for themselves about the best approaches to infant feeding in their own circumstances.

In-depth knowledge about the problems women experience with lactation needs recognition. Workable management strategies need to be devised. Because support for breastfeeding has been voiced by an array of health care disciplines and lay groups, and because breastfeeding counseling is now of high quality, breastfeeding should remain popular in the future. Continued attention should be given, however, to early childhood exposure to lactation along with effective educational programs for both boys and girls.

Review Questions

1. Diagram the structural components of the female mammary gland and define the process of human milk synthesis and movement through the system.
2. Describe the basic physiology of lactation referring to appropriate anatomic sites, hormonal contributions, and other significant details.
3. Outline the advantages and disadvantages of breastfeeding.
4. Define the significant characteristics of human milk that make it particularly suitable for human infants.
5. Outline a dozen concerns expressed by breastfeeding mothers and describe appropriate approaches to counseling women about these concerns.

References

1. Worthington-Roberts BS and Williams SR: Nutrition in pregnancy and lactation, ed 4, St Louis, 1989, Times Mirror/Mosby College Publishing.
2. Shaul DMB: The composition of milk from wild animals, Int Year Zoo Book 4:333, 1962.
3. Institute of Medicine, National Academy of Sciences: Nutrition during lactation, Washington, DC, 1991, National Academy Press.
4. Hartmann PE et al: Studies on breast-feeding and reproduction in women in Western Australia—a review, Birth Fam J 8:215, 1982.

5. Lovelady CA et al: Lactation performance of exercising women, Am J Clin Nutr 52:103, 1990.

6. Lawrence RA: Breastfeeding: a guide for the medical profession, ed 3, St Louis, 1989, The CV Mosby Co.

7. Lindblad BS and Rahimtoola RJ: A pilot study of the quality of human milk in a lower socio-economic group in Karachi, Pakistan, Acta Paediatr Scand 63:125, 1974.

8. Chavalittamrong B et al: Protein and amino acids of breast milk from Thai mothers, Am J Clin Nutr 34:1126, 1981.

9. Sturman JA: Taurine in development, J Nutr 118:1169, 1988.

10. Simopoulos AP: ω-3 Fatty acids in growth and development and in health and disease, Nutr Today 23:10, 1988.

11. Carroll JE et al: Carnitine deficiency revisited, J Nutr 117:1501, 1987.

12. Heitlinger LA et al: Mammary amylase: a possible alternate pathway of carbohydrate digestion in infancy, Pediatr Res 17:15, 1983.

13. McMillan JA et al: Iron sufficiency in breast-fed infants and the availability of iron from human milk, Pediatrics 58:686, 1976.

14. McMillan JA et al: Iron absorption from human milk, simulated human milk and proprietary formulas, Pediatrics 60:896, 1977.

15. Garry PJ et al: Iron absorption from human milk and formula with and without iron supplementation, Pediatr Res 15:822, 1981.

16. Owen GM et al: Iron nutriture of infants exclusively breast-fed the first five months, J Pediatr 99:237, 1981.

17. Casey CE et al: Availability of zinc: loading tests with human milk, cow's milk and infant formulas, Pediatrics 68:394, 1981.

18. Hollis BW et al: The effects of oral vitamin D supplementation and ultraviolet phototherapy on the antirachitic sterol content of human milk, American Society of Bone and Mineral Research Annual Meeting, 1982 (abstract).

19. Greer FR et al: Bone mineral content and serum 25-hydroxyvitamin D concentration in breast-fed infants with and without supplemental vitamin D, J Pediatr 98:696, 1981.

20. Greer FR et al: Bone mineral content and serum 25-hydroxyvitamin D concentrations in breast-fed infants with and without supplemental vitamin D: one year follow-up, J Pediatr 100:919, 1982.

21. Ozsoylu S and Hasanoglu A: Vitamin D supplementation in breast-fed infants, J Pediatr 100:1000, 1982.

22. Finberg L: Human milk feeding and vitamin D supplementation—1981, J Pediatr 99:228, 1981.

23. Bachrach S et al: An outbreak of vitamin D deficiency rickets in a susceptible population, Pediatrics 64:871, 1979.

24. Edidin DV et al: Resurgence of nutritional rickets associated with breastfeeding and special dietary practices, Pediatrics 65:232, 1980.

25. Byerly LO and Kirksey A: Effects of different levels of vitamin C intake on the vitamin C concentration in human milk and the vitamin C intakes of breast-fed infants, Am J Clin Nutr 41:665, 1985.

26. Felice JH and Kirksey A: Effects of vitamin B6 deficiency during lactation on the vitamin B6 content of milk, liver, and muscle of rats, J Nutr 111:610, 1981.

27. Borschel MW and Kirksey A: Relationship of plasma pyridoxal phosphate levels to vitamin B6 intakes during the first six months, Fed Proc 42:1331, 1983.

28. Sandberg DP et al: The content, binding, and forms of vitamin B12 in milk, Am J Clin Nutr 34:1717, 1981.

29. Specker BL et al: Vitamin B12: low milk concentrations are related to low serum concentrations in vegetarian women and to methylmalonic aciduria in their infants, Am J Clin Nutr 52:1073, 1990.

30. Kuhn T et al: Maternal vegan diet causing a serious infantile neurological disorder due to vitamin B12 deficiency, Eur J Pediatr 150:205, 1991.

31. Beerens H et al: Influence of breast-feeding on the bifid flora of the newborn intestine, Am J Clin Nutr 33:2434, 1980.
32. Reid B et al: Prostaglandins in human milk, Pediatrics 66:870, 1980.
33. Miranda R et al: Effect of maternal nutritional status on immunological substances in human colostrum and milk, Am J Clin Nutr 37:632, 1983.
34. American Academy of Pediatrics, Committee on Drugs: The transfer of drugs and other chemicals into human milk, Pediatrics 84:924, 1989.
35. Jacobson JL: Determinants of polychlorinated biphenyls (PBBs), polybrominated biphenyls (PBBs), and dichlorodiphenyl trichloroethane (DDT) levels in the sera of young children, Am J Pub Health 79:1401, 1989.
36. Savage EP et al: National study of chlorinated hydrocarbon insecticide residues in human milk, USA, Am J Epidemiol 113:413, 1981.
37. Le Guennec JC and Billon B: Delay in caffeine elimination in breast-fed infants, Pediatrics 79:264, 1987.
38. Binkiewicz A et al: Pseudo-Cushing syndrome caused by alcohol in breast milk, J Pediatr 93:965, 1978.
39. Little RE et al: Maternal alcohol use during breastfeeding and infant mental and motor development at one year, N Engl J Med 321:425, 1989.
40. Seitzer V and Benjamin F: Breastfeeding and the potential for human immunodeficiency virus transmission, Obstet Gynecol 75:713, 1990.
41. Belec L et al: Antibodies of human immunodeficiency virus in breast milk of healthy, seropositive women, Pediatrics 85:1022, 1990.
42. Davis MK: The role of human milk in human immunodeficiency virus infection. In Atkinson SA et al, editors: Breastfeeding, nutrition, infection and infant growth in developed and emerging countries, St Johns, Newfoundland, Canada, 1990, ARTS Biomedical Publishing and Distributing.
43. Mehta NR and Subramanian KNS: Human milk banking: current concepts, Indian J Pediatr 57:361, 1990.
44. Food and Nutrition Board, National Research Council: Recommended dietary allowances, ed 10, Washington, DC, 1989, National Academy Press.
45. English RM and Hitchcock NE: Nutrient intakes during pregnancy, lactation, and after the cessation of lactation in a group of Australian women, Br J Nutr 22:615, 1968.
46. Butte NF et al: Maternal energy balance during lactation, Fed Proc 42:922, 1983.
47. Manning-Dalton C and Allen LH: The effects of lactation on energy and protein consumption, postpartum weight change and body composition of well nourished North American women, Nutr Res 32:293, 1983.
48. Potter S et al: Does infant feeding method influence maternal postpartum weight loss? J Am Diet Assoc 91(4):441, 1991.
49. Popkin BM et al: Breast-feeding and diarrheal morbidity, Pediatrics 86:874, 1990.
50. Butte NF et al: Human milk intake and growth of exclusively breastfed infants, J Pediatr 104:187, 1984.
51. Perkin JE: Maternal influences on the development of food allergy in the infant, Top Clin Nutr 5:6, 1990.
52. Zeiger RS et al: Effect of combined maternal and infant food-allergen avoidance on development of atopy in early infancy: a randomized study, J Allergy Clin Immunol 84:72, 1989.
53. Gerrard JW: Allergy in breast-fed babies to ingredients in breast milk, Ann Allergy 42:69, 1979.
54. Lucas A and Cole TJ: Breast milk and neonatal necrotizing entero-colitis, Lancet 336:1519, 1990.
55. Auricchio S et al: Does breastfeeding protect against the development of clinical symptoms of celiac disease in children? J Pediatr Gastroenterol Nutr 2:428, 1983.
56. Riccardi G and Rivellese AA: Can diabetes mellitus be prevented by diet? Diab Nutr Metab 2:259, 1989.

57. Gielen AC et al: Maternal employment during early postpartum period: effects on initiation and continuance of breast-feeding, Pediatrics 87:298, 1991.

58. Kurinu N et al: Does maternal employment affect breast-feeding? Am J Pub Health 79:1247, 1989.

59. American Academy of Pediatrics, Committee on Nutrition: Nutrition and lactation, Pediatrics 68:435, 1981.

60. American Academy of Pediatrics: The promotion of breast-feeding, Pediatrics 69:654, 1982.

61. Pittard WB et al: Bacteriostatic qualities of human milk, J Pediatr 107:240, 1985.

62. Friend BA et al: The effect of processing and storage on key enzymes, B vitamins, and lipids of mature human milk, I. Evaluation of fresh samples and effects of freezing and frozen storage, Pediatr Res 17:61, 1983.

63. Bitman J et al: Lipolysis of triglycerides of human milk during storage at low temperature: a note of caution, J Pediatr Gastroenterol Nutr 2:521, 1983.

64. Bjorksten B et al: Collecting and banking human milk: to heat or not to heat? Br Med J 281:765, 1980.

65. Goldsmith SJ et al: IgA, IgG, IgM and lactoferrin contents of human milk during early lactation and the effect of processing and storage, J Food Protection 46:4, 1983.

66. Goldblum RM et al: Rapid high-temperature treatment of human milk, J Pediatr 104:380, 1984.

67. Paxson CL and Cress CC: Survival of human milk leukocytes, J Pediatr 94:61, 1979.

68. Goldblum RM et al: Human milk banking, I. Effects of container upon immunologic factors in mature milk, Nutr Res 1:449, 1981.

69. Carey WB: Am J Dis Child 135:973, 1981.

70. Frantz KB and Fleiss PM: Ineffective suckling as a frequent cause of failure to thrive in the totally breast-fed infant. In Freier S and Eidelman AI, editors: Human milk: its biological and social value, Amsterdam, 1980, Excerpta Medica.

Further Reading

Lawrence RA: Breast-feeding: a guide for the medical profession, St Louis, 1989, Times Mirror/ Mosby College Publishing.
   This manual provides a thorough review of the process of lactation, the composition of human milk, and counseling recommendations for breast-feeding women. The manual is especially aimed at physicians and other health care professionals.

Neville MC and Neifert MR, eds: Lactation: physiology, nutrition, and breast-feeding, New York, 1983, Plenum Press.
   This book provides a complete review of research related to lactation, human milk, and the breast-feeding experience.

Report of the Task Force on the Assessment of the Scientific Evidence Relating to Infant-feeding Practice and Infant Health: Pediatrics 4(suppl), October, 1984.
   This task force report gives a comprehensive overview of infant feeding practices around the world and their relationship to infant health.

US Department of Health and Human Services: Report of the Surgeon General's workshop on breast-feeding and human lactation, Washington, DC, 1984, US Government Printing Office.
   This report provides a summary of the recommendations of the expert committee that developed the policy of the US Surgeon General's office about breast-feeding.

US Department of Health and Human Services: Follow-up report of the Surgeon General's workshop on breast-feeding and human lactation, Washington, DC, 1986, US Government Printing Office.
   This follow-up report defines the impact of the Surgeon General's recommendations (1984) regarding breast-feeding.

Additional
New Readings

Black RF et al: Infant feeding decisions among pregnant women from a WIC population in Georgia, J Am Diet Assoc 90(2):255, 1990.

Commentary: Is supplemental water necessary for breast-fed babies? Clin Pediatr, p 669, Nov 1990.

Dusdieker LB et al: Prolonged maternal fluid supplementation in breast-feeding, Pediatrics 86:737, 1990.

Hayslip C et al: The effects of lactation on bone mineral content in healthy postpartum women, Obstet Gynecol 73:588, 1989.

Kistin N et al: Breast-feeding rates among black urban low-income women: effect of prenatal education, Pediatrics 86:741, 1990.

Martens WS et al: Failure of a nursing infant to thrive after the mother's gastric bypass for morbid obesity, Pediatrics 86:777, 1990.

Merchant K et al: Consequences for maternal nutrition of reproductive stress across consecutive pregnancies, Am J Clin Nutr 52:616, 1990.

Merchant K et al: Maternal and fetal responses to the stresses of lactation concurrent with pregnancy and short recuperative intervals, Am J Clin Nutr 52:280, 1990.

Motil KJ et al: Basal and postprandial metabolic rates in lactating and nonlactating women, Am J Clin Nutr 52:610, 1990.

Pabst HF and Spady DW: Effect of breastfeeding on antibody response to conjugate vaccine, Lancet 336:269, 1990.

Romero-Gwynn E et al: Breastfeeding intentions and practice among Hispanic mothers in Southern California, Pediatrics 84:626, 1989.

Posner AE and Schulman SK: Birth interval among breastfeeding women not using contraceptives, Pediatrics 86:747, 1990.

Sachdev HPS et al: Water supplementation in exclusively breastfed infants during summer in the tropics, Lancet 337:929, 1991.

Tate WH et al: Impact of source of drinking water on fluoride supplementation, J Pediatr 117:419, 1990.

Woolridge MW et al: Do changes in pattern of breast usage alter the baby's nutrient intake? Lancet 336:395, 1990.

Yamauchi Y et al: The relationship between rooming in/not rooming in and breast feeding variables, Acta Paediatr Scand 79:1017, 1990.

CHAPTER

6

Nutrition during Infancy

Peggy Pipes

*Basic
Concepts*

✔ *Early physical growth and maturation in the first year of life lays the foundation for continued development through the years.*

✔ *Individual energy and nutrient needs reflect rapid growth demands for the fuel, building materials, and basal metabolism.*

✔ *An appropriate milk source, breast milk or alternate formulas, with gradual solid food additions, supply both nutritional and developmental needs.*

✔ *Maturing oral structures and function determine developing infant eating skills and appropriate textures of food.*

✔ *Infant feeding behavior follows a defined developmental sequence.*

The first year after birth is one of dramatic change for normal human infants. The torso grows longer and subcutaneous fat accumulates. Infants progress from being newborns with no head control to being babies who pull themselves up to a standing position and begin to take steps. They change from securing their nourishment with a reflexive suck to picking up finger foods with a precise pincer grasp. They develop voluntary and independent movements of the tongue, lip, and jaw and begin rotary chewing. At 1 year they are beginning self-feeding and can drink from a cup if help is provided.

This chapter stresses the importance of an adequate energy and nutrient intake consumed in a loving and supportive environment. Milk and other foods supply the materials necessary for rapid linear growth and weight gain. Foods also support developmental progress. Adding appropriate textures and variety of food when infants are developmentally ready provides the stimulus for learning new skills, while feeding infants in a loving and nurturing environment helps them develop a sense of security and trust.

Human milk, or alternate formula if needed, is the baby's source of nutrients and energy for the first 4 to 6 months. The addition of semisolid foods progressing to "table foods" in the latter part of the first year provide important growth nutrients and support oral and fine motor development. Normal full-term infants fed on demand regulate their intake to consume precisely the amount they need to grow appropriately and soon establish their own schedule.

214

GROWTH AND MATURATION

From birth to 1 year of age, normal human infants triple their weight and increase their length by 50%. They progress from sucking a nipple reflexively to obtain food to beginning voluntary self-feeding in a sitting position. They change from a diet solely of milk to one that includes many finger and table foods, as well as beverages, that they will consume as adults. They bond with their parents and acquire a sense of trust, and each infant develops an ego identity as a unique person. Growth and maturation can be compromised or accelerated by undernutrition or overnutrition. Also, the stage of maturation determines the developmental readiness to progress in the acceptance of foods, texture, and self-feeding; for example, readiness to receive spoon foods and to self-feed with finger-foods. Throughout this important first year of life, infant feeding and nutrition influence both physical and psychosocial growth and development.

Physical Growth

In the 24 hours after birth, infants' adaptation to the out-of-placenta environment is critical. They begin to breathe; to receive oxygen for themselves and remove carbon dioxide from their tissues. They assume responsibility for their own circulation and temperature regulation, their own metabolic support. Digestion and absorption begin when they consume food.

Weight. Birth weight is determined by the mother's prepregnancy weight and her weight gain during pregnancy. After parturition, genetics, environment, and nutrition determine rates of gains in weight and height. Immediately after birth there is a weight loss due to a loss of fluid and some catabolism of tissue. This loss averages 6% of body weight, but occasionally exceeds 10%. Birth weight is usually regained by the tenth day. Thereafter, weight gain during infancy proceeds at a rapid but decelerating rate. Average weight gains for the first 4 months are 20 to 25 g per day, and during the next 8 months are 15 g per day. By 4 months of age, most infants weigh twice their birth weights, and by 12 months they usually weigh three times what they weighed at birth. Males increase in weight to twice their birth weights earlier than do females, and smaller newborns increase in weight to twice their birth weight sooner than do heavier neonates.

Length. Infants usually increase their lengths by 50% the first year, the average length being 25 to 30 cm (10 to 12 inches). But a period of "catch-up" or "lag-down" growth may occur. The majority of infants who are born small but are genetically determined to be longer shift **percentiles** on **growth grids** during the first 3 to 6 months. However, larger infants at birth, whose genotypes are for smaller size tend to grow at their fetal rates for several months before the lag-down in growth becomes evident. During this lag-down period, their length drops from a higher to a lower percentile rating on the growth chart. Often a new percentile rating is not apparent until the child is 13 months of age.[1] Figs. 6-1 and 6-2 depict catch-up and lag-down growth in the first year. Racial differences have been noted in rates of growth. American black males and females are smaller than Caucasians at birth, but they grow more rapidly during the first 2 years.[2]

Growth Charts

It is important that one concerned with infants' nutrient and energy intake be aware of how their growth is progressing. Height and weight data plotted on growth charts show how growth is proceeding. Measurements must be taken accurately, then weight and height values recorded on growth charts so that **growth velocity** as well as **acceleration** or **deceleration** can be monitored.

The most commonly used growth grids in North America are those prepared by an expert committee of the National Center for Health Statistics (NCHS).[3] Data collected

Growth velocity
(L *velocitas*, speed) Rapidity of motion or movement; rate of childhood growth over normal periods of development, as compared with a population standard.
Growth acceleration
Period of increased speed of growth at different points of childhood development.
Growth deceleration
Period of decreased speed of growth at different points of childhood development.

FIG. 6-1   Growth grid of a large infant who "lagged down" to her genetic potential. (Courtesy Ross Laboratories.)

FIG. 6-2 Growth grid of a small infant who "caught up" to his genetic potential. (Courtesy Ross Laboratories.)

by the Fels Research Institute from large numbers of a nationally representative sample of children were used to determine standards for children from birth to 36 months of age. The grids are prepared so that age values lie along the **axis** and height or weight values are plotted along the **abscissa.** Measurements at one age rank the baby's height or weight in relation to 100 other infants of the same age. Weight-height percentiles rank the baby's weight in relation to 100 other babies of the same length. Then sequential measurements plotted on the growth grid indicate if the baby is maintaining, reducing, or increasing the percentile rating as growth proceeds.

Changes in Body Composition

Changes during growth occur not only in height and weight but also in the components of the tissue. Increases in height and weight and skeletal maturation are accompanied by changes in body composition—water, lean body mass, and fat.

Body water. Total body water as a percentage of body weight decreases throughout infancy from approximately 70% at birth to 60% at 1 year of age. Reduction of body water is almost entirely extracellular. **Extracellular water** decreases from about 42% of body weight at birth to 32% at 1 year of age. At the same time **intracellular water** increases with the rapid growth of tissue its multiplying cells. This change results from decreases in the water content of **adipose tissue,** increases in adipose tissue, but largely from relative increases in lean body mass with its higher water content.[4]

Lean body mass. The fat-free mass of the body matures, the percentage of protein increasing as the percentage of total body water decreases. Fomon estimates that the protein content of the fat-free **lean body mass** gained increases from 12.5% at 1 month to 17% at 1 year in males and to 16.7% at 1 year in females.[4]

Body fat. The fat content of the body develops slowly during fetal life. Fat accounts for 0.5% of body weight at the fifth month of fetal growth and 16% at term. After birth, fat accumulates rapidly until approximately 9 months of age. Between 2 and 6 months of age the increase in adipose tissue is more than twice as great as the increase in the volume of muscle.[5] Sex-related differences appear in infancy, the female depositing a greater percentage of weight as fat than the male.

Changes in Body Proportions

Increases in height and weight are accompanied by dramatic changes in body proportions. The head proportion decreases as the torso and leg proportion increases (Fig. 6-3). At birth, the head accounts for approximately one fourth of the total body weight.

Extracellular water
Alternate term for collective body water or fluids outside of cells.

Intracellular water
Collective body water or fluids inside of cells; in body composition measures a large proportion assigned to total lean body mass, a vital component in cell metabolism.

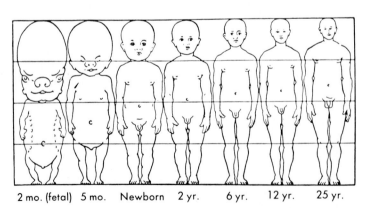

2 mo. (fetal)   5 mo.   Newborn   2 yr.   6 yr.   12 yr.   25 yr.

FIG. 6-3   Changes in body proportions from second fetal month to adulthood.
From Robbins WJ et al: Growth, New Haven, Conn, 1928, Yale University Press.

When growth has ceased, the head accounts for one eighth of the total body length. Between birth and adulthood, leg length increases from approximately three eighths of the newborn's birth length to one half of the adult's total body height.

Psychosocial Development

Healthy psychosocial development in the first year involves the development of trust. In early infancy babies do not tolerate delay of gratification. However, if their needs are quickly met in the early months, they accept delayed gratification later. In terms of feeding this means that in the first 2 to 3 months, infants need to be fed as soon as possible when hunger is noted. As they grow older, they can be expected to be more patient as preparation is made for feeding. **Tactile** stimulation is important in building trust and bonding. Infants need to be held and cuddled while feeding.

Tactile
(L *tactio*, to touch) Sense of touching, perception by the touch.

Digestion and Absorption

The digestive capacity of the infant matures and increases during the first year of life. The developing stomach and intestine provide an increasing ability to handle various nutrients and textures provided by the food. The full-term newborn is, however, prepared to digest and absorb an adequate supply of nutrients for normal growth and development. Table 6-1 indicates the percentage of adult-level factors needed for digestion that are present at birth.

Stomach actions. The stomach capacity at birth, 10 to 12 ml, increases to 200 ml by 12 months. The **gastric pH** is slightly alkaline at birth but within 24 hours acid secretion reaches a peak comparable to that of a 3-year-old child. It then declines to a low level, remaining lower than that of the adult for the first few months.[6] The stomach at birth empties in about 2½ to 3 hours. Newborns require small frequent feeds. As the infant matures, the emptying rate depends on the amount and composition of food consumed. Fat is the last of the macronutrients to leave the stomach, contributing to the satiety of the feed.

Gastric pH
(Gr *gaster*, stomach; *pH*, power of the hydrogen ion—H^+) Chemical symbol relating to H^+ concentration or activity in a solution; expressed numerically as the negative logarithm of H^+ concentration: pH 7.0 is neutral—above it alkalinity increases, and below it acidity increases. The hydrochloric acid (HCl) gastric secretions make gastric pH about 2.0.

TABLE 6-1 *Factors Necessary for Digestion Present at Birth*

Factors	% of Adult
H^+	<30
Pepsin	<10
Chymotrypsinogen	10 to 60
Procarboxypeptidase	10 to 60
Enterokinase	10
Peptidases	>100
Fat	
Lingual lipase	>100
Pancreatic lipase	5 to 10
Pancreatic colipase	?
Bile acids	50
Carbohydrate	
Alpha amylases	
Pancreatic	0
Salivary	10
Lactase	>100
Sucrase-isomaltase	100
Glucoamylase	<100 (?)

From Lebenthal E: Impact of development of the gastrointestinal tract on infant feeding, J Pediatr 102:1, 1983.

Intestinal actions. The intestines of newborns are larger in relation to body size than the adult and therefore have a larger surface area for absorption. **Reverse peristalsis** is common.

Enzymatic secretions provide the capacity for infants to digest and absorb the milk and food consumed.

Proteins. The newborn's concentrations of **trypsin** are near adult levels. Concentrations of **chymotrypsin** and **carboxypeptidase** in the duodenum are only 10% to 60% of the adult levels. Babies can digest adequate protein even though the quantity is limited. Newborns can completely digest about 1.95 g/kg/day of protein, 4-month-old babies about 3.75 g/kg/day.[6] In other words, a 3.5 kg newborn would be expected to digest 6.75 g of protein. An intake of 12.5 oz (369.6 ml) of human milk will meet the suggested energy intake and provide approximately 4.0 g protein. A formula-fed infant who consumes the same quantity will receive 5.54 g protein; either protein intake is adequately digested by the infant.

Fats. Pancreatic **lipase** activity is low in the newborn, especially in the premature infant. The bile acid pool, although present, is reduced. When compared to the adult on the basis of body surface area, the newborn, although able to synthesize **bile,** has a bile acid pool one half that of the adult.[7] Lingual and gastric lipase and milk lipases also contribute to the infant's ability to digest **lipids.** The fatty acid composition of the dietary fat influences how much of it will be digested and absorbed by the infant. **Triglycerides** with saturated fatty acids are not as well utilized as those with unsaturated fatty acids. Also, the position of a fatty acid on the fat's glycerol base affects absorption. Stearic acid is poorly absorbed in any position. Free palmitic acid **hydrolized** from positions 1 and 3 is poorly absorbed, whereas palmitic acid on position 2 of the glycerol base remains with the glycerol as a monoglyceride that appears to be well absorbed.[8] Fatty acids in human milk are better absorbed than those in cow's milk. Newborns absorb approximately 85% to 90% of the fat provided by human milk. Many infants absorb less than 70% of cow's milk fat.[9] Plant oils are more efficiently absorbed than animal fats. Mixtures of vegetable oils in commercially prepared infant formulas are well absorbed.

Carbohydrates. Sugars are well utilized. **Maltase, isomaltase,** and **sucrase** activity reach adult levels by 28 to 32 weeks gestation. Lactase, present in low levels at 28 weeks gestation, increases near term and reaches adult levels at birth.[10] Pancreatic **amylases** are low or absent up to 4 months of age. Salivary amylase, present at birth, rises to adult concentrations between 6 months and 1 year of age. Even though a large percentage of the salivary amylase is suspected of being inactivated by hydrochloric acid in the stomach, young infants do digest some starch. This is thought to be due to the presence of glycosidase and glucoamylase present in the **brush border** of the small intestines. These enzymes hydrolyze starch to glucose.

Renal Function

The newborn has an immature kidney. The functional development of the **nephron** is not complete until 1 month of age. The tubules are short and narrow and do not reach mature proportions until approximately 5 months. In addition, the pituitary gland produces only limited quantities of the antidiuretic hormone (ADH) **vasopressin,** which normally inhibits **diuresis.** These factors limit the newborn's ability to concentrate urine and to cope with fluid and **electrolyte** stress; i.e., electrolyte-dense formula, limited fluid intake, diarrhea. By 1 month of age, the normal infant can maintain water balance as efficiently as the adult.

Renal solute load. The major percentage of **solutes** presented to the kidney for excretion are the nitrogenous end products of protein metabolism, sodium, potassium, phosphorus, and chloride. If none of these elements were utilized in new body mass or lost by nonrenal

Trypsin
(Gr *tryein,* to rub; *pepsis,* digestion) Protein-splitting enzyme formed in the intestine by action of enterokinase on inactive precursor trypsinogen.

Chymotrypsin
(Gr *chymos,* chyme, creamy gruel-like material produced by gastric digestion of food) One of the protein-splitting and milk-curdling pancreatic enzymes, activated in the intestine from precursor chymotrypsinogen; breaks peptide linkages of the amino acids phenylalanine and tyrosine.

Carboxypeptidase
(L *carbo-,* coal, carbon, fundamental element in all organic compounds) The chemical group *carboxyl*—COOH—at the end of the carbon chain identifies the compound as an organic acid. The end of the word, *peptidase,* indicates a protein-splitting enzyme, which together with the first part means that this is an enzyme that acts on the peptide bond of the terminal amino acid having a free-end carboxyl group.

routes, such as perspiration, they would need to be excreted in the urine. They are therefore referred to as the potential **renal solute load.** The potential renal solute load can be calculated by assuming all nitrogen is excreted, dividing dietary nitrogen by 28 and adding sodium, potassium, chloride, and phosphorus in the feed expressed as **milliosmoles,** abbreviated **mOsm.**[11]

These solutes must be concentrated in water derived from that preformed in the diet and formed from the oxidation of protein and carbohydrates. Each milk for normal infants yields approximately 95 ml of water per 100 ml consumed. Some is utilized in new tissue, and some is lost in the feces or by evaporation. The solutes are dissolved in the remainder.

The concentrating capacity of some neonates has been reported to be as limited as 700 mOsm/L; of others as great as that of older children and adults, 1200 to 1400 mOsm/L.[12,13] Human milk has a potential renal solute load of 93 mOsm/L, commercially available cow milk-based formula of 133 mOsm/L, and soy formula of 177 mOsm/L.[11]

Difficulties with the renal solute load are unlikely in normal infants fed human milk or a correctly prepared formula. Problems may occur when elevated environmental temperature or fever increase evaporative loss, when diarrhea occurs, and/or when infants reduce the volume of fluids they consume.[11]

NUTRIENT NEEDS OF INFANTS

Individual differences of infants in nutrient reserves, body composition, growth rates, and activity patterns make defining actual nutrient requirements impossible. Estimates have been made from intakes of infants growing normally and from the nutrient content of human milk. **Nitrogen balance** studies have been conducted to establish amino acid requirements. Fat and calcium absorption have been examined. The Recommended Dietary Allowances (RDAs) are planned to provide a margin of safety to allow for maximum protection. Because of the declining growth rates during the latter part of the first year, recommended intakes have been set for two 6-month periods, from birth to 6 months and from 6 months to 1 year.[14]

Energy

The energy requirement in infancy is determined primarily by body size, physical activity, and rates of growth. Since large variations in these variables are seen among infants at any age and in any one infant from month to month, ranges of energy needs are large. Total energy needs (kcal/day) rise during the first year but energy needs per unit of body size decline in response to changes in rates of growth. The recommended **energy intake** (Table 6-2) falls from 108 kcal/kg in the first 6 months to 98 kcal/kg for 6 months to 1 year.[14] These figures were derived from estimates made by the World Health Organization (WHO) based on studies of intakes of healthy thriving infants in developed countries. They are about 15% higher than estimated energy expenditures, which indicate a requirement of 95 kcal/kg/day during the first 6 months and 84 kcal/kg/day in the last half of the first year.

Renal solute load
Collective number and concentration of solute particles in solution, carried by the blood to the kidney nephrons for excretion in the urine, usually nitrogenous products from protein metabolism, and the electrolytes Na^+, K^+, Cl^-, and HPO_4^-.

Milliosmoles (mOsm/L)
Osmole (Gr *osme*, small), standard unit of osmotic pressure; equal to the gram molecular weight of solute divided by the number of particles (ions) into which a substance dissociates in solution. Thus milliosmole would be a much smaller unit of measure of osmotic pressure—$\frac{1}{1000}$ of an osmole, equal to $\frac{1}{1000}$ gram molecular weight of a substance divided by the number of ions into which a substance dissociates in 1 liter (L) of solution. The term *osmolality* refers to this concentration of solutes per unit of solvent.

Energy intake
Energy value of carbohydrate, fat, and protein in food, measured in kilocalories.

TABLE 6-2 **Recommended Energy Intake for Infants**

Age	Energy (kcal)
≤6 months	kg × 108
6 months-1 year	kg × 98

It has been estimated that approximately 50% of the energy expenditure is due to the basal metabolic rate. Energy expended for growth declines from approximately 32.8% of intake during the first 4 months to 7.4% of intake from 4 to 12 months.[9] The contribution of physical activity to total energy expenditure is quite variable but can be expected to increase with age as motor skills develop. Some infants are quiet and cuddly while others spend a considerable amount of time crying, kicking, or just exploring with motor skills they have acquired. The most appropriate way to judge the adequacy of babies' energy intake is to monitor the adequacy of their linear growth and weight gain.

Protein and Amino Acids

Protein needs. Infants require protein for synthesis of new body tissue during growth, increases in the protein content of the body, as well as synthesis of enzymes, hormones, and other physiologically important compounds. Increases in body protein are estimated to average about 3.5 g/day for the first 4 months, and 3.1 g/day for the next 8 months.[4] The body content of protein increases from about 11.0% to 15.0% over the first year. The recommended intake is 2.2 g/kg for the first 6 months and 1.6 g/kg from 6 to 12 months. Fomon and associates have suggested that during infancy, amino acid and protein requirements expressed per unit of kilocalories consumed, reflecting both size and rate of growth, would be more meaningful than expressions of requirements on the basis of body weight alone.[15] They estimate the protein requirement to be 1.6 g/100 kcal for children 1 to 4 months of age, and 1.4 g/100 kcal for children 8 to 12 months of age. Protein intake of breastfed infants growing and gaining normally range from 2.43 g/kg/day in the first month to 1.51 g/kg/day in the fourth month.[16] The American Academy of Pediatrics has set minimum protein standards for infant formula of 1.8 g/100 kcal with a protein efficiency ratio equal to that of casein.[17]

Amino acid needs. Nine amino acids are dietary essentials in infancy. Amino acid requirements have been estimated by Holt and Snyderman from studies in which pure amino acids were supplied in proportions of amino acids in human milk.[18] The requirement of an amino acid was defined as the least amount required to maintain satisfactory nitrogen retention and weight gain when nitrogen levels and other amino acids were held constant. Fomon and Filer have estimated amino acid requirements from intakes of infants between the ages of 8 and 112 days who were fed whole protein in cow's milk formulas and soy formulas.[19] Satisfactory linear growth and weight gain, nitrogen balance, and serum concentrations of albumin equivalent to those of normal breastfed infants were used as criteria of adequacy.

TABLE 6-3 Estimated Amino Acid Requirements of Infants 3-4 Months of Age

Amino Acid	mg/kg/day
Histidine	28
Isoleucine	70
Leucine	161
Lysine	103
Methionine plus cystine	58
Phenylalanine plus tyrosine	125
Threonine	87
Tryptophan	17
Valine	93

From Energy and Protein Requirements, Report of a Joint FAO/WHO Ad Hoc Committee, World Health Organization technical report series No 522, FAO Nutr Meet Rep No 52, Geneva, 1973, World Health Organization.

Requirement standards. The FAO/WHO expert committee has suggested that a composite of the lower estimates of the data from the studies of Holt and Snyderman and from Fomon and Filer would provide estimates of the upper range of **essential amino acid** requirements of infants age 0 to 6 months.[17-20] The National Research Council has accepted these estimates as shown in Table 6-3.

Under certain conditions, other amino acids become essential. For example, the infant who has phenylketonuria cannot metabolize phenylalanine to tyrosine and tyrosine becomes essential. Premature infants require an external source of tyrosine and cystine.

Fat and Essential Fatty Acid

Fat needs. Fat, the most calorically concentrated energy nutrient, supplies between 40% and 50% of the energy consumed in infancy. The energy provided by fat spares protein for tissue synthesis. Its caloric concentration is an asset during periods of rapid growth when energy demands are great. Fat provides 45% to 50% of the energy content of commercial formula and 55% of the energy content of human milk. Commerical infant semisolid foods other than egg yolks are relatively low in fat.

Essential fatty acid. Polyunsaturated **linoleic acid** has been proved conclusively to be essential. One of the earliest manifestations of this fatty acid deficiency recognized in animals was an increased basal metabolic rate. Infants deficient in linoleic acid have an eczema-like dermatitis. Also, infants who are fed formulas low in this essential fatty acid consume greater numbers of kilocalories than do those who receive adequate amounts of linoleic acid to maintain normal growth. Caloric utilization has been reported to vary with intakes of linoleic acid up to 4% and 5% of the total kilocalories.[21] Minimal requirements for linoleic acid are considered to be approximately 1% of the total kilocalories consumed, and an optimal intake is thought to be 4% to 5% of the total kilocalories.[22] Approximately 5% of the total kilocalories in human milk and 1% of the kilocalories in cow's milk are provided by linoleic acid. Commercially available infant formulas contain blends of vegetable oils and contribute greater amounts of linoleic acid.

The Committee on Nutrition of the American Academy of Pediatrics has recommended that infant formulas contain a minimum of 300 mg of **18:2 fatty acids** per 100 kcal, or 1.7% of the energy content (total kilocalories).[17]

Water

Infants require more water per unit of body size than do adults. A larger percentage of water is located in the extracellular and **vascular spaces.** As noted before, young infants have an immature kidney. These two factors make the infant vulnerable to water imbalance. The water requirement is determined by water loss, water required for growth, and solutes derived from the diet.

Water is lost by evaporation through the skin and respiratory tract—**insensible water loss**—and through perspiration when the environmental temperature is elevated, and by elimination in urine and feces.[11] During growth additional water is necessary since water is needed as a constituent of tissue and for increases in the volume of body fluids. The amount of water required for growth, however, is very small. The body requirement for water is the sum of the above demands.

Water lost by evaporation in infancy and early childhood accounts for more than 60% of that needed to maintain homeostasis (see p. 67), as compared to 40% to 50% in the adult. At all ages approximately 24% of the basal heat loss is by evaporation of water through the skin and respiratory tract.[23] This amounts to 45 ml of insensible water loss per 100 kcal expended. Fomon estimates evaporative water loss at 1 month of age to average 210 ml/day and at age 1 year, 500 ml/day.[9] Evaporative losses increase with fever and increased environmental temperature. Increases in humidity decrease respiratory loss. Loss of water in the feces averages 10 ml/kg/day in infancy.[9]

Linoleic acid
The ultimate essential amino acid for humans.

18:2 fatty acid
Naming system for fatty acids according to structure: carbon chain length and number of double (unsaturated) bonds. Thus, an 18:2 fatty acid would have a long chain of 18 carbon atoms with two double bonds. This is the chemical shorthand for linoleic acid.

Vascular spaces
Spaces within fluid vessels in the body, blood vessels and lymph vessels; contain body fluids in transit, greater amount in blood and remainder in the interconnecting lymphatic system.

Insensible water loss
Daily water loss through the skin and respiration, so-named because a person is not aware of it. An additional smaller amount is lost in normal perspiration, the amount varying with the surrounding temperature.

TABLE 6-4 *Range of Average Water Requirements of Infants and Children under Ordinary Conditions*

Age	Amount of Water (ml/kg/day)
3 days	80-100
10 days	125-150
3 mo	140-160
6 mo	130-155
9 mo	125-145
1 yr	120-135
2 yr	115-125

Adapted from Behrman RE, Vaughan VC III, and Nelson WE, editors: Nelson textbook of pediatrics, ed 11, Philadelphia, 1987, WB Saunders Co.

Hyponatremia
Abnormally low levels of sodium (Na⁺) in the blood; can be easily caused by excess water intake to point of water intoxication, with resulting dilution of the major electrolyte (Na⁺) in extracellular circulating fluids.

The range of water requirements is shown in Table 6-4. The National Research Council recommends an intake of 1.5 ml/kcal of energy expenditure for infants.[14] Water intoxication resulting in **hyponatremia**, irritability, and coma can result if infants are fed too much water. Reported cases include infants fed 8 oz of water after each feeding or fed water instead of formula because of financial inability of parents to buy formula.[24] Under normal conditions, infants fed breast milk or infant formulas do not need additional water.

Minerals and Vitamins

Demands for minerals and vitamins are influenced by growth rates, mineralization of bone, increases in bone length and blood volume, and by energy, protein, and fat intakes. RDAs have been established for three major and four trace minerals and for 11 vitamins, as shown in Table 6-5. Ranges of safe intakes have been suggested for five trace minerals and two vitamins. Although all of these nutrients are essential, the discussion here focuses on those that are most commonly of concern during infancy.

Calcium. The recommended intake of calcium is planned to meet the needs of formula-fed infants who retain less than half of the calcium they consume. Breastfed infants retain two thirds of their calcium intake. The allowances are easily met by infants consuming commercially available formulas. The allowances are not applicable to breastfed infants. The calcium-phosphorus ratio, previously thought to be a factor in calcium absorption, is no longer a concern.

Iron. Infant iron needs are supplied from two different sources, prenatal reserves and food sources.

Prenatal reserves. Before birth, the fetus accumulates iron in proportion to body size. Premature and low-birth-weight infants have limited reserves that are quickly depleted. Even with the advantage of full-term iron stores, the rapidly growing infant is at risk for iron deficiency because of the increase in blood volume as the baby grows larger. The concentration of **hemoglobin** at birth averages 17 to 19 g/100 ml of blood. During the first 6 to 8 weeks of life it decreases to approximately 10 to 11 g/100 ml because of a shortened life span of the fetal cell and decreased **erythropoiesis.** After this age there is a gradual increase in hemoglobin concentration to 13 g/100 ml at 2 years of age.

Ferrous sulfate
Iron fortification compound in infant formulas used as needed to prevent anemia.

Food sources. Forty-nine percent of the iron in human milk, 10% of the iron in cow's milk, and 4% of the iron in iron-fortified formulas is absorbed.[25] Commercially available formulas are prepared both with and without the inclusion of **ferrous sulfate.** Iron-fortified commercial infant cereals are fortified with electrolytically reduced iron. Absorp-

TABLE 6-5   Recommended Dietary Allowances for Minerals and Vitamins for Infants

Age (yrs)	Calcium (mg)	Phosphorus (mg)	Iodine (μg)	Iron (mg)	Magnesium (mg)	Zinc (mg)	Selenium (μg)
0.0-0.5	400	300	40	6	40	5	10
0.5-1.0	600	500	50	10	60	5	15

Fat-Soluble Vitamins

	Vitamin A (μg RE)	Vitamin D (μg)	Vitamin E (mg α-TE)	Vitamin K (μg)
0.0-0.5	375	7.5	3	5
0.5-1.0	375	10	4	10

Water-Soluble Vitamins

	Thiamin (mg)	Riboflavin (mg)	Niacin (mg NE)	Vitamin B_6 (mg)	Folate (μg)	Vitamin B_{12} (μg)	Vitamin C (mg)
0.0-0.5	0.3	0.4	5	0.3	25	0.3	30
0.5-1.0	0.4	0.5	6	0.6	35	0.5	35

RE, retinol equivalent; α-TE, α-tocopherol equivalent; NE, niacin equivalent.
Reprinted with permission from Recommended dietary allowances, ed 10. © 1989 by the National Academy of Sciences. Published by National Academy Press, Washington, DC.

tion of this iron averages 5%. Many have recommended mixing this cereal with a fruit juice containing vitamin C to enhance the **iron absorption.** Normal full-term breastfed infants can maintain satisfactory hemoglobin levels without supplemental iron in early infancy. After 3 to 4 months, the addition of iron-fortified cereals or an iron supplement becomes important. If the infant is to be formula-fed, it is advisable to select a formula with iron.[26]

Zinc. The infant's zinc needs are met by a limited tissue supply at birth and early food sources.

Body stores. The infant is born without zinc body stores. Tissue concentrations at birth are similar to those of adults. Therefore, infants rapidly become dependent on a dietary source. Variations in concentrations of plasma zinc during growth reflect the continued utilization and depletion of body stores of zinc. Although there are not enough data to state a requirement, the RDA standard has been set for 5 mg during the first year. One study comparing hair zinc concentration of breastfed and bottle-fed babies during the first 6 months of life found that only male bottle-fed infants experienced a significant decline in hair zinc concentration, suggesting that males had a higher requirement for zinc during the period studied.[27]

Food sources. Colostrum contains 20 mg/L of zinc, three to five times as much as later milk. Human milk contains 4 mg/L of zinc in the first month declining to 0.6 mg/L at 6 months.[28] Cow's milk contains 3 to 5 mg/L of zinc. Formulas are supplemented and contain 5 mg/L. Animal studies suggest that the bioavailability of zinc is 59.2% in human milk, 43% to 53.9% in cow's milk, and 26.8% to 39.5% in infant formula.[29] The recommended intake of 5 mg/day is applicable for formula-fed infants.

Vitamins. The specific functions of vitamins in metabolic processes makes the require-

Iron absorption
Degree of iron absorption, relatively small at best, depends upon its acid reduction, either by accompanying food such as orange juice or by the gastric HCl secretions, from the ferric form (Fe^{+++}) in foods to the ferrous form (Fe^{++}) required for absorption. After absorption it is oxidized back to the ferric form required for incorporation in body metabolism.

ment for each vitamin dependent upon the related intakes of energy, protein, carbohydrates, and fats. Exact needs are difficult to define. Most vitamins cross the placenta and accumulate in the fetus at greater concentrations than in the mother. Maternal hypovitaminemia will be reflected in the fetus. Vitamins A, E, and beta-carotene (vitamin A precursor) concentrations are lower in the newborn infant's blood than in the mother's. The concentration of water-soluble vitamins in the blood of the neonate is higher than in that of the mother.[30]

Fat-soluble vitamins in excess of need are not excreted but are stored. Reserves can be accumulated. The toxicity of excessive intakes of vitamins A and D is well documented. In contrast to vitamins A, D, E, and K, the water-soluble vitamins are "stored" only in the sense of small degrees of tissue saturation that turn over rapidly so deficiencies can occur in a relatively short period if the nutrient is absent from dietary intake.

Fat-soluble vitamins. The infant's needs for the fat-soluble vitamins A, D, E, and K are met by food sources and in some instances added supplementation.

Vitamin A. The milk of well-nourished women contains 40 to 70 μg/dl **retinol** and 20 to 40 μg/dl of **carotenoids.** The recommended intake of 375 μg/retinol equivalents (RE) per day in the first year reflects the RE intake of an infant consuming 750 ml per day with a margin for the **coefficient of variation** between women.

Vitamin D. Although 2.5 micrograms (μg)(100 international units [IU]) of vitamin D prevents rickets and ensures adequate absorption of calcium and normal mineralization of bone in the infant, better calcium absorption and some increase in growth has been noted with intakes of 10 μg (400 IU)/day. Vitamin D can be formed by the action of sunlight on the skin. The amount formed depends on several variables, and amounts formed cannot be readily measured. To assure an adequate intake, the recommended intake as **cholecalciferol** is 7.5 μg (300 IU)/day for the first 6 months and 10 μg (400 IU)/day for the remainder of the first year. Breastfed infants who are not exposed to sunlight should receive a supplement of 5.0 to 7.5 μg (200 to 300 IU) daily. The U.S. RDA standards, as well as those of the international community, no longer use the former concept of *International Unit,* which was based on the biologic activity (in the case of vitamin D, 1 IU equals 0.025 μg) of a given amount of the vitamin to achieve its function, but now express RDAs in direct amounts needed for health.

Vitamin E. Defining appropriate intakes for vitamin E is complicated by large variations in the susceptibility to peroxidation of fatty acids in the diet and tissues. The recommended intake during infancy reflects the **tocopherol** concentration of human milk in which 6% of the kilocalories are provided by polyunsaturated fatty acid.

Vitamin K. Vitamin K, essential for the formation of **prothrombin** and other factors involved in blood clotting, is of particular concern for the breastfed infant. The newborn has low plasma prothrombin levels. The intestinal flora is very limited and human milk provides low levels of vitamin K (2 μg/L). If the breastfed infant does not receive supplements, the infant is at risk for intracranial hemorrhage.[31] A **prophylactic** intramuscular dose of 0.5 to 1 mg of vitamin K or an oral dose of 1 to 2.1 mg of vitamin K is usually given to infants at birth in the hospital.[32] Home-delivered infants who are to be breastfed need the same supplement.

Water-soluble vitamins. The current RDAs set standards for six of the B vitamins—thiamin, riboflavin, niacin, B_6, B_{12}, and folate—and for vitamin C. Only safe and adequate estimates for two additional B vitamins, biotin and pantothenic acid, are possible at this time.

Thiamin. Requirements for thiamin are related to energy intake since it functions as a vital coenzyme factor in energy metabolism. One study, based on the consumption of 1 L of human milk, suggests that the minimum requirement for thiamin during infancy

---

Retinol

Chemical name for vitamin A derived from its function relating to the retina of the eye and light-dark adaptation. Daily RDA standards are stated in retinol equivalents (RE) to account for sources of the preformed vitamin and its precursor provitamin A beta-carotene.

Tocopherol

(Gr *tokos,* childbirth; *pherein,* to carry) Chemical name for vitamin E, so-named by early investigators because their initial work with rats indicated a reproductive function, which did not turn out later to be the case with humans, in whom it functions as a strong anti-oxidant to preserve structural membranes such as cell walls.

Prothrombin

(Gr *pro-,* before; *thrombos,* clot) Blood-clotting factor (number II), synthesized in the liver from glutamic acid and CO_2, catalyzed by vitamin K.

is 1.7 mg/day. The Academy of Pediatrics estimates the allowance of thiamin for infants as 0.4 mg/1000 kcal consumed.[31]

Riboflavin. Requirements for riboflavin are also related to energy intake, reflecting its coenzyme role in energy metabolism. An intake of 0.4 mg of riboflavin per day has been noted to maintain blood and urine levels in infants weighing 5.9 to 9.0 kg. The average breastfed infant who consumes 750 ml/day of breast milk receives 0.26 mg of riboflavin, or 0.48 mg/1000 kcal.

Niacin. The fact that the amino acid tryptophan can be converted to niacin makes basic requirements for niacin difficult to determine. Human milk contains 1.5 mg of niacin and 210 mg of tryptophan per liter. Minimum requirements for niacin appear to be 4.4 mg/1000 kcal. The allowance for infants before 6 months of age is 8 **niacin equivalents (NE)**/1000 kcal. For infants older than 6 months, allowances are based on the same standard as that for adults, 6.6 NE/1000 kcal.

Vitamin B_6. Vitamin B_6 **(pyridoxine)** functions as an essential coenzyme factor in the metabolism of amino acids and lipids, as well as nucleic acid, a key component of the genetic structure in the cell nucleus deoxyribonucleic acid (DNA). The requirement for this vitamin increases as the protein intake increases. The recommended intake, 0.3 mg/day during the first 6 months of life and 0.6 mg/day the last half of the first year, is based on experience with commercial infant formulas.

Vitamin B_{12}. Vitamin B_{12} **(cobalamin)** functions as a coenzyme in the degradation of certain amino acids and of fatty acids with **odd-numbered carbon chains.** It is essential, along with folate, in metabolic processes that transfer single carbon fragments from one compound to another in amino acid metabolism and nucleic acid synthesis. Deficiency of either vitamin results in growth retardation. The allowances for vitamin B_{12} are based on 0.3 µg/day for the young infant and 0.5 µg/day for the infant over 6 months of age. Symptoms of B_{12} deficiency have been found in a few breastfed infants whose mothers had followed a strict vegan diet or who had **pernicious anemia.**

Folate. Body stores of folate at birth are small and rapidly depleted. Serum and **erythrocyte** levels fall below adult levels by two weeks of age and remain there during the first year of life. The allowance for folate is 3.6 mg/kg per day for the first year. The folate needs of infants are adequately met by both human and cow's milk. Goat's milk is folate deficient for the human infant.

Vitamin C. Newborn infants consuming 7 to 12 mg/day of vitamin C **(ascorbic acid)** have been protected from scurvy. An intake of 30 mg/day, based on the amount provided by human milk, is recommended during the first 6 months of life, and 35 mg/day for the next 6 months. Infants who are fed human milk or commercial infant formula will receive adequate vitamin C.

Vitamin and mineral supplements. Full-term infants who receive milk from a well-nourished lactating mother will receive all the vitamins they need, with the exception of vitamin D. Breastfed infants should receive vitamin D supplements by 2 months of age. Infants who receive a commercially available formula that is properly prepared will be adequately nourished with vitamins.

Cow's milk contains 0.03 to 0.1 µg/L of fluoride; human milk contains less than 0.05 µg/L.[32] Infant formulas are not prepared by the manufacturer with fluoridated water. Unless the infant receives a formula prepared at home with fluoridated water, supplements are appropriate. Table 6-6 shows recommended fluoride intakes.

The need for supplemental iron depends on the composition of the diet consumed. Solely breastfed infants should receive a supplement by 4 to 6 months of age. Those who receive iron-fortified cereals will probably not need supplements. Infants receiving iron-fortified formula will need no supplemental iron.

Niacin equivalent (NE)
Current international measure for recommended amounts of the B-vitamin niacin that accounts for the preformed vitamin and the amino acid precursor tryptophan, from which the vitamin can be synthesized. Thus, 1 NE equals 1 g niacin or 60 mg of dietary tryptophan.

Pyridoxine
Chemical name for vitamin B_6, derived from its ring-like structure. In its active form, pyridoxal phosphate, it acts as a coenzyme in many types of transamination and decarboxylation reactions in amino acid metabolism.

Cobalamin
Chemical name for vitamin B_{12}, from its structure as a complex red crystalline compound of high molecular weight, with a single cobalt atom at its core. Its food sources are of animal origin, but the ultimate source is from the colonies of synthesizing microorganisms inhabiting the gastrointestinal tract of herbivorous animals.

Erythrocyte
(Gr *erythro-, red; cyte,* hollow vessel) Red blood cell.

TABLE 6-6   *Supplemental Fluoride Dosage Schedule (mg/day*)*

	Concentration of Fluoride in Drinking Water (ppm)		
Age	<0.3	0.3-0.7	>0.7
2 weeks to 2 years	0.25	0	0
2 to 3 years	0.50	0.25	0
3 to 16 years	1.00	0.50	0

*2.2 mg of sodium fluoride contains 1 mg of fluoride.
From Committee on Nutrition: Pediatrics 63:150, 1979. Reproduced by permission of Pediatrics, © 1979.

MILK FOR INFANTS
Human Milk and Formulas

The advantages of human milk for feeding human infants are numerous and breast-feeding is encouraged by most health care professionals. Many mothers breastfeed their infants for a few months and then offer them a formula. Most normal full-term infants who are not breastfed receive a cow's milk–based formula. Infants who do not tolerate cow's milk may receive a soy or hydrolyzed casein formula.

Differences in human and cow's milk were discussed in Chapter 5. From such comparisons it soon becomes apparent that if cow's milk is offered to infants, it must be modified. Products prepared for infant feeding do indeed modify cow's milk. In fact, most attempt to simulate human milk.

AAP Standards

The Committee on Nutrition of the American Academy of Pediatrics (AAP), concerned about the composition of proprietary infant formulas, issued a policy statement on standards for these products.[17] These standards are based on the composition of human milk from a healthy mother. The minimum amount for each nutrient is close to that of human milk and thus is the preferable quantity. The maximum amount is given for formulas intended for low-birth-weight or sick infants who take less formula and thus need the higher nutrient content (Table 6-7).

Modified Cow's Milk Formulas

Commercially manufactured formulas prepared from nonfat cow's milk are readily available and are generously used for feeding in infancy. The protein and mineral content is decreased to reduce the solute load. The curd tension is reduced by **homogenization** and heat treatment to produce an easily digested protein. Three manufacturers combine whey with nonfat milk to produce a product with a whey-casein ratio similar to that in human milk. Combinations of vegetable oils, a high percentage of which are absorbed by infants, are added, and carbohydrate is added to increase the caloric concentration to approximately that of human milk and cow's milk. Vitamins and minerals are added. Formulas are marketed both with and without ferrous sulfate in amounts that provide 12 mg of iron per quart. Pediatricians encourage the use of formulas with iron.

Hypoallergenic Formulas

Soy formulas. The most commonly used products for infants who have conditions that contraindicate the use of cow's milk are the soy milks. These formulas are constructed of protein isolated from soy meal fortified with methionine, corn syrup or sucrose, and soy

Homogenization
(Gr *homos*, same; *genos*, kind) Process of forming a permanent milk emulsion by breaking up fat portion into fine globules and dispersing them equally throughout the milk for uniform quality.

TABLE 6-7 *Nutrient Levels of Infant Formulas (per 100 kcal)*

Nutrient	CON 1976 Recommendations	
	Minimum	Maximum
Protein (g)	1.8	4.5
Fat		
(g)	3.3	6.0
(% cal)	30.0	54.0
Essential fatty acids (linoleate)		
(% cal)	3.0	—
(mg)	300.0	—
Vitamins		
A (IU)	250.0 (75 μg)*	750.0 (225 μg)*
D (IU)	40.0	100.0
K (μg)	4.0	—
E (IU)	0.3 (with 0.7 IU/g linoleic acid)	—
C (ascorbic acid) (mg)	8.0	—
B_1 (thiamin) (μg)	40.0	—
B_2 (riboflavin) (μg)	60.0	—
B_6 (pyridoxine) (μg)	35.0 (with 15 μg/g of protein in formula)	—
B_{12} (μg)	0.15	—
Niacin		
(μg)	250.0	—
(μg equiv)	—	—
Folic acid (μg)	4.0	—
Pantothenic acid (μg)	300.0	—
Biotin (μg)	1.5	—
Choline (mg)	7.0	—
Inositol (mg)	4.0	—
Minerals		
Calcium (mg)	50.0†	—
Phosphorus (mg)	25.0†	—
Magnesium (mg)	6.0	—
Iron (mg)	0.15	—
Iodine (μg)	5.0	—
Zinc (mg)	0.5	—
Copper (μg)	60.0	—
Manganese (μg)	5.0	—
Sodium (mg)	20.0 (6 mEq)‡	60.0 (17 mEq)‡
Potassium (mg)	80.0 (14 mEq)‡	200.0 (34 mEq)‡
Chloride (mg)	55.0 (11 mEq)‡	150.0 (29 mEq)‡

*Retinol equivalents.
†Calcium to phosphorus ratio must be no less than 1.1 nor more than 2.0.
‡Milliequivalent for 670 kcal/L of formula.
From Committee on Nutrition: Pediatrics 57(2):278, 1976. Reproduced by permission of Pediatrics, © 1976.

Trypsin inhibitor
A natural substance in raw soybeans that is responsible for a toxin in the bean. Fortunately this substance is destroyed by heat and rendered inactive.

Goitrogens
Natural substance in certain foods such as soybeans that cause hypothyroidism and a compensatory enlargement of the thyroid gland, producing symptoms of iodine-deficiency goiter; effect diminished by adequate heating of the soy meal and adding iodine supplementation.

Casein hydrolysate formula
Infant formula with base of hydrolyzed casein, major milk protein, produced by partially breaking down the casein into smaller peptide fragments, making a product that is more easily digested.

Elemental formula
Infant formula produced with elemental, ready to be absorbed, components of free amino acids and carbohydrate as simple sugars.

or other vegetable oils to which vitamins and minerals have been added. The **trypsin inhibitor** in raw soybean meal is inactivated during heat processing. The **goitrogenic** effect of soy is diminished by heating and the addition of iodine.

Casein hydrolysate formulas. Three other formulas are marketed for infants who do not tolerate either soy or cow's milk. Nutramigen, prepared from a casein hydrolysate and corn oil; Progestimil, which contains a casein hydrolysate and medium-chain triglycerides; and Alimentum which contains free amino acids, **elemental formula** components. All three formulas have an unpleasant odor and taste and are rarely accepted by infants if not introduced before 8 to 9 months of age. The composition of non-cow's milk–based formulas is given in Table 6-8.

Formula and Milk for Older Infants

Two manufacturers market cow's milk-based formula for older babies. These formulas, designed to accompany the feeding of semisolid foods, are higher in protein and lower in fat than formula for the younger infant. However, examination of the nutrient intakes of infants from 6 months to 1 year reveals that their intakes are completely adequate without the additional protein. Pediatricians feel there is no justification for the use of these milks.[33,34]

The use of whole, 2%, 1%, or nonfat cow's milk in the first year is strongly discouraged. It has been noted to contribute to the incidence of anemia. Not only is there no iron in this milk, it may cause a very tiny blood loss from the intestinal tract. If a test of the baby's feces is done with paper impregnated with guaiac solution and/or a fecal hemoglobin test is performed, small amounts of blood may be found. Over time, this may lead to anemia.[35]

Formulas prepared for younger infants are perfectly adequate for the first year.

Substitute and Imitation Milks

Feeding infants formulas made from recipes that have not been proved to support adequate nutrition should be strongly discouraged. Malnutrition was observed in infants fed a barley water, corn syrup, and whole milk formula suggested in a magazine for mothers.[36] Kwashiorkor, an advanced protein-deficiency state of malnutrition, has been reported in infants fed a nondairy creamer as a substitute for milk.[37]

Substitute or imitation milks should not be offered to infants. Substitute milk is defined by the Food and Drug Administration as nutritionally equivalent to whole or nonfat milk based on their content of only 14 or 15 nutrients. It does not include all nutrients recommended as components of infant formulas. Imitation milk simulates milk but does not meet the standard of identity for substitute milk.[38]

Formula Preparation

Types of formula available. Manufacturers market three basic types of formulas, each of which is prepared according to its form: (1) *liquid concentrates* prepared for feeding by mixing equal amounts of the liquid and water; (2) *ready-to-feed* formulas that require no preparation are available in an assortment of sizes (4-, 6-, and 8-oz bottles and 32-oz containers); and (3) *powdered* formulas that are prepared by mixing 1 level tablespoon of powder for each 2 oz of water. All of these formulas, when properly prepared and adequately supplemented, provide the nutrients important for the infant in an appropriate caloric concentration and present a solute load reasonable for the full-term infant (Table 6-9). Errors in dilution caused by lack of understanding of the proper method of preparation, improper measurements, adding extra water to make the formula last longer, or the belief of the parents that their child should have greater amounts of nutritious food can lead to problems.

TABLE 6-8   *Nutrient Content of Soy Formulas and Other Milk Substitutes for Infants*

Nutrient Source	Prosobee	Isomil	Nutramigen	Progestimil	Alimentum
Protein	Soy protein	Soy protein	Casein hydrolysate	Casein hydrolysate	Cystine, tyrosine, tryptophan
Fat	Soy oil	Coconut oil, soy oil	Corn oil	Corn oil, medium-chain triglycerides	Medium-chain triglycerides, safflower and soy oils
Carbohydrate	Corn syrup solids	Corn syrup solids, sucrose	Modified tapioca starch, sucrose	Corn syrup solids, modified tapioca starch	Sucrose, modified tapioca starch
Nutrients per 100 ML — normal dilution					
Energy (kcal)	67	68	67	68	68
Protein (g)	2.0	2.0	1.9	1.9	1.9
Fat (g)	3.1	3.6	2.7	2.8	3.7
Carbohydrate (g)	7.1	6.8	9.4	9.4	6.9
Vitamin A (IU)	210	203	210	250	203
Vitamin D (IU)	42.0	41.0	42.0	51.0	41.0
Vitamin E (IU)	2.2	2.0	2.1	2.5	2.1
Vitamin C (mg)	6.0	5.5	5.5	7.9	6.0
Thiamin (µg)	52.0	41.0	52.0	52.0	41.0
Riboflavin (µg)	63.0	61.0	63.0	63.0	61.0
Niacin (mg) (equiv.)	0.8	0.9	0.8	0.8	0.9
Pyridoxine (µg)	42.0	41.0	42.0	42.0	41.0
Vitamin B_{12} (µg)	0.2	0.3	0.2	0.2	
Folic acid (µg)	11.0	10.0	10.6	10.6	10.0
Calcium (mg)	63.0	71.0	63.0	63.0	71.0
Phosphorus (mg)	50.0	51.0	42.0	42.0	51.0
Magnesium (mg)	7.4	5.1	7.4	7.4	5.1
Iron (mg)	1.3	1.2	1.3	1.3	1.2
Zinc (mg)	0.5	0.5	0.5	0.5	0.5
Copper (µg)	63.0	51.0	63.0	63.0	63.0
Iodine (µg)	7.0	10.0	4.8	4.8	4.8

TABLE 6-9 *Nutrient Content of Commercially Available Cow's Milk-Based Formula*

Nutrient Source	Similac	Enfamil	S.M.A.	Gerber	Good Start
Protein	Casein	Reduced mineral whey, casein	Demineralized whey, casein	Nonfat milk	Hydrolyzed, reduced-mineral whey
Fat	Soy oil, coconut oil, corn oil	Soy oil, coconut oil	Oleo; soybean, safflower, and coconut oils	Soy oil, coconut oil	Palm, safflower, and coconut oil
Carbohydrate	Lactose	Lactose	Lactose	Lactose	Lactose, corn syrup
Nutrients per 100 ML — normal dilution					
Energy (kcal)	68	67	67	67	67
Protein (g)	1.5	1.5	1.5	1.5	1.6
Fat (g)	3.6	3.8	3.6	3.6	3.4
Carbohydrate (g)	7.2	6.9	7.2	7.1	7.4
Vitamin A (IU)	200	207	240	200	200
Vitamin D (IU)	40	42	42	40	40
Vitamin E (IU)	2	2	1	2	8
Vitamin C (mg)	5.5	5.5	5.8	6.0	5.3
Thiamin (µg)	65	53	71	67	40
Riboflavin (µg)	10	11	11	10	9
Niacin (mg) (equiv.)	0.7	0.8	1.0	0.7	0.5
Pyridoxine (µg)	40	42	40	40	40
Vitamin B_{12} (µg)	0.15	0.16	0.11	0.16	0.17
Folate (µg)	10	10.5	5.3	10	6
Calcium (mg)	51	46	44	50	42
Phosphorus (mg)	39	31.7	33	38	24
Magnesium (mg)	4	4	5	3.3	4.5
Iron (mg)	Trace	Trace	Trace	Trace	Trace
Zinc (mg)	0.5	0.5	0.37	0.5	0.5
Copper (µg)	60.0	63.4	48	60	53
Iodine (µg)	10	6.8	7	5.3	5.6

Results of errors in formula preparation. Failure to gain appropriately in height and weight has been observed as a result of dilution of ready-to-eat formulas in the manner that concentrated formulas are prepared. Mothers have been known to add extra water in the belief that more dilute formula might reduce spitting up by their infants. Also, overdiluting formula or offering water as a substitute for milk or as a pacifier can lead to serious consequences.

Feeding undiluted concentrated formula increases kilocalories, protein, and solutes presented to the kidneys for excretion and may predispose the young infant to hypernatremia and **tetany** as well as obesity. Problems of improper formula preparation have most frequently been reported with the use of powdered formula and occur most often when an increased need for water caused by a fever or infection is superimposed on consumption of an already high-solute formula. Infants fed concentrated formula during such illnesses may become thirsty, demand more to drink, or refuse to consume more liquid because of anorexia secondary to the illness. When presented with more milk concentrated in the protein and solutes, the **osmolality** of the blood increases and **hypernatremic dehydration** may result. Cases of cerebral damage and gangrene of the extremities have been reported to be the result of hypernatremic dehydration and **metabolic acidosis.**[39]

Anticipatory guidance of parents of young infants should include information on the variety of formulas available, differences in methods of preparation of each product, and the dangers of overdiluted formula and excessive water intake.

Sterilization of formulas. Although terminal sterilization may be recommended for infant formulas, most parents do not follow this practice but prepare formulas by the clean technique, one bottle at each feeding time, and immediately feed the infant. No differences have been found in incidence of illness or infection of infants fed formulas prepared by the clean technique or by terminal sterilization regardless of socioeconomic background or housekeeping practices.[40,41] Formulas prepared by both methods result in milk that produces aerobic bacteria.

To prepare formula by the clean technique, the hands of the person preparing the formula should be washed carefully. All equipment to be used during preparation, including the cans that contain the milk, the bottles, and the nipples, must be thoroughly washed and rinsed. Once opened, cans of formula must be covered and refrigerated. The formula is prepared immediately before each feeding as described above. After the formula has been heated and the infant has been fed, any remaining milk should be discarded. Warm milk is an excellent medium for bacterial growth.

SEMISOLID FOODS IN THE INFANT'S DIET

In spite of the fact that no nutritional or developmental advantage can be expected from the early introduction of semisolid foods, many families feed them in the first month of infant life. Some parents add semisolid foods hoping that the added foods will encourage their infants to sleep through the night, a commonly held belief that has proved to be untrue. Other parents feed semisolid foods because they think that their infants are hungry or because they consider the acceptance of these foods a developmental landmark.

Many infants receive foods with texture such as baked potato or drained tuna fish by the time they can sustain a sitting posture. When they reach out and secure foods with a pincer grasp, finger foods such as zwieback and arrowroot cookies can be offered.

Age of introduction. The age of introduction of semisolid foods to infants in the United States declined between 1920, when these foods were seldom offered before 1 year of age, and the period between 1960 and 1970 when they were frequently offered in the first weeks and months of life. Concern that this early introduction of semisolid

Osmolality
(Gr *osmos*, impulsion through a membrane) Property of a solution that depends on the concentration of the particles (solutes) in solution per unit of solvent base; measured as milliosmoles per liter (mOsm/L).

Hypernatremic dehydration
An abnormally high sodium ion concentration in the extracellular fluid, due to water loss or restriction, drawing cell water to restore osmotic balance, causing dangerous cell dehydration.

Metabolic acidosis
Abnormal rise in acid partner of the carbonic acid-base bicarbonate buffer system by excess of organic acids, which displace part of the base bicarbonate in the buffer system and cause the H+ concentration to rise.

foods predisposed infants to obesity and allergic reactions caused many healthcare professionals in the pediatric community to reexamine the appropriate age to introduce these foods. It is currently recommended that the feeding of semisolid foods be delayed until the consumption of food is no longer a reflex process and the infant has fine, gross, and oral motor skills appropriate to consume them, that is, at approximately 4 to 6 months of age.

FEEDING BEHAVIORS
Developmental Readiness

Illingworth and Lister have defined a "critical or sensitive" period of development in relation to eating.[40] This is a time at which a specific stimulus, solid food, must be applied to the organism to learn a particular action, accepting and eating table foods. They point out that infants learn to chew at about 6 or 7 months of age, thus at this point they are developmentally ready to consume food. If solid foods are withheld until a later age, the child will have considerably more difficulty in accepting them.

In 1937 Gesell and Ilg published their now classic observations made during extensive studies of the feeding behavior of infants.[41] Their observations are as valid today as they were then. **Cineradiographic** techniques developed since then have permitted more detailed descriptions of the actions involved in sucking, suckling, and swallowing.[42,43]

Development of Oral Structures and Functions

It is important to recognize that even though the normal neonate is well prepared to suck and swallow at birth, the physical and motor maturation during the first year alter both the form of the oral structures and the methods by which the infant extracts milk from a nipple. Each of these changes influences the infant's eating skills. At birth the tongue is disproportionately large in comparison with the lower jaw and essentially fills the oral cavity. The lower jaw is moved back relative to the upper jaw, which protrudes over the lower by approximately 2 mm.[44] When the mouth is closed, the jaws do not rest on top of each other; the tip of the tongue lies between the upper and lower jaws. There is a "fat pad" in each of the checks. It is thought that these pads serve as a prop for the muscles in the cheek, maintaining rigidity of the cheeks during suckling.[45] The lips of the neonate are also instrumental in suckling and have characteristics appropriate for their function at this age. A mucosal fold disappears by the third or fourth month, when the lips have developed muscular control to seal the oral cavity.[45] The newborn infant sucks reflexively, the young infant beginning at 2 or 3 weeks of age suckles, and as infants grow older they learn mature sucking. Some description of these two processes therefore seems important.

Suckling

Studies by Ardran, Kemp, and Lind have shown that the processes of breast and bottle suckling are similar.[42] The nipple of the breast becomes rigid and elongated during breast-feeding so that it resembles a rubber nipple in shape, and both assume a similar position in the infant's mouth. The infant grasps the nipple in the mouth. The oral cavity is sealed off by pressure from the middle portions of the lips assisted by the mucosal folds of the jaws. The nipple is held in the infant's mouth with the tip located close to the junction of the hard and soft **palate.**

During the first stage of suckling, the lower jaw and tongue are lowered while the mouth is closed, thus creating a negative pressure. The tip of the tongue moves forward. The lower jaw and tongue are next raised, compressing the beginning base of the nipple. The compression is moved from the beginning base to the tip of the nipple as the tip of the tongue withdraws, thus stroking or milking the liquid from the nipple. The moved

Cineradiographs
(Gr *cine-*, *kinesis*, movement; L *radius*, ray; Gr *graphein*, to write) Fluoroscopic motion film records of internal structures and their functions.

Palate
(L *palatum*, palate) The partition separating the nasal and oral cavities, with a hard bony front section and a soft fleshy back section.

back position of the lower jaw maximizes the efficiency of the stroking action.[42,43] As the tongue moves back, it comes in contact with the tensed soft palate, thus causing liquid to squirt into the side food channels. The location of the **larynx** is further elevated by the muscular contractions during swallowing. As the liquid is squirted back in the mouth, the **epiglottis** functions as a breakwater during swallowing. As the liquid is squirted back in the mouth, the epiglottis is positioned so that it parts the stream of liquid, passing it to the sides of the larynx instead of over it. Thus liquid does not pass over the laryngeal entrance during early infancy because of the relatively higher position of the larynx and the parting of the stream of liquid by the epiglottis.

Sucking

Mature sucking is an acquired feature of the **orofacial muscles.** It is not a continuous process. Upon accumulation of sufficient fluid in the mouth, sucking and breathing are interrupted by a swallowing movement. The closure of the nasopharyngeal and laryngeal sphincters in response to the presence of food in the **pharynx** is responsible for the interruption of the nasal breathing.[46]

During swallowing the food lies in the swallow preparation position on the groove of the tongue. The farther back portion of the soft palate is raised toward the **adenoidal pad** in the roof of the **epipharynx.** The tongue presses upward against the nipple so that the swallow of milk follows gravity down the sloping tongue and reaches the pharynx. As the milk in the mouth moves downward, the rear wall of the pharynx comes forward to displace the soft palate toward the back surface of the tongue and the larynx is elevated and arched backward. The accumulated milk is expressed from the pharynx by peristaltic movements of the pharyngeal wall toward the back of the tongue and the larynx. The milk spills over the joining folds of the pharynx and epiglottis folds into the side food channels and then into the esophagus.[43]

The **tonsils** and **lymphoid tissue** play an important role as infants swallow. They help keep the airway open and the food away from the rear pharyngeal wall as the infant is held in a reclining position, thus delaying nasopharyngeal closure until food has reached the pharynx.[45]

As the infant grows older the oral cavity enlarges so that the tongue no longer fills the mouth. The tongue grows differentially at the tip and attains motility in the larger oral cavity. The elongated tongue can be protruded to receive and pass solids between the gum pads and erupting teeth for mastication. Mature feeding is characterized by separate movements of the lip, tongue, and gum pads or teeth.[45]

Sequence of Development of Feeding Behavior

The sequence of development of feeding behavior is related to the individual maturation of the infant.

Newborns. The "rooting reflex" caused by stroking of the perioral skin including the cheeks and lips causes an infant to turn toward the stimulus, so that the mouth comes in contact with it. Stimulus placed on the lips causes involuntary movements toward it, closure, and pouting in preparation for sucking.[47] These reflexes thus enable the infant to suck and receive nourishment. Both rooting and suckling can be elicited when the infant is hungry but are absent when the infant is satiated.[44] During feeding the neonate assumes a tonic position, the head rotated to one side and the arm on that side fisted. The infant seeks the nipple by touch and obtains milk from the nipple with a rhythmic suckle.[41] Semisolid foods, introduced by spoon at an early age into the diets of many infants, are secured in the same manner as milk, by stroking movements of the tongue with the tongue projecting as the spoon is withdrawn. Frequently, the food is expelled from the mouth.

Age 16 to 24 weeks. By 16 weeks of age the more mature suckling pattern becomes

Larynx
(Gr *larynx*, upper part of windpipe) Structure of muscle and cartilage lined with mucous membrane, connected to top part of the trachea and to the pharynx; essential sphincter muscle guarding the entrance to the trachea and functioning secondarily as the organ of the voice.

Orofacial muscles
(L *os, oris*, mouth) Adjoining muscles of the mouth and face.

Pharynx
(Gr *pharynx*, throat) The muscular membranous passage between the mouth and the posterior nasal passages and the larynx and esophagus.

Adenoidal pad
(Gr *adenos*, gland; *eidos*, form) Normal lymphoid tissue in the nasopharynx of children.

Epipharynx
(Gr *epi*, on; *pharynx*, throat) Nasopharynx; the part of the pharynx that lies above the level of the soft palate.

Lymphoid tissue
(L *lympha*, water) Tissues related to the body system of lymphatic fluids.

evident, with the tongue moving back and forth as opposed to the earlier up-and-down motions. Spoon feeding is easier because the infant can draw in the lower lip as the spoon is removed. The tonic neck position has faded and the infant assumes a more symmetric position with the head at midline. The hands close over the bottle.[41] By 20 weeks of age the infant can grasp on tactile contact with a palmar squeeze. By 24 weeks of age the infant can reach for and grasp an object on sight. In almost every instance the object goes into the mouth.

Age 24 to 28 weeks. Between 24 and 28 weeks of age chewing movement, an up-and-down movement of the jaws, begins. This movement, coupled with the ability to grasp and the hand-to-mouth route of grasped objects, as well as sitting posture, indicates a readiness of the infant to finger feed. Infants at this age grasp with a **palmar grasp.** Therefore, the shape of the food presented to the child to finger feed is important. Cookies, melba toast, crackers, and teething biscuits are frequently introduced at this stage.

Age 28 to 32 weeks. Between 28 and 32 weeks of age the infant gains control of the trunk and can sit alone without support. The sitting infant has greater mobility of the shoulders and arms and is better able to reach and grasp. The grasp is more digital than the earlier palmar grasp. The infant is able to transfer items from one hand to the other and learns to release and resecure objects voluntarily. The beginning of chewing patterns, up-and-down movements of the jaws, is demonstrated. The tongue shows more maturity in regard to spoon feeding than in drinking. Food is received from the spoon by pressing the lips against the spoon, drawing the head away, and drawing in the lower lip. The infant is aware of a cup and can suck from it. Milk leaks frequently from the corners of the mouth as the tongue is projected before swallowing.[41]

Age 6 to 12 months. The introduction of soft mashed, but not strained, foods is appropriate at this stage of development. In fact, it is at this stage of development that Illingworth and Lister believe it is critical to introduce the infant to harder-to-chew foods. Between 6 and 12 months of age the infant gradually receives greater amounts of food from the family menu and less and less of the pureed and strained items. Foods should be carefully selected and modified so that they are presented in a form that can be manipulated in the mouth without the potential of choking and aspirating, as may occur with small grains of rice or corn. Many parents mash well-cooked ground meat dishes, such as ground meat in gravies or sauces, which appear to be easily accepted, as are liverwurst, minced chicken livers, and drained tuna fish. Custards, puddings, and ice cream soon become favorites.

By 28 weeks of age infants are able to help themselves to their bottle in sitting postures, although they will not be able to tip the bottle adaptively as it empties until about 32 weeks of age. By the end of the first year they can completely manage bottle-feeding alone.

By 32 weeks of age infants bring their heads forward to receive the spoon as it is presented to them. The tongue shows increased motility and allows for considerable increased manipulation of food in the mouth before swallowing. At the end of the first year, infants are able to manipulate food in the mouth with definite chewing movements.

During the fourth quarter of the first year, the child develops an increasingly precise **pincer grasp.** The bottle can be managed alone and can be rescued if it is lost. The child can drink from a cup only if help is provided. Infants at this age are increasingly conscious of what others do and often imitate the models set for them.[41] By 1 year of age the patterns of eating have changed from sucking to beginning rotary chewing movements. Children understand the concept of the container and the contained, have voluntary hand-to-mouth movements and a precise pincer grasp, and can voluntarily release and rescue objects. They are thus prepared to learn to feed themselves, a behavior they learn and refine in the second year.

This development of feeding behavior is summarized in Table 6-10 and is shown in the sequence of illustrations in Fig. 6-4.

Palmar grasp
Early grasp of the young infant, clasping an object in the palm and wrapping whole hand around it.

Pincer grasp
Later digital grasp of the older infant, usually picking up smaller objects with a precise grip between thumb and fore-finger.

TABLE 6-10   *Sequence of Development of Feeding Behavior*

Age	Reflexes	Oral, Fine, Gross Motor Development
1-3 months	Rooting and suck and swallow reflexes are present at birth Tonic neck reflex present	Head control is poor Secures milk with suckling pattern, the tongue projecting during a swallow By the end of the third month, head control is developed
4-6 months	Rooting reflex fades Bite reflex fades Tonic neck reflex fades by 16 weeks	Changes from a suckling pattern to a mature suck with liquids Sucking strength increases Munching pattern begins Grasps with a palmar grasp Grasps, brings objects to mouth and bites them
7-9 months	Gag reflex is less strong as chewing of solids begins and normal gag is developing Choking reflex can be inhibited	Munching movements begin when solid foods are eaten Rotary chewing begins Sits alone Has power of voluntary release and resecural Holds bottle alone Develops an inferior pincer grasp
10-12 months		Reaches for a spoon Bites nipples, spoons, and crunchy foods Grasps bottle and foods and brings them to the mouth Can drink from a cup that is held Tongue is used to lick food morsels off the lower lip Finger feeds with a refined pincer grasp

Modified from Gessell A and Ilg FL: Feeding behavior of infants, Philadelphia, 1937, JB Lippincott Co.

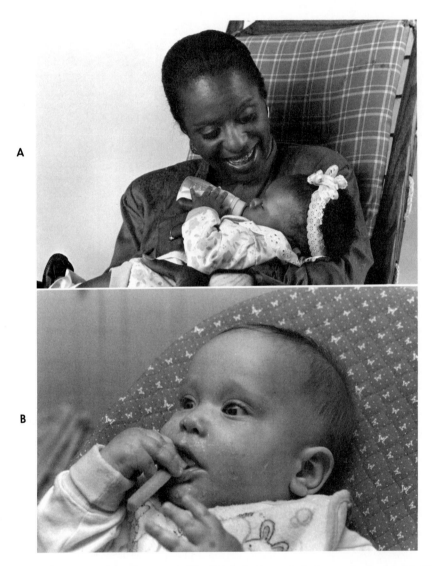

FIG. 6-4 Sequence of development of feeding behaviors. **A,** Infant sucks liquids. **B,** Five-month-old infant begins to finger feed.

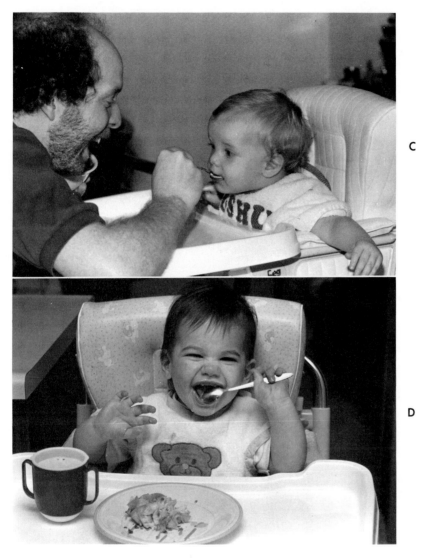

C

D

FIG. 6-4, cont'd   **C,** Eight-month-old infant is fed table food. **D,** Eleven-month-old infant begins to feed himself.

Continued.

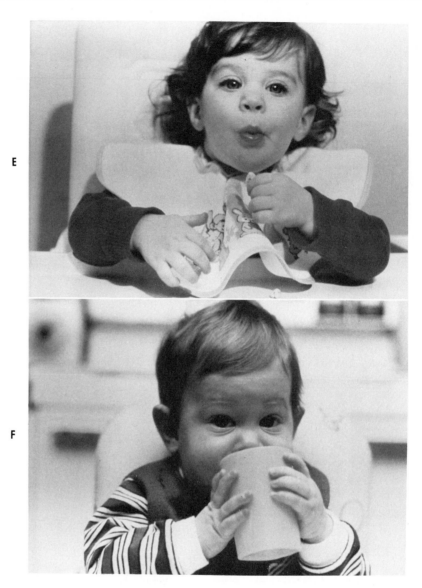

FIG. 6-4, cont'd   E, Ten-month-old infant purses her lips. **F,** Twelve-month-old infant drinks from a cup.

FOOD CHOICES
Commercially Available Infant Foods

A vast number of commercially prepared flaked (freeze-dried), canned, and frozen foods are marketed for feeding the infant. The new mother may select organically grown products or products prepared from farms and vineyards that probably use fertilizers and insecticides. She will find jarred single foods and juices and dinners of vegetables mixed with meat, several juices mixed together, and can choose from 2½ oz, 4 oz, or 6 oz jars (first foods, second foods, third foods). Some may find toddler meals interesting. In the freezer there are complete frozen meals of two or three foods for babies in varying textures. Flake (freeze-dried) baby foods might also be on the grocers' shelves. Juices are marketed

FIG. 6-5   Many varieties and mixtures of infant foods are available in multiple-size containers.

in 4 oz, 8 oz, and 25.3 oz bottles, some prepared from fresh fruit, others from concentrates. This wide range of choice among current products in the U.S. baby food market may at first appear confusing to the new mother (Fig. 6-5), and she may choose to prepare some of the basic foods herself from fresh produce (p. 243).

Foods as Sources of Nutrients

The range of nutrients found in any group of foods for infants is quite wide, as indicated in Table 6-11. Ready-to-serve dry infant cereals are fortified with electrically reduced iron. Three level tablespoons of cereal will provide about 5 mg of iron, or from one half to one third of what the infant requires. Therefore, cereal is usually the first food added to the infant's diet. Cereal and fruit mixtures in jars are fortified with ferrous sulfate to provide 7 to 9 mg of iron per 4.5 oz jar.

Strained and junior vegetables and fruits provide carbohydrate and variable amounts of vitamins A and C. Vitamin C is added to a number of the fruits and all of the fruit juices. Several fruits, including apricots, have sugar added and are marketed as fruit desserts. Tapioca is added to a number of the fruits. Milk is added to creamed vegetables and wheat is incorporated into mixed vegetables.

Strained and junior meats and egg yolk are prepared with only water, except for lamb which has lemon juice added. Strained meats, which have the highest caloric density of any of the commercial baby foods are an excellent source of high-quality protein and **heme iron.** Water is the most abundant ingredient in meat and vegetable combinations and high-meat dinners. The introduction of these products should be delayed until it has been determined that the infant has no allergic reactions to any of the wide variety of ingredients they contain.

A number of dessert items are also available, including puddings and fruit desserts. The nutrient composition of these products varies, but all contain sugar and modified corn or tapioca starch.

Home Preparation of Infant Foods

In spite of the fact that the manufacturers of infant foods no longer add salt or sugar to most of their commercially prepared products, many parents prefer to make their own infant foods at home with a food grinder, blender, or strainer. The foods should be

Heme iron
Dietary iron from animal sources, from heme portion of hemoglobin in red blood cells. More easily absorbed and transported in the body than non-heme iron from plant sources, but supplying the smaller portion of the body's total dietary iron.

TABLE 6-11 *Ranges of Selected Nutrients Per Ounce in Commercially Prepared Infant Foods*

Food	Energy (kcal)	Protein (g)	Iron (mg)	Vitamin A (IU)	Vitamin C (mg)
Dry cereal	102-114	2.0-10.2	17.0-21.0	0-20	0-1.4
Strained and junior fruits	11-23	0.0-0.2	0.0-2.0	3-206	0.2-35.3
Strained and junior vegetables	7-18	0.2-1.0	0.1-0.4	9-3348	0.6-3.6
Strained and junior meats	27-42	3.6-4.4	0.3-1.5	8-10811	0.3-0.7
Strained egg yolks	58	2.8	0.8	355	0.4
Strained and junior meat and vegetable dinners	20-33	1.6-2.6	0.0-0.3	22-237	0.1-0.5
Strained and junior vegetables and meat dinners	9-70	0.1-1.5	0.1-0.3	4-1114	0.2-1.2
Strained and junior desserts	17-25	0.0-0.8	0.0-0.1	4-71	0.2-8.9

From Gebhardt SE, Cutrufelli R, and Matthews RH: Composition of food, baby foods, raw, processed, prepared. Agriculture handbook No 8-3, Washington, DC, 1978, US Department of Agriculture

carefully selected from high-quality fresh, frozen, or canned fruits, vegetables, and meats, and prepared so that nutrients are retained. The preparation area and all utensils used must be meticulously cleaned. Salt and sugar should be used sparingly, if at all. When the food has been cooked, then pureed or strained, it should be packaged in individual portions and refrigerated or frozen so that a single portion can be heated and fed without compromising the quality and bacterial content of the entire batch (Fig. 6-6). The box on p. 243 provides directions for the home preparation of infant foods. Care must be taken not to use additional seasoning, as home-prepared infant foods usually have a greater caloric content than the commercial products do, and many have a higher salt content.

Table Food

Cultural influence. Food from the family menu is introduced at an early age in the diets of many infants. The age of introduction and type of food offered will reflect cultural practice. For example, crumbled cornbread mixed with pot liquor (the liquid from cooked vegetables) may be fed to infants in the southern states by 3 months of age, "sticky" rice may be fed to Oriental infants in the Pacific Northwest by 6 to 7 months of age, mashed beans with some of the cooking liquid are often given to Hispanic American infants at 2 to 4 months of age, and mashed potatoes are offered to many infants by 3 to 4 months of age. Examples of nutrient content of some selected table foods commonly fed to older infants are given in Table 6-12.

Form and texture. Solid foods offered to infants should be in a form easily masticated and not given in small pieces. Choking and aspiration can occur if small pieces of hot dogs, grapes, hard candy, nuts, and other food in small, hard pieces are consumed.

Honey. Sometimes honey is used as a sweetener for home-prepared infant foods and formulas. Honey is also recommended for use on pacifiers to promote sucking in hypotonic infants. However, honey has been implicated as the only food source of spores of *Clos-*

FIG. 6-6 **A,** Mother prepares food for her infant. **B,** After the food is frozen in ice-cube trays, she removes the cubes and stores them in individual portions for later use.

ONE STEP FURTHER

Directions for Home Preparation of Infant Foods

1. Select fresh, high-quality fruits, vegetables, or meats.
2. Be sure all utensils, including cutting boards, grinders, knives, etc., are thoroughly clean.
3. Wash your hands before preparing the food.
4. Clean, wash, and trim the foods in as little water as possible.
5. Cook the foods until tender in as little water as possible. Avoid overcooking, which may destroy heat-sensitive nutrients.
6. Do not add salt. Add sugar sparingly. Do not add honey to foods for infants less than 1 year of age.*
7. Add enough water so that the food has a consistency that is easily pureed.
8. Strain or puree the food using an electric blender, a food mill, a baby food grinder, or a kitchen strainer.
9. Pour puree into ice cube tray and freeze.
10. When food is frozen hard, remove the cubes and store in freezer bags.
11. Unfreeze and heat in serving container the amount of food that will be consumed at a single feeding (in water bath or microwave oven).

---

*Botulism spores have been reported in honey, and young infants do not have the immune capacity to resist this infection.

From Pipes PL: Nutrition in infancy. In Krause MV and Mahan LK, editors: Food, nutrition, and diet therapy, ed 7, Philadelphia, 1984, WB Saunders Co.

TABLE 6-12   *Nutrient Content of Selected Table Foods Commonly Fed to Infants*

Food	Portion Size	Energy (kcal)	Protein (g)	Iron (mg)	Vitamin A (IU)	Vitamin C (mg)
Cooked cereal (farina)	¼ cup	26	0.8	Dependent on level of fortification		
Mashed potato	¼ cup	34	1.1	0.2	10	5
French fried potato	3, 1 to 2 inches	29	0.4	0.2		
Spaghetti	2 tbsp	19	0.6	0.2		
Macaroni and cheese	2 tbsp	54	2.1	0.2	107	
Liverwurst	½ oz	45	2.1	0.8	925	
Hamburger	½ oz	41	3.4	0.5	5	
Eggs	1 medium	72	5.7	1.0	520	
Cottage cheese	1 tbsp	5	1.9		23.7	
Green beans	1 tbsp	3	0.15	0.2	43	1
Cooked carrots	1 tbsp	2.81			952	
Banana	½ small	40	0.5	0.35	90	5
Pudding	¼ cup	70	2.2	Trace	102	
Lollipop	1 oz hard candy	109				
Saltine crackers	1	12	0.2			
Vanilla wafer	¼ inch thick, 1¾ inch diameter	18	0.2			
Cheese strips	¼ oz	28	1.78		92	

From Adams CF: Nutritive value in American foods in common units, Agriculture Handbook no 456, Washington, DC, 1975, US Department of Agriculture.

Botulism
A serious, often fatal, form of food poisoning from ingesting food contaminated with the powerful toxins of the bacteria *Clostridium botulinum*. The toxin blocks transmission of neural impulses at the nerve terminals, causing gradual paralysis and death when affecting respiratory muscles. Most cases result from eating carelessly home-canned food, so all such food should be boiled at least 10 minutes before eating. Cases reported in infants have been related to eating spore-containing honey, so it should not be used.

tridium botulinum during infancy. These spores are extremely resistant to heat and are not destroyed by present methods of processing honey. **Botulism** in infancy is caused by ingestion of the spores, which germinate into the toxin in the lumen of the bowel. Honey should not be fed to infants less than 1 year of age.[48]

Feeding the Infant

Presented with the breast of an adequately fed lactating mother, or the nipple on a bottle of properly prepared formula, the hungry infant receives both biochemical and psychosocial nurturance.

Feeding schedule. The infant held in a semireclining position who is offered the nipple sucks and receives the major portion of nourishment in 20 minutes. Newborn infants will initially feed six to eight times a day at intervals of 2 to 4 hours and will consume 2 to 3 oz at a feeding. By 2 weeks of age most infants will have increased the amount of milk consumed at a feeding and reduced the number of feedings to six. By 2 months of age most infants are fed five times a day and sleep through the night. By 6 months of age most babies consume three meals and four milk feedings a day.

Intakes of infants. Volume of intake and energy consumption is influenced not only by the infant's requirements for maintenance, growth, and activity, but also by the parents'

CASE STUDY

Rachel's First Solid Foods

Rachel is attending well-baby clinic with her mother for her regular visit. She is now 5.5 months old, weighs 7.3 kg and is 65.3 cm long. She is currently breastfed and receives no other foods. Her mother feels it is time to add other foods to her diet.

Questions for analysis
1. List developmental landmarks that should be reached before other foods are added.
2. What foods should be introduced to the baby first? Why?
3. How should foods be added to identify any possible food allergies or intolerances?

---

sensitivity to and willingness to accept cues of hunger and satiety, eagerness for the infant to feed, and skill at feeding. Infants eat differently, and mothers vary in their sensitivity to the child's cues. Thoman found that mothers with their first baby spent more time stimulating their infants during feeding than did mothers who had several children, yet their infants spent less time sucking during breastfeeding and consumed less from bottles at feeding than did infants of multiparous mothers.[49] The stimulation prolonged the pauses between sucking and reduced the total consumption of food (see box above).

Growth Response to Feeding

Formula-fed newborn infants have been reported to regain to their birth weights more rapidly than breastfed infants.[9] Thereafter, weight gains until 3 months appear similar in breastfed and bottle-fed babies, after which bottle-fed infants gain more rapidly.[50]

Energy intakes. Per unit of size, infants consume the greatest number of kilocalories between 14 and 28 days of age, a time referred to by many pediatricians as the "hungry period." After this time, although total quantity of energy intake increases, intakes per unit of size decrease. Infants consume greater amounts of food and nutrients as they grow older but less and less per unit of body size.

Wide ranges of volume of intake and energy consumption throughout the first year of life have been noted in formula-fed infants by several researchers. Quantities of milk consumed by breastfed and bottle-fed infants are similar during the first 3 months. By the fourth month of age, the formula-fed infants consume significantly more milk than breastfed babies. Males and females tend to consume similar quantities during these early months.

Texture progress. Stages of development of feeding behavior indicate readiness for the addition of semisolid and table foods. Ages at which these stages occur and when foods other than milk are offered are shown in Table 6-13.

Food Selection

Because of the great variability in energy and nutrients provided by foods offered to infants, selection of foods and the amounts offered should be based on the infant's rate of gain in height and weight as well as on nutrient needs. Iron-fortified infant cereals are usually the first foods added to the infant's diet. It makes little difference whether fruits or vegetables are introduced next. New foods should be added singly, no more than one new food every 3 days. The introduction of vegetables containing nitrates—for example,

TABLE 6-13   Suggested Ages for the Introduction of Semisolid Foods and Table Food

Food	Age (months)		
	4 to 6	6 to 8	9 to 12
Iron-fortified cereals for infants	Add		
Vegetables		Add strained	Gradually delete strained foods, introduce table foods
Fruits		Add strained	Gradually delete strained foods, introduce chopped well-cooked or canned foods
Meats		Add strained or finely chopped table meats	Decrease the use of strained meats, increase the varieties of table meats
Finger foods such as arrow-root biscuits, oven-dried toast		Add those that can be secured with a palmar grasp	Increase the use of small-sized finger foods as the pincer grasp develops
Well-cooked mashed or chopped table foods, prepared without added salt or sugar			Add
Juice by cup			Add

carrots, beets, and spinach—is usually delayed until the infant is at least 4 months of age, because nitrate can be converted to nitrite in the stomach of the young infant, resulting in methemoglobinemia. It is generally recommended that the introduction of fruit juice be delayed until it can be consumed by cup. Examples of foods and milks that might be consumed by infants at various ages are shown in Table 6-14.

During feeding both the mother and the infant receive satisfaction and pleasure. The infant is pleased because hunger is satiated. The mother is pleased because she has fulfilled the needs of her infant. Successful feeding provides the basis for the warm, trusting relationship that develops between infants and their mothers. Infants swallow air as well as milk during feeding. Holding the child in an upright position and gently patting the back encourages expulsion of swallowed air and prevents distension and discomfort.

Feeding-Related Concerns

Colic. Parents of colicky babies—those who are otherwise healthy and well-fed but who cry constantly for several hours, draw their legs onto their abdomens, and pass large amounts of gas—often request changes in their infants' formulas. This rarely resolves colic and frequent change in formulas should be discouraged. It has been suggested that colic in some breastfed babies may be resolved by eliminating milk from the mother's diet.[51,52] A casein hydrolysate formula may alleviate symptoms in some but not all bottle-fed infants.[53]

Spitting up food. Spitting up can occur in infants and usually causes concern for parents. During the early months of life, some otherwise healthy infants spit up a small amount of any milk or food digested at each feeding. Although the infants do not fail to thrive, parents may seek help in resolving the situation. There is no therapy. The problem usually resolves itself by the time the infant can sustain a sitting position.

TABLE 6-14   *Sample Menus for Infants at Various Ages*

Age	Weight (kg)	Energy Needs (kcal/kg)	Menu
2 months	5	540	26-28 oz human milk or infant formula
6 months	7.75	775	3 oz human milk or infant formula
			4 tbsp strained applesauce
			½ cup iron-fortified infant cereal
			4 tbsp strained pears
			1 piece zwieback
10 months	9.5	925	24 oz formula or human milk
			½ cup iron-fortified cereal
			½ cup applesauce
			1 piece melba toast
			1 oz finely chopped chicken
			½ mashed baked potato + ½ tsp oleo
			3 oz junior vegetable
			1 arrowroot cookie
			¼ oz cheese strip
			1 6-oz beef noodle dinner
			2 tbsp well-cooked broccoli
			¼ cup vanilla pudding
			2 saltine crackers

Nursing bottle syndrome. A characteristic pattern of tooth decay in infants and younger children of all the upper and sometimes the lower posterior teeth, known as nursing bottle syndrome, is often observed in children who are given sweetened liquid by bottle at bedtime or who are breastfed frequently when they sleep with their mothers.[54] As children suck, the tongue protrudes slightly from the mouth, covering the lower front teeth. Liquids are spread over the upper teeth and the lower posterior teeth. Sucking stimulates the flow of saliva, which washes the debris from the teeth and promotes the secretion of compounds that buffer the acids in the plaque. When children are awake they swallow the liquid quickly. However, if they fall asleep, sucking stops and the salivary flow and buffering are reduced. The sweetened liquid pools around the teeth not protected by the extended tongue, and the bacterial plaque has contact with the carbohydrates during the hours of sleep.

Infant formulas, fruit juice, human milk, and cow's milk consumed when infants are falling asleep may cause this decay. To prevent this dental destruction it has been suggested that infants be held when feeding and burped and put to bed as soon as they fall asleep.

Infant obesity. In the past, there has been speculation that formula feeding and the early introduction of semisolid foods might be factors in excessive intakes of energy and the development of infant obesity, and that obese infants very often become obese adults. However, a number of studies have shown that neither breastfeeding nor bottle-feeding nor the age of introduction of semisolid foods are causes of obesity in infancy.[55,56] Obesity in infancy has not been found to be predictive of obesity in later life. One study found measures of fatness at 8 years of age no greater in children who had been bottle-fed as compared to those who had been breastfed.[57] A longitudinal study of children found that infants who were obese at 6 months and 1 year of age became progressively thinner as they grew older. Weight gain in infancy was not found to be predictive of obesity at 9 years of age (see box on p. 248).[58]

CASE STUDY

Danny's Grandmother Wonders about His Weight

Danny is 6 months old, a happy and healthy baby. However, his grandmother seems worried about his weight. At well-child clinic today, his mother says she feels that Danny is doing well, but she asks for some answers to questions raised by her mother-in-law. Danny's chart shows his weight/height record:

	2 weeks	2 months	4 months	6 months
Weight (kg)	5.34	7.60	9.59	10.60
Height (cm)	57.10	62.50	67.10	72.60

Danny was solely breastfed until 4 months of age. At that time semisolid foods were added to his diet and he was given a cow's milk–based formula. Now, at 6 months of age, his usual intake is:

Formula, commercially prepared (20 kcal/oz)	32-40 oz
Rice or oatmeal baby cereal	8 tablespoons dry
Strained pears or applesauce	½ cup
Strained squash or carrots	½ cup

Questions for analysis
1. In what percentile do his height, weight, and weight-height plot on his growth chart?
2. Is there any reason for concern about Danny's rate of weight gain?
3. Is this diet appropriate for him? How would you counsel his mother?

Summary

Adequate nourishment for infants can be achieved through consumption of a variety of combinations of milks, supplements, and semisolid foods. Maturation of the oral and fine motor skills indicates appropriate stages for the introduction of semisolid and solid foods. Current recommendations include breastfeeding by an adequately nourished mother and the introduction of semisolid foods at 4 to 6 months of age, and of finger foods when the infant reaches out, grasps, and brings items to his mouth.

If the mother is unable or unwilling to breastfeed her child, a variety of properly constructed infant formulas are marketed that have been proven to support normal growth and development in infants. It is to the formula-fed baby's advantage to receive a formula with iron.

Infants should be permitted to establish their own feeding schedule and be fed to satiety. When they develop a voluntary mature sucking pattern, the introduction of semisolid foods is appropriate. When munching and rotary chewing begin, the use of soft-cooked table foods is appropriate. Infants can begin to drink from a cup with help between 9 and 12 months of age.

Review Questions

1. Why is there such a wide range of acceptable intakes of energy during infancy?
2. Under what circumstances should the infant's water intake be carefully monitored?

3. What is the difference in fat absorption of human and cow's milk?
4. What supplements should be given to a solely breastfed 3-month-old male infant?
5. Describe the difference between sucking and suckling.
6. What developmental landmarks indicate a readiness for semisolid foods to be added to the infant's diet?
7. At what age is it reasonable to feed whole cow's milk?
8. Why is it important for a baby to go to sleep without a bottle?

References

1. Smith D et al: Shifting linear growth during infancy, J Pediatr 89:225, 1976.
2. Smith DW: Growth and its disorders, Philadelphia, 1977, WB Saunders Co.
3. National Center for Health Statistics: NCHS growth charts, 1976, Monthly vital statistics report, vol 25, no 3, suppl (HRA) 76-1120, Rockville, Md, 1976, Health Resources Administration.
4. Fomon SF et al: Body composition of reference children from birth to 10 years, Am J Clin Nutr 55:1169, 1982.
5. Widdowson EM and Spray CM: Chemical development in utero, Arch Dis Child 62:205, 1951.
6. Lebenthal EL, Lee PIC, and Heitlinger LA: Impact of development of the gastrointestinal tract on infant feeding, J Pediatr 102:1, 1983.
7. Watkins JB: Bile acid metabolism and fat absorption in newborn infants, Pediatr Clin North Am 2:501, 1974.
8. Filer LJ, Mattson FH, and Fomon SJ: Triglyceride configuration and fat absorption by the human infant, J Nutr 99:293, 1969.
9. Fomon SJ: Infant nutrition, ed 2, Philadelphia, 1974, WB Saunders Co.
10. Bayless TM and Christopher NL: Disaccharidase deficiency, Am J Clin Nutr 22:181, 1969.
11. Ziegler E and Fomon J: Potential renal solute load of infant formulas, J Nutr 119:1785, 1989.
12. Edelman CM, Barrett HL, and Troupkon V: Renal concentrating mechanisms in newborn infants. Effect of dietary protein and water content, role of urea and responsiveness to antidiuretic hormone, J Clin Invest 39:1062, 1960.
13. Polack E and others: The osmotic concentrating ability in healthy infants and children, Arch Dis Child 40:291, 1965.
14. Food and Nutrition Board, National Research Council, National Academy of Sciences: Recommended Dietary Allowances, ed 10, Washington, DC, 1989, National Academy Press.
15. Fomon SJ et al: Requirements for protein and essential amino acids in early infancy, Acta Paediatr Scand 62:33, 1973.
16. WHO (World Health Organization): Energy and protein requirements. Report of a joint FAO/WHO/UNU Expert Consultation, Technical Series 724, World Health Organization, 1985.
17. Committee on Nutrition, American Academy of Pediatrics: Commentary on breast-feeding and infant formulas, including proposed standards for formulas, Pediatrics 57:279, 1976.
18. Holt LE Jr and Snyderman SE: The amino acid requirements of infants, J Am Nurs Assoc 175:100, 1961.
19. Fomon SJ and Filer LJ: Amino acid requirements for normal growth. In Nyhan WL, editor: Amino acid metabolism and genetic variation, New York, 1967, McGraw-Hill Book Co.
20. Report of a Joint FAO/WHO Ad Hoc Expert Committee: Energy and protein requirements, World Health Organization Technical Series No 522, FAO Nutr Meet Ser No 52, Geneva, 1973, World Health Organization.
21. Wesson LJ and Burr GO: The metabolic rate and respiratory quotients of rats on fat-deficient diets, J Biol Chem 91:525, 1931.
22. Holman RJ, Caster WO, and Weise HF: The essential fatty acid requirement of infants and the assessment of their dietary intake on linoleate by serum fatty acid analysis, Am J Clin Nutr 14:70, 1964.

23. Hey EN and Katz G: Evaporative water loss in the newborn baby, J Physiol 200:605, 1969.

24. Partridge JC et al: Water intoxication secondary to feeding mismanagement, Am J Dis Child 135:38, 1981.

25. McMillan MA, Landau SA, and Oski FA: Iron sufficiency in breast milk and the availability of iron from human milk, Pediatrics 58:686, 1976.

26. Committee on Nutrition, American Academy of Pediatrics: Iron-fortified infant formulas, Pediatrics 84:114, 1989.

27. MacDonald LD, Gibson RS, and Miles JE: Changes in hair zinc and copper concentrations of breast-fed and bottle-fed infants during the first six months, Acta Paediatr Scand 71:758, 1982.

28. Cavell PA and Widdowson EM: Intakes and excretion of iron, copper, and zinc in the neonatal period, Arch Dis Child 39:496, 1964.

29. Johnson PE and Evans GW: Relative zinc availability in human breast milk, infant formulas, and cow's milk, Am J Clin Nutr 31:416, 1978.

30. Baker H et al: Vitamin profile of 174 mothers and newborns at parturition, Am J Clin Nutr 28:59, 1975.

31. American Academy of Pediatrics: Composition of human milk: normative data, Appendix K, ed 2, Elk Grove, Ill, 1985, American Academy of Pediatrics.

32. Dirks OB et al: Total and free ionic fluoride in human and cow's milk as determined by chromatography and fluoride electrode, Caries Res 8:181, 1974.

33. Fomon SJ, Sanders KD, and Ziegler E: Formulas for older infants, J Pediatr 16:690, 1990.

34. Committee on Nutrition, American Academy of Pediatrics: Follow-up of weaning formulas, Pediatrics 88:1067, 1989.

35. Ziegler EE et al: Cowmilk feeding in infancy: Further observations on blood loss from the gastrointestinal tract, J Pediatr 116:11, 1990.

36. Fabius RJ et al: Malnutrition associated with a formula of barley water, corn syrup, and whole milk, Am J Dis Child 135:615, 1981.

37. Sinatra FR and Merritt RJ: Iatrogenic kwashiorkor in infants, Am J Dis Child 135:21, 1981.

38. Committee on Nutrition, American Academy of Pediatrics: Imitation and substitute milks, Pediatrics 73:876, 1984.

39. Comay SC and Karabus CD: Peripheral gangrene in hypernatraemic dehydration of infancy, Arch Dis Child 50:616, 1975.

40. Illingworth RS and Lister J: The critical or sensitive period with special reference to certain feeding problems in infants and children, J Pediatr 65:839, 1964.

41. Gesell A and Ilg FL: Feeding behavior of infants, Philadelphia, 1937, JB Lippincott Co.

42. Ardran GM, Kemp FH, and Lind J: A cineradiographic study of breast feeding, Br J Radiol 31:156, 1958.

43. Ardran GM, Kemp FH, and Lind J: A cineradiographic study of bottle feeding, Br J Radiol 31:11, 1958.

44. Subtelny JD: Examination of current philosophies associated with swallowing behavior, Am J Orthod 51:161, 1965.

45. Peiper A: Cerebral function in infancy and childhood, New York, 1963, Consultant's Bureau.

46. Gwynne-Evans E: Organization of the oro-facial muscles in relation to breathing and feeding, Br Dent J 91:135, 1952.

47. Ingram TTS: Clinical significance of the infantile feeding reflexes, Dev Med Child Neurol 4:159, 1962.

48. Arnon SS et al: Honey and other environmental risk factors for infant botulism, Pediatrics 94:331, 1979.

49. Thoman EB: Development of synchrony in mother-infant interaction in feeding and other situations, Fed Proc 34:1587, 1975.

50. Butte NF, Smith EO, and Garza C: Energy utilization of breast-fed and formula-fed infants, Am J Clin Nutr 51:350, 1990.

51. Jakobsson I and Lindberg T: Cow's milk as a cause of infantile colic in breast-fed infants, Lancet 2:437, 1978.

52. Jakobsson I and Lindberg T: Cow's milk proteins cause infantile colic in breast-fed infants: a double-blind crossover study, Pediatrics 71:268, 1983.

53. Lothe L, Lindberg T, and Jakobsson I: Cow's milk formula as a cause of infantile colic, Pediatrics 70:7, 1982.

54. Finn SB: Dental caries in infants, Curr Dent Concepts 1:35, 1969.

55. Dubois S, Hill DE, and Benson GN: An examination of factors believed to be associated with obesity, Am J Clin Nutr 32:1997, 1979.

56. Ferris AG et al: The effect of diet on weight gain in infancy, Am J Clin Nutr 33:2635, 1980.

57. Fomon SJ et al: Indices of fatness and serum cholesterol at eight years in relation to feeding and growth during infancy, Pediatr Res 18:1233, 1984.

58. Shapiro LR et al: Obesity prognosis: a longitudinal study of children from the age of 6 months to 9 years, Am J Public Health 74:968, 1984.

Further Reading

Bare RG et al: Feeding and temperament as determinants of early infant crying/fussing behavior, Pediatrics 84:514, 1989.

This study was designed to determine if breast or bottle feeding and early infant temperament were predictors of crying at 6-week frequency or crying was predicted only by socioeconomic status, temperament, and frequency of feeding. Later fussing/crying behavior was not predicted by initial feeding. Infants who had been initially breastfed, then weaned to formula, cried for shorter periods in the evening but longer periods in the morning than breastfed infants.

Agras WS et al: Does a rigorous feeding style influence early development of adiposity? J Pediatr 110:799, 1991.

This study investigated certain factors and feeding behavior that might influence adiposity from birth to 2 years of age. A vigorous sucking style, including rapid eating, was associated with higher calorie intake and greater than average adiposity.

Walter T et al: Iron deficiency anemia: adverse effects on iron psychomotor development, Pediatrics 84:7, 1989.

This study assessed the relationship between iron deficiency and psychomotor development from birth to 15 months of age. Infants who were anemic received lower scores on mental and psychomotor development than iron-deficient infants. Oral iron supplements did not improve test scores after 10 days or 3 months. A hemoglobin concentration less than 10.5 g/dl resulted in lower mental and motor scores, especially in language capabilities and body balance coordination.

Committee on Nutrition, American Academy of Pediatrics: Hypoallergenic infant formulas, Pediatrics 83:1068, 1989.

Much effort has been devoted to the identification of infants who are at risk for allergic immune-mediated reaction to cow's milk and to the identification of appropriate milks for these babies. Neither soy nor goat's milk has been effective in the prevention or treatment of adverse reactions to cow's milk. Casein hydrolysate formula has been used with rare treatment failures. A whey hydrolysate formula recently available might be a successful alternative for infants who are intolerant but not allergic to cow's milk.

Nutrition in Childhood

Peggy Pipes

✔ *A generally slowed and erratic growth rate between infancy and adolescence and a child's individual needs affect nutrient requirements.*

✔ *Numerous family and community factors determine a child's food choices.*

✔ *Food availability and food choices govern nutrient intake and developing food patterns in young children.*

✔ *Meeting the physical and psychosocial needs guide considerations in feeding young children.*

✔ *Nutrition concerns during childhood relate to growth and development needs for positive health.*

*A*fter the infant's first year of rapid growth, the interval between infancy and adolescence is a period of slower growth. This interval is a time for the acquisition of skills that permit independence in eating and feeding and the development of individual food preferences. The development of gross motor skills makes increased activity possible. Preschool children learn to control body functions, to interact with others, and to behave in a socially acceptable manner. School-age children attempt to develop personal independence and establish a scale of values. Individual variations in children become more noticeable in such areas as rates of growth, activity patterns, nutrient requirements, personality development, and food intakes.

There is a wide range of nutrient requirements of children at any age during this period. Body size and composition, activity patterns, and rates of growth influence basic needs. The foods available to and accepted by the child are determined not only by parental food selection but also by the mealtime environment, peer pressures, advertising, and the child's food experiences. If appropriate support is provided by parents, food patterns that support normal growth and weight, ensure good dental hygiene, and prevent iron-deficiency anemia can be established.

PHYSICAL GROWTH DURING CHILDHOOD
Growth Rate

The rapid rate of growth during infancy is followed by a deceleration during the preschool and school-age years. Weight gain approximates 4 to 6 lb (1.8 to 2.7 kg) per year. Length increases approximately 3 inches (7.6 cm) per year between 1 year and 7 to 8 years of age, then increases 2 inches (5.1 cm) per year until the pubertal growth spurt. Between 6 years of age and the adolescent growth spurt, sex differences can be noted. At age 6 boys are taller and heavier than girls. By age 9 the height of the average female is the same as that of the 9-year-old male and her weight is slightly more.

Racial differences have been noted in rates of growth. American black infants are smaller than American white infants at birth. However, they grow more rapidly during the first 2 years of life, and from 2 years of age through adolescence are taller than American white children of the same age. Asian children tend to be smaller than black children and white children.[1]

Body Composition

Muscle mass accounts for an increasingly greater percentage of body weight during the preschool years. Children become leaner as they grow older. Fatfold measurements decrease. Females, however, have more subcutaneous fat than males.

Brain growth is 75% complete by the end of the second year; by 6 to 10 years of age brain growth is complete. This results in a decrease in head size in relation to body size.

Body fluid proportion is similar to that of an adult by the time the child is 2 to 3 years of age. Rapid shifts in fluid between intracellular and extracellular compartments are less likely. The child is less vulnerable to dehydration than the infant. The extracellular fluid continues to decrease while intracellular fluid increases because of the growth of new cells. The approximate percentage of total body fluid is 59% in the toddler compared with 64% in the adult male.

Bone growth results from elongation of the legs. However, bone is not an inert tissue but is constantly being remodeled by destruction and renewal of collagen and the addition and loss of mineral. Increases in skeletal length are achieved by this process of dissolution and reshaping of bone. The school-age child with longer legs appears more graceful and slimmer than the preschooler.

Growth Charts

Normal differences in individual children become apparent in the percentile channel of growth followed by each child. Once the percentile ranking is established on the growth grid, children can be expected to maintain **growth channels** when sequential measurements over time are recorded. However, physicians will not predict later height from growth grids before a child is 2 years of age. It is more important to know that a child is maintaining his height and weight in relation to other children and in the weight-height percentile than it is to know that they are tall or short.

The infant growth charts, as described in Chapter 6 (p. 215), are constructed to 36 months of age and should be used until the child is at least 24 months old. The growth grids for children from 2 to 18 years of age were prepared from data from the National Health and Nutrition Examination Surveys (NHANES).[2] It should be noted that length measurements on the infant grid are recumbent lengths and those on the children's grid are standing height measurements. Children should be weighed in stocking feet and standard examination clothing on a beam balance scale. Standing height is measured using a hard board while the heels, buttocks, and shoulders touch a flat wall (see Chapter 2). It is not unusual for small changes to occur in length percentile ratings on growth grids when changing from recumbent to upright measurement.

Growth channel
The progressive regular growth pattern of children, guided along individual genetically controlled channels, influenced by nutritional and health status.

FIG. 7-1 The growth grid of a female whose weight remained in the 90th percentile over time but who became anorexic at 4½ years. She did not consume enough food to support an appropriate weight gain.

Courtesy Ross Laboratories.

FIG. 7-2 The growth grid of a male who began eating excessive amounts of high calorie food at age 4½ years. His rate of weight gain increased.

Courtesy Ross Laboratories.

Excesses or inadequacies in energy and nutrient intakes will be reflected in patterns of growth. The child who is not eating sufficient food will show a drop on channel of growth grids (Fig. 7-1). If food deprivation is severe enough and lasts long enough, rates of linear growth will be reduced or growth will cease. Intakes of energy in excess of expenditure will be noted by increases in weight percentile (Fig. 7-2).

Feeding Skills

The child's rate of physical growth will also be reflected in the development of self-feeding skills. Children learn to feed themselves independently during the second year of life. The 15-month-old child will have difficulty scooping food into the spoon and bringing food to the mouth without turning the spoon upside down and spilling its contents because of lack of wrist control. By 2 years of age spilling seldom occurs.

By 16 to 17 months of age a well-defined **ulnar deviation** of the wrist occurs and the contents of the spoon may be transferred more steadily to the mouth. By 18 months of age the child lifts the elbow as the spoon is raised and flexes the wrist as the spoon reaches the mouth so that only moderate spilling occurs, in contrast to earlier stages of self-feeding.

Handedness is not established at 1 year of age. Children may grasp the spoon with either hand and find when they try to fill the spoon that the bowl is upside down.

A refined pincer grasp will have been developed in the first year. Finger-feeding is easy and often preferred. Foods that provide opportunities for finger-feeding should be provided at each meal (Table 7-1), avoiding inappropriate ones that may cause choking. Young children, especially preschoolers, are at risk of choking on food. Death from asphyxiation resulting from intakes of small pieces of food has been described in 102 children over a 2 year period. Children less than 2 years of age were most affected. Foods most often responsible include hot dogs, hard candy, nuts, and grapes.[3] Children will often place food in the spoon with their fingers and may finger-feed foods that are commonly spoon-fed, such as vegetables and pudding.

Ulnar deviation
Turning and articulation of the *ulna* (inner and larger bone of the forearm on the side opposite the thumb) with the wrist joint to accomplish coordinated movement of the wrist and hand.

TABLE 7-1   Appropriate Finger Foods for Young Children with a Refined Pincer Grasp

Appropriate Foods (no skins or peeling)	Inappropriate Foods (may cause choking or gagging)
Dry cereal: Cheerios, Kix	
Banana slices	Dried fruits: raisins, coconut, dates
Soft cut-up fruit	Small fruit with skin or peel: grapes
Mealy apple	Raw vegetables
Canned or well-cooked vegetables (green beans, broccoli, carrots)	
Cheese sticks, hard cheese (cheddar, Monterey Jack)	Processed American cheese
Large curd cottage cheese	
Small pieces tender meats (small meatballs, chicken, liver)	Hot dogs
Scrambled eggs	Nuts, including peanuts
Fish sticks (no bones)	Peanut butter
Oven-dried toast	Popcorn
Zwieback toast	Potato chips
Arrowroot biscuits	Corn chips
Graham crackers	Tortilla chips

By 15 months of age children can manage a cup, but will have difficulty in lifting, tilting, and lowering it. The cup is tilted, using the palm, often too rapidly. By 18 to 24 months of age the cup will be tilted by manipulation of the fingers.

Children refine the rotary chewing movements that began at 1 year of age. The ability to chew hard and fibrous foods will increase through the school years.

NUTRIENT NEEDS OF CHILDREN

Recommendations for energy intakes for children have been derived from intakes of normal healthy children growing satisfactorily. Recommendations for nutrient intakes are based on only a few balance studies, mostly extrapolated from requirements for infants and adults. It is important to remember that the range of adequate intakes is quite wide among groups of children. The Recommended Dietary Allowances (RDAs) provide guidelines for studying groups of children but not for evaluating diets of individual children.[4]

Energy

Individual needs. The energy requirements for individual children are determined by resting energy expenditure (REE), rate of growth, and activity. REE varies with the amount and composition of **metabolically active** tissue, which varies with age and sex. However, sex differences are relatively small until children reach 10 years of age and no sex differences have been made in recommended energy intakes before these ages. The average energy cost of growth after infancy is small, about 5 kcal/g of tissue gained. The energy needs of individual children of the same age, sex, and size vary. Reasons for these differences remain unexplained. Differences in physical activity, in the metabolic cost of minimal and excessive protein intakes at equivalent levels of energy intake, and in the efficiency with which individuals utilize energy have all been hypothesized to exert an influence. The RDA standards established by the Food and Nutrition Board of the National Research Council are given in Table 7-2.[4] These allowances reflect the standards of international agencies.

Physical activity. The contribution of physical activity to total energy expenditure is quite variable among children and in individual children from day to day. At all ages activity patterns among children show wide ranges both in the time spent in the various activities and in the intensity of the activities. Some children may engage in sedentary activities such as looking at books or watching television, whereas their peers may be engaged in physical activities that demand running, jumping, and general body movements. Spady estimated the energy expenditure for physical activity of fourth- and fifth-grade school children, for example, to be 31.2% and 25.3% of total energy expenditure for males and females, respectively.[5]

Metabolic activity
Sum of biochemical actions and reactions in the body that build and maintain tissue, regulate body functions, and require a constant energy source. The most metabolically active body tissue is the lean body mass.

TABLE 7-2   *Recommended Energy Intakes for Children*

Age (years)	Weight (kg)	Height (cm)	Energy Allowances/Day (kcal)	Energy Allowances/kg/Day (kcal)
1-3	13	90	1300	102
4-6	20	112	1800	90
7-10	28	132	2000	70

Reprinted with permission from Recommended dietary allowances, ed 10. ©1989 by the National Academy of Sciences. Published by National Academy Press, Washington, DC.

Studies indicate that the actual energy intakes of children agree with the recommended intakes.[6] However, wide-ranging intakes will be noted among individual children. The most appropriate evaluation of adequacy of a child's energy intake is based on observation of rates of growth as depicted on growth grids and on measurements of body fat.

Catch-up growth. During a period of catch-up growth, the requirements for energy and nutrients will be greatly increased. Daily intakes of 150 to 250 kcal/kg of body weight have been recommended for children of preschool age. An intake of 200 kcal/kg/day should produce a weight gain of 20 g/day.[7]

Protein

Basis of need. The protein needs of children include those for maintenance of tissue, changes in body composition, and synthesis of new tissue. During growth, the protein content of the body increases from 14.6% at 1 year of age to 18% to 19%, which are adult values, by 4 years of age. Estimates of protein needs for growth range from 1 to 4 g/kg of tissue gained. As the rate of growth falls, maintenance requirements gradually represent an increasing proportion of the total protein requirement.

Recommended intakes. The recommended protein intake, calculated on the maintenance requirements of the adult, growth rates, and body composition, gradually decreases from 1.3 g/kg at 1 year of age to 1.0 g/kg at 10 years of age (Table 7-3).[4] This intake approximates 4% to 5% of the total kilocalories, less than most children consume. Protein provided 13% to 15% of the energy intake in the average child's diet.

An evaluation of a child's protein intake must be based on the adequacy of growth rate, the quality of protein in the foods eaten, combinations of foods that provide **complementary amino acids** when consumed together, and the adequacy of those nutrients, vitamins and minerals, and energy that are necessary for protein synthesis to proceed.

Inadequate protein intakes are rarely noted in North America. Some children have such limited energy intakes that part of the protein consumed must be used for body fuel. Children who consume a **vegan diet** have been reported to be shorter and leaner than the average child.

Minerals and Vitamins

Minerals and vitamins are necessary for normal growth and development. Inadequate intakes will be reflected in slow growth rates, inadequate mineralization of bones, insufficient iron stores, and anemia. The RDAs are shown in Tables 7-4 and 7-5.

Calcium. Attempts to establish recommended intakes of calcium have caused considerable controversy for many years. Populations that have adapted to intakes of 200 to 400 mg/day without effects have been identified. Absorption of calcium fluctuates from 30% to 60% of intake. Lactose increases absorption. Binders such as **phytic acid** and **oxalic acid** reduce absorption. The level of dietary protein affects the urinary excretion of calcium. As levels of protein intake increase, levels of urinary calcium increase.

Osteomalacia, which improved rapidly with calcium supplements, was identified in three South African black children (4-year-old female, 6-year-old male, and 13-year-old male).[8] Recommendations for children are set at 800 mg/day since growing children may need two to four times as much calcium per unit of body weight as adults require.

Milk and other dairy products are the primary sources of calcium. Thus, children who consume limited amounts of these products risk a deficient calcium intake.

Zinc. The trace mineral zinc is essential for normal protein synthesis and growth. Variations in plasma zinc concentrations during growth reflect the continual use and depletion of body stores of zinc. The steepest decline occurs at 10 to 11 years of age in the female and at 12 to 13 years of age in the male, when growth is most rapid.[9] Zinc intakes of children 1 to 3 years of age have been estimated to average 5 mg/day; those of children 3 to 5 years of age average 5 to 7 mg/day.[10]

Complementary amino acids
Combinations of amino acids from a variety of combined protein foods that complement one another according to their relative amounts of the individual amino acids, in order to meet growth requirements for the nine essential amino acids that the body does not sufficiently synthesize.

Vegan diet
Strict vegetarian diet that does not allow any animal protein; requires careful food combinations of incomplete plant proteins to complement one another and achieve an overall adequacy of essential amino acids for growth needs.

Phytic acid
A compound in certain grains, such as wheat, that binds calcium and hinders its absorption.

Oxalic acid
A compound in a variety of foods, including green leafy vegetables, corn, soy products such as tofu, and wheat germ, that binds calcium in the food mix and hinders its absorption.

Many preschool and school age children from low- and middle-income families may not be ingesting adequate amounts of zinc. Supplements of zinc sulfate that provided 0.2 mg of zinc per kilogram of body weight given to five school children with **hypogeusia** and low hair zinc levels resulted in normalization of taste perception and substantial increases in hair zinc content.[11]

There is speculation that poor linear growth in early childhood in some low-income populations may result from a growth-limiting zinc deficiency state. A study of Hispanic American children 2 to 6 years of age who consumed 5 to 6 mg of zinc per day and

Hypogeusia
(Gr *hypo-*, under; *geusis*, taste; *aisthesis*, perception) An abnormally diminished acuteness of the sense of taste.

TABLE 7-3   *Recommended Dietary Allowances of Protein*

Age (years)	Protein (g/kg)	Protein (g/day)
1-3	1.2	16
4-6	1.1	24
7-10	1.0	28

Reprinted with permission from Recommended dietary allowances, ed 10. ©1989 by the National Academy of Sciences. Published by National Academy Press, Washington, DC.

TABLE 7-4   *Recommended Daily Dietary Allowances for Minerals*

Age (years)	Calcium (mg)	Phosphorus (mg)	Iodine (μg)	Iron (mg)	Magnesium (mg)	Zinc (mg)	Selenium (μg)
1-3	800	800	70	10	80	10	20
4-6	800	800	90	10	120	10	20
7-10	800	800	120	10	170	10	30

TABLE 7-5   *Recommended Dietary Allowances of Vitamins*

Vitamin	Age (years)		
	1-3	4-6	7-10
Fat-Soluble			
Vitamin A (μg RE)	400	500	700
Vitamin D (μg)	10	10	10
Vitamin E (mg α-TE)	6	7	7
Vitamin K (μg)	15	20	30
Water-Soluble			
Thiamin (mg)	0.7	0.9	1.0
Riboflavin (mg)	0.8	1.1	1.2
Niacin (mg)	9	12	13
Vitamin B_6 (mg)	1.0	1.1	1.4
Folate (μg)	50	75	100
Vitamin B_{12} (μg)	0.7	1.0	1.4
Ascorbic acid (mg)	40	45	45

Reprinted with permission from Recommended dietary allowances, ed 10. ©1989 by the National Academy of Sciences. Published by National Academy Press, Washington, DC.

whose linear growth was below the 10th percentile found low hair and plasma zinc levels. Increasing their zinc intake to 10 mg/day increased rates of linear growth.[12]

Small amounts of zinc are more efficiently absorbed than large amounts. Children in poor zinc status absorb zinc more efficiently than those in good status. High intakes of phytate and fiber depress zinc absorption. The bioavailability of zinc varies with the food source. Meats are a good source of available zinc; cereal grains contain a less available form of zinc. The average toddler in the United States consumes 8.5 mg zinc per day.

Iron. Iron deficiency is the most common nutritional deficiency in North America. It occurs most frequently in children 4 to 24 months of age, in adolescent males, and in females in their childbearing years. It may result from inadequate iron intake, impaired absorption, a large hemorrhage, or repeated small blood losses.

The RDA standards of the National Research Council assume 10% iron absorption and are planned to meet variations of need in individuals.[4] Iron requirements of individual children vary with rates of growth and increasing total iron mass, iron stores, variations in menstrual losses of iron in adolescent females, and the timing of the growth spurt of adolescents. Larger, more rapidly growing children have the greatest requirements for iron because they are increasing their blood volumes more rapidly.

Nonheme iron
The larger portion of dietary iron, including all of the plant food sources and 60% of the animal food sources, that lacks the more easily absorbed and bioavailable heme iron in the remaining 40% of the animal food sources that contain hemoglobin residues of iron-containing heme.

Prevention of anemia. Many younger preschoolers do not have the oral motor strength to masticate meat and prefer **nonheme** plant sources of iron. The consumption of foods or a supplement containing vitamin C along with the foods containing nonheme iron can help increase the amount of the iron absorbed. Absorption can also be increased by consuming meat when nonheme iron is ingested. Iron absorption is decreased by antacids, bran, and tea. Also, directing parents to use more foods containing heme iron that are easier to chew, such as ground beef, can increase iron intake. For children whose iron intake is limited, a supplemental maintenance dose of iron (10 mg/day) may be indicated. Children with diagnosed iron-deficiency anemia will receive therapeutic doses of iron, 3 mg/kg/day, for 3 months.

Vitamins. The function of vitamins in metabolic processes means that their requirements are determined by intakes of energy, protein, and saturated fats. Exact needs are difficult to define. The RDA standard for most vitamins and for some trace minerals (Table 7-6)

TABLE 7-6A   Estimated Safe and Adequate Daily Dietary Intakes of Selected Trace Minerals for Children

Age (years)	Copper (mg)	Manganese (mg)	Fluoride (mg)	Chromium (µg)	Molybdenum (µg)
1-3	0.7-1.0	1.0-1.5	0.5-1.5	20-80	25-50
4-6	1.0-1.5	1.5-2.0	1.0-2.5	30-120	30-75
7-10	1.0-2.0	2.0-3.0	1.5-2.5	50-200	50-150
11+	1.5-2.5	2.0-5.0	1.5-2.5	50-200	75-250

TABLE 7-6B   Estimated Minimum Requirements of Electrolytes

Age (years)	Sodium (mg)	Potassium (mg)	Chloride (mg)
2-5	300	1400	500
6-9	400	1600	600
10-18	500	2000	750

Reprinted with permission from Recommended dietary allowances, ed 10. ©1989 by the National Academy of Sciences. Published by National Academy Press, Washington, DC.

is interpolated from infant and adult allowances or calculated on the basis of energy and protein allowances.

Vitamin Supplementation

Dietary evaluation. Vitamin supplementation of diets of children should be recommended only after careful evaluation of the child's food intake. Diets of children who restrict their intake of milk because of real or imagined allergies, lactose intolerance, or for psychosocial reasons should be monitored for riboflavin and vitamin D. Diets of infants and children receiving goat's milk should be carefully monitored for food sources of folate. Diets of children who consume limited amounts of fruits and vegetables should be checked for sources of vitamins A and C.

Children at risk. The Committee on Nutrition of the American Academy of Pediatrics has defined four groups of children at particular risk and for whom vitamin supplementation may be appropriate.[13]

1. Children from deprived families, especially those who suffer from parental neglect or abuse
2. Children who have anorexia, poor and capricious appetites, poor eating habits, and who are on regimens to manage obesity
3. Pregnant teenagers
4. Children who consume vegan diets

Any vitamin supplements, especially those that are colored and sugar coated, should be stored in places inaccessible to young children.

The importance of appropriate vitamin supplementation of breastfed infants is discussed in Chapter 6. After infancy, however, the percentage of toddlers who are given vitamin supplements declines. But over half of the preschool and school-age children receive multivitamin-mineral preparations.

Cook and Payne found that use of vitamin supplements significantly increased the percentage of second-grade and sixth-grade children who meet 67% of the RDA compared with nonsupplemented children.[14] Thus they consider vitamin supplementation advisable. However, Breskin noted no significant differences in biochemical indices with the exception of red blood cell folate of children who used supplements compared with those who did not, even though mean intakes of vitamin B_6 of the nonsupplemented group were 30% below the RDA.[15] Many of the nonsupplemented children did not ingest two thirds of the RDA for folate. All blood values were in the range of accepted standards.

FACTORS THAT INFLUENCE FOOD CHOICES

The adequacy of children's food intake depends not only on the foods available to them but also on a number of cultural, environmental, interactional, and societal factors. Most investigators who have studied food choices have focused on preschoolers because groups of children can be found in preschools and day-care settings. Also, it is at this stage of development that parents often become confused about the children's food selections and concerned that their children are not eating the kinds and amounts of foods they should. Food acceptance and factors that influence it assume increasing attention.

Food Acceptance

Acceptance of food is affected by a number of factors that include nutritional status, degree of satiation, taste, previous experiences and beliefs about specific foods. Infants have a preference for sweetened water, a preference that can be extinguished by offering only beverages that are not sweetened.[16] Young infants seem to have an aversion to bitter tastes and an indifference to salty tastes. Tastes for salt change from neutral to preferred at 4 months of age when the salt taste is combined with other tastes in food. Preschoolers reject salty beverages but prefer a higher level of salt in soup than do adults.[17]

Parental Influences

Nutrition knowledge. The nutrition knowledge of parents and other caregivers appears to be an important factor in children's food choices. The degree to which knowledge of nutrition is incorporated into family meal planning seems to be related to positive attitudes toward self, problem-solving skills, and family organization. This relationship held in spite of a professed concern all mothers interviewed about the total diet offered to young children and the importance of mealtime with children.[18] The ordinal position of the preschool child in the family appears to influence choices of specific foods regardless of equivalent knowledge of nutrition between groups of mothers.[19] When a preschool child is the youngest child in the family, the mothers appear to be less susceptible to the child's requests for new products. Mothers are willing, however, to accommodate that preference when the preschooler is the oldest child in the family.

Models. The models set for children by their families and other persons close to them exert a strong influence on their developing food patterns. Parental food preferences exert a definite influence. Food habits of siblings exert an influence equal to that of parents. Parents report that they know little about nutrition but think it is important.

Parent-child interactions. Children's interactions with their parents influence their acceptance of foods and the food patterns they develop. If parents accept casually the food jags and transient food dislikes preschoolers develop, these passing food behaviors are soon forgotten. However, parents who find these behaviors difficult to accept and give much attention to them by trying to bribe or encourage the child to eat, discussing the children's dislikes in front of them, or providing a preferred food when they refuse to eat may pattern that behavior into a permanent food habit. A study in Nebraska found that a child's social-emotional environment was directly related to the adequacy of the child's dietary intake. Companionship at mealtime, a positive home atmosphere, and appropriate food-related parenting behaviors were strongly associated with improved quality of diet.[20]

The parent-child interaction also has an important influence on the amount of food consumed. There appear to be differences between the interactions of thinner children and their mothers and fatter children and their mothers both in food and nonfood situations. Thinner children and their mothers talk more with each other and eat less food more slowly than fatter children and their mothers.[21] Preferences for foods are enhanced when foods are offered as a reward or with a brief positive social interaction with adults.[22]

Contingencies. It is also a common practice for parents to use rewards such as "Clean your plate and you can have dessert" to achieve a child's acceptance of foods. While this practice often achieves its immediate goal, the long-term effects are often negative. Children understand that external pressure is usually applied to get them to eat a less-preferred food. When the contingency is removed they eat less of the food.[23] The ability of the child to recognize hunger and satiation has also been studied by Birch.[24] Of all the children in the study, 95% ate less lunch after a high-caloric density preload than a low-caloric density preload. Only 60% of the adults followed the same pattern.

Quantities of food consumed. If normal well-nourished children are offered a variety of nutritionally appropriate foods and permitted to eat just those foods they select in the amounts they wish, they will consume an appropriate energy intake. Studies conducted in the 1920s and early 1930s on 6-month-old to 4-year-old foundlings in a Chicago hospital presented the children with 10 unprocessed foods at each meal. The children were permitted to self-select the foods and amounts they ate at any meal. A more recent study by Birch with 15 children in a day-care center used the same menu for 2 days each week for 3 weeks in the day-care center and at home. Foods included in the menu would provide appropriate nutrient intake. In both studies there was considerable variability in the quantity of food each child consumed from one day to the next. However, the children self-selected an appropriate energy intake when the study days were averaged.[25] It is important to note that both researchers utilized a laboratory setting and controlled for a variety of parent-child interaction issues that influence food acceptance. These studies do, however, provide a model of an optimal method of achieving the acceptance of a nutritionally appropriate diet by children.

Influence of Television on Children

Food attitudes and requests. In addition to the many familial, cultural, and psychosocial influences on children's food habits, mass media have an impact on children's attitudes toward food and their requests for particular products. Of all the forms of mass media, television has the greatest impact on children because it reaches many children before they are capable of verbal communication and because it engages much of their time. Children spend more time in front of a television set than they do in any other activity except for sleeping. Children from low-income families watch more television than do children from moderate- to high-income families. It has been estimated that children watch television 22 to 25 hours per week. At this rate, by age 70, 7 years of their life will have been spent watching television.[26]

Lifestyle. Extensive television viewing can be detrimental to growth and development by encouraging sedentary and passive activities, thus promoting a lifestyle that may lead to obesity. An association between obesity and time spent watching television has been documented in 6- to 11-year-old children and in adolescents.[27] The unhealthy depiction of body types and eating behavior on television may also contribute to anorexia. Television viewing by children is also correlated with between-meal snacking. Advertisers attempt to use children to influence their parents' purchasing behavior. They present frequent cues for food and drink and often encourage consumption of a wide variety of sugared products. Television programs, as well as advertising, present models of behavior children may imitate. One study of prime-time television noted 5.31 food-related behaviors of characters per program. The behaviors that involved more nutritious food were almost equal in number to those that involved nonnutritious food.[28]

Television advertising. It is estimated that the average child watches 3 hours of television advertising per week, or 19,000 to 22,000 commercials per year. Kindergarten children often are unable to separate commercials from the program and frequently explain them as part of the program. Younger school-age children 5 to 10 years of age watch commercials more closely than do older children 11 to 12 years of age.[29] Older children are more conscious of the concept of commercials, the purpose of selling, and the concept of sponsorship and are less likely to accept advertisers' claims without question. They perceive that television commercials are designed to sell products rather than entertain or educate. Children in the second grade have been found to have a concrete distrust of commercials based on experience with advertised products. Children in the sixth grade have been found to have global mistrust of all commercials.[30]

Food manufacturers and fast-food establishments use the greatest percentage of advertising time on television. A classic study of children's programs on Saturday and Sunday in Boston revealed that 68.5% of the advertisements were for food.[31] Of these advertisements, 25% were for cereal, 25% were for candy and sweets, and 8% were for snacks and other food. Quick meals and eating places were the subject of 10% of the advertisements. Only a few commercials were broadcast for milk, bread, or fruit. Advertisements for sugared cereals outnumbered those for unsugared cereals by a ratio of 3 to 1.

Certain attributes of food are promoted by television advertising as being superior to others. The main characteristics presented positively are "sweetness," "chocolatey," and "richness."[32] Many food manufacturers, in other words, deemphasize the physiologic need for nutrients and encourage selection on the basis of sweet flavor. Exposure to such messages may distort a child's natural curiosity toward other characteristics of food such as the fresh crispness of apples or celery.

There has been ongoing concern about the influence of television on the growth and health of young children. It has been demonstrated that television influences the eating habits and thus the nutritional status of children in three significant ways: (1) television advertising influences family food purchases and the snacking patterns of young children, (2) the use of food as depicted by television programs shows food being used for many activities other than the satiation of hunger, and (3) the few overweight children used on television programs suggests that inappropriate use of foods has no impact on health or nutritional status. In addition, Dietz and Gortmaker outline other aspects of television watching that are of concern: (1) the relationship between increased television watching and snacking, (2) the increased consumption of foods advertised on television as watching time increases, (3) the direct association of increased viewing time with the number of attempts of the young child to influence the supermarket purchases of the parent. The foods advertised on weekend children's programs are usually ones of high-caloric density, that if purchased and consumed without an increase in activity can lead to inappropriate weight gain and poor food habits. The larger intake of highly concentrated sweets and fat foods plus the decrease in activity that is associated with excess television watching has led to an increase of obesity among children in the United States.[27]

Parental response. Children are influenced by television commercials and attempt to influence their parents' buying practices. Commercials for food have the strongest influence and mothers are more likely to yield to requests for food than for other products. Parents have a greater tendency to respond to requests from older children, but certainly do not ignore those of younger children.[33] Highly child-centered mothers are less likely to buy children's favorite cereals than are mothers who are not as child-centered. Crawford, Hankin, and Huenemann reported that two thirds of the mothers interviewed stated that food choices were influenced by television commercials by the time the child was 4 years of age.[34]

PRESCHOOL CHILDREN

Although clinical signs of malnutrition are rarely found in preschool children in North America and many low-income families are showing good management of scarce economic resources for food, there is evidence that some children are receiving diets that are limited in some nutrients and in some cases energy. A survey of preschool children's diet quality in Nebraska found that the overall quality of the diets was adequate. However, 25% of the children had low intakes of iron and vitamin C. A Canadian study found energy intakes sufficient to support growth, but intakes of all nutrients except iron were considered inadequate.[35] A study of low-income Mexican American preschoolers in Colorado also found that the children consumed an adequate nutrient intake.[36]

Both longitudinal and cross-sectional studies of nutrient and energy intakes of children have shown large differences in intakes between individual children of the same age and sex. Some children consume two to three times as much energy as others.[37] After a rapid rise in intake of all nutrients during the first nine months of life, reductions can be expected in the intakes of some of the nutrients as increases occur in intakes of others. Several researchers have noted sex differences in intakes of energy and nutrients. In all studies males consumed greater quantities of food, thus greater amounts of nutrients and energy.

The Preschool Years

During the preschool years there is a decrease in intake of calcium, phosphorus, riboflavin, iron, and vitamin A because of discontinued use of iron-fortified infant cereals in the diets of children, a reduction in milk intakes, and a disinterest in vegetables. During this period children increase their intake of carbohydrate and fat. Protein intakes may plateau or increase only slightly.[37] Between 3 and 8 years of age there is a slow, steady, and relatively consistent increase in intake of all nutrients. Since intakes of vitamins A and C are unrelated to energy intakes, greater ranges of intakes of these nutrients have been noted. Black preschoolers in California have been reported to have higher intakes of sodium than do whites because of their frequent intake of undiluted commercially prepared soups. Between ages 2 and 4, they were also found to have greater energy intakes than whites.[34]

Normal Food Behaviors of Preschool Children

Food jags and rituals. Few children pass through the preschool years without creating concern about their food intake.[38] Between 9 and 18 months of age children display a disinterest in food that lasts from a few months to a few years. Food jags are common. Likes and dislikes may change from day to day and week to week. For example, a child may demand only boiled eggs for snacks for a week and completely reject them for the next 6 months. Rituals become a part of food preparation and service. Some children, for example, accept sandwiches only when they are cut in half, and when parents quarter the sandwich the children may throw tantrums. Others demand that food have a particular arrangement on the plate or that dishes be placed only in certain locations on the table.

Appetites. During this period appetites are usually erratic and unpredictable. The child may eat hungrily at one meal and completely refuse the next. The evening meal is generally the least well received and is one of the most concern to the majority of parents. It is possible that children who have consumed two meals and several snacks have already met their needs for energy and nutrients before dinner time.

Food preferences. Parents report that preschool children enjoy meat, cereal grains, baked products, fruit, and sweets. They frequently ask for dairy products, cereal, and snack items such as cookies, crackers, fruit juice, and dry beverage mixes.[39] Food preferences during the preschool years seem to be for the carbohydrate-rich foods that are easiest to masticate. Cereals, breads, and crackers are selected often in preference to meat and other protein-rich foods. The use of dry **fortified cereals** as a primary source of many nutrients is increasing.[34] Yogurt and cheese appear to be increasing in popularity among young children.

Fortified cereal
Cereal food products enriched by addition of minerals such as iron and zinc, and vitamins such as thiamin, riboflavin, niacin, folate, B_6, and B_{12}.

Frequency of Eating

Huenemann has pointed out that we are raising a generation of nibblers.[40] Nearly 60% of children 3 to 5 years of age eat more than 3 times a day. They consume food on an average of 5 to 7 times a day, although ranges of 3 to 14 times a day have been noted. Crawford, Hankin, and Huenemann found that by 6 years of age 50% of children ate 5 times a day.[34] Eppright and others noted that the frequency of food intakes was unrelated to nutrient intakes except when children consumed food less than four or more than six times a day.[41] Children in this study who consumed food less than 4 times a day consumed fewer kilocalories and less calcium, protein, ascorbic acid, and iron than the average intakes of other children their age. Those who consumed food more than 6 times a day consumed more energy, calcium, and ascorbic acid than average intakes of children their age. Farris and others found that snacks contributed 33% of the daily energy, 20% of the protein, 33% of the fat, and 40% of the carbohydrate consumed each day by 10-year-old children.[42]

The Preschool Child

In spite of the reduction of appetite and erratic consumption of food, preschool children do enjoy well-prepared and attractively served food. If simply prepared foods are presented in a relaxed setting, children will consume an appropriate nutrient intake. Meals and snacks should be timed to foster appetite. Intervals necessary between meals and snacks may vary from one child to another. Rarely can the clock be depended on to know appropriate intervals and times when it may be important for a child to eat. However, indiscriminate snacking dulls the appetite and such patterns should be discouraged.

Foods for young children. Children accept simple unmixed dishes more willingly than casseroles, and prefer most of their food at room temperature, neither hot nor cold. Food preparation is important. Children recognize poorly prepared food and are likely to refuse it. Most children eat most easily those foods with which they are familiar. Small portions of new foods can be introduced with familiar and popular foods. Even if the child only looks at the new food or just feels or smells it at first, this is a part of learning about it and accepting it.

Dry foods are especially hard for preschool children to eat. In planning a menu always balance a dry food with one or two moist foods. For example, it is wise to put a slice of meat loaf, relatively dry, with mashed potatoes and peas in a little cream sauce. Also, combinations of sharp, rather acid-flavored foods with mild-flavored foods are popular with young children, and they are pleased to find colorful foods such as red tomatoes, green peppers, and carrot sticks included in their meals.

Ease of manipulation. Foods eaten easily with the unskilled and seemingly clumsy hands of a young child are very important. Many small pieces of foods such as cooked peas or beans are difficult for a child to spoon up. Foods can be prepared so that a child can eat them with the fingers. Hard-cooked eggs may be served in quarters, cooked meat can be cut in small strips, and cooked green beans can be served as finger foods. Children like oranges that have been cut in wedges, skin and all, much better than peeled and diced oranges. Mixed-up salads, when there are layers of food to be eaten, are much more difficult to eat than simple pieces of raw vegetables with no salad dressing. Cottage cheese or similar foods should be served separate from the lettuce leaf on the child's plate. Creamed foods served on tough toast are difficult for children to manage.

Relatively small pieces of food that can be handled with the child's eating tools are best for preschool children. The problem of handling silverware and conveying food to the mouth at this early age is a greater task than many adults realize. Pieces of carrots that slide across the plate and are too small to remain on the fork are frustrating. On the other hand, cubes of beets so large that they must be cut into smaller pieces before they can be eaten exhaust the patience of a 2- or 3-year-old child. Most foods for these children should be served in bite-size pieces. When the child is 4 years of age and older, the skills to cut up some foods may have been developed. If, however, difficulty in managing food is noticed, small pieces should be served, with occasional encouragement to cut up some easier to manage foods. Canned pears and other soft fruits, for example, are usually easy to cut into bite-size pieces.

In general, the aim is to support the young child's early efforts at self-feeding and many creative adaptations can be helpful. Stringy spinach or tomatoes, for example, are a trial for anyone to eat. Much can be done with food shears in the kitchen to make these foods easier to eat. Finger foods such as pieces of lettuce or toast can be used in meals where some of the foods are difficult to handle. Small sandwiches, that is, a large one cut into four small squares, are popular with young children.

Food characteristics. Three general food characteristics affecting taste, acceptance, and self-feeding skills development are important considerations in early feeding of young children. These aspects are texture, flavor, and portion sizes.

Texture. It is wise to serve one soft food for easy chewing, one crisp food for easy chewing and enjoyment of the sounds in the mouth, and one chewy food for emerging chewing skills without having too much to chew in each meal for young children. Pieces of meat seem to be hard for a young child to eat, which explains why children often prefer hamburgers to frankfurters. Most children's meat can be served as ground meat. Ground meat should be cooked only long enough for the color to change to brown, and not be allowed to become dry and crusted, which makes it hard for a child to eat. Some children may prefer moderately rare meat, which is even more moist, but care must be taken that it is cooked sufficiently to be safe.

Flavor. In general, young children reject strong flavors. Many children, however, do seem to like pickles and some spicy sauces, which may seem to contradict this. In general, it has been found that children like food only mildly salted. Pepper and other sharp spices and acids such as vinegar should also be used sparingly on children's food.

Portion sizes. Children are easily discouraged by large portions of food. Offer less than the child usually eats and permit seconds, rather than discourage him with portions that are too large. Appropriate portion sizes are shown in Table 7-7.

Parental concerns. Occasionally anxious or concerned parents need help with food sources of nutrients usually supplied by food refused or in establishing limits to the preschooler's food intakes and feeding behavior. Of the commonly expressed concerns, limited intakes of milk, refusal of meat and vegetables, eating too many sweets, and limited intakes of food appear to cause the most problems.

Milk. It is important to recognize that 1 oz of milk supplies 36 mg of calcium, and many children receive 6 to 8 oz of milk on dry cereal daily. Although they consume only 1 to 2 oz at a time, their calcium intakes may be acceptable when they consume milk with meals and snacks. When abundant amounts of fruit juice or sweetened beverages are available, children may simply prefer to drink them instead of milk. Other dairy products can be offered when milk is rejected. Cheese and yogurt are usually accepted. Powdered milk can be used in recipes for soups, vegetables, and mixed dishes.

Meat. Parents' perceptions of children's dislike of meat may need to be clarified, or an easier to chew form used. If in fact preschoolers do consistently refuse all food sources of heme iron, their daily intake of iron should be carefully monitored.

Vegetables. When vegetables are consistently refused, wars between parents and children should not be permitted to erupt. Small portions of 1 or 2 teaspoons should continue to be served without comment and should be discarded if the child does not eat them. Preschool behavior modification programs that included token rewards when children consumed vegetables served at mealtime have been found to increase children's acceptance and intake of them.[37]

Sweets. Parents concerned about children's excessive intakes of sweets may need help in setting limits on amounts of sweet foods they make available to their children. It may be important also to help them convey their concern and the need to set limits on the availability of these foods to other family members, day care operators, and teachers (see box below).

Food intake. If children's food intakes are so limited that their intakes of energy and nutrients are compromised, parents may need help in establishing guidelines so that the children develop appetites. They should provide food often enough so that children do not get so hungry that they lose their appetite, yet not so often that they are always satiated. Intervals of 3 to 4 hours are often successful. Very small portions of foods should be offered, and second portions permitted when they consume the foods already served. Attention should always be focused on children when they eat, never when food is refused.

CASE STUDY

A Preschooler's View of Milk and Vegetables

During a well-child clinic visit the mother of a 3-year-old boy expresses concern about his nutrient intake. She tells the clinical nutritionist, "He doesn't like to drink milk and refuses vegetables."

Questions for analysis
1. How does his food behavior compare with that of other preschool children?
2. What nutrients should be assessed in the food that he does eat?
3. What nonfood parameters should be evaluated?

TABLE 7-7 A Feeding Guide for Children

This is a guide to a basic diet. Fats, desserts, and sauces will contribute additional kilocalories to meet the needs of the growing child.

Food	1 year old		2-3 years old		4-6 years old		7 years to Puberty		Comments
	Portion Sizes	No. of Servings	Portion Sizes	No. of Servings	Portion Sizes	No. of Servings	Portion Sizes	No. of Servings	
Milk	½ cup	4-5	¼-¾ cup	4-5	½-¾ cup	3-4	1 cup	3	The following may be substituted for one-half cup of liquid milk: ½-¾ oz cheese; ¼-½ cup yogurt; 2½ tbsp non-fat dry milk powder
Meat and meat equivalents	¼-1 oz, 2-4 tbsp	1	1-2 oz	2	1-2 oz	2	2-3 oz	3	The following may be substituted for one ounce of meat, fish, poultry: 4-5 tbsp cooked legumes; 1 egg; 2 tbsp peanut butter
Fruit and vegetables Vegetables		4-5		4-5		4-5		4-5	Include one green leafy or yellow vegetable, e.g., spinach, broccoli, carrots, winter squash
Cooked	1-2 tbsp		2-3 tbsp		3-4 tbsp		½ cup		
Raw	1-2 tbsp		few pieces		few pieces		½ cup		
Fruit Canned	2-4 tbsp		2-4 tbsp		4-6 tbsp		½ cup		Include one vitamin C–rich fruit or juice per day
Raw	2-4 tbsp (chopped)		½-1 small		½-1 small				
Juice	2-4 oz		3-4 oz		4 oz		4 oz		
Grains and grain products	½ slice	3	¼-1 slice	3	1 slice	4	1 slice	6	The following may be substituted for one slice of bread: ½ cup cooked cereal; ½ cup spaghetti or other pasta; ½ cup rice; 5 saltines. Whole grain products provide additional bulk to the diet

Adapted from Lowenberg ME: The development of food patterns in young children. In Pipes P: Nutrition in infancy and childhood, ed 3, St Louis, 1985, Times Mirror/Mosby College Publishing.

Group Feeding

Increasing numbers of mothers of young children are working outside the home. Many children of these women receive care and meals in family day care homes or child care programs. Children whose mothers work fulltime are often in a child care facility for 9 to 10 hours 5 days a week and receive both meals and snacks in this setting.[43] Kindergartens and preschools also offer snacks and meals along with food experiences that are often included as part of the learning activities.

Family day care homes and day care centers are licensed by state agencies that mandate the meal pattern and types of snacks to be provided for the children, as well as the percentage of the recommended daily allowances that must be included in the menus. In general, a child in day care for 8 hours should receive at least one third the RDA from food and snacks, a child in day care for more than 8 hours should receive one half to two thirds the RDA. Assistance is available to nonprofit, licensed day care programs from the U.S. Department of Agriculture. This assistance includes reimbursement for meals in addition to donated foods.

Breakfast should be provided for children who receive none at home. Snacks should be planned to complement the daily food intakes. Small portions of food should be served, and children should be permitted second servings of those foods they enjoy. Disliked or unfamiliar foods may be offered by the teaspoonful, and the child's acceptance or rejection received without comment. Children who eat slowly will need to be served first and permitted to complete the meals without being rushed to other activities. Teachers and caretakers should eat with the children without imposing their attitudes about food.

A new setting provides an opportunity for children to have exposure to many new foods. Day care centers, kindergartens, and preschools can provide an important educational setting for both children and their parents. Children learn to prepare food, how food grows, how it smells, and what nutrients it contains. Parents learn through participation, observation, and conversation with the staff. An organized approach to feeding children must include parents, teachers, and other staff who offer food to children. Teachers and day care workers can provide important information to parents about how children successfully consume food, the nutrients children need, and the foods that provide these nutrients. Parents offer important information to the centers about their children's food acceptance and needs. Each needs to be reinforced positively by the other for their efforts to provide food for the children to be successful.

A study of 48 day care and Head Start programs found that all participating children consumed appropriate intakes of nutrients. Total daily energy intakes were similar for all children regardless of whether one meal and one snack or two meals and two snacks were provided. In fact, when children consumed one meal and one snack, 82% of their energy intake was provided, but when two meals and two snacks were provided, 84% of the energy intake was consumed in this setting.[44]

SCHOOL-AGE CHILDREN

Studies of the school-age population have found that most children are adequately nourished. One will, however, find groups in which an inadequate food and nutrient intake is of concern. Biochemical evidence of vitamin B_6 deficiency has been reported in 9% of children studied in Virginia.[45] There have been several reports of failure-to-thrive and delayed onset of puberty because of very zealous parents' efforts to prevent obesity and cardiovascular disease caused them to allow their children only inadequate energy intake, insufficient for normal growth.[46,47] It is clear that the children who eat regular meals in preference to only snacking do better nutritionally. Studies have also revealed that currently the fat in children's diets is the same as in the diets of adults, lower in fat than they were several years ago.[48]

School entrance provides an opportunity to identify children whose growth parameters may indicate nutrition concerns, such as growth failure, obesity, underweight. Feeding programs such as the school lunch and breakfast programs contribute significantly to children's nutrient intake.

Patterns of Nutrient Intake

By school age most children have established a particular pattern of nutrient intake relative to their peers. Although wide ranges of food intake, and thus of energy and nutrients, continue to be observed, those who consume the greatest amount of food consistently do so, whereas those consuming smaller amounts maintain these lesser intakes relative to their peers. Differences in intake between males and females gradually increase to age 12 and then become marked. Boys consume greater quantities of food, thus energy and nutrients, than girls.[37]

Physical and Social Development

The school-age period is one of few apparent feeding problems. A natural increase in appetite creates normal increases in food intake. Because children spend their days at school, they adjust to a more ordered routine. As they explore the environment of school and peers, children will be influenced by these experiences (Fig. 7-3). Often the credibility of parents is questioned, in the face of advice from teachers, peers, or peers' parents. The school-age child has more access to money, to grocery stores and vending machines, and therefore to foods with questionable nutrient value. Many school-age children have some responsibility for preparing their own breakfasts or sack lunches and arrive home from school looking for a snack.

Food Patterns

Although school-age children usually increase the amount they eat and the varieties of food they accept, many continue to reject vegetables, mixed dishes, and liver. The range of food they voluntarily accept may be small. Sugar contributes 24% to 25% of the total kilocalories in the diets of many school-age children. Milk is the primary contributor. Sweetened beverages, fruits, fruit juice, cakes, cookies, and other dessert items are also significant contributors.

Food dislikes of older children consistently include cooked vegetables, mixed dishes, and liver. Children accept raw vegetables more readily than cooked ones but often take only a limited amount. Sweetness and familiarity are significant factors that influence food preferences in all children.

A common difficulty for parents is finding a time when school-age children are willing

FIG. 7-3   Food habits are part of both physical and psychosocial development.

Steve Fritz.

to sit down and eat a meal. Frequently they are so involved with other activities that it is difficult to get them to take time to eat. Often they satisfy their initial hunger and rush back to their activities and television programs, returning later for a snack.

Meal Patterns

Breakfast is an important meal. Even so, estimates of children who do not eat breakfast range from 8% to 29%.[49] Children will have to rise earlier to eat an unhurried and balanced meal and may have to prepare it themselves. Early morning school activities may make preplanning necessary. Some may find a glass of milk and fruit juice important before early sports activities. Studies have shown that when breakfast is consumed, children have a better attitude and school record compared with when it is omitted.[50] Pollitt, Leibel, and Greenfield found that 9- to 11-year-old well nourished children who skipped breakfast showed a decrease in accuracy of response in problem-solving but an increase in immediate memory in short-term accuracy.[51] The effect was attributed to a heightened arousal level, which in turn had a qualitative effect on cognitive function.

Actually, most children do eat breakfasts that contribute at least one fourth of the RDA standard.[49] A larger percentage of children in the lower grades eat breakfast than those in the middle and upper grades. Reasons for skipping breakfast included "not hungry," "no time," "on a diet," "no one to prepare food," "do not like food served for breakfast," and "foods are not available."[40] Morgan, Zabik, and Leville[49] found that children who consumed ready-to-eat cereals three or four times a week skipped breakfast less frequently than did children who ate non-ready-to-eat hot cereal. The school-age child often participates in the School Breakfast and Lunch Program administered by the Department of Agriculture, which provides cash reimbursement and supplemental foods to feeding programs that comply with federal regulations. Low-income children may receive reduced prices or free meals.

Children who do not participate in the school lunch program generally bring a packed lunch from home. Studies have indicated that, compared with the school lunch, these meals provide significantly fewer nutrients, but do supply energy. Little variety is seen in the lunches since favorite foods tend to be packed and repacked and lack of refrigeration limits the kinds of foods that can be carried.

The evening meal provides an opportunity for family interaction and socialization, as well as one of food and nutrient intake. Children should be expected to participate in both activities. It is important that parents not cater to children's food idiosyncrasies but offer them the family menu.

The emotional environment at the dinner table may influence nutrient intake. The evening meal is not the place for family battles or punitive action toward children. If eating is to be successful and enjoyable it must occur in a setting that is comfortable and free from stress and unreasonable demands. Lund and Burke found that mealtime criticism about non-food-related activities reduced the level of food consumption and adversely affected intakes of vitamins A and C in 9- to 11-year-old children.[52]

School Meals

School feeding and nutrition education programs, when adequately implemented, provide not only important nutrients for children, but also an opportunity to learn to make responsible food choices. These feeding programs contribute significantly to the nutrient and energy intake of many low-income children. In fact, such feeding programs may provide motivation for children to go to school.

Since its inception in 1946, the school lunch program has been administered by the U.S. Department of Agriculture, which provides cash reimbursement and supplemental foods to feeding programs that comply with federal regulations. Federal regulations require that school lunches and breakfasts be sold at reduced prices or be given free to

TABLE 7-8   School Lunch Pattern — Approximate Per Lunch Minimums

Components		Minimum Quantities				Recommended Quantities for
		Group I: Age 1-2; Preschool	Group II: Age 3-4; Preschool	Group III: Age 5-8; K-3	Group IV: Age 9 and Older; 4-12	Group V: 12 Years and Older; 7-12*
Milk	Unflavored, fluid lowfat, skim or buttermilk must be offered†	¾ cup (6 fl oz)	¾ cup (6 fl oz)	½ pint (8 fl oz)	½ pint (8 fl oz)	½ pint (8 fl oz)
Meat or meat alternate (quantity of the edible portion as served)	Lean meat, poultry, or fish	1 oz	1½ oz	1½ oz	2 oz	3 oz
	Cheese	1 oz	1½ oz	1½ oz	2 oz	3 oz
	Large egg	½	¾	¾	1	1½
	Cooked dry beans or peas	¼ cup	⅜ cup	⅜ cup	½ cup	¾ cup
	Peanut butter or an equivalent quantity of any combination of any of above	2 tbsp	3 tbsp	3 tbsp	4 tbsp	6 tbsp
Vegetable or fruit	2 or more servings of vegetable or fruit or both	½ cup	½ cup	½ cup	¾ cup	¾ cup
Bread or bread alternate (servings per week)	Must be enriched or whole-grain — at least ½ serving ‡ for group I or one serving ‡ for groups II-V must be served daily	5	8	8	8	10

*The *minimum* portion sizes for these children are the portion sizes for group IV.
†If a school serves another form of milk (whole or flavored), it must offer its children unflavored fluid lowfat milk, skim milk, or buttermilk as a beverage choice.
‡Serving 1 slice of bread; or ½ cup of cooked rice, macaroni, noodles, other pasta products, other cereal product such as bulgur and corn grits; or as stated in the *Food Buying Guide* for biscuits, rolls, muffins, and similar products.
From Food and Nutrition Service, Department of Agriculture: National School Lunch Program Regulations, Nov. 16, 1982, Federal Register.

children whose families cannot afford to buy them. The lunch menus must be planned to meet the guidelines established for the National School Lunch Program. Table 7-8 shows minimum quantities of food required for the various age groups in a school lunch.

To provide variety and to enlist participation and consumption, schools are encouraged to provide a selection of foods. Senior high school students may be permitted to decline up to two items. Students below the senior high school level may decline up to two or only one item at the discretion of the local school food authority. Breakfast must include liquid milk, fruit or vegetable juice, and bread or cereal. Schools are encouraged to keep fat, sugar, and salt at moderate levels.

Current regulations require that schools involve students and parents in planning the school lunch program. They may be included in such activities as menu planning, enhancing the eating environment, program promotion, and related student community support activities.

Foods sold in competition with school lunch in snack bars or vending machines must provide at least 5% of the recommended dietary allowances for one or more of the following nutrients: protein, vitamin A, vitamin C, niacin, riboflavin, thiamin, calcium, and iron. This regulation eliminates the sale of soda water, water ices, chewing gum, and some candies until after the last lunch period. It should also encourage the offering of more fruits, vegetables, and fruit and vegetable juices in places that compete with the school lunch. Concentrated sources of sucrose have been a concern of many interested in dental health, the control of obesity, and the development of sound food habits for all children. Sufficient concern has been created in some school districts that only machines that provide fruit, milk, nuts, and seeds have been made available to students. Initially, sales have been found to decrease, but ultimately they increase. One school discovered that they made a greater profit on apples than on chocolate bars.

Many persons concerned about the prevention of atherosclerosis and obesity have made statements about the quantity and saturation of fats as well as the caloric density of foods in these school lunches. Indeed, some schools have responded to these concerns and provided low-fat menu options.

Although elementary school children are making more decisions regarding food selection, supervision and supportive guidelines may be necessary at lunchtime. Children may give priority to activities other than eating and rush through their meals. Some may refuse to eat the food on the menu. Children who need therapeutic diets will need guidance in the foods they should and should not eat.

PREVENTION OF NUTRITION AND HEALTH PROBLEMS

Nutrition concerns during childhood include iron-deficiency anemia, overweight and obesity, and dental caries. In addition some persons are worried about children's intakes of specific foods and food constituents such as artificial flavors and colors and sugar and their possible effect on behavior. Also, it is important to recognize that many risk factors for cardiovascular disease can be modified by changes in dietary patterns. Identification of children at risk and modifying fat and salt intakes as well as other contributing factors are important health promotion actions.

The prevention of iron-deficiency anemia has been discussed earlier in this chapter (p. 260). Any discussion on childhood nutrition should include attention to these other concerns as well.

Weight Management

An excessive rate of weight gain and deposition of fat occurs when energy intake exceeds energy expenditure. Over time this situation can lead to obesity. By monitoring rates of growth and deposition of adipose tissue, children who are accumulating more fat than would be anticipated can be identified, and measures to increase activity and decrease excessive caloric intakes can be taken.

Family attitudes. Adolescents make their own decisions about what and when they eat. Counseling must be directed to the teenagers themselves. But parents control the food available to younger children, create the environment that influences their acceptance of food, and can influence energy expenditure by the opportunities they create for physical activity for their children. It may be important to explore first with parents their reasons for encouraging their children to consume amounts of food that result in rapid weight gain. Some parents may not recognize that their expectations for the quantity of food they encourage their children to consume are excessive and that the "chubby" child is not necessarily the healthy child.

Parents may need help in developing appropriate parenting skills. They may need to learn how to respond to hunger and other needs of their infants and how to interact with their children. They may need help in identifying ways to help their children develop initiative and to cultivate friends and outlets in the community.[53]

Physical activity. The activity pattern of both the child and the family should be explored. It may be important to help parents find ways of increasing their child's level of activity. Parents who live in apartments often reinforce sedentary activities to reduce the noise level and complaints from neighbors. Those who live in one-family dwellings may have limited space for children's activities. City park departments, preschools, and schools frequently have programs that offer opportunities for increasing children's activities.

Appropriate energy intake. It is important to remember that at any age the range of appropriate energy intakes is large. Overweight children and children with familial trends to obesity may need fewer kilocalories than do their peers. Griffith and Payne found that normal weight 4- to 5-year-old children of obese parents expended 1174 kcal/day as compared with 1508 kcal/day expended by children of the same size and age of normal weight parents.[54] It was interesting that the children of normal weight parents expended twice as much energy in physical activity as did those of obese parents. Families of children with a familial tendency to obesity may require help in identifying the kinds and amounts of food that provide an energy intake that will support normal growth and weight gain.

Nutrition counseling. Programs of nutrition counseling should be family oriented and based on normal nutrition, emphasizing foods that provide a balance of nutrients as well as appropriate kilocalorie intakes. Families will need to realize that these efforts are directed at reduction in rates of weight gain and are not intended to effect weight loss. They must recognize that the food available and the models set for their child will determine the child's response to efforts to control weight gain. Family meals may need to be modified to include fewer fried foods, less gravy, and fewer rich desserts. Parents and siblings may have to modify their own eating practices to set appropriate examples. Teachers, baby-sitters, and day care workers should be alerted to and included in programs designed to control weight. Food experiences at school may need to be modified to exclude corn dripping with butter and chocolate cupcakes so frequently provided for special occasions. Low caloric snacks such as raw fruits and vegetables can be provided instead of cookies, candy, and hot dogs.

It is important to recognize that school-age children are very concerned about size. In fact, many are on self-imposed diets because they worry about becoming overweight. Weight control programs should be planned carefully so that they do not become the cause of an eating disorder in adolescence (see box on p. 275).

CASE STUDY

> ### *Wise Weight Management for a School-Age Girl*
>
> At the regular pediatric clinic visit of a 7-year-old girl, the pediatrician and pediatric nutritionist found that the girl's weight-for-height on the growth grid was above the 95th percentile. Her rate of weight gain had increased in the past year, crossing from the 50th to the 90th percentile.
>
> #### Questions for analysis
> 1. What factors that influence her food intake and energy expenditure should be assessed?
> 2. What is a reasonable goal to correct her overweight status?
> 3. Outline a daily food plan to achieve this goal.

Dental Caries

Dental caries, one of the most common nutritional diseases, affects children of all ages and family income levels. As with other tissues, nutrition plays an important role during development in the acquisition of sound teeth and the surrounding structures that hold them and in the later susceptibility of the teeth to caries. Once the tooth has erupted, the composition of the diet, the presence of acid-producing bacteria, and the **buffering capacity** of the saliva interact and result in control or development of dental caries. Calcified dental tissues, unlike the long bones, which are subject to constant remodeling and repair, do not have the ability to repair themselves. Tooth destruction by decay is permanent.

Etiology. Dental plaque, a prerequisite for dental caries, has been described as a sticky, gelatinous mixture that contains water, salivary protein, **desquamated cells,** and bacteria.[44] The plaque bacteria, using energy derived from the catabolism of dietary carbohydrate, synthesize several toxic substances including enzymes that have the potential to degrade the **enamel** and **dentin** and are precursors of acidic fermentation products. *Streptococcus mutans* appears to be the primary bacteria. These acids and enzymes cause demineralization of the **hydroxyapatite** of the enamel followed by **proteolytic** degradation and demineralization of the enamel and dentin. It has been proposed that when the acidic environment falls below 5.5, cariogenic bacteria invade the tooth and caries results. The saliva, the **pH** of which is 6.5 to 7.0, acts as a buffer and provides mechanical cleansing of the teeth.

Sugar. It has been well documented from animal studies and studies of humans in institutions and as outpatients, that when intakes of sugar could be controlled sucrose is the most cariogenic carbohydrate. The incidence of caries can be reduced when the intakes of sugar are reduced.[55] Glucose is thought to be the next most cariogenic sugar, and maltose, lactose, and fructose have been found to have equal effect. Starch can also cause the production of large amounts of plaque acid because the carbohydrate, once attacked by salivary amylase, is broken down into sugar and attacked by plaque bacteria.

Frequency of eating. The presence of sucrose, or even the total amount of sucrose in the diet, may not be the determining factor in the incidence of dental caries. An often quoted study in an institution for the mentally handicapped in Sweden showed that the more important factors were the frequency with which the sugar is consumed and the adhesiveness of the food to the teeth.[55] The researchers who conducted this 5-year study showed that the consumption of sticky candy between meals produced a high increase in

Buffering capacity
Function of the body's main buffer system of two balancing partners, an acid partner (carbonic acid) and a base partner (sodium bicarbonate), that act together to buffer or neutralize any incoming acid or base to maintain the necessary degree of acidity and alkalinity in the body fluids that is compatible with life and health.

Desquamation
(L *de-*, from; *squama*, scale) The shedding of epithelial tissue, mainly the skin and oral mucosa, in scales or small sheets.

Hydroxyapatite
An inorganic compound of calcium and phosphorus found in the matrix of bones and teeth; gives rigidity and strength to the structure.

the incidence of dental caries, whereas the increase in incidence of caries from the addition of sugar sweetened water at mealtime was small. When sucrose was fed in chocolate or bread, an intermediate increase in the incidence of caries was noted. Other studies have not supported these findings. Many researchers have found no difference between meal eating habits of caries-free and caries-prone individuals.

Snacking at bedtime is especially effective in increasing dental caries. Reduction of the flow of saliva, which occurs during sleep, reduces the natural cleansing mechanism and permits greater fermentation of cariogenic material. The ingestion of foods that alter the buffering capacity of the saliva, for example, milk and fats, which form a protective oily film on the tooth surface, may offer some protection for the teeth.[56]

Control. The less frequently sucrose-containing foods are consumed and the less ability the foods have to adhere to the teeth, the more positive will be the outlook for the control of dental caries.

Fluoride. It has definitely been proven that fluoride can reduce the incidence of dental caries. Fluoride suppresses sugar metabolism by bacteria, makes enamel more resistant to acid, and stimulates remineralization of the teeth. A fluoridated water supply is an important approach to the prevention of dental caries. Other approaches to ensuring adequate fluoride that are under investigation include sodium fluoride capsules that can be chewed and swallowed, the use of an aerosol that causes fluoride-containing organisms to adhere to the teeth and enhances fluoride uptakes by the plaque and enamel, and the use of a small device attached to the teeth that releases fluoride at a predetermined rate for at least 6 months.[57]

Diet: foods and frequency. Dietary control continues to be a most important and effective approach to the control of dental caries. The frequency of eating breads, rolls, and cereals has not been associated with an increase in dental caries, whereas the frequency of eating candy and chewing gum has been shown to increase the number and incidence of dental caries. Cookies, cakes, pies, and candies have been shown to cause profound falls in pH levels of the plaque. It is interesting that the researchers found that the more acid-carbonated beverages depress the pH less than apple and orange juice.[58] A study of 147 junior high school students' snacking patterns in relation to caries production showed chocolate candy to be the most carious snack food selected. Children who consumed fruit drinks, cookies, or apples at bedtime and between meals had a significant caries increment during the year studied. No carious lesions developed in 47 children who had higher intakes of fruit juice and oranges and lesser use of sugar-sweetened chewing gum than the other children. As the amount of a child's spending money increased, the frequency of snacking increased.[59]

Plaque control. Researchers have studied the cariogenicity of foods in rats by noting the caries experience after food comes in contact with the teeth for designated periods of time, and in humans by noting changes in the plaque pH before and immediately after a food is eaten. The box on p. 277 shows foods that cause the plaque pH to fall below 5.5 and are considered to be cariogenic. Certain foods do not cause the plaque pH between the teeth to fall to levels at which demineralization will occur. These foods have a relatively high protein content with basic amino acids, a moderate fat content, a strong buffering capacity, a high mineral content including calcium and phosphorus, and a pH greater than 6.0. They also stimulate saliva flow. Meats, nuts, and cheese have been found to be noncariogenic. In fact, they have a beneficial effect when consumed with other foods. Cheddar cheese has been observed to block caries formation caused by sweet snacks when sweets and cheese have been eaten alternately.[60]

Nutrition education. Children should be taught to select foods that provide the essential nutrients and to limit their consumption of cariogenic foods. It is important that they learn to include noncariogenic protective foods in their snacking patterns, especially

ONE STEP FURTHER

A Partial List of Foods That Cause the pH of Human Interproximal Plaque to Fall Below 5.5

Apples, dried	Cola, beverage	Oranges
Apples, fresh	Cookies, vanilla sugar	Orange juice
Apple drink	Corn flakes	Pasta
Apricots, dried	Corn starch	Peanut butter
Bananas	Crackers, soda	Peas, canned
Beans, baked	Cream cheese	Potato, amylose
Beans, green, canned	Doughnuts, plain	Potato, boiled
Bread, white	Gelatin, flavored dessert	Potato chips
Bread, whole wheat	Grapes	Raisins
Caramel	Milk, whole	Rice, instant cooked
Carrots, cooked	Milk, 2%	Sponge cake, cream-filled
Cereals, nonpresweetened	Milk, chocolate	Tomato, fresh
Cereals, presweetened	Oatmeal, instant cooked	Wheat flakes
Chocolate, milk	Oats, rolled	

From Schachtele CF: Nutr News 42:13, 1982. Courtesy Nutrition News, National Dairy Council.

when sucrose-containing foods are included in the menu. The important between meal snacks can be carefully planned to contribute nutrients without creating an oral environment conducive to tooth decay. Sweet foods such as dessert items should be consumed as infrequently as possible within the framework of acceptability to the child and to the family.

Food and Behavior

There has been considerable speculation that certain additives and food constituents such as sugar and caffeine may play a part in the etiology of hyperactivity in childhood. This condition is characterized by inattention, excess motor activity, impulsiveness, and poor tolerance for frustration; the onset of hyperactivity occurs before 7 years of age. It affects 5% to 10% of school age children.

Additives. In recent years the hypothesis that artificial flavors and colors and naturally occurring **salicylates** cause hyperactivity in as many as 50% of children so affected has been popular. Many persons have felt that a diet that eliminated these constituents was indicated. But research has not supported this hypothesis. A very small percentage of children, however, have been identified to be "responders" to the additives.

Salicylates
Compound salts of salicylic acid, found in certain plants and in drugs such as common aspirin (acetylsalicylic acid—ASA).

Open clinical trials have indicated behavioral improvements in as many as 50% of hyperactive children. They have also reported that diet improved behavior in nonhyperactive children, suggesting that behavioral changes may be due to changes in the parent-child interactions and family dynamics.[61] A recent study using a total dietary replacement design once again looked at dietary manipulations in 24 preschool hyperactive boys. All children received both the experimental and control diets. Food dyes, food flavorings, preservatives, monosodium glutamate, chocolate, and caffeine were eliminated from the diet. Specific foods that the family felt to be detrimental to the child's behavior were also eliminated. Almost 50% of the boys showed some behavioral improvement using the accepted rating scales. Sleep patterns also were better.[62]

Double-blind studies suggest that food additives do not play a major role in the etiology

Placebo
(L "I will please") An inactive substance or preparation used in controlled drug or nutrient studies to determine the efficacy of an agent under study.

Atherosclerosis
(Gr *athere*, gruel; *skleros*, hard) Condition characterized by gradual formation, beginning in childhood in genetically predisposed individuals, of fatty cheese-like streaks then harder plaques in the intima or inner lining of major blood vessels such as coronary arteries, eventually in adulthood cutting off blood supply to the tissue served by the vessel; the underlying pathology of coronary heart disease.

Atherosclerotic lesions
Characteristic lesions, called *athromas,* the fatty raised streaks and plaques that signal atherosclerosis, the underlying cardiovascular disease associated with elevated levels of serum lipids, especially cholesterol, and related risk factors such as smoking, obesity, and hypertension.

Aorta
Main large trunk blood vessel from the heart, leading down the center of the body through the chest and into the abdomen, from which the systemic arterial blood system proceeds.

of hyperactivity in the majority of cases. Interestingly, two different researchers found an order effect. In one study parents noted a slight effect if the additive-free diet had been given first, and in another study teachers noted the same effect when it was given first.[61] Studies that have challenged hyperactive children on an additive-free diet with a food containing additives or a **placebo** have indicated that one in 25 hyperactive children who respond to the additive-free diet show behavioral response when challenged with the constituents.[63]

Sugar. Sugar has also been hypothesized to play a role in the etiology of behavioral difficulties in children. Most of the reports that have indicted sugar have been based on clinical assessment, with few on controlled studies. A retrospective review of glucose tolerance curves of hyperactive children found 75% of the 261 hyperkinetic children had abnormal glucose tolerance curves following a 5-hour glucose tolerance test. Other studies have not found abnormal glucose tolerance curves.[64]

Several double-blind challenge studies have not found sugar to contribute to hyperactivity even in children whose mothers felt they were responders. However, speculation that sugar is an offender in the etiologies of the disorder continues on the basis of observations of behavior and food intake. An association was suggested between destructive aggressive behavior and sugar intake of 4- to 7-year-old hyperkinetic but not normal children on the basis of 7-day food diaries kept by the mothers and videotaped observations of behavior by trained observers.[65] Another study noted an inverse relationship in the percentage of sugar in the children's diets suggested by a 1-day dietary recall and standardized measures of intelligence and school achievement.[66] It should be noted that none of the above studies has shown a cause and effect relation between sugar and behavior.

One hyperkinetic 5-year-old male and his mother were both found to become frustrated, hyperactive, and difficult to control after a double-blind challenge with sugar in lemonade.[67] However, not one of 50 other hyperkinetic children tested in the same way responded to a sugar challenge. Definitive evidence that sugar causes behavioral problems in children has not been found.[68,69] However, there may be some children who are sensitive to sugar and further investigation using a double-blind crossover design is appropriate.

Prevention of Atherosclerosis

Risk factors. Major risk factors associated with **atherosclerosis** and its resulting cardiovascular disease include obesity, a strong family history of heart disease, a sedentary lifestyle, hypertension, and elevated blood lipids, especially low-density lipoprotein (LDL) cholesterol. These risk factors are independent and continuous variables. Studies of adults have shown a significant relation between elevated serum cholesterol, blood pressure, and the extent of **atherosclerotic lesions.** The extent of the raised lesion is associated with total fat, saturated fat, cholesterol, and animal protein intakes.

Evidence that the atherosclerotic process leading to adult coronary heart disease begins in childhood includes (1) observations at autopsy of children and young adults who died of noncoronary events, and (2) epidemiologic studies of adult relatives of children with elevated plasma cholesterol levels. Findings at autopsy have described fatty streaks in the **aortas** of preschool children and fibrous plaques in coronary arteries of 20- to 22-year-old American soldiers who died in the Korean and Vietnam wars. Epidemiologic studies indicate that blood lipids and lipoproteins track from birth to the young adult years.[70-72] It is also known that food habits developed in childhood continue into the adult years.

Because of these findings, it is becoming increasingly clear that the origin of atherosclerosis, especially in genetically predisposed persons, is in early childhood. Several groups have recommended changing the diet of all children over 2 years of age. The recommendation includes reduction of total dietary fat to less than 30% of the day's total kilocalories, saturated fat reduced to less than 10% of the total kilocalories, and cholesterol limited to 300 mg/day.[73,74]

ONE STEP FURTHER

NCEP Report: Recommended Cholesterol Levels for Children and Adolescents

	Total cholesterol		Low-density lipoprotein cholesterol	
	mmol/L	mg/dl	mmol/L	mg/dl
Acceptable	<4.4	<170	<2.8	<110
Borderline	4.4-5.1	170-199	2.8-3.3	110-129
High	≥5.2	≥200	≥3.4	≥130

The National Cholesterol Education Program, Report of the Expert Panel on Blood Cholesterol Levels in Children and Adolescents, Bethesda, Md, 1991, National Heart, Lung and Blood Institute.

Many pediatricians disagree with this universal recommendation, feeling that such diets may not provide sufficient energy and essential nutrients for normal growth and development. In fact, children of some conscientious parents trying to implement the recommendations have been diagnosed with growth deficits and failure to thrive.[46,47] The American Academy of Pediatrics states that the recommendation should be followed with moderation.[75]

Panel report. A panel from the National Institutes of Health also recommends screening of high-risk children. Children, they indicate in their report, should be selected by their pediatricians for cholesterol screening if they have high-risk families, with parents or grandparents with diagnosed cardiovascular heart disease or a cardiac event before age 55, or if one or both parents have had elevated serum cholesterol levels over 240 mg/dl. The panel recommended dietary intervention for children with borderline low-density lipoprotein (LDL) cholesterol levels of 110 to 129 mg/dl, and drug therapy for children over 10 years of age who have very high serum cholesterol levels over 200 mg/dl or LDL cholesterol level above 130 mg/dl that does not respond to dietary intervention.[76,77]

The American Academy of Pediatrics recommends cholesterol testing only for children over age 2 who have a family history of **hyperlipidemia** or early **myocardial infarction.** If an elevated serum cholesterol is confirmed in the child, dietary counseling is advised. Drug therapy is advised only for children with serum cholesterol levels greater than 200 mg/dl and for those who do not respond to dietary intervention in a reasonable period of time.[78] The new guidelines in the National Cholesterol Education Program (NCEP) report for blood total cholesterol and LDL-cholesterol limits for children, shown in the box above, are consistent with the American Academy of Pediatrics recommendations, as well as national health guides and objectives of the American Heart Association, National Academy of Sciences, and the U.S. Surgeon General, and are supported by the American Dietetic Association.[79-81]

Hyperlipidemia (Gr *hyper,* above; *lipos,* fat; *haemia,* blood) General term for elevated concentrations of any or all of the lipids in the blood plasma.

Summary

Children between 1 year and the onset of puberty grow at a steady rate. They acquire new skills, learn much about their environment, and test the limits of behavior the environment will accept. All of these factors influence the food they accept and the frequency with which they eat. As they grow older, children's food intakes become more influenced by peers, activities, and stimuli in their environment.

Prevention of nutrition problems is important during childhood. Of particular concern is the prevention of iron deficiency anemia, obesity, and dental caries, as well as reducing later adult risks for cardiovascular coronary heart disease in identified children of high-risk families.

Review Questions

1. Why do energy needs of children vary so widely at any age?
2. What independent feeding skills would you expect a normal 18-month-old child to have?
3. What factors influence food acceptance by children?
4. List food and feeding behavior concerns of most importance to mothers of preschool children.
5. List snack foods appropriate for children that are supportive of a program to prevent excessive weight gain and dental caries.
6. Describe the family history and blood lipid levels that would identify a child at risk for development of arteriosclerotic heart disease.

References

1. Smith DW: Growth and its disorders, Philadelphia, 1977, WB Saunders Co.
2. National Center for Health Statistics: NCHS growth charts, 1976, Monthly Vital Statistics Report, vol 25, no 3, suppl (HRA) 76-1120, Rockville, Md, 1976, Health Resources Administration.
3. Harris CS et al: Childhood asphyxiation by food: a national analysis and overlook, JAMA 251:2231, 1984.
4. Food and Nutrition Board, National Research Council: Recommended dietary allowances, ed 10, Washington, DC, 1989, National Academy of Sciences.
5. Spady DW: Total daily energy expenditure of healthy, free ranging school children, Am J Clin Nutr 33:766, 1980.
6. Food and nutrient intakes of individuals in 1 day in the United States, 1977, USDA Nationwide Food Consumption Survey, 1977-1978, Preliminary report number 2, Washington, DC, 1980, Science and Education Administration.
7. Ashworth A and Millward DJ: Catch-up growth in children, Nutr Rev 44:157, 1986.
8. Marie PJ et al: Histological osteomalacia due to dietary calcium deficiency in children, N Engl J Med 307:584, 1982.
9. Butrimonitz GP and Purdy WC: Zinc nutrition and growth in children, Am J Clin Nutr 31:1409, 1978.
10. Schlage C and Wortberg B: Zinc in the diet of healthy preschool and school children, Acta Paediatr Scand 61:421, 1972.
11. Hambidge KM et al: Low levels of zinc in hair, anorexia and poor growth and hypogeusia in children, Pediatr Res 6:868, 1972.
12. Walravens PA et al: Zinc supplementation in infants with a nutritional pattern of failure to thrive: a double-blind, controlled study, Pediatrics 83:1089, 1989.
13. Committee on Nutrition, American Academy of Pediatrics: Vitamin and mineral supplement needs of normal children in the United States, Pediatrics 66:1015, 1980.
14. Cook CC and Payne IR: Effect of supplements on the nutrient intake of children, J Am Diet Assoc 74:130, 1979.
15. Breskin MW et al: Water soluble vitamins: intakes and indices in children, J Am Diet Assoc 85:49, 1985.
16. Beauchamp GK and Coward BJ: Congenital and experimental factors in the development of human flavor preferences, Appetite 6:357, 1985.

17. Cowart BJ and Beauchamp GK: The importance of sensory content in young children's acceptance of salty tastes, Child Dev 57:1034, 1986.
18. Swanson-Rudd J et al: Nutrition orientations of working mothers in the North Central Region, J Nutr Educ 14:132, 1982.
19. Phillips DE, Bass MA, and Yetley E: Use of food and nutrition knowledge by mothers of preschool children, J Nutr Educ 10:73, 1980.
20. Stanek K et al: Diet quality and the eating environment of preschool children, J Am Diet Assoc 90:1582, 1990.
21. Birch LL et al: Mother-child interaction patterns and the degree of fatness in children, J Nutr Educ 12:17, 1981.
22. Birch LL et al: The influence of social-affective context on the formation of children's food preferences, J Nutr Educ 13:115, 1981.
23. Birch LL et al: Eating as a "means" activity in contingency: effect on young children's food preferences, Child Dev 55:431, 1984.
24. Birch LL and Deysher M: Caloric compensation and sensory specific satiety: evidence for self regulation of food intake by young children, Appetite 7:323, 1986.
25. Birch LL et al: The variability of young children's energy intake, N Engl J Med 324:232, 1991.
26. Strasburger VC: Children, adolescents, and television: the role of pediatricians, Pediatrics 83:446, 1989.
27. Dietz WH and Gortmaker SL: Do we fatten our children at the television set? Obesity and television viewing in children and adolescents, Pediatrics 75:807, 1985.
28. Way WL: Food-related behaviors on prime-time television, J Nutr Educ 15:105, 1983.
29. Blatt J and others: A cognitive developmental study of children's reactions to television advertising. In Rubinstein EA et al, editors: Television and social behavior, vol 4, Television in day to day life: patterns of use, Washington, DC, 1972, US Government Printing Office.
30. Ward S et al: Children's attention to television commercials. In Rubinstein EA et al, editors: Television and social behavior, vol 4, Television in day to day life: patterns of use, Washington, DC, 1972, US Government Printing Office.
31. Television, 1976, North Brook, Ill, 1976, AC Neilson Co.
32. Gussow J: Counternutritional messages of TV ads aimed at children, J Nutr Educ 4:48, 1972.
33. Wackman DB and Ward S: Children's information processing of television commercial messages, manuscript based on a symposium at the American Psychological Association Convention, Montreal, 1973. (Cited in Sheikh)
34. Crawford PB et al: Environmental factors associated with preschool obesity, J Am Diet Assoc 77:589, 1978.
35. Leung M et al: Dietary intakes of preschoolers, J Am Diet Assoc 84:551, 1984.
36. Sanjur D et al: Dietary patterns and nutrient intake of toddlers from low-income families in Denver, J Am Diet Assoc 90:823, 1990.
37. Beal VA: Dietary intake of individuals followed through infancy and childhood, Am J Pub Health 51:1107, 1961.
38. Beal VA: On the acceptance of solid foods and other food patterns of infants and children, Pediatrics 20:448, 1957.
39. Lamkin G et al: Food purchasing practices of young families, J Home Econ 62:598, 1970.
40. Huenemann RL: Environmental factors associated with preschool obesity, J Am Diet Assoc 64:489, 1974.
41. Eppright ES et al: The North Central Regional Study of diets of preschool children. III. Frequency of eating, J Home Econ 62:407, 1970.
42. Farris RP et al: Macronutrient intake of 10-year-old children, 1973 to 1982, J Am Diet Assoc 86:765, 1986.
43. Office of Human Development Services, US Department of Health and Human Services: Family day care in the United States, executive summary, National Day Care Home Study, DHHS Pub No (OHD5) 80-30287, 1981.

44. Williams S et al: Contribution of food service programs in preschool centers to children's nutritional needs, J Am Diet Assoc 71:610, 1977.
45. Fries ME et al: Vitamin B6 status of a group of preschool children, Am J Clin Nutr 34:2706, 1981.
46. Pugliese MM et al: Parental health beliefs as a cause of non-organic failure to thrive, Pediatrics 80:175, 1987.
47. Lifshitz F and Moses N: Growth failure, Am J Dis Child 143:537, 1989.
48. McPherson RS et al: Intake and food sources of dietary fat among school children in the Woodlands, Texas, Pediatrics 86:520, 1990.
49. Morgan KJ et al: The role of breakfast in nutrient intake of 5- to 12-year-old children, Am J Clin Nutr 34:1418, 1981.
50. Tuttle WW et al: Effect on school boys of omitting breakfast, J Am Diet Assoc 30:674, 1974.
51. Pollitt EL et al: Brief fasting stress and cognition in children, Am J Clin Nutr 34:1526, 1981.
52. Lund LA and Burk MC: A multidisciplinary analysis of children's food consumption behavior, Technical Bull No 265, St Paul, 1969, University of Minnesota, Agricultural Experimental Station.
53. Hertzler AA: Obesity impact of the family, J Am Diet Assoc 75:525, 1981.
54. Griffith M and Payne PR: Energy expenditure in small children of obese and nonobese parents, Nature 260:698, 1976.
55. Gustafson BE et al: The Vipeholm dental caries study: the effect of different levels of carbohydrate intake on dental caries in 436 individuals observed for five years, Acta Odontal Scand 11:232, 1954.
56. Weiss ME and Bibby BG: Effects of milk on enamel solubility, Arch Oral Biol 11:49, 1966.
57. Mirth DB and Bowen WH: Chemotherapy antimicrobials and methods of delivery in microbial aspects of dental caries. In Styles HM et al, editors: Microbial aspects of dental caries, Washington, DC, 1976, Informational Retrieval.
58. White-Graves MV and Schiller MR: History of foods in the caries process, J Am Diet Assoc 86:241, 1986.
59. Clancy KL et al: Snack food intakes of adolescents and caries development, J Dent Res 56:568, 1977.
60. Schachtele CF: Changing perspectives on the role of diet in dental caries formation, Nutr News 42:13, 1982.
61. Levitsky DA and Strump BA: Nutrition and the behavior of children. In Walker WA and Watkins WF, editors: Nutrition in pediatrics, Boston, 1985, Little Brown and Co.
62. Kaplan BJ et al: Dietary replacement in preschool hyperactive boys, Pediatrics 83:7, 1989.
63. Connors CK et al: Food additives and hyperkinesis: a controlled double-blind experiment, Pediatrics 58:154, 1976.
64. Langseth L and Dowd J: Glucose tolerance and hyperkinesis, Food and Cosmetics Toxicology 16:129, 1978.
65. Printz RJ et al: Dietary correlates of hyperactive behavior in children, J Consult Clin Psych 48:760, 1980.
66. Lester MB et al: Refined carbohydrate intake, hair cadmium levels, and cognitive function in children, Nutrition and Behavior 1:3, 1982.
67. Gross MD: Effect of sugar on hyperkinetic children, Pediatrics 74:876, 1984.
68. Ferguson HB et al: Double-blind challenge studies of behavioral and cognitive effects of sucrose-aspartame ingestion of normal children, Nutr Rev (suppl) p 144, May 1986.
69. Rapoport JL: Diet and hyperactivity, Nutr Rev (suppl) p 158, May 1986.
70. Berenson GS et al: Serum high density lipoprotein and its relationship to cardiovascular disease risk factor variables in children—the Bogalusa Heart Study, Lipids 14:91, 1979.
71. Enos WF et al: Coronary disease among United States soldiers killed in action in Korea, JAMA 152:1090, 1952.
72. McNamara JJ et al: Coronary artery disease in combat casualties in Vietnam, JAMA 216:1185, 1971.

73. Department of Health and Human Services, National Heart, Lung, and Blood Institute, The National Cholesterol Education Program: Report of the Expert Panel on Population Strategies for Blood Cholesterol Reduction, DHHS Pub No (NIH) 90-3046, Washington, DC, 1990, US Government Printing Office.

74. National Institutes of Health: Consensus conference, JAMA 253:2080, 1985.

75. Committee on Nutrition, American Academy of Pediatrics: Prudent lifestyles for children. Dietary fats and cholesterol, Pediatrics 78:521, 1986.

76. Department of Health and Human Services, National Heart, Lung, and Blood Institute, The National Cholesterol Education Program: Report of the Expert Panel on Blood Cholesterol Levels in Children and Adolescents, Bethesda, Md, 1991, National Heart, Lung, and Blood Institute.

77. Nutrition Week, Community Nutrition Institute, vol 21, no 15, Washington, DC, April 12, 1991.

78. American Academy of Pediatrics, Committee on Nutrition: Indications for cholesterol testing in children, Pediatrics 83:141, 1989.

79. National Academy of Sciences, National Research Council, Food and Nutrition Board: Diet and health, implications for reducing chronic disease risk, Washington, DC, 1989, National Academy Press.

80. US Department of Health and Human Services, Public Health Services: Healthy people 2000, national health promotion and disease prevention objectives, DHHS Pub No (PHS) 91-50212, Washington, DC, 1990, US Government Printing Office.

81. ADA Reports: Timely statement on NCEP report on children and adolescents, J Am Diet Assoc 91(8):983, 1991.

Further Reading

Gattas V et al: Protein-energy requirements of prepubertal school-age boys determined by using the nitrogen balance response to a mixed diet, Am J Clin Nutr 52:1037, 1990.

A nitrogen-balance study of eight male children 8 to 10 years of age was conducted in Chili using a mixed vegetable protein and a controlled milk and egg diet. The study validates the protein intakes recommended by FAO/WHO and the RDAs.

Kumanyika SK et al: Stature and weight status of children in an urban kindergarten population, Pediatrics 83:783, 1990.

This survey conducted in Washington, DC, to assess growth problems at school entrance provides comparative data on growth status among hispanic, black, and white children.

Maloney MJ et al: Dieting behavior and eating attitudes in children, Pediatrics 84:482, 1989.

This survey of school-age children in grades 3 through 6 found a preoccupation with dieting, with 45% wanting to be thinner, 37% having tried to lose weight, and 9% of the girls being anorexic. The authors recommend focusing study on the early development of dieting behavior and atypical attitudes of young children to understand the roots of eating disorders.

Satter E: How to get your kid to eat but not too much, Palo Alto, Calif, 1987, Bull Publishing Co.

This book presents parenting issues related to feeding children. Written especially for parents by a practicing nutritionist-therapist and mother, it emphasizes a healthy feeding relationship that results in an appropriate nutrient-energy intake. The last four chapters discuss practical approaches to children's eating problems.

Nutrition in Adolescence

Jane M. Rees

Basic Concepts

++

✔ *Adolescent growth and development include both rapid physical growth and dramatic psychosocial development with sexual maturing.*

✔ *Normal adolescent growth and development require increased nutritional support.*

✔ *Adolescent physical activities and health problems lead to specific nutritional needs.*

✔ *Personal needs guide approaches to adolescent nutrition assessment, counseling, and management.*

---

*A*dolescence is a phase of the life cycle that has long puzzled individuals and their parents as well as health professionals. An awareness of the characteristics and needs of this special group, however, can contribute to a greater appreciation for teenagers in general and for those who have special nutritional needs. Knowledge from other disciplines in the physical and social sciences must be integrated to provide a comprehensive basis for understanding nutritional issues. The unique characteristics of adolescent growth and development, both physical and psychologic, are relevant not only to theoretical discussions of the specific topics but also to clinical protocols, in which results from controlled studies are synthesized to derive solutions to long-term problems arising in uncontrolled real life situations.

In this chapter we see that typical eating habits of adolescents are affected by environment, life style, and normal development. We also understand why counseling techniques useful in helping adolescents improve their nutritional practices include the most sophisticated ones available from the social sciences today. Specifically planned nutritional support for growth and development is required for such diverse circumstances as eating disorders, fitness activities and competitive sports, chronic disease, and pregnancy. Current research is beginning to shed light on the theories and myths that surround nutritional influence on adolescent behavior. While many questions related to adolescent nutrition remain unanswered, a body of sound practical knowledge exists to guide adolescents in maintaining positive nutrition and health.

ADOLESCENT GROWTH AND DEVELOPMENT
Physiologic Growth

Puberty. The process of physically developing from a child to an adult is called puberty. Puberty, referring to maturation of the total body, is initiated by poorly understood physiologic factors. During late childhood growth begins to accelerate with pubescence until the rate is as rapid as that of early infancy. Fig. 8-1 shows that linear growth in centimeters per year during the teen years compares with that for the second year of life. The individual will gain about 20% of adult height and 50% of adult weight during pubertal growth.[1] Most of the body organs will double in size.

Initiation of puberty. What causes the upsurge in hormonal activity that initiates pubertal development? Current **radioimmunoassay** techniques allow the measurement of hormonal concentrations that previously were below the sensitivity limits of earlier assays. This advance allows the hormonal changes to be measured as they occur chronologically. However, even with the development of these refined laboratory techniques, the exact factor or combination of factors that triggers these changes is still unknown.[1] Many theories have been suggested. One popular theory proposes that there is a "gonadostat," an area in the brain that is extremely sensitive to the sex steroids estrogen, testosterone, and progesterone. This "gonadostat" governs the release of these hormones by a feedback mechanism that allows increased production with the onset of puberty.

Radioimmunoassay
(L *radius,* ray; *immunis,* free, exempt; *assay,* examine, analyze) Technique using radioactive labeling of the material being studied; used for measuring minute constituent quantities of antigen or antibody, hormones, certain drugs, and other substances.

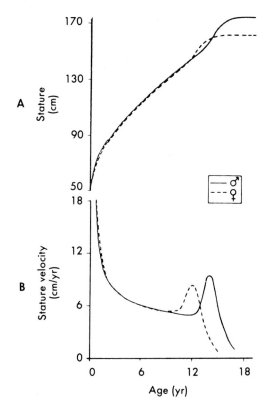

FIG. 8-1 **A,** Growth in stature of typical boy *(solid line)* and girl *(dashed line).* **B,** Growth velocities at different ages of typical boy *(solid line)* and girl *(dashed line).*

From Marshall WA: Clin Endocrinol Metab 4:4, 1975.

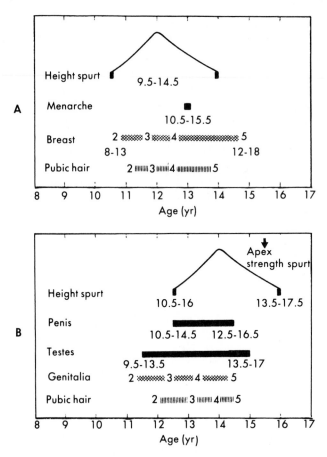

FIG. 8-2   Diagram of sequence of events at puberty in girls **(A)** and boys **(B)**. *Cross-hatched and small vertical line bars with numbers* refer to developmental stages described in Table 8-1.

Reprinted by permission of The New England Journal of Medicine, Marshall WA, and Tanner JM: Arch Dis Child 45:13, 1970.

Other theories relate pubertal onset to a change in body composition. An association between menarche and the attainment of a critical body weight has been observed in North American and most European females. It has been theorized that the achievement of the critical body weight of 47.8 kg (105 lb) causes a change in metabolic rate that in turn triggers menarche and initiates the adolescent growth spurt in girls. Another way of stating this relationship is that the attainment of a minimal level of body fatness (17% of body weight) is necessary for the onset of menstruation. Other researchers acknowledge an association between change in body composition and the onset of menarche, but do not view it as a triggering factor of puberty.

Sequence and stages of growth and development. Adolescent growth is characterized by a predictable sequence of stages in sexual maturity, increased height and weight, and changes in body composition. The timing and milestones of pubertal development are summarized in Fig. 8-2. The range of initiation and completion of milestones is listed in years.

Sexual maturity. Beginning with the enlargement of genitalia in males and breast development in females and accompanied by pubic hair distribution, the sexual maturation of humans can be observed and compared with norms. Table 8-1 describes the detailed

TABLE 8-1   Stages of Sexual Maturation (Sexual Maturity Ratings)

Boys	Pubic Hair	Genitalia
Stage 1	None	No change from childhood
Stage 2	Small amount at outer edges of pubis; slight darkening	Beginning penile enlargement; testes enlarged to 5 ml volume; scrotum reddened and changed in texture
Stage 3	Covers pubis	Longer penis; testes 8-10 ml; scrotum further enlarged
Stage 4	Adult type; does not extend to thighs	Larger, wider, and longer penis; testes 12 ml; scrotal skin darker
Stage 5	Adult type; now spread to thighs	Adult penis; testes 15 ml

Girls	Pubic Hair	Breasts
Stage 1	None	No change from childhood
Stage 2	Small amount; downy on labia majora	Breast bud
Stage 3	Increased; darker and curly	Larger; no separation of nipple and areola
Stage 4	More abundant; coarse texture	Increased size; areola and nipple form secondary mound
Stage 5	Adult type; now spread to thighs	Adult distribution of breast tissue; continuous outline

Modified from Tanner JM: Growth at adolescence, ed 2, Oxford, 1962, Blackwell Scientific Publications, Ltd.

stages of that development. In Fig. 8-2 these stages are depicted by the crosshatched and multilined bars with sequence of milestones that make up puberty. The onset of menses (menarche) in females and the completion of genitalia growth in males corresponds with stage 5, or adult status of sexual maturity.

Data have been accumulated to show that during the last century young women have gradually come to experience the menarche at younger ages, the so-called "secular trend." Total maturation probably occurs earlier for males as well. The theory is generally accepted, though records of menstrual age are scarce enough that the basis for its formulation has been questioned.

Height and weight. Throughout the approximately 5 to 7 years of pubertal development, rapid growth continues although a great percentage of height will be gained during the "growth spurt." Like the initiation of puberty, the 18 to 24 month period of the peak **growth velocity** will occur at different ages for different individuals fitting into the sequence of overall sexual development. It occurs earlier for girls than for boys.[1] Following the achievement of sexual maturity, linear growth and weight acquisition continue at a much lower rate and then cease, as shown by the downward slope of the height-spurt curve in Fig. 8-2. For rare females it will continue into the late teens and for males into the 20s. Most females will gain no more than 2 to 3 inches (5.1 to 7.6 cm) after the onset of menses. The rate of weight gain following the menarche is discussed in the later section on adolescent pregnancy (p. 335).

Body composition. The composition of the body changes in the process of maturation. In the prepubertal period the proportion of fat and muscle in males and females tends to be similar (body fat about 15% and 19% respectively) and lean body mass is about equal for both sexes. During puberty females gain proportionately more fat so that as adults the normal percentage of body fat is about 23% for females while for males it is about 12%. Males during this time gain twice as much muscle as females do. This striking difference in adolescent growth between males and females influences nutritional needs. Because the adolescent male experiences greater gain in bone and lean tissue than the female does, he requires more protein, iron, zinc, and calcium than the female for development of these tissues. Another reason for the male's larger requirements for these nutrients is his greater rate of growth.

Measurement of growth. Knowing the relationship between the milestones of sexual development and physical growth will enable the clinician to assess the progress of growth in an adolescent at a particular time, and give some indication of the extent of future growth. Thus **pubertal development** can be monitored clinically by using weight and height tables and **sexual maturity ratings.** For example, a 16-year-old female who has experienced her menarche and progressed beyond stage 4 of breast development, but who is not as tall as her peers would be considered to be close to her adult height. Excessive or less than normal growth can be detected by plotting height changes on the standard growth grids (see Appendix A). If her height corresponded to the 25th percentile for her age, the physical maturation of the young woman in the example above would be considered to be normal. The major cause of short stature during adolescence is genetically late initiation of puberty, though such conditions as chronic disease and skeletal and chromosomal abnormalities also account for certain children being shorter than normal. Hormonal imbalances leading to abnormal growth are rare.[1] In the United States malnutrition as a primary cause of short stature is also rare.

Weight can be plotted on a similar grid as height to determine whether or not an individual is keeping pace with peers, or exceeding them in total weight at a particular year of age. Because of the wide variation in weights seen in sample individuals in the adolescent period, some of whom were obese, the frequency distribution represented by the grids cannot be used for evaluation of weight-for-height proportion as it is used for younger children. Evaluation of weight-for-height proportion in adolescents is described here in the assessment section (p. 297).

Acne. Initiated by the influence of hormones on the sebaceous glands, **acne** is a normal characteristic of adolescent development. It occurs in varying degrees of severity in individual teenagers, mediated by factors such as stress and phase of the menstrual cycle. Almost all adolescents have acne, and as many as half of all adolescent contacts with health professionals are associated with dermatologic complaints. Traditionally, dietary factors have been blamed for the appearance of acne. But studies have shown no correlation between ingestion of foods and the appearance or degree of this condition.

Education about the physiologic basis for the development of acne supports teenagers in their efforts to control it. Systematic antibiotics given orally and topical applications of benzoyl peroxide and **tretinoin,** as well as special cleansing agents, have been shown to be effective.

It has been suggested that pharmacologic levels of zinc and vitamin A derivatives are useful in treating acne. Low levels of serum zinc have been found in one study among persons suffering most, suggesting that zinc deficiency makes the condition worse. In general, while no research is available to confirm the effect, it would seem that the optimally nourished body will be best able to cope with the development of acne as with many conditions.

Psychosocial Development

Span and scope of adolescence. Adolescence is the term applied to the period of maturation of both mind and body and therefore may be applied to humans before and after as well as during puberty. Along with physical growth, emotional, social, and intellectual development are rapid during adolescence.[2] Milestones in psychologic development of humans are shown in Table 8-2. The ability to use abstract thinking as opposed

Pubertal development
Rapid physical growth and sexual development of puberty

Sexual maturity ratings
Scale defining stages of sexual maturation during puberty.

Tretinoin
A form of retinoic acid, a vitamin A derivative, used as a drug in the medical treatment of chronic acne as a topical keratolytic agent (Gr *keras,* horn; *lysis,* dissolution). Keratin is a hard protein; it is the principle constituent of skin, hair, nails, and scar tissue.

TABLE 8-2   *Comparison of Erikson's and Piaget's Models for Emotional and Cognitive Development*

Age (years)	Erikson (emotional)	Piaget (cognitive)
0-2	**Phase I** Basic trust versus mistrust	**Sensorimotor period** Learning through senses and manipulation
2-4	**Phase II** Autonomy versus shame and doubt	**Preconceptual period** Classification by a single feature (e.g., size); no concern for contradictions
4-8	**Phase III** Initiative versus guilt	**Initiative thought period** Intuitive classification (e.g., awareness of conservation of mass concept)
8-12	**Phase IV** Industry versus inferiority	**Concrete operations period** Logical thought development; learning to organize
12-20	**Phase V** Ego identity versus role confusion	**Formal operations period** Comprehension of abstract concepts; formation of "ideals"
20 onward	**Phase VI** Intimacy versus isolation	—
Middle adulthood	**Phase VII** Generativity versus stagnation	—
Late adulthood	**Phase VIII** Integrity versus despair	—

to the concrete thought patterns of childhood, which the adolescent develops, enables the individual to accomplish these tasks. Planning ahead and connecting facts into integrated ideas becomes possible. With the accomplishment of the developmental "tasks of adolescence" as seen in Fig. 8-3, the person is prepared for a role in adult society.

Implications for nutritional issues. Many of the tasks of adolescence relate to the nutritional health of the individual. For example, emotional maturity allows teenagers to develop their own value system. As a result they can choose foods that will enhance their health rather than making their choices by responding to less healthful characteristics of foods as they may have done in childhood. They may go through a time of experimentation while they are learning to make wise choices.

Body image. Developing an image of the physical self that includes an adult body is an intellectual and emotional task intertwined with nutritional issues. Adolescents often feel uncomfortable with rapidly changing bodies. At the same time, being very much affected by influences outside themselves, they want to be like their most perfect peers and the idols of their culture. Stereotypes in the mass media reinforce such images. Teenagers may wish certain body parts were larger and other parts were smaller. They may want to

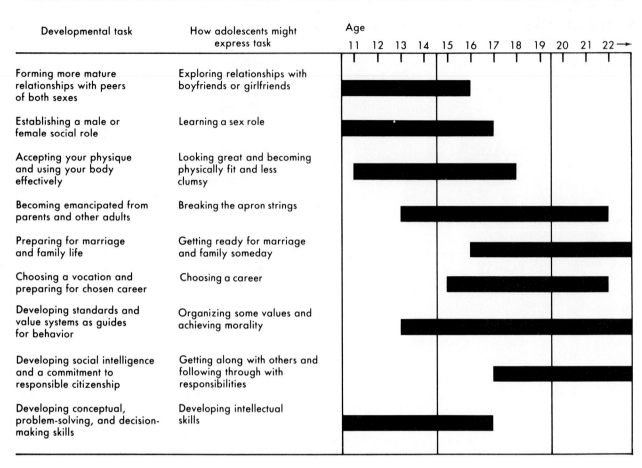

FIG. 8-3   Developmental tasks in adolescence.

Adapted from Thornburg H: Contemporary adolescence: readings, ed 2, Monterey, Calif, 1975, Brooks/ Cole Publishing Co.

grow faster or slower. These feelings can lead them to try to change their bodies by manipulating their diets, an impulse that certain commercial interests are quick to exploit. Young women who have not developed a mature body image may unnecessarily restrict the amount of food they eat in response to weight gained with the development of secondary sex characteristics. Hoping to achieve the muscular appearance of adult males, young men are tempted to use nutritional supplements.

NUTRITIONAL REQUIREMENTS
Growth as a Basis for Nutritional Requirements

Limitations of the RDA standard. Studies of the nutritional requirements of adolescents must take into account not only age but also stage of physical maturity.[3] Since such studies are not generally available, the research base on which recommendations are made is limited. The Recommended Dietary Allowances (RDAs) are stated for three adolescent age groups, not related to stages of maturity. The highest levels of nutrients are recommended for the group assumed to be growing at the most rapid rate. Adolescents

TABLE 8-3   *Daily Increments in Body Content Due to Growth*

		Average for Period 10-20 years (mg)	At Peak of Growth Spurt (mg)
Calcium	M	210	400
	F	110	240
Iron	M	0.57	1.1
	F	0.23	0.9
Nitrogen*	M	320	610 (3.8 g protein)
	F	160	360 (2.2 g protein)
Zinc	M	0.27	0.50
	F	0.18	0.31
Magnesium	M	4.4	8.4
	F	2.3	5.0

*The maintenance needs (2 mg/basal calorie) at 18 years of age are 3500 mg and 2700 mg for males and females, respectively.

From Forbes GB: Nutritional requirements in adolescence. In Suskind RM, editor: Textbook of pediatric nutrition, New York, 1981, Raven Press.

at the peak of their growth velocity will require large quantities of nutrients. They have been shown to incorporate twice the amount of calcium, iron, zinc, magnesium, and nitrogen into their bodies during the years of the growth spurt compared with that of other years (Table 8-3).

Calculation of needs by height. Dividing the RDA total of nutrient by the centimeters of the reference individual's height provides a quantity of nutrient in units per centimeter that can be applied to any teenager. For example, the RDA for protein for 11- to 14-year-old males is 45 g/day. The reference height is 157 cm. Thus 0.29 g/cm would be recommended. Then the total protein need would be 39 g for the 135 cm male and 54 g for the 185 cm male. This example of variation in size during the teenage years is quite realistic, since persons experience the growth spurt at different ages. Nutrient recommendations will come closest to meeting needs when the largest quantity of nutrient per centimeter is suggested for those experiencing the most rapid growth, even if the age does not coincide with the age at which the highest RDA standard is made.

Specific Nutrient Needs

Energy. The recommended energy intake in the RDA standard for adolescents as shown in Table 8-4 reflects the needs of teenagers. As well as growth rate, level of exercise will need to be considered in determining the needs of the individual.[4]

Protein. The protein requirement of adolescents has been studied the least of all the age groups. The recommendation is that the energy value of the protein intake should make up 7% to 8% of the total energy consumed. Sex, age, nutritional status, and quality of the dietary protein must be considered in estimating the amount an individual will need. The range of total protein need will be about 39 to 56 g. These amounts are usually obtained in the normal diet, so protein consumption should not be overly emphasized. Protein stores of adolescents should be carefully monitored and supported in situations where nutritional depletion may occur so that physical development will not be impaired.[4]

Calcium. Calcium is an important nutrient in adolescence since the requirement is based on the amount of the mineral needed for skeletal growth. Forty-five percent of total bone

TABLE 8-4   Recommended Dietary Allowances for Energy for Children and Adolescents (kilocalories per day)

Age (years)	Allowance	Reference Height (cm)	Energy (kcal/cm height)
Children			
7-10	2000	132	15.2
Males			
11-14	2500	157	15.9
15-18	3000	176	17.0
Females			
11-14	2200	157	14.0
15-18	2200	163	13.5

Adapted from Recommended dietary allowances, ed 10. ©1989 by the National Academy of Sciences. Published by National Academy Press, Washington, DC.

TABLE 8-5   Calculated Iron Requirements for Males and Females at the 3rd, 25th, 75th, and 97th Percentile for Body Weight (from 10-16 years of age)

Percentile Rating	Calculated Iron Requirements (mg)					
	Daily Dietary Need*		Peak Daily Dietary Need*		Cumulative Need†	
	Male	Female	Male	Female	Male	Female
3rd	6.6	5.1	13.2	10.3	966	751
25th	9.3	5.2	18.6	10.4	1360	772
75th	11.0	5.5	21.9	11.0	1610	794
97th	12.9	5.7	25.8	11.9	1885	836

*Period of adolescent growth spurt.
†Total body iron increment represented by muscle tissue increase during 10-16 year interval.
From McKigney JI and Munro HN, editors: Nutrient requirements in adolescence, Cambridge, Mass, 1978, The MIT Press. Copyright © 1978 The MIT Press.

growth occurs during this period. The total recommendations are the same for both sexes though accumulations are higher for males than for females because of the larger frame males will develop.[4]

Iron. Both males and females have high requirements for iron, as seen in Table 8-5. Males require more iron during adolescence because the buildup of muscle mass is accompanied by greater blood volume. Adolescent females require more than children because they will begin to lose iron monthly with the onset of menses.

Zinc. Zinc is known to be essential for growth as well as sexual maturation and therefore of great importance in adolescence. The retention of zinc increases especially during the growth spurt leading to more efficient use of the nutrient in the diet.[4]

Other minerals. The roles of other minerals in the nutrition of adolescents are not well studied. However, magnesium, iodine, phosphorus as well as copper, chromium, cobalt, and fluoride are important. The possibility of interactions between these nutrients cannot be overlooked. The recommendations for safe levels should be followed with moderation so that imbalances will not develop.

Vitamins. Adolescents require high amounts of thiamin, riboflavin, and niacin because of their high energy requirements. Vitamin D is especially needed for rapid skeletal growth. Recommended amounts of vitamins A, E, C, folate, and B_6 are the same as those for adults. Often the quantity of vitamins recommended for adolescents are of necessity **interpolated** from studies in adults and children.[4]

EATING BEHAVIOR
Typical Nutritional Patterns

Surveys of nutrient intake have shown that adolescents are likely to be obtaining less vitamin A, thiamin, iron, and calcium than recommended. They also ingest more fat, sugar, protein, and sodium than is currently thought to be optimum.[5,6]

While concern is often expressed over the habit of eating between meals, it has been shown that teenagers obtain substantial nourishment from foods eaten outside traditional meals. The choice of foods they make is of greater importance than the time or place of eating. Emphasis should be placed on fresh vegetables and fruits as well as whole grain products to complement the foods high in energy value and protein that they commonly choose.[7]

Irregular Meals

The number of meals teenagers miss and eat away from home increases from early adolescence to late adolescence, reflecting the growing need for independence and time away from home. The evening meal appears to be the most regularly eaten meal of the day. Females are found to skip the evening meal, as well as breakfast and lunch, more often than males.

Breakfast is frequently neglected and is omitted more by teenagers and young adults under 25 years of age than by any other age group in the population. A likely explanation as to why females are more apt to miss breakfast than are males is the pursuit of thinness and frequent attempts at dieting. Many teenage girls believe that they can control their weight by omitting breakfast or lunch. Young women who are dieting should be counseled that this approach is likely to accomplish just the opposite. By midmorning or lunchtime they may be so hungry that they eat more than if they had had at least simple foods in the early morning.

Factors Influencing Eating Behavior

By the time a person reaches adolescence, the influences on eating habits are numerous and the formation of those habits is extremely complex as shown in Fig. 8-4. The growing independence of adolescents, increased participation in social life, and a generally busy schedule of activities have a decided impact on what they eat. They are beginning to buy and prepare more food for themselves and they often eat rapidly and away from home.

Advertising. While the basic foundation for eating habits is found in the family, the influences on eating behavior originating outside the home in modern America are great. Teenagers are very vulnerable to the kind of advertising messages seen in Fig. 8-5. By the time Americans become adolescents they have been influenced by 10 years of television food commercials and the eating habits portrayed in television programs. The average teenager will have watched over a million food commercials, the majority of which are for products with a high concentration of sweetness and fat (p. 263).

Interpolation
(L *interpolare*, to make new) Process of injecting new interpretation or application of data to expand meaning or use, as in deriving data from one age group and applying it to another.

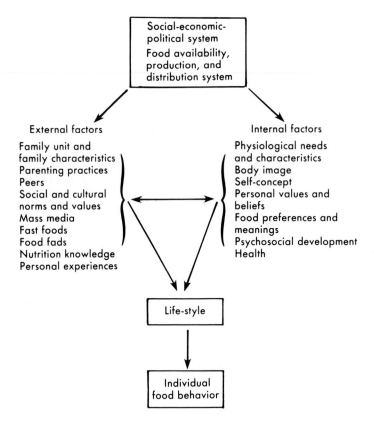

FIG. 8-4   Schematic diagram of factors influencing adolescent food behavior.

Ease of obtaining ready-to-eat foods. The ease of obtaining food that is ready to eat also influences the eating habits of teenagers. Through vending machines, at movies and sporting events, and at fast-food outlets and convenience groceries food is available at numerous times throughout the day. During the time of their peak growth velocity, adolescents may need to eat often and in large amounts and are able to use foods with a high concentration of energy. However, they will usually need to be more careful of amounts and frequency once growth has slowed.

Nutritional limitations of fast foods. The following factors appear to be the major nutritional limitations of fast-food meals:

- **Calcium, riboflavin, vitamin A.** These essential nutrients are low unless milk or a milkshake is ordered. Extensive use of soft drinks contributes to low intakes of these nutrients in addition to magnesium and vitamin C.[8]
- **Folate, fiber.** There are few sources of these key factors.
- **Fat.** The percent of body fat is high in many meal combinations.
- **Sodium.** The sodium content of fast-food meals is high.
- **Energy.** Common meal combinations are excessive in kilocalories when compared with the amounts of nutrients provided.

Although fast foods can contribute nutrients to the diet, they cannot completely meet the nutritional needs of teenagers. Both adolescents and health professionals should be aware that fast foods are acceptable nutritionally when they are consumed judiciously and as a part of a well-balanced diet.[7] When they become the mainstay of the diet there is cause for concern.[9] A nutrient imbalance may not appear to be a problem until a number

FIG. 8-5 Examples of enticements and advertisements for weight-loss products featured in popular magazines.

of years have gone by, unless some specific problem such as a chronic disease exists. However, evidence is accumulating to show that food intake patterns of teenagers affect their health in later life.[4]

Hypertension and hyperlipidemia. If an adolescent is hypertensive or there is a strong family history of the disease, a diet controlled in sodium and total energy is a part of long-term nutritional care. In the case of hyperlipidemia, fat and energy intake should be controlled. All adolescents should be cautioned against a high intake of sodium, fat, and energy because of the suspected link with cardiovascular disease and should be screened for hyperlipidemia once during adolescence. The following is a guide to the risks of particular levels of blood lipids for ages 2 to 19 years by sex:

	Total cholesterol (mg/dl)	Risk	LDL-cholesterol (mg/dl)	Risk
Males	175-190	Moderate	110-130	Moderate
	>190	High	>130	High
Females	178-200	Moderate	115-140	Moderate
	>200	High	>140	High

Recommended guidelines for monitoring total cholesterol and LDL cholesterol of children and adolescents from high-risk families have recently been issued by the National Cholesterol Education Program (NCEP) and a National Institutes of Health expert panel (see Chapter 7, p. 279).

Dental Caries and Periodontal Disease

Dental caries
(L *caries*, "rottenness") Molecular decay or death of hard tissue; disease of the calcified tissues of the teeth resulting from action of microorganisms on carbohydrates, characterized by disintegration of hard outer enamel, followed by breakdown of softer inner dentin material, leaving cavities and exposed soft tissue.

Gingivitis
(L *gingiva*, "gum of the mouth") Inflammation of the gum tissue in the mouth surrounding the base of the teeth.

Periodontal disease
(Gr *peri*, around; L *dens*, tooth) General term for disease of tissues surrounding the tooth, affecting its integrity and stability and contributing to tooth loss.

It is becoming apparent that the cause of **dental caries** is a complex process involving the interaction of several factors. The minerals of the tooth enamel are in constant equilibrium with the oral environment. It is necessary therefore to consider not only the presence of fermentable carbohydrate but also such factors as food solubility, mineral composition, and the buffering capacity of the oral environment. Adolescents' propensity to snack on refined carbohydrates is conducive to tooth decay. Since 80% of the average person's total incidence of dental lesions occur in the teenage years, this is the time to encourage habits built on choosing alternatives to sugar-containing foods.

Gingivitis increases in prevalence during the teenage years, and **periodontal disease** often follows. Little is known about the role of nutrition in periodontal disease, although nutritional deficiency, widespread in underdeveloped countries with high incidence of periodontal disease, has also been implicated. Inadequate intake of these nutrients in the teenage years can have an adverse effect on the health of the gums in later life.

Role of Parents

In order to encourage adolescents to form reasonable eating habits parents should give their children increased responsibility and choice within the range of nourishing foods as they are growing up. By the time they are teenagers they will need some freedom to use the kitchen. This is true for young men as well as for young women.

Substance Use and Abuse

Substance abuse in adolescence is a public health problem of major significance and concern. The substances most widely abused by adolescents are tobacco, smokeless tobacco, alcohol, marijuana, and cocaine. The strongest predictor of drug use by an adolescent is association with a peer group that uses drugs, although poor parenting and drug use by parents is also a strong influence. Adolescents who are left alone for long periods of time are more likely to use drugs and to start using them earlier than those who are with families or other positive supervised group activity more of the time. Over 90% of high school seniors have consumed alcohol; in one study one out of seven seniors admitted they had been inebriated once a week. The use of marijuana has been declining in recent years while there has been a steady increase in cocaine use throughout the 1980s. While rates of tobacco use have remained stable since the early 1980s, the rate among females has increased and the age of beginning use has declined for all teenagers. Smokeless tobacco, in the form of chewing tobacco and snuff, is typically used by male adolescents in rural areas and by young white male athletes, from 7% to 25% in populations studied. It has caused significant oral damage including cancer and thus is cyclical in its relationship to nutritional status.

Overall about 10% to 15% of teenagers have had no experience with drugs and alcohol, 70% to 80% have experimented, 10% to 15% have definable problems, and somewhat less than 1% are chemically dependent, addicted. Cognitive, emotional, and social development is likely to be retarded in the last group.[10]

Impact on nutritional status. Two small studies have been published of nutritional status in drug- or alcohol-abusing teenagers: one study was of a racially mixed group and the other was of a Native American population.[11,12] Deficient nutrient levels were not found in blood samples from either group, and neither reported consuming less of the nutrients studied than they needed or than nonusing peers. However, in the study that reported food choices, the nutrient levels of abusers were different from those of controls in that most of the nutrients they consumed came from snack foods and meat products. Fruits, vegetables, and milk were left out of their usual dietary patterns. Thus, though the adolescents studied did not have deficiencies that were measured either biochemically or in reported consumption, the long-term effects of their characteristic dietary habits, coupled with exposure to alcohol, would account for the development of the nutritional disorders seen in adult abusers. Studying the nutritional status of 18- to 25-year-old drug abusers would be most useful in the exploration of the natural history of deficiency diseases among alcohol and drug abusers. In summary, it can be said that the effect of substance abuse on nutritional status of any individual depends on the substance, the amount, duration and frequency of use, prior health and nutritional status, stage of physical growth, and nutritional adequacy of the diet consumed.

Identification and referral. Since the incidence of greatest abuse is among 18- to 25-year-old individuals, all health professionals need to be aware of the indicators of drug use so that they can refer adolescents with a definable problem for treatment before they reach a more advanced stage of chemical dependency. These indicators include:

Rash	Dyspnea on exertion
Muscle weakness	Faintness
Vomiting	Hangover
Diarrhea	Blackouts
Stomach pain	Nervousness
Nausea	Depression
Indigestion	Tiredness
Bleeding gums	Insomnia
Sore tongue	Somnolence
Taste loss	Headache
Appetite loss	Seizures
Memory loss	

Nutritional assessment, intervention, and support are components of the comprehensive physical and psychologic rehabilitative process of adolescent substance abusers.

ASSESSMENT OF NUTRITIONAL STATUS

Teenagers are in a fluctuating state of balance between supplying their bodies with needed nutrients and using up the nutrients. At any one time, this flow is the teenager's nutritional status. Assessment of **nutritional status** is described in Chapter 2 (p. 41). Modification for the adolescent requires use of the sexual maturity ratings and a specific data base with which to compare height, weight, and weight-height proportion.

Anthropometric Data

To evaluate the relationship between the weight and height of an individual adolescent, the detailed tables of the National Health and Nutrition Examination Survey (NHANES),

Nutritional status (L *status,* condition, situation) Condition of an individual's body tissues and health, especially as related to the nutrients that are essential to the structure, function, and maintenance of body tissues.

TABLE 8-6 *Weight in Kilograms of Girls Aged 17 Years at Last Birthday, United States, 1966-1970*

| Height (cm) | \| | Percentile | | | | | |
	5th	10th	25th	50th	75th	90th	95th
145-149.9	38.6	38.8	40.1	45.1	45.7	51.1	51.2
150-154.9	41.6	42.3	44.6	48.9	53.5	59.2	64.1
155-159.9	44.4	45.5	48.7	53.2	57.7	61.6	76.2
160-164.9	46.8	48.0	50.2	55.4	61.5	72.3	82.3
165-169.9	47.9	50.3	55.1	59.3	65.1	69.4	71.6
170-174.9	50.6	52.9	55.5	60.2	65.7	76.1	82.7
175-179.9	54.9	56.7	60.1	61.7	75.2	75.9	83.0

Modified from National Center for Health Statistics: Height and weight of youths 12-17 years, United States. In Vital and health statistics, series 11, no 124, Health Services and Mental Health Administration, Washington, DC, 1973, US Government Printing Office. Data from the national health survey, US Department of Health, Education, and Welfare, 1973.

National Center for Health Statistics can be used. An example is shown in Table 8-6; full tables are given in Appendix B. For each 2 cm increment in height at a particular year of age, a range of weights is given. Weight-height values for age and sex between the 25th and the 75th percentiles can be considered to be in the normal range. This range allows for the normal differences in body build of individuals.

In addition, **anthropometric data** from a skinfold evaluation will yield a more precise assessment of the proportion of fat to muscle and therefore weight to height. For example, a low value for triceps skinfold measurement (p. 43) in an individual above the 75th percentile for weight-height indicates that the adolescent is overweight but not overfat. An assessment of midarm circumference and arm muscle area (pp. 43, 44) will confirm the muscular body composition. This type of evaluation is plotted in Fig. 8-6. Anthropometric reference tables are given in Appendixes D, E, and F.

Sexual Maturity Rating

The evaluation of sexual maturity is an essential factor in making a valid nutrition assessment of an adolescent in a normal clinical setting. By knowing the stage of sexual maturity of the adolescent (see Fig. 8-2), it is possible to determine whether the full height has been reached or growth can still occur. Also, it is possible to determine whether the proportion of fat to muscle seen is that which the individual has developed as an adult or has obtained at one stage as a still-developing adolescent. Thus, if a young woman at stage 1 of sexual maturity is at the 90th percentile weight-for-height, she will continue to grow in height and has a greater potential to stay within the bounds of normal body composition than has a female of the same age, the same weight-for-height, but who has experienced menarche and is at stage 4 of sexual maturity.

Nutrition Environment

The **nutrition environment,** the combination of factors that influence the nutritional status, is also an important consideration. Such factors as general medical history, socioeconomic status, medications, alcohol or tobacco use, family attitudes, and peer group food practices all contribute to the adolescent's food choices. Table 8-7 summarizes the significance of each of these influences. **Nutrition assessment** includes the study of both the nutritional status and the nutrition environment of the individual adolescent. The

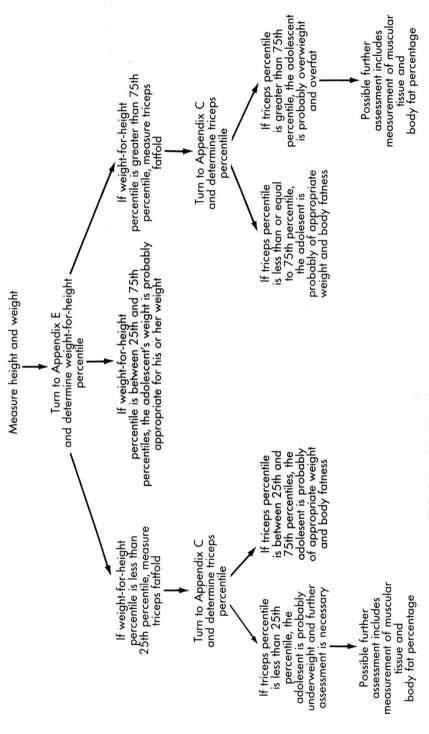

FIG. 8-6   Algorithm for evaluating an adolescent's weight.

TABLE 8-7 **Nutrition Environment Evaluation Guide**

Influences	Key Issues	Significance
Likes and dislikes	Does patient dislike any particular food that is a major source of a specific nutrient (for example, milk is a major source of calcium; citrus fruits of vitamin C; meat of high-quality protein)?	Points out need to explore alternative ways to supply nutrients (for example, substitute cheese and yogurt for milk; broccoli and green peppers for citrus fruit; proper combinations of plant foods for meat)
Environment and attitudes Individual	Does patient express interest in his or her diet?	Gives clues to attitude toward role of nutrition in health care
	Are there any behavioral problems that influence patient's food choices?	May indicate need to work with other health team members to resolve problem that temporarily precludes nutrition intervention
	Has patient ever followed a special diet? If so, who prescribed it, what type of diet was it, and when was it prescribed? What instructions did patient receive?	Self-prescribed diet may signal inappropriate or unreliable approach toward control of health by diet; points out medical and educational considerations needed in design of care plan
	Does patient think he or she has been following the diet? Is there evidence to substantiate this?	If discrepancy exists, indicates lack of understanding of diet by patient or unwillingness or inability of patient to make dietary changes
	What difficulties if any does patient see in making dietary changes?	Focuses on issues that need consideration in design of individualized care plan
Family	Who purchases and prepares food in home (that is, partially controls patient's food supply)?	Sets scene for type of action plan suitable to patient and family
	Does patient have adequate cooking facilities and equipment or access to other resources?	May indicate need to provide basic nutrition guidelines, including personalized menu plan
	Are there any cultural, regional, or religious factors that affect patient's food choices?	Requires consideration to tailor care plan to individual needs
Peers	How often does patient eat away from home? Where and with whom does patient eat? Are there specific food intake patterns related to peer influences?	Indicates potential influences of peers on food choices; points out potential efficacy of patient- versus family-oriented care plan

TABLE 8-7   Nutrition Environment Evaluation Guide—cont'd

Influences	Key Issues	Significance
Schools	Does patient eat at school? Does patient participate in school feeding programs?	School feeding programs with their standardized composition assure minimal nutrient availability and provide reference for accuracy of reported information
	Is there anything about school schedule or cafeteria environment that may discourage appropriate nutrient intake?	"Too little time for lunch" or "no one to eat with" may necessitate consultation with other team members or school to resolve life-style problems
	Is patient in appropriate grade in school? Has patient received food and nutrition information in school courses?	Gives clues to current knowledge of nutrition and level of intellectual functioning; allows practical planning for educational aspects of care plan
Limited food funds	Is patient or family eligible for food stamps; Women, Infants, and Children program (WIC); or reduced-price or free school lunch? Do they participate in programs? Does patient or family receive other social assistance?	Indicates family has limited income and may need assistance with food buying and preparation to assure nutritionally adequate diet; points out need to consider referral to appropriate food program or nutrition education resource
Health-related concerns	Does patient have any food allergies or intolerances (as distinguished from dislikes)?	Excludes foods from diet; indicates need to plan and assure adequacy with alternative food choices
	Are there any physical conditions affecting ability to consume adequate nutrients (for example, mouth sores, swallowing problems, taste abnormalities)?	Indicates need to consider flavor, consistency, and temperature of food in care plan
	Are there any problems in digestion, absorption, or metabolism that will interfere with nutrient utilization? Will any other therapy (drugs, exercise, radiation) affect nutrient needs?	Indicates need to address these problems in diet preparation

methods described in Chapter 2 will be used to help the health professional understand the effect they have on the adolescent's eating habits. A probing interview by a sensitive nutritionist who has had experience communicating with adolescents will also be required to find out how an individual teenager feels about and manages food.

Nutritional Care Plan

Assessment of all factors in the environment that may influence nutriture is essential if appropriate action to meet needs is going to be initiated as a personal **nutritional care plan.** The extent to which the total nutrition environment is studied depends on the projected use of the nutrition assessment. For example, a great deal of detailed information reflecting nutritional status is needed for a 13-year-old male with Crohn's disease who is scheduled for a course of **parenteral nutrition.** Information about the nutrition environment would be less vital at this time. However, nutritional care planning for a newly diagnosed 15-year-old female with insulin-dependent diabetes mellitus (IDDM) would require both nutritional status evaluation and assessment of the nutrition environment. Without both components, the care plan cannot adequately address physiologic nutritional needs and the adolescent's ability to meet them.

NUTRITIONAL COUNSELING FOR ADOLESCENTS
Facilitating Change

Attempts to help adolescents improve their nutritional status must be approached with skill, especially because of their growing independence.[13] Nutrition counselors must know adolescents' physical and psychologic development, life styles, and habits as well as appropriate methods of communicating with them.

Strategies for change. Sophisticated strategies to add knowledge, alter attitudes, and change behavior must be used in any setting if the objective is to influence an adolescent's eating habits. Providing knowledge or teaching can be done in a variety of settings from the classroom to the hospital bedside. Altering attitudes is much more difficult and usually demands an individualized experience. Facilitating the adoption of new behavior is even more difficult and requires a lengthy period of time. The adolescent will have to feel positive about any plan before it can succeed. In fact, much effort must be directed toward encouraging the person to want to change before introducing steps to bring the change about.

Personalized counseling. Besides changes in attitude the counselor must impart knowledge in an especially meaningful and individualized manner. Finally, behavior change can be approached in increments that are sufficiently realistic to ensure personal success.

Role of parents. Parents must be appropriately involved in the counseling process. They need help in being supportive, as opposed to being intrusive, as the adolescent makes changes. Both adolescents and their parents must be helped to see the importance of focusing on the process of making change rather than solely on the desired goal of self-care. A sure understanding of both the physical and social sciences, along with a liberal injection of art, are needed in nutrition counseling for adolescents and their parents. It is indeed a challenging field.

The Health Care Team

Adolescent health care is one of the most demanding of clinical problems. As such, it is best handled as a team effort. Any one professional will generally not possess the skills to meet all the client's needs. For example, Table 8-8 lists some of the types of issues that will arise throughout the course of teenage pregnancies with a suggested list of professionals to guide clients in managing these issues. This does not mean that certain

Nutritional care plan
The person-centered care plan, based on nutritional assessment data and evaluation, for individual nutritional care and education to promote health and prevent or treat disease.

Parenteral nutrition
(Gr *para,* beyond, beside; *enteron,* intestine) Nourishment received not through the gastrointestinal tract but rather by an alternate route such as injection into a vein; intravenous feeding of elemental nutrients.

TABLE 8-8 *Suggested Members of Health-Care Team to Guide Adolescents in Issues Arising in Pregnancy*

Issues	Obstetrician	Adolescent Medical Specialist	Nurse	Nutritionist	Social Worker	Psychologist
			Discipline			
General health and planning of continuous care		×	×	×	×	
Complications of pregnancy	×	×	×	×		
Labor and delivery preparation	×	×	×			
School program					×	×
Economic resources			×		×	
Substance abuse (cessation and education)		×	×	×	×	×
Psychologic adjustment and stress	×	×	×	×	×	×
Developmental delay			×		×	×
Infant-care education		×	×	×		
Relinquishment counseling			×		×	×
Nutritional care		×	×	×		
Education		×	×	×		
Resource coordination			×	×	×	
Family or marital conflict					×	×

problems are the responsibility of any one profession to the exclusion of others. Each professional team member can support and reinforce the messages and guidance provided by other team members. Team conferences aid in coordination of care and team efficiency in meeting identified needs and noting the client's progress in solving various problems. Nutritionists and other professionals who are in positions to influence program planning can help develop clinical teams for the care of adolescents.

EATING DISORDERS

Although recent precise figures are not available, as many as 30% of American teenagers are said to be obese. The number with diagnosed anorexia nervosa or bulimia is growing, and many adolescents with eating disorders remain undiagnosed and untreated. Because these disorders are so common among adolescents, health professionals interested in adolescent nutrition must understand them. Eating disorders provide good models for study of other adolescent nutrition problems and their treatment. Therefore, it is valuable to study these disorders in depth.

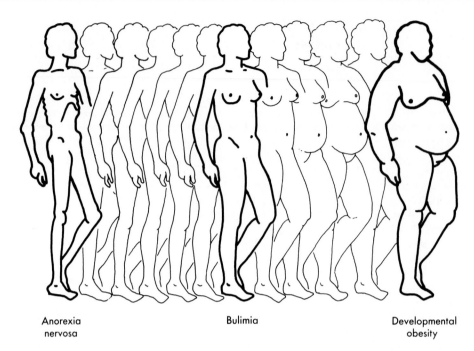

Anorexia
nervosa

Bulimia

Developmental
obesity

FIG. 8-7   The spectrum of eating disorders. Although physical conditions vary, underlying psychologic characteristics are held in common across the spectrum.

Spectrum of Eating Disorders in Adolescence

Common characteristics. Eating disorders can best be studied when the physical symptoms are viewed as a spectrum, with developmental obesity at one end and anorexia nervosa at the other (Fig. 8-7). In between are persons at normal and abnormal weights. Along the spectrum these persons hold in common basic underlying psychologic problems that interfere to varying degrees with normal functioning. In developing responses to life, these persons often use food inappropriately. Food-related behaviors and the resulting deviation in weight, the two most obvious aspects of these disorders, are usually the main focus of attention of the person affected, the public, and often the health professional. It is the underlying neurophysical and psychodevelopmental mechanisms, however, that are the essential features of more fundamental study needed by clinicians who are treating the disorders.

Rapid adolescent growth and body image. Because of rapid physical growth and body-image development in adolescence, eating disorders are of special concern at this stage of life. These changes intensify associated self-esteem problems. Anorexia nervosa, for example, is a disorder so tied to body image distortion that it is most commonly seen in adolescence, the period when a person is struggling with self-identity and is most vulnerable to body image problems. Progress in adopting a normal adult body image will be interrupted for the teenager with an eating disorder. Bruch and others have provided classic descriptions of distorted body images in both anorexic and obese adolescents.[14]

Autonomy
(Gr *autos*, self; *nomos*, law) State of functioning independently; self-determination.

Developmental tasks. Teenagers with severe eating disorders fail in varying degrees to accomplish the development tasks of adolescence. The development problems of these persons are summarized in the box on p. 305. The most striking of their problems is failure to develop **autonomy**.

Developmental Problems Associated with Eating Disorders in Adolescents

Inability to develop and use formal operational thought processes, especially in reference to themselves

Inability to experience bodily sensations originating within themselves as "normal" and "valid"

Unrealistic perceptions of body size

Preoccupation with weight and food, reflecting dependence on social opinion and judgment

Failure to normalize eating and exercise patterns

Unrealistic expectations for themselves

Failure to develop autonomy

Difficulty in accomplishing the normal tasks of adolescence

Based on Bruch H: Eating disorders, New York, 1973, Basic Books, Inc.

Family interaction. In recent years studies of factors contributing to the origin of eating disorders have turned to the structure and interaction of the adolescent's family. Although obese teenagers are a much less homogeneous group than anorexic persons, the family patterns have much in common. Minuchin has described such families as being psychotic.[15] These families are **enmeshed,** rigid, and overprotective with a low tolerance for conflict.

Enmeshed
To catch, as in a net, and entangle; intertwined family relationships that capture and diminish individual autonomy or self-regard.

Multifaceted origin. Eating disorders are very complex and may have developed throughout life or appear in the chaotic time of change that is adolescence. Individual and familial, biologic, and psychologic characteristics influenced by the modern social milieu contribute to their origin.

ANOREXIA NERVOSA
Symptoms

The term anorexia nervosa is actually a misnomer.[14] The implication that affected persons have a lack of appetite has been shown to be invalid. Superficially, the motivation to be thin keeps the person with anorexia nervosa from eating.[15] In over 100 years of description in the literature, however, a combination of symptoms has come to be recognized as characteristic of the disorder. Although certain of these symptoms may be seen in other disorders, the combination is unique in **anorexia nervosa.** This unique combination of symptoms has been defined by the American Psychiatric Association[16] as follows:

Anorexia nervosa
(Gr *anorektos*, without appetite; L *nervosa*, nervous or emotional disorder) A severe psychophysiologic eating disorder, usually seen in girls and young women, in which the person does not lack appetite, as the label would indicate, but is psychologically unable to eat and refuses food, becoming extremely emaciated; a form of self-starvation.

- Refusal to maintain body weight over minimal normal for age and height: Loss or failure to gain with maintenance 15% below expected
- Fear of gaining weight or becoming fat though underweight
- Disturbance in body weight, size, or shape perception: Feels fat or that body parts are fat though underweight
- Absence of three consecutive menstrual cycles

The above criteria focus more on physical symptoms at the crisis stage than on the underlying psychologic symptoms. Recognition of the psychologic symptoms, however, is of equal importance. The principal psychologic features of anorexia nervosa are "a relentless pursuit of thinness" and "a misuse of the eating function in efforts to solve or camouflage problems that otherwise would appear insolvable," that is, problems resulting from arrested normal development.[14]

Incidence

The majority of persons with anorexia nervosa are adolescents, although it has been seen in other age groups. About 10% of young women are thought to be affected. The disorder has not been commonly seen in males; only 5% to 10% of anorexic teenagers are male. Males who develop the disorder appear to experience anorexia nervosa in essentially the same form as females. Because of the predominance of females in the population seen with anorexia nervosa, the feminine pronoun will be used in this discussion.

Anorexia nervosa occurs predominantly in affluent classes and nations and is supported by a cultural paradox in which food is abundant. Food is used lavishly for purposes other than survival, yet slimness is highly valued. These cultural values are strong internal messages that have great impact on a young adolescent who has not developed autonomy. The lack of a similar value on slimness in males probably accounts for the small number of males seen with the disorder, though the influence of rock stars and other celebrities with excessively thin bodies is beginning to impact the ideals of young males.

Etiology

Theories about the etiology of anorexia nervosa have evolved from the initial psychoanalytic idea that the disease stemmed from an inability to deal with innate sexual drives; through periods when it was ascribed to endocrine deficits and then disturbed patterns of family interaction; to the present when a combination of these biologic, psychologic, and social factors is thought to contribute to the development of the disorders.

Mother-daughter relationship. Bruch's work was the first to incorporate a broader focus than simply the patient and her symptoms.[14] An interaction pattern prevails in which the mother misperceives the needs of her child from infancy on or the child fails to express her needs clearly. In any case the child acquiesces to the mother's misguided ministrations. During the period of infancy and childhood, the daughter is so controlled by her mother that she does not develop a true sense of self as distinguished from mother.

Effect of adolescence. As adolescence approaches, the body develops and demands for decisions and performance in many areas increase. The teenager panics at her lack of ability to cope independently. She develops rituals related to eating in an effort to be thin and "good." To gain her "independence," the teenager regresses to the period when independence ordinarily begins. In this early stage the principal way of demonstrating growing independence is eating behavior.

Family system. Minuchin's more recent approach describes how not only relationships with the mother but also interrelationships within the family system foster anorexia nervosa.[15] If family members are enmeshed in a system that does not allow development of appropriate roles, the system can produce a variety of psychosomatic problems. The particular direction toward anorexia nervosa may be determined when the main themes of family interaction are related to food, fitness, and appearance.

Biochemical process. The possibility that a biochemical process may be responsible for development of anorexia nervosa continues to be investigated. Although various mechanisms have been proposed, so far none has shown to be primary or causative. These mechanisms appear to result from psychologic stress, malnutrition, and starvation. The fact that patients and their families fit such characteristic and complex patterns would raise doubt that a single primary physiologic cause exists in most cases. However, it may be found that biochemical factors contribute to development of the disorder.

Psychologic State

The physical manifestations of anorexia nervosa may be sudden, although unrecognized underlying characteristics may have been present previously. Intervention strategies must address both the psychologic and physiologic states of the patient.

Progressive development. From the family's point of view, the anorexic teenager is usually a "model child" until she begins to develop a compulsive attitude about her weight. She has fit into the family unit and met their high expectations. She has worked extremely hard at school, being satisfied with nothing less than excellent grades.

Suddenly the whole family erupts in conflict over her eating behavior. The teenager herself has become troubled about her role in life. She is unable to sustain peer friendships and she is very anxious about relationships with males. She is confused by the need to establish more adult behavior patterns and clings to the rigid standards of childhood. She isolates herself. Life appears to be out of her control. She has conflicting feelings about living as her parents direct, is hurt by their critical comments, and begins to realize that she must assert herself. She takes a stand and will not compromise on her eating and exercise habits. She feels that she is too fat and must be slim to prove that she is a worthy person. She is increasingly preoccupied with her rituals and is angry when her family interferes. She denies her illness.

Distorted perceptions. A wide range of distorted perceptions have been noted, related specifically to body size, sex, hunger, rest, satiety, body temperature, pleasure, control, and to "feeling states" in general. The anorexic teenager has often been described as wishing to stave off adulthood. But the question remains as to whether she wishes to avoid maturation or whether maturation eludes her.

Family problems. Although most families with anorexic teenagers would describe themselves as normal and without problems until the manifestations of anorexia nervosa, these families often have a multitude of problems. The parents may have been dominating and intrusive. They may have overlooked the actual (including nutritional) needs and emotions of their children, even in times when the children have been ill. By adopting a "helpless" stance, the affected children may be thoroughly manipulative and involved in their parents' conflicts. Both parents and children become locked into a system where problems go unresolved and responses are stereotyped.[15]

Physiologic State

In the initial stage of anorexia nervosa, physical symptoms are related to weight, diet, exercise, menses, and nutritional status.

Weight. In some cases the anorexic teenager is overweight when the disorder begins. The anorexic young woman is typically hypersensitive to developing breasts and hips. These young patients often recall a chance statement about their needing to lose weight by a relative or close friend, or a weight reduction plan suggested by a health professional, as the trigger for their initial weight loss behavior.

Diet. The anorexic adolescent usually develops a personal philosophy about her diet, limiting herself by eating food only from certain categories and in certain ways. She may manipulate the fluid or sodium content of her intake. In addition, she may force herself to vomit and misuse laxatives or diuretics to rid herself of food energy and weight. Vomiting may follow episodes of gorging.

Exercise. Exercise rituals are equally varied. Anorexic teenagers include excessive calisthenics and other strenuous activities in their schedules. They may limit rest and use stimulants. They are so frequently involved in junior and senior high school athletics and dancing that coaches and teachers should be educated about the disorder. Good coaches should recognize which of their students may be exercising to their detriment by compulsively training beyond reasonable endurance while losing weight at a rapid rate.

Menses. Although a young woman in a state of starvation would be expected to become amenorrheic, indications are that cessation of the menses occurs in most patients with anorexia nervosa before they have lost sufficient weight and body fat to cause an interruption of the cycle, and lasts beyond the time they have regained weight and body fat.[17,18]

Psychologic factors probably contribute to the problem, as well as hormonal disturbances, since stressful states are known to interfere with the endocrine system regulating the menstrual cycle.

Nutritional status. During the initial phase of an anorexic teenager's energy restriction, the body does not exhibit the effects of malnutrition to a measurable degree other than to decrease in weight. Infections are not generally seen. Deficiencies in specific nutrients have not been reported, but they may exist subclinically depending on the food habits of the individual. If weight loss continues unchecked, however, the symptoms of severe starvation may become apparent and additional nutritional problems listed in the box on p. 305 begin to undermine basic health. This state indicates an onset of a crisis.

Intervention Strategies

Initial intervention strategies include early recognition of symptoms, psychotherapy, and nutritional support.

Early recognition of symptoms. A recognition of the developing symptoms is the most important early intervention strategy. A **protocol** for assessing anorexia nervosa and bulimia is provided in Table 8-9. Friends, school personnel, family, and health professionals are among those who observe the growing problems and can take steps to initiate treatment.

Psychotherapy. Individual and family psychotherapy by experienced therapists will enable both the affected adolescent and her family to adopt more appropriate roles. It will also help the anorexic teenager to complete the psychologic developmental processes that have been arrested.[14]

Nutritional support. Other than general monitoring of the height and weight, it may not be necessary to treat the patient physically at this stage. Refocusing her attention on the primary emotional and interactional problems rather than the power struggle over food and exercise patterns will often enable the patient to abandon her compulsive striving for thinness. The patient should have access to a professional who can answer her questions about nutrition and make sure that she has the information she needs to begin to regulate her eating patterns to meet her physical needs. Information should be given in the context of the adolescent's desire to change rather than imposed as a rigid system of dietary planning by a professional. The overall disorder should not be defined as solely a nutritional problem, although nutrition counseling is an important component of therapy.

Crisis Stage: Psychologic State

Overall, a lack of progress toward positive family interaction patterns during the initial therapy or continuing avoidance of intervention will often lead to physical and mental deterioration. When the crisis stage of anorexia nervosa develops, severe psychologic and physiologic symptoms appear and intervention must be directed toward the deteriorating condition.

Psychologic effects of starvation. The anorexic teenager in crisis can cause panic in family, friends, and professionals. The family generally sees the adolescent's bizarre eating behavior as the problem and fails to understand the extent of developmental and interactional patterns. As a result, they often seek treatment that does not demand their involvement with the patient in therapy. As she becomes truly **cachectic,** the psychologic changes inherent in starvation, described by Keys in his classic studies, become evident[17]:

- Cognitive processes center around food. Thoughts of food intrude constantly; the major part of the waking hours are spent in contemplating it.
- Behavior around food includes toying with it and hoarding, especially during renourishment.

Protocol

(Gr *protokollon,* leaf or tag attached to a rolled papyrus manuscript containing notes as to its contents) A set of governing rules; the plan and procedures for carrying out a scientific study or a person's treatment regimen.

Cachexia

(Gr *kakos,* bad, ill; *hexia,* habit) A profound and grave state of body disorder and deterioration, as seen in cases of advanced malignant disease or starvation, causing gross body weight loss to cadaverous proportions as a result of disordered metabolism.

TABLE 8-9   *Issues to Address in a Clinical Assessment of Eating Disorder*

Motivation
Appropriateness of weight goals
Desire to change unhealthful habits
Insight into problem

Emotional/psychological status
Depression
Locus of control
Body image
Self-esteem
Oral expression
Coping skills
Compulsivity
Perfectionism
Independence

Mental function
Intellectual ability
School performance
Attitude toward school
Ability to articulate

Family characteristics
Eating disorders
Other diseases
Natural or other parent
Intrusiveness
Enmeshment
Rigidity
Conflict resolution
Role of food
Exercise patterns
Perceptions of problem
Attempts to intervene
Willingness to participate in
  therapy

Social relationships
Friends
Social habits
Social skills
Attitude of peers

Eating behavior
Knowledge/acknowledgment of nutritional
  needs
Meal pattern
Bizarre eating habits
Personal philosophy toward eating
Nutritional adequacy
Control over food supply

Physical status
Signs of bulimia
Signs of starvation
Terminal signs of starvation
Thyroid status (obesity)
Resting heart rate (HR)
Exercise to reach 60% maximum HR

Growth and adiposity
Weight/height/age percentile
Triceps skinfold/age percentile
Arm muscle area/age percentile
Weight/height history
Growth velocity
Maturational stage
Age

Physical activity
Exercise patterns
Hobbies/interests
Personal feeling about exercise

- Coherent creative thinking is impaired.
- Mental function is characterized by apathy, dullness, exhaustion, and depression.
- Interest in sexual function is lacking.

These effects of starvation are superimposed on the anorexic teenager's already disturbed psychologic state. The behavior pattern, distorted perceptions, and weight phobia become more pronounced.

Behavior pattern. Many patients resist what they see as intrusions by professionals. They are secretive and protect the fact that they are carrying out their rituals. Their behavior may otherwise reflect the apathy typically seen in starving people. In obsessional preoccupation they plan menus, read recipes, cook and serve food to others, cut or manipulate food before eating it, and record all that they eat. They usually have a detailed knowledge

Cheilosis

(Gr *cheilos,* lip) A general symptom of tissue inflammation and breakdown producing swelling and reddening of the lips, a chapped appearance, and fissures at the corners of the mouth; associated with general malnutrition, especially a deficiency of riboflavin.

Hirsutism

(L *hirsutus,* shaggy hair) A condition marked by abundant and excessive hair; abnormal hairiness, especially an adult male pattern of body hair distribution in women.

Alopecia

(Gr *alopekia,* disease in which hair falls out) Baldness; absence of hair from skin areas where it normally is present.

Acrocyanosis

(Gr *akron,* extremity; *kyanos,* blue) Condition due to excessive concentration of reduced hemoglobin in the blood, resulting in arterial unsaturation with oxygen; characterized by cyanosis of extremities with persistent mottled blue or red discoloration of skin on fingers, wrists, toes, and ankles, accompanied by coldness of fingers and toes.

of the energy value of foods. When forced, they may pretend to eat and then hide and dispose of the food. The disturbed adolescent's fear of gaining weight becomes increasingly evident as her weight phobia intensifies.

Crisis Stage: Physiologic State

In the crisis stage of anorexia nervosa, the physiologic state deteriorates with physical signs of starvation, endocrine abnormalities, and undeniable signs of approaching terminal starvation.[19]

Physical signs of starvation. As the crisis stage develops, the individual is unable to take care of herself. The physical state of starvation is now superimposed on the other problems inherent in the disorder. These physical signs of starvation include:

Fat-store depletion	**Hirsutism**
Muscle wasting	Thin, dry, brittle hair
Amenorrhea	**Alopecia**
Cheilosis	Degradation of fingernails
Desquamation	**Acrocyanosis**
Dry skin	Postural hypotension

Additional nutritional problems. In addition to the clinical signs, recent research has focused on zinc nutriture, bone mineralization, growth failure, and structural changes in the brain, which result from severe long-term malnutrition in anorectic patients.[20,21] The possibility that bone demineralization, growth retardation, and brain structure may prove irreversible to some degree is especially troublesome and warrants further examination.[22-24] The relationship of depressive symptoms and sex role and body image distortion to lowered body weight, and the suggestion that less than the expected number of children are born to patients formerly diagnosed with anorexia nervosa are equally disturbing long-term effects of chronic malnutrition. These relationships have serious implications for dancers, gymnasts, and other athletes who keep themselves in a state of starvation, as well as for anoretics.[25-27]

Endocrine abnormalities. The endocrine abnormalities in anorexia nervosa are such that the body essentially reverts to a prepubertal hormonal state. As a result of hypothalamic change, the anorexic adolescent is amenorrheic, is unable to adapt to heat and cold, suffers sleep disturbances, and is unable to conserve body water. There is no interest in sex.

Terminal starvation signs. During the crisis, professionals must monitor the physical state of the patient and take remedial action when there are signs that starvation is approaching a terminal state. The most outstanding of these signs include:

- Fluid and electrolyte imbalance indicating inability of the body to maintain homeostasis (dehydration and edema)
- Severe cardiac abnormalities in the absence of electrolyte imbalances, indicating a wasted **myocardium**
- Absence of **ketone bodies** in the urine, indicating a lack of fat stores for metabolic fuel
- Concurrent infection, indicating increasing nutritional needs

Crisis Intervention Strategies

When the anorexic adolescent's condition reaches the crisis stage, hospitalization is necessary to provide comprehensive care involving nutritional therapy.

Hospitalization. For some clinicians, the decision to hospitalize an anorexic patient depends on her reaching a life-threatening physical state. However, if the goal is to renourish the individual so that she will be able to benefit from psychotherapy without semistarvation neurosis, as many authoritative therapists recommend, the anorexic patient must be hospitalized before a critical stage has been reached. The patient can be released from the hospital when she has been nutritionally rehabilitated, usually confirmed by reaching a particular weight-for-height goal (Fig. 8-8).

Comprehensive treatment. Nutritional components of therapeutic regimens for anorexia nervosa in crisis are intertwined with the psychologic aspects of the treatment, and team care is essential. Certain principles can be observed that will apply regardless of the treatment modality. Renourishment obviously will begin with a gradual increase in energy intake.

Diet therapy. In some programs the patient will be allowed to choose anything available on the hospital menu. Other programs impose rules, make additions to what is ordered, or serve a set menu. If a diet is prescribed following the principles established for renourishing malnourished individuals, it should have adequate protein to meet basic needs with additional energy made up of complex carbohydrates and a small amount of fat.

Nutritional supplements. If a patient refuses food, a nutritional supplement, which is prescribed and dispensed as a medicine, has been used. If a life-threatening state is reached at any time, with the patient refusing oral feeding, nourishment by nasogastric tube or parenteral methods may be necessary. These methods will be presented as life-saving procedures and not as punishment for refusing to eat. Nourishment by mouth is the preferred route and is possible in most cases.

Renourishment edema and body image. Edema generally appears with the renourishment and can be a problem because of the anorexic patient's phobia of weight gain. The edema is seen as proof to her that she will "expand" as she feared. Some anticipatory guidance can help her accept such development. Assurance that professionals will aid her in gaining appropriate weight, which is strengthening for her but not forming excess fat, can help desensitize the issue.

Role of the clinical nutritionist. The inclusion of a clinical nutritionist/dietitian on the therapeutic team gives attention to nutritional support care in a manner that does not subvert the psychotherapeutic goal of redirecting the focus of the patient's concern. The nutritionist's knowledge of energy balance as it applies to the individual is needed in determining appropriate weight goals throughout therapy and especially for termination of the hospitalization.

Long-Term Therapy

Psychologic state. The anorexic teenager who has recovered from a starvation crisis by gaining a certain amount of weight to improve her physical state will still have to deal with the developmental arrest that brought her to the crisis, a process that usually requires several years. There will continue to be problems concerning vocational choices and preparation, economic stability, relationships with peers and especially with the opposite sex, weight management, and body image.

Physiologic state. In the long term the anorexic young woman will often experience wide swings in weight from extreme thinness to obesity before she will be able to bring her life into control. She may see herself as somewhat detached from her body and experiment with various food habits before putting food into a more normal perspective. She may keep herself sufficiently thin that she will not resume her menses. She may feel bloated and have bouts of edema, physical responses to starvation and refeeding, and **carotenemia,** a symptom found in anorexia.

Intervention strategies. In the recovery period the psychotherapeutic goal will be to facilitate normal development in the anorexic teenager, to prepare her for a full adult role in society, and to enable her to function without depending on bizarre eating and exercise habits. She will need information and retraining about food and the physical aspects of

Carotenemia
Condition associated with excess intake or impaired metabolism of carotenoid pigments, especially beta-carotene, resulting in excess carotene in the blood, sometimes to the extent of producing yellowing of the skin resembling jaundice.

FIG. 8-8   A, Anorexic woman before treatment.

Courtesy Sycamore Hospital, a division of Kettering Medical Center, Dayton, Ohio.

life. Many of the techniques described in the section on obesity (p. 319) will be useful. Issues such as the state of nourishment necessary to maintain the menstrual cycle will resurface from time to time as development proceeds. Returning to such issues will enable her to deal more capably with them as time goes on. Guided food experiences in cafeterias, grocery stores, cooking, and entertaining help ready the person for managing food in her environment. The objective is to help the individual put food in a reasonable perspective and give up overfocusing on food out of ignorance. A team consisting of medical, psychologic, and nutrition specialists may provide care, or the care may be left to a single therapist who will be responsible for all aspects of therapy in consultation with other team members.

Outcome. Common features of anorexia nervosa are the strong resistance to treatment and the high incidence of relapse and partial recovery. Some of these patients will manifest varying degrees of the anorexic symptoms in adulthood. Though follow-up criteria have been inconsistently used by researchers, results reported to date indicate that in spite of the fact that weight-for-height proportion improved in about 75% of the patients, menstrual cycles were often unsatisfactorily maintained, ideas about food and weight were disturbed, and psychosocial maladjustment was common.

FIG. 8-8, cont'd **B,** Same patient after *gradual* refeeding, nutritional management, and psychologic therapy.

BULIMIA

First called bulimarexia, **bulimia nervosa** is the most recently recognized eating disorder and is characterized by gorging followed by self-induced vomiting or diarrhea. Although these symptoms may be a part of anorexia nervosa, they also comprise a separate syndrome.

Symptoms

The person suffering from bulimia generally maintains close to normal weight (Fig. 8-7), while gorging (bingeing, eating abnormally large amounts of food) and vomiting or purging (forcing bowels to empty) on a regular basis. The bulimic teenager may have somewhat less severe distortions in body image and less restrictive weight goals than the adolescent with anorexia nervosa. She is often older at age of onset.

APA Criteria

The official diagnostic criteria established by the American Psychiatry Association (APA) includes the following behaviors[16]:

Bulimia nervosa

(L *bous,* ox; *limos,* hunger; *nervosa,* nervous or emotional condition) A psychophysiologic eating disorder, seen mainly in girls and young women, marked by alternate gorging on large amounts of food followed by self-induced vomiting and purging with laxatives; weight usually remains fairly stable at a normal amount.

- Recurrent episodes of binge eating, rapid consumption of a large amount of food in a discrete period
- Lack of control over binges
- Regular self-induced vomiting, use of laxatives or diuretics, strict dieting or fasting, or vigorous exercise
- Average of two binge-eating episodes a week for at least 3 months
- Overconcern with body shape and weight

Incidence

The syndrome of bulimia should be differentiated from the recent behavior of many normal adolescent females who occasionally use self-induced vomiting as a means of controlling weight.[28] As many as 20% of college-age females may engage in bulimic behaviors with an estimated 2% to 4% meeting the criteria for diagnosis of bulimia nervosa. A serious condition will be uncontrollable, and the psychologic features of the disorder will impair normal functioning. Bulimia sometimes develops after a serious bout with anorexia nervosa or obesity. The bulimic person is more likely to be fertile than the individual with anorexia nervosa. Therefore, certain young women will be bulimic during pregnancy.

Psychologic State

Separation anxiety is one of the important issues for the bulimic teenager. Her self-esteem is extremely low and is tied to her feelings about her body. She demonstrates excessive need for control and approval. She thinks of herself as physically unattractive, although she is well groomed and has a normally attractive physique. She develops guilt over her habits and her secret feelings of inadequacy. Superficially, she may be very responsible and keep a heavy social schedule. In reality she has few close friends and feels that no one really knows her. In contrast to the more rigid anorexic adolescent, the young woman with bulimia often demonstrates poor impulse control, abuses substances, and becomes easily enraged. By all accounts, the gorging, vomiting, and purging serve to release tension for the sufferers. However, the residual guilt brings renewed tension that perpetuates an uncontrolled cycle. Social isolation is also perpetuated because of the fear that the secret will be found out. If she is pregnant, the bulimic teenager may be committed to protecting the fetus but retain ideas that inhibit normal nourishment of herself, her fetus, and the child after birth.

Physiologic State

Food behavior. The bulimic teenager periodically eats large amounts of food and then voluntarily vomits and purges. Each person with bulimia defines what a binge is for herself. Because of distortions in thinking about food, as little as one doughnut may be thought of as a binge by one person while as much as an entire package of doughnuts may constitute a binge for another. As the duration of the habits extends, it becomes easier for her to vomit. Eventually, the vomiting is a nearly automatic response. In addition, she may take laxatives to purge herself of the energy she has ingested or use diuretics to remove body fluid.

Physical symptoms. As a result of these behaviors, physical symptoms of the bulimic adolescent will include:

- Damage to the teeth
- Irritation of the throat
- Esophageal inflammation (all of the above symptoms from exposure of unprotected tissues to acidic vomitus)
- Swollen salivary glands (from acidic reflux or constant stimulation)

- Broken blood vessels in face (from force of vomiting)
- Cracked, damaged lips
- Rectal bleeding (from overuse of laxatives)

Life-threatening situations are more rare than in anorexia nervosa. They are:

- Dehydration, electrolyte imbalance
- Fistulas or ruptures in upper gastrointestinal tract
- Kidney damage

Concerns during pregnancy are the adverse biochemical environment for the mother and fetus, the mother's abnormal weight gain pattern (weight loss, lack of weight gain, inordinate gain), and the mother's unrealistic ideas about infant feeding.

Intervention Strategies

The techniques most frequently reported in treating bulimia are similar to those used in the long-term recovery period of the person with anorexia nervosa (p. 308). Psychotherapy, nutritional therapy, and care of any pregnancy that may occur must be included.

Psychotherapy. The emphasis of therapy is on freeing the person from guilt, facilitating gains in self-esteem, and helping her deal with anxiety as well as challenging distorted goal-setting based on perfection. Ideally, the young woman's family or partner will be included in the therapy.

Nutritional therapy. While she deals with the psychologic problem, the bulimic individual will still have an eating disorder and will need reeducation to nourish herself properly. Physical and nutritional education can fill gaps in knowledge these teenagers have about their body functions. Over time, myths about weight management can be dispelled and more normal eating habits developed. Because of distorted feelings about food, the bulimic person may feel guilty every time she eats, despite the fact that food is necessary for life. The family often reinforces the guilt by a misguided overfocus on food, thinness, and the physical aspects of life. The bulimic teenager usually restricts her food intake to match the ideal plan she conceives for herself. Binges may thus arise from the natural need for adequate food and the desire for additional gratification.[28]

Role of clinical nutritionist. The clinical nutritionist on the professional team will help the young person with bulimia to see food in a more appropriate context and accept more realistic weight goals using the techniques described in the obesity section (p. 319). Helping her understand the physiologic processes of energy balance and nutrient functions as well as the effects of bingeing, vomiting, and purging as they affect her personally is especially useful. This education, however, must be done gradually in a counseling mode allowing time for alteration of her own rigid system of beliefs. Family and individual psychotherapy will continue concurrently, and it is necessary to deal with the underlying causes of the obsessional food behavior. Group therapy is also used.

Pregnancy care. The bulimic teenager who is pregnant can be helped to accept the idea that the baby she wants must be nourished. She can then be supported in learning to retain those foods that the fetus needs even if she cannot totally give up bingeing and vomiting. She should also be helped in learning to recognize natural hunger signals from her baby after he is born.

OBESITY

At the other end of the physical spectrum of eating disorders is the very obese teenager. Unlike anorexic adolescents, persons who are abnormally heavy do not fit into a homogeneous group and may be carrying excessive weight for a variety of reasons. Factors leading to obesity can be broadly divided into those that are psychologic and those that are physiologic. In any individual a combination of these factors may operate in the development and maintenance of obesity. Because of the cultural response to obesity, the adolescent whose obesity may be physiologically based will generally be subject to many of the same problems as those whose obesity is more psychologically based.

Psychologic Factors

Various psychologic factors are associated with adolescent obesity, whether it develops during earlier childhood or is related to more severe psychiatric disorders.

Developmental obesity. Bruch has described a form of obesity that primarily results from psychologic factors within the family.[14] Thus, it is termed developmental obesity. It is an eating disorder comparable to anorexia nervosa in that it originates in the early life of the child. The families of developmentally obese teenagers fit descriptions of the psychosomatic family. The family's attitudes and behavior thus stunt the child's psychologic development and serve as primary causes of the obesity. The obesity itself further inhibits normal development, and this in turn leads to maintenance or increase of body weight. The affected children are made to feel pressure, inappropriate responsibility, and specialness to an abnormal degree in family interactions. They become rigid, isolated, and enmeshed. They develop misperceptions about their basic physical needs and rely on coping skills based on **food abuse.** As obese teenagers, these persons may not develop their full potential as self-competent, well-functioning adults, but they are less likely to experience the complete developmental arrest that the anorexic teenager does.

Body image. The teenager who is overweight is vulnerable to body image disturbances. The type and extent of the disturbance depend on the length of time the person has been heavy, the amount of excessive weight carried, the person's sex, and the life situation surrounding the individual's unique development. For example, teenagers who have been heavy from childhood may react differently than those who have gained weight only during later adolescence. Like anorexic teenagers, many tie thoughts of success or failure to their weight status.

Associated psychologic disorders. In some teenagers, obesity may be associated with severe psychiatric disorders. In others, the overeating behavior may act as an emotionally stabilizing influence helping to maintain the person at a functioning level. Interference in such a situation without substantial support provided can cause the disintegration of the person into an anxious or depressed state.

Cultural and Family Influences

The abundance of food and lack of necessity to expend energy in our society make it very easy for children to gain unwanted weight. In families where food intake and exercise patterns are not appropriate for dealing with this situation, an overweight state can result without other specific psychologic or physiologic origins.

Behavior Patterns in Obese Teenagers

The usual overweight or obese teenager is passive in interactions with others and with the environment. This response further reinforces the weight problem and leads to social isolation, lack of exercise, and disturbed patterns of eating and family interaction.

Social isolation. The passive response pattern of the obese adolescent in contact with others creates social isolation and an increased dependence on the family for relationships, even though the family interaction patterns may be unpleasant and the parents constantly exhibit intrusive and negative attitudes. Adolescents often react to the stigma of obesity by adopting a stereotyped life style with a narrow range of activities.

Sedentary lifestyle. The eating and exercise functions in the lives of obese teenagers generally become distorted. They may never feel comfortable eating in social situations. Their isolation leads them to opt out of many activities that would expend energy. They

Food abuse
Misuse and excess eating of food as a reflection of underlying personal needs or problems, rather than in normal quantity and nature as an essential part of good health and enjoyment.

fear being seen wearing gym clothes or swim suits or doing physical activities because they feel they are the object of attention and even ridicule. Instead they usually spend an inordinate amount of time in passive pursuits such as watching television or reading. Both of these activities may be paired with eating. Commercial television, especially, fosters this behavior with frequent food-related cues.

Eating patterns. Although many studies of teenagers after they have become obese have shown that on the average they eat no more, and sometimes less, than their normal weight peers, they often have disturbed unstructured patterns of eating. They may eat only in the latter part of the day, feeling nausea when eating earlier, and eat rapidly and indiscriminately.

Family patterns. Parents in some families may be locked into power struggles with their children, attempting in vain to control what they eat. Overanxiety regarding even slight overweight may actually contribute to growing obesity. In other families overeating may be the main theme with most interactions revolving around food.

Physiologic Factors

In certain individuals physiologic factors are principally responsible for their obesity. These factors are summarized in Table 8-10. Two of these underlying factors deserve note here.

TABLE 8-10   *Processes Leading to and Sustaining Obesity: Therapeutic Implications*

Process	Therapeutic Implications
Genetic predisposition Certain inherited biochemical, morphologic, and histologic features foster excess storage of energy as fat.	Teach individual to control energy intake and output and to exert any possible control; emphasize the need to be vigilant even if unable to avoid being greater than normal size.
Sodium pump activity Less activity in cells of obese individuals decreases energy usage, making more energy available for storage.	No direct intervention; not known if process is reversible.
Body temperature differences Defect in regulation with failure to maintain normal core temperature by obese individuals increases energy available for storage.	As above.
Adipose tissue lipoprotein lipase activity Rate-limiting enzyme in triglyceride storage is more active in the obese individual, enhancing adipose tissue synthesis.	As above.
Brown adipose tissue activity Responsible for increased facultative thermoclines in animals; also being investigated in humans to no avail so far.	

Continued.

TABLE 8-10 *Processes Leading to and Sustaining Obesity: Therapeutic Implications—cont'd*

Process	Therapeutic Implications
Insulin resistance Obese bodies are less sensitive to insulin. Resulting hyperinsulinemia tends to maintain obese state.	Exercise improves sensitivity to insulin even without weight loss; insulin resistance is also reversible with weight loss.
Thermogenesis Less energy is spent in obligatory (food processing) or facultative (response to sympathetic nervous system) thermoclines in obese individuals.	Complex carbohydrate increases obligatory thermoclines in some individuals; timing exercise before or after meals increases facultative thermoclines in some.
Adipocyte hypertrophy When energy is available for storage, fat cells enlarge.	Decrease energy available by changing intake/output. Cell size is reduced with energy deficit.
Adipocyte hyperplasia When fat cells are filled, new cells will be formed if energy continues to be available for storage.	Already obese individuals can decrease energy available to prevent formation of even more cells. Cell number does not decrease even with energy deficit.
Regional distribution of adipose tissue Typically, males have more central (abdominal) adipose tissue with higher waist/hip ratios than females who have more peripheral (femoral and gluteal) fat with lower waist/hip ratios. Male distribution is associated with diabetes, hypertension, and cardiovascular disease; female distribution is more difficult to change. Difference in cell size and lipoprotein lipase activity in various sites may be important.	Assessing waist/hip ratio helps determine difficulty of achieving weight loss and the harm in remaining obese.
Set point weight Bodies of certain individuals defend high body weights. Others defend low weights or no particular weight.	Decrease excess energy through exercise and substituting complex carbohydrates for fat, so as to reverse any processes that are reversible. If obese adolescents have control of energy intake and output, psychologic support for physiologically sustainable weight is reasonable.

Set-point theory. One theory that cannot be overlooked is that certain individuals may be subject to a body weight "set-point." A certain body weight may be physiologically normal for each person, and body characteristics may be tuned to keep the body at that weight.

Lower basal energy need. A decreased requirement for the amount of energy used in biochemical reactions may increase the amount of energy available in the systems of some people for storage as fat. Based on present theory, the longer the teenager has been obese and the greater the extent of the obesity, the greater the effect of these factors. The adolescent whose obesity was originally caused by other factors such as social, psychologic, or family influences will, as time passes, have added problems of physiologic obesity. This pattern increases the complexity of the obese state.

Intervention Strategies

An effective program for working with obese teenagers and their families will provide personalized care, giving attention to identifying individual needs and attitudes, setting realistic goals, developing related strategies within a comprehensive approach (see box on p. 320), and evaluating outcome.

Assessment. The individual combination of psychologic and physiologic circumstances by which an individual teenager has become obese must be identified so that intervention can be directed toward specific aspects of the problem. The degree of overweight must be considered. The material in the assessment section (p. 299), especially Fig. 8-6, may be used to evaluate the size of heavy adolescents. Generally they will be (1) *overweight,* only moderately above weight-height midranges for health; (2) *obese,* about 20% or more above normal weight-height ranges with a higher degree of fatness; and (3) *morbidly obese,* much higher weight for height and a greater amount of fat tissue, associated with multiple health problems. Some of these persons will suffer from hidden eating disorders such as bulimia or anorexia nervosa (recovery stage). The information needed to assess adolescent obesity (Table 8-11) may best be gathered by a team of professionals. Many of these aspects cannot be assessed immediately but will need to be explored over time. Basic initial steps assess physical status and personal attitude.

Physical status. A physical examination will disclose the stage of puberty and rule out any endocrine abnormalities or complications of the obese state. Endocrine disorders are rarely found. Most physiologic abnormalities indicated by clinical laboratory measures that are associated with obesity will respond to weight reduction.

Personal attitude. The most important aspect of initial evaluation is whether or not the individual is committed to making changes. The teenager's feelings must be assessed initially and at each visit. It is of no value for other persons to have goals related to weight management if the teenager is not ready to change the status quo. The question needs to be, "Are you ready to make changes?" rather than, "Do you want to lose weight?" Many teenagers will answer "yes" to the second question but remain totally passive, the implication being that the process of weight management for them is a passive one in which the professional administers treatment.

Reasons for not starting a weight loss program. A weight loss program should not be instituted if (1) the adolescent has not reached full height, (2) there is a lack of commitment, (3) it is likely to be another in a series of failures harmful to the individual's self-esteem, or (4) the individual is obviously predisposed to obesity by overwhelming physiologic factors. If obese teenagers keep fit, maintain energy equilibrium, and are emotionally healthy, they will be candidates for weight loss only if they understand the physiologic aspects of obesity and are determined to test these aspects in a healthful manner. Those adolescents who are still growing in height should not be encouraged to lose weight because the level of energy restriction required to do so is inadequate to support growth.

Text continued on p. 324.

ONE STEP FURTHER

Fitness: Testing and Planning Improvement Programs

1. a. Have client sit quietly and relax for 3 to 5 minutes.
   b. Take pulse for 10 seconds.*
   c. Record *resting heart rate (RHR):* _____
2. a. Find intensity of exercise required to reach *training heart rate (THR)*† immediately after exercise. THR for teens is 20 to 22 beats/10 sec.‡
   Stop with the exercise that achieves 20 to 22 beats/10 sec. This is the exercise to use initially in the improvement program.

   Intensity increases →

	Run for 5 minutes
	Jog for 5 minutes
	Jog for 2 minutes—walk for 2 minutes—jog for 2 minutes
	Walk uphill or upstairs for 2 to 3 minutes
	Walk for 5 minutes at a more rapid pace
START	Walk for 5 minutes at a moderate pace

   b. Monitor pulse return toward RHR after each exercise level—it should be below 16 beats/10 sec by 5 minutes.

   _____ _____ _____ _____
   Immediate → 1 minute → 2 minutes → 5 minutes → . . .

3. *Improvement program:* To maintain THR for 15 minutes 4 to 5 days/week:
   a. Work with client to design an individualized program that is comfortable for him or her.
   b. Plan 5-minute warm-up—move at level below the level that maintains THR.
   c. Exercise at intensity that maintains THR.
   d. Five-minute cool down—back to warm-up speed—client should not sit or lie down immediately.
   e. Use a combination of exercise levels and types, if necessary.
   f. If the client is ill, he or she should begin after illness at lower intensity and return slowly to intensity achieved before illness.
4. a. Retest every 3 to 4 weeks.
   b. Increase intensity of exercise to maintain THR.
   c. Client can increase time spent doing the exercise by 5-minute increments, up to 30 minutes.
   d. When client has reached jogging level and maintained it for 6 to 8 weeks, increase THR to 22 to 25 beats/10 sec.
   e. Client can use any aerobic activities (for example, jogging, bicycling, skating, dancing) or combinations that the client prefers.

NOTE: Contraindications for testing and initiating fitness program will be revealed by routine medical history and physical examination.
* 10-second time segment is easiest to measure and use.
† *Maximum heart rate (MHR)* is approximately 200 beats/min for persons under 20 years of age (Cumming GR, Everatt D, and Hastman L: Am J Cardiol 41:69, 1978). THR is 60% of MHR for persons with poor initial fitness, 75% of MHR for persons who are fit (that is, 60% of 200 = 120 beats/min = 20 beats/10 sec [20 to 22 beats/10 sec for normal variation]).
‡ An adolescent of normal weight and in reasonable shape may want to start at 22 to 25 beats/10 sec.
From Pipes PL: Nutrition in infancy and childhood, St Louis, 1981, Times Mirror/Mosby College Publishing; developed by Scott B and Rees J, Adolescent Program, University of Washington, Seattle, Wash.

TABLE 8-11* *Weight Management Assessment

Rate on Scale of 0 to 5 the Contribution to Weight Management
(0 = minimum, 5 = maximum)

	0	1	2	3	4	5

NOURISHMENT

1. Knowledge of
    Meaning of term "calories"
    Role of food in life
    Relationship of energy intake/output
    Major nutrients
        Physiologic role
        Energy value
        Amount needed
        Food sources
        Amount of food needed
    Choosing food in a variety of situations
    Behavior modification techniques
    Appropriate weight/height/age/genetic heritage

2. Attitude
    Acceptance of responsibility for nourishing self
    Commitment to health-promoting habits
        Obtaining appropriate foods
        Nutrition education

3. Eating behavior
    Control of food supply
        Fat content
        Types of food
        Amounts
        Meal pattern
        Between meal eating
        Binges/night eating/other aberrations
    Uses behavior modification techniques
    Eats in social situations
        With family
        Peers

4. Family
    Eating meals together
        Place
        Distractions (TV)
    Serving methods
    Support for weight control via
        Use of food
        Knowledge
        Autonomy allowed to patient to choose food

Continued.

TABLE 8-11 *Weight Management Assessment—cont'd*

	0	1	2	3	4	5

ENERGY TIME MANAGEMENT

1. Knowledge of
         Exercise in energy balance
         Fitness
               Cardiorespiratory
               Muscular
         Exercise
               Aerobic
               Anaerobic
         Monitoring pulse

2. Attitude
         Commitment to exercising regularly
               Without others, equipment, or money if necessary
         Interest in fitness education
         Pleasure in moving

3. Behavior
         Fitness tested
               Program planned
               Program maintained
         Level of fitness
         Relaxation
         Rest/sleep
         Activities shared
               With friends
               With family
         Consciously plans exercise/relaxation/rest

4. Family
         Support of activities
         Family activities
         Understanding of exercise in weight management

PSYCHOSOCIAL HEALTH

1. Knowledge of
         Emotional factors in weight management
         Cues to eat
               Internal
               External
         Impact on emotional health of
               Physical activity
               Nourishment
         Responsibility for weight management
         Need to seek guidance for unsolvable problems

TABLE 8-11 *Weight Management Assessment—cont'd*

	0	1	2	3	4	5
2. Attitude						
Commitment to mental health						
Learning about weight control						
Solving problems						
3. Behavior						
Pleasurable experiences						
Relationships						
Peers						
Family						
Teachers						
Counselors						
School activities						
Social skills						
Intellect						
Insight						
Communication						
Problem solving						
School performance						
Goal setting						
Short term						
Long term						
Self rewards						
4. Emotional Status						
Body image						
Self efficacy						
Locus of control						
Depression versus nondepression						
Sense of humor						
Oral gratification						
Coping skills						
Compulsivity						
Perfectionism						
Independence						
5. Parental						
Perception of weight problem						
Support versus intrusion						
Emotional						
Financial						
Rigidity						
Conflict resolution						
Commitment to treatment						

Continued.

TABLE 8-11 *Weight Management Assessment—cont'd*

OBJECTIVE

Age _____ yr

Length of obesity

	Infancy	Toddler	Early Child-hood	Elementary School	Senior High	Junior High
Reduction attempts	Yo-yo Anorexia	Severe Bulimia	Diets	Exercise	0	Reasonable
Parents	Natural Anorexia	Adoptive Bulimia	Obesity	Overweight		
Grandparents	Natural Anorexia	Adoptive Bulimia	Obesity	Overweight		
Maturation (stage)	0	1	2	3	4	5
Menarche	0	+1yr	+2yr	+3yr	+4yr	+5yr
Thyroid screen						

Cholesterol (mg/dl) _____   HDL mg/dl _____   LDL mg/dl _____

	Infancy	Toddler	Early Child-hood	Elementary School	Senior High	Junior High
Weight percentile*	>95	95	95-75	75	75-50	50
Height percentile*	95	90	75	50	25	10
Weight/Height	100-50 lb	50-25 lb				
percentile*	>95	>95	>95	95	95-75	75
BMI						
TSF percentile†	>95	95	95-75	75	75-50	50
SSF percentile† (male)	>95	95	95-75	75	75-50	50
MAC percentile†	>95	95	95-75	75	75-50	50
AMC percentile†	>95	95	95-75	75	75-50	50

Waist circumference _____ inches

Hips circumference _____ inches

Waist/hip ratio _____

BMI, body mass index (kg/m^2) >30 considered obese, 24-27 [females] and 25-27 [males] considered over-weight); TSF, triceps skinfold; SSF, subscapular skinfold; MAC, midarm circumference; RHR, resting heart rate; AMA, arm muscle area.

*National Center for Health Statistics: Height and weight of youths 12-17 years, United States. In Vital and health statistics, series 11, no 124, Health Services and Mental Health Administration, Washington, DC, 1973, US Government Printing Office. Above 75th percentile weight/height/age/sex considered obese if TSF also greater than 75th percentile; 25th-75th percentile weight/height/age/sex considered in normal range (Mahan LK and Rees JM: Nutrition in adolescents, St Louis, CV Mosby Co, 1984, p 51).

†Standards in Frisancho AR: Am J Clin Nutr 34:2540, 1981.

From Rees JM: Management of obesity in adolescence. In Farrow JA, editor: Adolescent medicine, Med Clin North Am 74:1285. Reprinted with permission.

Goals. Realistic planning of goals includes a series of short-term steps to the long-term goal.

    Short-term goals. Short-term goals need to be based not on changes in weight but on positive changes in food- and exercise-related attitudes and behaviors with appropriate rewards built in. It is especially necessary to build a program around short-term manageable goals related to behavioral change since physiologic factors may make actual weight loss

TABLE 8-11   *Weight Management Assessment—cont'd*

Exercise to reach 120 beats/min	Slow walk	Moderate walk	Fast walk	Walk up hill	Walk/ jog	Jog
Entry Date _____		+3 mo _____	+6 mo _____	+12 mo _____	+18 mo _____	+24 mo _____
Weight _____ lb	+10 _____					
	+5 _____					
	−2.5 _____					
	−5 _____					
	−10 _____					
	−15 _____					
Percent body fat _____	+3 _____					
	+2 _____					
	−2 _____					
	−5 _____					
RHR _____	+5 _____					
	+3 _____					
	−3 _____					
	−5 _____					
Height _____ inches	+3 _____					
	+2 _____					
	+1 _____					
AMA _____ mm²	+500 _____					
	+200 _____					
	+100 _____					
	−100 _____					
	−200 _____					

a difficult, long-term achievement. The teenager should be made aware that over the long term an energy deficit will eventually lead to weight loss, however slowly. Working toward improved knowledge, attitudes, or behaviors listed in Table 8-11 is a worthy short-term goal.

Weight goal. The initial weight goal in a weight management program is usually maintenance, that is, cessation of weight gain. In certain situations an even more basic change from rapid gain to slow gain is the more appropriate goal. Immature adolescents who have not completed linear growth can bring weight and, more specifically, percentage of body fat into better proportion with height by holding their weight stable or by reducing gains to a lower rate as height increases. This pattern eliminates nutritional risk to the individual from severe diet restrictions at a time of rapid growth and development. For teenagers who have stabilized their weight and are no longer gaining in height, the next step will be a slow steady loss based on reeducation in the use of energy. A loss of 0.9

kg/week (2 lb/week) should not be exceeded. If this rate appears insignificant to the teenager, point out that it would add up to more than a 45 kg (100 lb) loss over 1 year. Improvement in any of the physical measures of Table 8-11 constitutes achievement of a long-term goal.

Intervention Strategies: Physiologic Factors

Strategies planned to deal with the physiologic factors of obesity must be based on the laws of **energy exchange** and **balance,** address positive changes in personal food behaviors, avoid the dangers of "crash diets" and life-threatening situations, and increase physical activity and fitness.[29]

Basic individual energy balance. Whatever the reasons for a teenager being overweight, the method for altering the situation remains the same: decreasing the body's energy intake and increasing the energy output until the appropriate deficit state is established. There is no way of knowing the exact use of energy by a particular body except by testing it over time. To lose weight an energy deficit must be achieved at the cellular level. Because this state is not measurable under normal clinical circumstances, there is no set formula that assures weight loss. It is an error to count kilocalories of food energy being eaten and assume that this amount of energy will be available within the biochemical system. Thus a deficit of 3500 kilocalories calculated at the point of intake does not necessarily lead to a loss of 1 lb of body weight. This does not imply that the second law of **thermodynamics** is inoperative, but simply that energy from food may be used in a variety of ways once it is in the body, as indicated previously (Table 8-10). Thus both the physiologic and the psychologic aspects of weight management are unique to the individual.

Eating habits. Each individual teenager must be guided in learning the level of energy intake and output that produces weight gain, loss, and maintenance for them if the treatment is to be effective. An understanding of physiologic factors must be incorporated. The teenager must be made aware that however bleak the physiologic situation appears, the possibility of weight management has not been tested until the individual has control over energy intake and output. There is usually some potential for improvement in the diet that will help even those persons who are physiologically prone to obesity to become more fit and healthy, and to stabilize and perhaps to reduce their weight—in small amounts.

Dietary change. Strategies for dietary change must address the issues of (1) energy and nutrient content of the food intake; (2) circumstances of eating related to timing, place, accompanying social factors, and emotions; and (3) principles of nutrition regarding weight management.

Food use retraining. Specific diets have rarely achieved long-term changes in eating behavior. This result is especially true for teenagers, who tend to rebel against authoritarian techniques and hold a number of negative views about diets. Food use retraining, a series of habit changes planned jointly by the teenager and the therapist and instituted in succession over time, will be more acceptable to most adolescents and is a more realistic way to approach a complex problem.

Time factor. Because eating habits have been developed over a number of years, it is logical that the teenager will need considerable time to make changes. A person cannot suddenly pick up a musical instrument and play it well but will need education, practice, and support to become proficient. Similarly, most teenagers will not be able to learn a new food pattern or "diet" and perfect it immediately. Usually intensive treatment will need to be continued for a year or more to accomplish major dietary changes. Breaking down the problem of food misuse into small components makes change more probable.

Energy balance
Physiologic aspect of weight management, based on balance between energy intake in food and energy output in physical activity and internal metabolic work.

Laws of thermodynamics
(Gr *therme,* heat; *dynamis,* power) Basic three laws of physics relating to heat-energy balance: (1) energy like matter is neither created nor destroyed, only constantly transformed and recycled, thus conserving energy in any process; (2) there is always an increase in *entropy* (Gr *entrope,* a turning inward), a measure of the part of heat or other energy form in a system that is not available to perform work, thus entropy increases in all natural (spontaneous and irreversible) processes; and (3) absolute zero in energy balance is unattainable.

What habit will be the initial focus, how change will be accomplished, what foods will be eaten, and what motivations and rewards will be effective are developed and clarified in counseling sessions between the therapist and the teenager.

Therapy objective. The nutritional therapist's objective is eventually to focus on each time and point of day and environment where teenagers meet with food and to help them to retrain themselves in the use of food. Most teenagers will have some reasonable habits that can be supported and used as a foundation for the emerging positive patterns.

Self-responsibility. Teenagers will need help at every step to take responsibility for their actions. Coupled with psychologic support, the process can lead to effective change. Even those who are unsuccessful in retraining themselves during the adolescent period will have a model for the future, when they may be able to take greater control. Education regarding the physiologic factors of obesity will help teenagers avoid the harmful quick loss plans to which they are so vulnerable.

Dangers of "crash" diets. A very important component of programs in weight management education involves helping the teenager understand that rapid weight loss by either starvation or too low an energy intake is ineffective. Since the loss is in lean body mass and fluids, inevitably weight will be regained when usual eating is resumed, and muscle (and the ability to use energy) not fat will have been lost. The deprivation in such a regimen often leads to even greater overeating. Thus, the final result of a "crash" diet is often a net gain. It is not difficult to convince those who have had the experience a few times that such practices are ineffective, but it is important to support their impressions by teaching them the physiologic reasons. Teenagers who will not be convinced that such methods and "diet aids" are unhealthy will be deterred from using them by the knowledge that they will not lose *fat*.

Morbid obesity. There are certain life-threatening situations for very obese persons when drastic intervention will be necessary. The physical condition should be monitored to detect any rapid deterioration. The following conditions warrant hospitalization:

- Sudden changes in cardiac or respiratory function
- Inability to move, maintain balance, or travel
- Rapid weight increase because of the above factors
- Inability to fit into furniture and having to rest on floor
- Ulcerations at pressure points and friction areas

As with the anorexic teenager, a period of separation from the family may break up a pernicious cycle leading to physical deterioration. Comprehensive treatment using a modified fast as the dietary component is at present the most practical therapy. Although it is still controversial whether lean body mass can be spared, such dietary methods appear less objectionable than other radical procedures.

Physical activity and fitness. One of the most important concepts of weight management is that energy output must be increased. Individualized exercise programs need to be developed with the obese teenager in order to achieve a gradual increase in physical activity.

The fitness test shown in the box on p. 320 is designed to be a conservative tool that can safely be used with even an extremely obese person. It can be used with or without professional help. Physically, it appears that increasing activity can be rewarding in itself, whereas denying oneself an accustomed food may be more like punishment. Besides fitness testing and improvement, various strategies can be directed toward increasing energy output by increasing physical activity. These guidelines should be followed. Activities should (1) be built into everyday life, (2) be something the person enjoys or finds useful, (3) not depend on help from others or complex equipment, and (4) not be stressful by causing embarrassing exposure of the body or awkwardness.

Intervention Strategies: Psychologic Factors

Weight management for teenagers should be a total rehabilitation program. It demands a significant length of time and must be individualized. Like the physiologic component, the psychologic component of any weight management problem cannot be overlooked. Activities planned to meet these needs include motivational support, psychotherapy, and counseling.

Motivation. In a short-term situation where the teenager has only a few pounds to lose, the problem is one of motivation. This support can be provided in settings such as schools and many other community settings.

Psychotherapy. With extreme developmental obesity, changes usually require extensive psychotherapeutic intervention. This includes the family when the teenager is living at home.

Counseling. For teenagers falling between these two extremes, a variable degree of supportive counseling will be needed to increase self-acceptance, to decrease stress, to facilitate development, and to enable adolescents to carry out weight management strategies. Teenagers need help in learning to experience the body's signals related to hunger and satiety and to adopt nondestructive coping mechanisms to replace the misuse of food.

Comprehensive Approach

To provide a comprehensive approach to a weight management program for teenagers, attention must be given to additional resources available. These resources include group activities applied with professional guidance, parent education and counseling, and school and community support.

Group activities. Strategies such as camp settings, support groups, peer counseling, social skills and assertiveness training, body awareness experience, physical fitness training, and behavior modification can be used successfully with some individuals. Groups and preplanned programs will help those adolescents with mild, relatively simple problems. *Camps and other groups that provide only for short-term weight loss are detrimental and should be avoided.*

Professional guidance. None of the group settings, however, provide a solution for all aspects of obesity. To be effective, weight management techniques must be applied within the context of ongoing supportive counseling by professionals who assess the specific problems of the individual over time and choose appropriate treatment methods. A team of professionals will be best able to carry out a comprehensive program as described here.

Parent education and counseling. Counseling will enable parents to support their teenagers in learning to manage weight. Education about the physiologic factors involved and rational approaches to management will help dispel myths parents hold. Helping them develop a nonintrusive attitude toward their teenagers is of extreme importance. The counselor can demonstrate this by stressing the need for teenagers, not counselors or parents, to establish their own goals.

School and community support. Although they are rarely in the position to carry out therapy because of the complexity of the problem, teachers, school counselors, nurses, coaches, and other community leaders of adolescents have many opportunities to educate and support overweight teenagers. Curriculum materials such as those in Fig. 8-9 have been designed to help adolescents understand the complexity of weight management.

Outcome

Reviews of the outcome of weight management therapies for teenagers are uniformly gloomy. In general such programs are designed as studies of weight loss, when informed

BE SIZEWISE

Don't Lose
Your Balance

Nourishment	**Activities**	**Feelings**
Be good to your body—give it what it needs	Do interesting things—quiet as well as energetic	Learn to know and like yourself
Don't starve or stuff yourself	Take time to relax every day	Have realistic goals for yourself
Know what's in the food you eat	Don't let eating be your only recreation	Don't substitute food for love and companionship
	Do some strenuous activity every day	Build satisfying relationships with your family and friends
	Share active and quiet time with friends	Get help for problems you can't cope with alone

FIG. 8-9   Be sizewise—materials for clinicians, educators, and teenagers.
© American Heart Association of Washington.

workers in the field of adolescent health have stressed the importance of focusing on the other benefits of weight management programs such as increased self-esteem. Added knowledge, increased readiness to work for change, and improved practices are important outcomes of weight management programs for adolescents.

Summary—Eating Disorders

The spectrum of eating disorders affects adolescents physically, psychologically, personally, and socially. Intervention strategies must be directed toward both the nutritional and developmental aspects of these disorders to be effective. Goals must be established in relation to all aspects. Helping teenagers put food into reasonable perspective in their lives will be a principal goal of nutritional therapy. A recognition of the amount of time required for effective intervention is essential for a basic understanding of eating disorders.

PHYSICAL FITNESS AND ATHLETICS
Benefits of Physical Fitness

All teenagers should be encouraged to exercise in ways best suited to their lives. The exercised body is more likely to remain healthy than one that remains sedentary, because historically the human required great energy exchange to obtain food, protect itself, and to survive the elements. Physical activity has many benefits[30]:
- It helps maintain optimal body composition.
- It improves the possibility of weight loss when that is necessary.
- It increases the efficiency of muscle fibers to produce energy.
- It increases the efficiency of hormones (insulin, lipoprotein lipase, epinephrine) to regulate energy metabolism.

- It decreases the production of lactic acid, which interferes with energy production.
- It strengthens the heart, lungs, and circulatory system.
- It increases levels of HDL over LDL and decreases levels of some triglycerides.
- It raises rates of basal metabolism.
- It helps control appetite.

Lack of Fitness

Health care workers are increasingly called upon to help teenagers incorporate fitness into their lives as the energy requirements of modern life decrease.[31] Only about 50% of young people today are regularly involved in vigorous exercise. When tested, 30% of males and more than 50% of females 6 to 17 years of age cannot do one pull-up.[31]

Elements of Fitness

Each teenager should participate in activities that maintain the elements of fitness: body composition; cardiorespiratory function; and muscular strength, endurance, and flexibility. Raising the heart rate to at least 50% but no more than 75% of maximum for 15 minutes, with 5 minutes warm-up and cool-down, at least 3 days a week will maintain cardiorespiratory fitness. This process is incorporated in the testing and improvement protocol given here (see box on p. 320). The maximum heart rate of adolescents has been shown to be about 200. This number can be used until age 20, when the usual calculation for adults, substracting the age from 220 to derive the maximum heart rate, can begin. Stressful exercise is unnecessary and undesirable. Continuous gradual improvement and maintenance are effective. A few well-chosen calisthenics will maintain muscular strength, flexibility, and endurance. Adolescents who participate in sports as well as those who do not should develop personal programs to assure fitness is maintained between seasonal participation in organized programs.

Nutritional Requirements for Athletics

Adolescent athletes require specific nutritional support, primarily to maintain normal growth and physiologic maturation in spite of the physical stress. Energy is the basic factor in this process. The amount of additional energy needed will depend on the intensity, duration, and type of exercise being done.

Carbohydrate fuel
Basic organic carbon compound in food (starches and sugars) that is the primary and most efficient form of body fuel for energy, especially for building body muscles.

Sources of energy. Energy is best utilized if it is supplied as **carbohydrate.** An additional 6 to 7 g of protein per day is sufficient in a muscle building phase. Thereafter 2 to 3 g of protein per day above the daily recommended allowance will support body maintenance in most athletes. Abnormally high levels of protein are counterproductive, leading to dehydration as the body rids itself of nitrogenous waste products. The need for carbohydrate rather than protein as fuel to build muscle is one of the most misunderstood principles among adolescent athletes.

Weight management. Weight should be gained or lost following safe effective methods described here. To support normal growth successfully, weight should be maintained at an optimal level long term rather than be subjected to seasonal, or especially, weekly manipulation as is often urged by coaches of wrestling teams and crew teams during competition. The development pattern of skeletal growth and weight gain must be considered. Two problems in this area are common among teenage athletes who become too thin in trying to reduce the percentage of body fat: (1) females interrupt their menses, and (2) males stunt their **linear growth.** Anabolic steroids taken by males to increase weight cause stunting of growth and disturbed development of secondary sex characteristics.

Linear growth
(L *linearis,* a line) Linear measure of growing body length; height.

Supplements. An increased dietary intake should provide sufficient amounts of nutrients making supplements unnecessary. Supplementation of nutrients in amounts above those recommended has not resulted in benefits during competition. Of the vitamins and minerals, iron is particularly important to young athletes because "sports anemia" is associated with reduced oxygenation; the B vitamins are essential in energy production.[32]

Anabolic steroids. Many young adolescents (estimated at 5% to 10% by those studying the incidence) use **anabolic steroids.** Use is apparently greater among male athletes who say they use them to increase muscle, size, strength, speed, and to improve personal appearance and athletic performance. The research shows that young people who use these substances lack appropriate knowledge of the profound effects they have on the whole body.[33] Studies of the effects on adolescents are not available.

Short-term events. A light workout one day before competition, combined with increased dietary carbohydrate, mainly starches, will assure a supply of liver and muscle glycogen to support the athlete during a short-term event. On the day of competition eliminate roughage, fats, and gas-forming foods from the diet to decrease discomfort and untimely need for elimination. If several short-term events are held in one day, additional carbohydrate will provide energy. Otherwise stores should be sufficient. Fluid replacement follows the same principles given below for long-term events.

Long-term events. For longer events that last at least 1 hour, supplies of body fuel and fluids will need attention.

Body fuel stores. Modified **glycogen loading** before a long-term event will improve not only liver storage but also muscle reserves. Glucose can be taken after the event begins to spare liver glycogen stores, but it should not be ingested just before an event because it impairs lipid mobilization.

Fluids and electrolytes. Body fluid–electrolyte balance is very important during long-term events, indeed throughout athletic training and competition.[30] Exaggerated shifts in fluids and electrolytes due to strenuous exercise are intensified by environmental temperatures and the sweat of exertion. Water must be replaced at the level of 1 pint for each pound of body weight lost in any exercise or training session. Thus, fluid must be available to keep up with thirst during events and may have to be replaced at levels beyond thirst in the post-event period. Electrolytes and additional glucose can be obtained by using natural juices and fluids made with specified concentrations. The maximal sugar content for an efficient replacement drink is 2.0 to 2.5 g of sugar per decaliter. The need for replacing fluids will vary according to loss due to the event and climate. It is unnecessary for athletes trying to keep warm on the sidelines of a soccer game in a cold northern climate to drink electrolyte-rich fluids designed for sweat-inducing events in tropical conditions.

Overall nutritional goals. Maintaining appropriate weight for height is a good general guide to dietary adequacy as long as the foods eaten to attain that weight are nutrient rich. Obtaining sufficient food may prove difficult for teenage athletes whose days may be filled from early morning to late evening with practices as well as normal activities including classes and study assignments. Parents, coaches, and school officials need to support teenagers by helping them plan specifically to obtain adequate acceptable foods at times when rigorous schedules allow them to eat.

ADOLESCENT PREGNANCY
Developmental Issues

Teenage pregnancy must be studied in the light of the highly dynamic nature of adolescence. Both the psychologic and the physical status of the adolescent have implications for the course of any pregnancy. The many interactions of factors in adolescent

Anabolic steroids
(Gr *anabole,* a building or construction) Any of a group of synthetic derivatives of testosterone, the male sex hormone, having pronounced anabolic (tissue building) properties; a drug used in clinical medicine to promote growth and repair body tissues in debilitating illness. Widespread illegal abuse of the drug by some athletes and body builders harms health.

Glycogen loading
Practice among athletes in endurance events of increasing intake of complex carbohydrates in days before the event to increase glycogen storage for energy reserve fuel during the event.

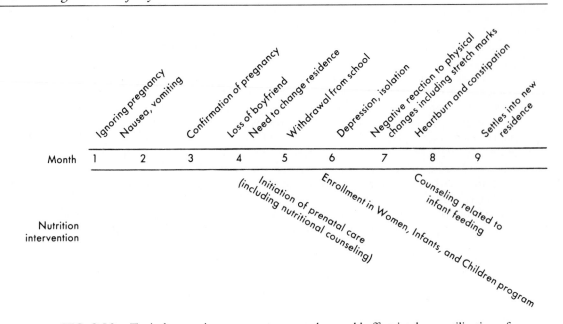

FIG. 8-10 Typical events in teenage pregnancy that could affect intake or utilization of nutrients.

development and in reproduction have great clinical significance for all aspects of the pregnancy, including the nutritional aspect.[34] Indeed, adolescents are changing so profoundly that pregnancy for the younger, less mature teenager will be different from that of the older, more mature adolescent.

Less mature teenagers will be more dependent on others and less able to act and make decisions on their own. They will be more **narcissistic** and less able to comprehend the needs of others. These young women will be less realistic, engage in more fantasy and wishful thinking, and have less insight into their own behaviors and motives. In general, younger teenagers will have fewer intellectual and physical skills to cope with any situation, especially a complex reproductive experience. Many of the difficulties related to pregnancy in adolescence stem from this immaturity. As development advances, a person is able to carry out reproduction and child rearing in a more normal, less problem-fraught way. As seen in Fig. 8-10, the timeline of events in teenage pregnancy has great potential for affecting the nutritional well-being of the adolescent.

Reproduction during Adolescence

The pregnant adolescent's nutritional needs are influenced by many factors. Primary influences are her growth and nutrient stores, her **gynecologic age,** and her preconception nutritional status.

Adolescent growth and nutrient stores. The assumption that pregnant adolescents need a supply of nutrients to support their own growth along with that of the growing fetus has been questioned. Because hormone levels are high in pregnancy, even the slower adolescent growth that usually follows menarche may not occur. According to recent studies growth does continue to some degree during adolescent pregnancy.[35] Whether or not actual growth continues for an adolescent who becomes pregnant, she will have

Narcissism

Self-love; drawn from Narcissus, a character in Greek mythology who saw his image mirrored in a pool of water and fell in love with his own reflection.

Gynecologic age

(Gr *gynaikos*, women) Length of time from onset of menses to present time of conception.

experienced rapid growth more recently than her adult counterparts. There will have been less opportunity for storage of nutrients. Thus, there may be greater physiologic risk to young women who conceive in the early years of menarche.

Gynecologic age. The number of years between the onset of menses and conception is calculated to derive the gynecologic age. Those adolescents who are more sexually mature, that is, of greater gynecologic age, share a vulnerability to physiologic stresses but appear to have no more physically based complications than do adult women. It is the young women of lower gynecologic age who carry more risk and need more nutritional support. The number of adolescents who become pregnant in the first 2 years following menarche will be relatively small because most of them will not be ovulating during that time even though they are menstruating. Those who do become pregnant, however, are of great concern to clinicians and researchers in this area.

Nutritional status at conception. Pregnant adolescents who are of young gynecologic age and malnourished at the time of conception are at double risk. They appear to have the greatest need for nutrients to support a pregnancy and maintain optimal health themselves.[36]

Hazards to the Mother

Given the complexity of pregnancy in the adolescent period, it is logical to question how these young women fare during pregnancy. They have more complications, a higher risk of maternal mortality, and more problems in personal psychologic development and education that carry implications for economic well-being.

Complications. The variety of complications often described for the teenage mother during gestation include:

- First and third trimester bleeding
- Anemia
- Difficult labor and delivery
- **Cephalopelvic disproportion**
- Pregnancy-induced hypertensive disorders including **preeclampsia** and eclampsia
- Infections

Of these complications, the most common physical problem is infection, while the most common serious complication is preeclampsia. Preeclampsia usually occurs in the third trimester and is manifested in increased weight gain, fluid retention, high blood pressure, and proteinuria; it does not appear to run a different course in pregnant teenagers than in older women. Some researchers point out that it is a disease of first pregnancies. By and large, data support this observation. In addition, the harmful effects of preeclampsia, or the more serious state of eclampsia, may be greater in teenagers. Damage to the cardiovascular and renal systems initiated with a first pregnancy early in life and intensified by insults such as other pregnancies can increase the risk of developing renal and cardiovascular problems with increasing age.

Maternal mortality. The serious burden of maternal mortality is also a problem. The rate is 2½ times greater for mothers under 15 years of age than for those 20 to 24 years of age.

Effect on normal developmental steps. Apart from the physical sequelae, pregnancy often affects teenagers' psychologic development, education, and ability to gain economic independence. Clearly these developmental steps are difficult to achieve in any case, and for many adolescents pregnancy is not a cause of failure but a coinciding event. The situations responsible for early pregnancy often remain unresolved, and many teenage mothers have additional pregnancies before the adolescent years are over.

Cephalopelvic disproportion
(Gr *kephale*, head; *pyelos*, an oblong trough, pelvis) Relationship of fetal head to size of the maternal pelvis.

Preeclampsia
(Gr *pre-*, before; *eklampein*, to shine forth) Abnormal condition of late pregnancy marked by rather sudden hypertension and increased edema, usually accompanied by proteinuria; may progress to more severe stage of eclampsia with convulsions and coma.

Hazards to the Infant

Infants born to teenage mothers suffer a higher incidence of morbidity and mortality in the perinatal period than infants of older mothers. Problems seen more frequently include[36]:

- Prematurity
- Stillbirth
- Low birth weight (the major hazard in adolescent pregnancy)
- Perinatal and infant deaths
- Physical deformities

It is difficult to compare the likelihood of these problems occurring in infants born to teenage versus older mothers, or to younger versus older teenage mothers. But it is generally agreed that the problems do occur in a considerable number of teenage pregnancies. For example, the incidence of low birth weight is far greater when the mothers are adolescent.

Weight Gain

Specific requirements. There is evidence that adolescents need to gain substantial weight during gestation to deliver optimal weight infants. Their infants will be somewhat smaller than the infants born to adult women with the same gestational weight gain.[37,38] For example, when adolescents gain from 26 to 35 lb, the incidence of low birth weight (under 2500 g, or 5.5 lb) is 6.3%, equivalent to the incidence for adult women who have gained 21 to 25 lb.[39] The incidence of fetal mortality and morbidity are thus linked to weight gain, because they are linked to low birth weight.

The continuing growth and development of the adolescent may account for the extra weight that is needed. Table 8-12 shows the amount of weight a young woman could be expected to gain in the 9 month period corresponding to her gynecologic age if she were not pregnant. That amount plus the amount she would have to gain to be normal weight for her height and age if she is underweight probably constitute the extra amount she will gain in pregnancy.[40] Some authors refute this idea, theorizing (1) that teenagers may retain extra weight following delivery if they gain more than adult women, and (2) that their infants may be small in a natural adaptation to the less mature maternal biologic state of the adolescent and therefore not at risk simply because their birth weights are lower.[41,42] Many questions about the gestational weight gain of adolescents remain to be answered by future research:

- Is delivery of an infant weighing 3000 to 4000 g between 39 and 41 weeks gestation an optimal outcome for adolescent as well as adult young women?

TABLE 8-12   *Approximate 9-Month Increments in Weight of Postmenarcheal Women*

Postmenarcheal Year	lb	kg
1	8	3.45
2	5	2.0
3	2	.90
4 and 5	1.32	.60

Data from Frisch RE: Hum Biol 48:353, 1976.

- Is weight gain controlled by the biologic make-up in adolescence so it would not be possible for a young woman to gain more weight even if it was well known that achieving a certain range of weight gain would allow her to deliver an optimal weight infant?
- If adolescent mothers retain larger amounts of body fat as a result of gaining at a higher rate than adult women, is the adverse effect to the mother of potentially retaining 5 lb extra, for example, more serious than the actual risk to an infant born at a lower than optimal birth weight after a pregnancy during which the adolescent mother gained less than optimal weight?

Rate of gain. The latest recommendations from the National Academy of Sciences suggests that, depending on their prepregnant weight status, women gain at the following rates in the last two trimesters of pregnancy:

Normal weight	.361-.529 (.440 average) kg/week
Underweight	.386-.588 (.490 average) kg/week
Overweight	.218-.386 (.300 average) kg/week

The committee recommended that adolescents gain at the upper end of these ranges, but felt there was not sufficient evidence to make separate recommendations for teenage mothers. Other recommendations of this report are discussed in Chapter 4.[43]

Evidence is accumulating to show that the average rate of gain by adolescents in the final trimesters of pregnancy are on the average above .500 kg/week. In one study a group of multiethnic adolescent mothers who delivered term infants with a mean birth weight of 3258 g (calculated from data given) gained at the rate of .505 to .531 kg/week (50th percentile) during the last 18 weeks of pregnancy. The 75th percentile was .692 to .893 kg/week.[44] To decrease the number of infants weighing less than optimal, the average rate would have to be greater. As it was, 5% of the term infants following relatively uncomplicated pregnancies weighed under 2500 g, in the category of high risk.

In summary, the evidence does not suggest that the natural gain of adolescents should be restricted to levels recommended for adult women. The upper limit of optimal needs to be established because some young women will need to exercise control in order not to gain in excess of that needed to improve infant size at birth.

Assessment and Management of Nutrition

Risk factors. In order that nutrition services can be provided efficiently and effectively, pregnant teenage clients should be screened for those risk factors most closely linked to poor outcomes. At this point, significant factors include:

- Low gynecologic age
- Low prepregnancy weight for height, or other significant evidence of malnutrition
- Low pregnancy weight gain
- Infections during pregnancy
- Excessive pregnancy weight gain
- Excessive weight-for-height at conception
- Anemia

Other risk factors gathered from history include:

- Unhealthy lifestyle (including use of tobacco, drugs, and alcohol)
- Unfavorable reproductive history
- Chronic diseases or eating disorders

Overall assessment of the pregnant teenager follows more or less the general pattern for assessment of all pregnant women, as discussed in Chapter 4.

TABLE 8-13   Recommended Dietary Allowances for Pregnant Adolescent Females

| | Age (reference height) | | | |
| | 11-14 years (157 cm) | | 15-18 years (163 cm) | |
Nutrient	RDA	RDA/cm	RDA	RDA/cm
Energy (kcal)*	2500	15.9	2500	15.3
Protein (g)	56	0.38	54	0.36
Calcium (mg)	1200	7.6	1200	7.4
Phosphorus (mg)	1200	7.6	1200	7.4
Iron (mg)	30	0.19	30	0.18
Magnesium (mg)	300	2.0	320	2.1
Iodine (μg)	175	1.1	175	1.1
Zinc (mg)	15	0.09	15	0.09
Vitamin A (μg RE)	800	5.1	800	4.9
Vitamin D (μg)	10	0.06	10	0.06
Vitamin E (mg α-TE)	10	0.06	10	0.06
Ascorbic acid (mg)	60	0.38	70	0.43
Niacin (mg NE)	17	0.11	17	0.10
Riboflavin (mg)	1.6	0.01	1.6	0.01
Thiamin (mg)	1.5	0.01	1.5	0.01
Folate (μg)	400	2.3	400	2.5
Vitamin B_6 (mg)	2.0	0.01	2.1	0.01
Vitamin B_{12} (μg)	2.2	0.01	2.2	0.01

*Second and third trimester.
Modified from Food and Nutrition Board, National Research Council: Recommended dietary allowances, ed 10, Washington, DC, 1989, National Academy of Sciences.

Nutrient needs. A summary of recommended amounts of nutrients is provided in Table 8-13. It combines the allowance for pregnancy in adult women with the amounts recommended for nonpregnant adolescents. A clinically practical way of assuring nutrient adequacy is to encourage the pregnant adolescent to gain the recommended amount of weight by consuming nutrient-rich foods. Sources of protein, calcium, iron, micronutrients, and dietary fiber are important. Contact with health professionals during prenatal care provides many important opportunities to teach adolescents about feeding themselves and their families. A clinical protocol for nutritional management of adolescent pregnancy is provided in the box on p. 337.

Economic and psychosocial needs. The economic instability of pregnant adolescents makes it impossible to assume that they will have an adequate food supply. The impact of lifestyle, economics, and other stressful issues on the nutritional well-being of young pregnant women is great and must be acknowledged in any program to improve their nutritional status. A summary of these issues is provided here (see box on p. 338). Above all, the stage of social and emotional development will determine the mother's ability to cope with all aspects of reproduction.

Involving the father of the infant. When the partner of the young pregnant woman is available, he should be included in counseling sessions to build mutual nutritional

ONE STEP FURTHER

Protocol for Assessment and Management of Normal Teenage Pregnancy

Initial evaluation (if possible)

Review intake material, social and lifestyle history

Review clinical data
  Height and weight
  Gynecologic age
  Physical signs of health
  Expected delivery date

Review laboratory data
  Hematocrit or hemoglobin
  Urinalysis

Begin to build relationship with the client (and partner if available)

Assess client's perspective of nutrition issues

Assess attitude about, and acceptance of, prepregnancy with and feelings about weight gain during pregnancy

Assess intake patterns using dietary methodology best suited to client and professional

Make preliminary assessment of food resources and refer to supportive agencies if necessary

Check for nausea and vomiting and suggest possible remedy

Discuss supplemental vitamins and minerals

Make initial plan that sets priorities for issues

Come to agreement with patient about any initial changes and steps to take; have client state plan as she perceives it

Determine client understanding of relation between nutrition and health

Do initial anthropometrics, calculate reasonable weight gain

Second visit

Check on referrals to other agencies

Discuss results of initial evaluation and suggest any changes necessary in dietary patterns (use printed materials as appropriate)

Do any further investigations when necessary

Laboratory studies
  For specific diagnosis of anemia:
    Protoporphyrin heme or serum ferritin
    Serum or red cell folate

Serum vitamin B_{12}
  Further probing of dietary habits if necessary

Monitor weight gain; discuss projected weight gain for following visit and total for gestation

Assess and address issues affecting nutritional status in order of priority for the individual
  Activity level
  Appetite changes
  Pica, food cravings, and aversions
  Allergies/food intolerances
  Supplementation practices (prescribed and self-selected)

Subsequent visits

Monitor and support appropriate weight gain; include discussion of fitness and encourage habitual safe exercise

Support upgrade in nutritional pattern in support of the woman and the developing infant; augment knowledge of principles of nutrition; continue to address issues affecting nutritional status

Check for heartburn, small food-intake capacity, and elimination problems; suggest dietary interventions

Begin preliminary discussion and comparison of advantages/disadvantages of breastfeeding and formula feeding

Final prenatal visit(s)

Discuss infant feeding if client will keep infant

If breastfeeding is chosen, provide preliminary guidance about breastfeeding practices

If formula feeding is chosen, discuss product selection and preparation; define important details about feeding techniques

Postpartum visits

Help client to understand safe methods of managing weight following delivery

Review infant feeding practices and infant growth; provide assistance when problems are identified

ONE STEP FURTHER

Issues in Adolescent Pregnancy That Influence Nutritional Well-Being

Acceptance of the pregnancy

Desire to carry out successful pregnancy
Acceptance of responsibility (even if child is to be relinquished)
Clarification of identity as mother separate from her own mother
Realistic acceptance versus fantasy and idealization

Food resources

Family meals (timing, quantity, quality, responsibility)
Self-reliance
School lunch
Fast-food outlets
Socially related eating
Food assistance (WIC program and others)
Mobilization of all resources

Body image

Degree of acceptance of an adult body
Maturity in facing bodily changes throughout pregnancy

Living situation

Acceptance by living partners and extended family
Role expectations of living partners
Financial support
Facilities and resources
Ethnic group (religious, cultural, and social patterns)
Emancipation versus dependency
Support system versus isolation

Relationship with the father of child

Presence or absence of father
Quality of relationship
Influence on decision making
Contribution to resources
Influence on mother's nutritional habits and general lifestyle
Understanding of physiologic processes
Tolerance of physical changes in pregnancy and physical needs of mother and child
Influence on child feeding

Peer relationships

Support from friends
Influence on nutritional knowledge and attitudes
Influence on general lifestyle

Nutritional state

Weight-for-height proportion
Maturational state
Tissue stores of nutrients
Reproductive and contraceptive history
Physical health
History of dietary patterns and nutritional status, including weight-losing schemes
Present eating habits
Complications of pregnancy (nausea and vomiting)
Substance use
Activity patterns
Need for intensive remediation

Prenatal care

Initiation of and compliance with prenatal care
Dependability of supporting resources
Identification of risk factors

Nutritional attitude and knowledge

Prior attitude toward nutrition
Understanding of role of nutrition in pregnancy
Knowledge of foods as sources of nutrients and of nutrients needed by the body
Desire to obtain adequate nutrition
Ability to obtain adequate nutrition and to control food supply

Preparation for child feeding

Knowledge of child-feeding practices
Attitude and decisions about child feeding
Responsibility for feeding
Understanding the importance of the bonding process
Support from family and friends

support for the pregnancy. Specific outreach to the father can be beneficial. If he is employed or in school, an effort should be made to see him at least occasionally. This effort will be especially important if for some reason he is interfering with the young woman's ability to nourish herself. Sharing what is known about the father's contribution to the outcome of pregnancy helps some adolescent males become more interested in maintaining healthy living habits.

Individualized counseling. To be effective, the clinician must work within the context of an individualized counseling relationship with the young pregnant adolescent and her partner.[36] The counselor will not "prescribe" but make practical suggestions and give support for changing of the teenagers' habits, usually in small increments, throughout the pregnancy.

Benefits of nutrition counseling. The benefits of nutrition counseling will generally be seen more in the long term than in a particular pregnancy. Prenatal care is one of the best opportunities to present sound nutritional information to a vulnerable group of teenagers. Even if they seek care late in pregnancy and miss appointments, for most of them these contacts constitute the greatest input of health care during their adolescence.

Energy and nutrient intake. Helping pregnant adolescents follow the suggested rate of gain can ensure sufficient energy intake to support the pregnancy and the mother's own developmental needs. Following the guidelines dramatically demonstrates in just a few months the possibility of exerting personal control over eating, as well as the effect on both weight and nutritional status, in a way the teenager can understand. There is great appeal in discussing with adolescents the effects of various events on their bodies and on the growing fetus. Learning about the physiologic needs of both her own body and her developing infant can be the teenager's impetus for upgrading the quality of her diet to keep pace with the increase in energy intake needed to support adequate weight gain. Repeated counseling sessions to review those needs may motivate the young mother to try new foods to obtain additional sources of nutrients. Attention to nutritional health in the prenatal period can become a model for taking responsibility for feeding a family. The young woman can gain experience in the use of community resources to obtain food for herself and her family.

CASE STUDY

Two Teenage Pregnancies

Two adolescent females in the same grade become pregnant. One is 16.5 years of age: her menses began at age 14, and her weight for height is below the 5th percentile. The other pregnant adolescent is 15 years of age: her menses began at age 9, and her weight for height is at the 50th percentile.

Questions for analysis
1. Describe the theoretical difference in nutritional needs of the two adolescents.
2. Which one should be given clinical priority? Why?
3. If neither young woman sought prenatal care, what might you expect as outcome for the respective infants? Why?

In summary, nutrition counseling in prenatal care for teenagers can accomplish the following goals:

1. Serve as a model for exerting control over what a person eats with visible results in terms of the optimal weight gain pattern and the quality of foods contributing to it.
2. Be an impetus for trying new foods.
3. Serve as a model for taking responsibility and using community resources to feed a family.

The nutrition counselor will be most effective when working within a clinical program designed specifically for adolescents. Such programs have been shown to improve overall outcome in adolescent pregnancy.[36] A case study of two teenage pregnancies is provided in the box on p. 339.

Summary

The physical and psychosocial gains in development are rapid and all encompassing in the adolescent period of human life. The parameters of physical growth are the basis for determining nutritional needs. Eating behavior is influenced to a great extent at this time by the developing body image and, as a result of breaking ties with the family, by the total culture. Thus if health professionals hope to help adolescents improve their nutritional patterns they must use appropriate tactics. They will need to sort out fact and reality in terms of the realistic role of nutrition in health and behavior. Emphasis must be placed on physical fitness as an important way to help all adoelscents balance energy intake and output.

In eating disorders the overall objective is to help the individual put the eating function into proper perspective. The athlete must obtain sufficient nourishment to support a growing body that is subjected to stress. In chronic diseases the diet must eliminate nutrients that cause symptoms and be supplemented if necessary to allow growth to continue. If a pregnancy should occur, the adolescent will need support in nourishing herself and her developing infant during a chaotic time. While a great deal is still unknown about nutritional needs of adolescents, the growing interest in this age group should stimulate the research necessary to close gaps in our knowledge.

Review Questions

1. Define the terms *adolescence* and *puberty*. Explain how they are related.
2. Draw the growth velocity curve for males and females from birth to adulthood and describe the implications of different stages on the nutritional needs of humans.
3. Discuss the reasons for not using commonly available growth grids to assess weight/height proportion in adolescents and the alternate database that is appropriate.
4. Describe ways in which psychologic development influences nutritional status of adolescents.
5. Discuss the commonalities and differences of specifically recognized syndromes across the spectrum of eating disorders.
6. Describe how you would set up a comprehensive weight management program for teenagers in a community where none had ever existed before.
7. It has been proposed that adolescents need to gain more weight during pregnancy than adult women do. What aspects of adolescent growth and development lead to the idea that these larger gains are beneficial?

References

1. Tanner JM: Foetus into man, Cambridge, Mass, 1978, Harvard University Press.
2. Newman B and Newman P: Adolescent development, Columbus, Ohio, 1986, Merrill Press.
3. McKigney JI and Munro HN, editors: Nutrient requirements in adolescence, Cambridge, Mass, 1976, Massachusetts Institute of Technology Press.
4. Gong E and Heald FT: Diet, nutrition, and adolescence. In Shils M and Young VR, editors: Modern nutrition in health and disease, ed 7, Philadelphia, 1987, Lea & Febiger.
5. Witschi JC et al: Sources of fat, fatty acids, and cholesterol in the diets of adolescents, J Am Diet Assoc 90:1429, 1990.
6. Read MH et al: Adolescent compliance with dietary guidelines: health and education implications, Adolescence 23:567, 1988.
7. Bigler-Doughten S and Jenkins MR: Adolescent snacks: nutrient density and nutritional contribution to total intake, J Am Diet Assoc 87:1678, 1987.
8. Guenther PM: Beverages in the diets of American teenagers, J Am Diet Assoc 86:493, 1986.
9. Portnoy B and Christenson GM: Cancer knowledge and related practices: results from the National Adolescent Student Health Survey, J School Health 59:218, 1989.
10. Farrow JA: Adolescent chemical dependency. In Farrow JA, editor: Adolescent medicine, Med Clin North Am 74:1265, 1990.
11. Farrow JA et al: Health, developmental, and nutritional status of adolescent alcohol and marijuana abusers, Pediatrics 79:218, 1987.
12. Story M and Van Zyl York P: Nutritional status of Native American adolescent substance users, J Am Diet Assoc 87:1680, 1987.
13. Story M and Resnick MD: Adolescents' views on food and nutrition, J Nutr Educ 18:188, 1986.
14. Bruch H: Developmental considerations of anorexia nervosa and obesity, Can J Psychiatry 26:212, 1981.
15. Minuchin S et al: Psychosomatic families: anorexia nervosa in context, Cambridge, Mass, 1978, Harvard University Press.
16. Diagnostic and statistical manual of mental disorders, ed 3, Washington, DC, 1980, American Psychiatric Association.
17. Keys A et al: The biology of human starvation, Minneapolis, 1950, University of Minnesota Press.
18. Meyer AE et al: Psychoendocrinology of remenorrhea in the late outcome of anorexia nervosa, Psychother Psychosom 45:174, 1986.
19. Commerci G: Eating disorders. In Farrow JA, editor: Adolescent medicine, Med Clin North Am 74:1293, 1990.
20. Bachrach LK et al: Decreased bone density in adolescent girls with anorexia nervosa, Pediatrics 86:440, 1990.
21. Nussbaum M et al: Cerebral atrophy in anorexia nervosa, J Pediatr 96:867, 1980.
22. Rigotti NA et al: The clinical course of osteoporosis in anorexia nervosa: a longitudinal study of cortical bone mass, J Am Diet Assoc 265:1133, 1991.
23. Nussbaum MP et al: Blunted growth hormone responses to clonidine in adolescent girls with early anorexia nervosa: evidence for an early hypothalmic defect, J Adol Med 18:145, 1990.
24. Dolan RJ et al: Structural brain changes in patients with anorexia nervosa, Psychol Med 18:349, 1988.
25. Laessle RG et al: Depression as a correlate of starvation in patients with eating disorders, Biol Psychiatry 23:719, 1988.
26. Steiger H et al: Relationship of body-image distortion to sex-role identification, irrational cognitions, and body weight in eating-disoriented females, J Clin Psychol 45:61, 1989.
27. Brinch M et al: Anorexia nervosa and motherhood: reproduction pattern and mothering behavior of 50 women, Acta Psychiatr Scand 77:611, 1988.

28. Polivy J and Herman CP: Diagnosis and treatment of normal eating, J Consulting Clin Psychol 55:635, 1987.
29. Rees JM: Management of obesity in adolescents. In Farrow JA, editor: Adolescent medicine, Med Clin North Am 74:1275, 1990.
30. McArdle WD et al: Exercise physiology: energy, nutrition, and human performance, ed 2, Philadelphia, 1986, Lea & Febiger.
31. Gortmaker SL et al: Inactivity, diet, and the fattening of America, J Am Diet Assoc 90:1247, 1990.
32. American Medical Association and American Dietetic Association: Targets for adolescent health: adolescent nutrition and physical fitness, Chicago, 1991, Am Med Assoc.
33. Johnson MD et al: Anabolic steroid use by male adolescents, Pediatrics 83:921, 1989.
34. Story M, editor: Nutrition management of the pregnant adolescent: a practical reference guide, Washington, DC, 1990, MCH National Clearinghouse.
35. Scholl TO et al: Maternal growth during pregnancy and decreased infant birth weight, Am J Clin Nutr 51:790, 1990.
36. Rees JM et al: Position of the American Dietetic Association: nutrition management of adolescent pregnancy, and technical support paper, J Am Diet Assoc 89:900, 1989.
37. Haiek L and Lederman SA: The relationship between maternal weight for height and term birth weight in teens and adult women, J Adol Health Care 10:16, 1988.
38. Frisancho AR et al: Developmental and nutritional determinants of pregnancy outcome among teenagers, Am J Physical Anthro 66:247, 1985.
39. Taffel S, National Center for Health Statistics: Maternal weight gain and the outcome of pregnancy, United States, 1980, Vital and Health Statistics, Series 21, No 44, DHHS Pub No (PHS) 86-1922, Washington, DC, June 1986, US Government Printing Office.
40. Rosso P and Lederman SA: Nutrition in the pregnant adolescent. In Winick M, editor: Adolescent nutrition, New York, 1982, John Wiley & Sons.
41. Garn SM and Petzold AS: Characteristics of the mother and child in teenage pregnancy, Am J Dis Child 137:365, 1983.
42. Stevens-Simon C and McAnarney ER: Adolescent maternal weight gain and low birth weight: a multifactorial model, Am J Clin Nutr 47:948, 1988.
43. Institute of Medicine, National Academy of Sciences: Nutrition during pregnancy, Washington, DC, 1990, National Academy Press.
44. Hediger ML et al: Rate and amount of weight gain during adolescent pregnancy: associations with maternal weight-for-height and birth weight, Am J Clin Nutr 52:793, 1990.

Further Reading

Arquitt AB et al: Dehydroepiandrosterone sulfate, cholesterol, hemoglobin, and anthropometric measures related to growth in male adolescents, J Am Diet Assoc 91:575, 1991.

This study investigates the relationship of nutritional status and biochemical and physical markers of maturation in adolescent males.

Expert Panel on Population Strategies for Blood Cholesterol Reduction, National Cholesterol Education Program: executive summary, NIH Pub No 90-3047, Washington, DC, 1990, US Department of Health and Human Services.

This expert panel report provides recommendations for promoting healthy eating patterns in all Americans including adolescents, with the goal of lowering blood cholesterol of individuals and reducing the average cholesterol level throughout the population, in turn reducing risks of atherosclerosis and coronary heart disease.

Heald FP: Atherosclerosis during adolescence. In Farrow JA, editor: Adolescent medicine, Med Clin North Am 74:1321, 1990.

This author reviews the evidence for development of atherosclerotic lesions in early life and discusses the need to assess and treat adolescents in order to prevent further damage.

Moore DC: Body image and eating behavior in adolescent girls, Am J Dis Child 142:1114, 1988.

Moore DC: Body image and eating behavior in adolescent boys, Am J Dis Child 144:475, 1990.

In these twin articles, the author reports results of surveys regarding dissatisfaction with weight and shape, and the attempts by both males and females to change their bodies.

Thibault L and Roberge AG: The nutritional status of subjects with anorexia nervosa, Int J Vit Nutri Res 57:447, 1987.

These authors report the relationship of nutritional deficiencies in the diets of 25 anorectic patients and discuss these findings in relation to symptoms of the disorder.

Nutrition for
Aging and the Aged

Eleanor D. Schlenker

Basic Concepts

✦✦

✔ *Persons 60 years of age and older—the fastest growing segment of the population—sometimes need nutrition support services to maintain independent healthy living.*

✔ *Aging brings a gradual decline in normal physiologic functions.*

✔ *Energy needs decrease with age but protein, vitamin, and mineral needs remain the same, making nutrient density important in meal planning.*

✔ *Vitamins and minerals are the nutrients most likely to be lacking in an older person's diet; they are also most adversely affected by multiple medications, both over-the-counter and prescription drugs.*

✔ *Numerous social, physiologic, and economic factors can influence food and nutrient intake in older people.*

---

*T*he numbers of older people in our society will increase significantly over the next few years. One in eight Americans is now age 65 or older. By the year 2030 one in four will be in that age range.[1] The actual number of older people will double and the fastest growing segment in that age group will be those over age 85. As older consumers increase in number, businesses will expand their products and services to meet the demands of older groups. Food manufacturers will enlarge the print now used on food labels as more people undergo age-related changes in vision. As the number of older workers reaching retirement age begins to exceed the number of younger workers entering the work force, older workers will be encouraged to remain on the job.

As the increasing lifespan places greater responsibility on older workers and older family members, those in the health care field will face the challenge of providing health and nutrition education that will promote well-being and assist older persons in maintaining their independence. At the same time it will be necessary to plan appropriate nutrition services for those individuals in declining health who require specialized care. These projections are more than just numbers. This information concerns the lives of real people with particular needs and resources who will require health and nutrition services that are not practiced or even understood in our society today.[2]

In this chapter we look at the changing nutrient needs of the aging population. We explore the environmental, personal, and health factors that influence them. We seek effective intervention strategies based on sensitive evaluation of each older person as an individual.

DEMOGRAPHIC ASPECTS OF AGING
Population Trends

In the United States age 65 is frequently used as a benchmark to characterize the older population—the "retired" generation. **Chronologic age,** however, is not always a measure of physical health or zest for life. Also, individuals continue to change as they age so that 65-year-olds differ markedly from 90-year-olds. To mark these changes United States population reports classify older Americans in three subgroups[1]:

- age 65 to 74—the young-old
- age 75 to 84—the old-old
- age 85 and over—the oldest-old

Most census reports group older adults in these ranges.

As the total over-65 group increases from about 12% to 21% of the general population, it will also increase in diversity. The number of persons above age 85 will triple. Ethnic diversity will also change because the number of nonwhite elderly are increasing at a faster rate than white elderly.

Changes in Life Expectancy

Nature of changes. **Life expectancy** is the average remaining years of life for a person of a given age. The dramatic increase in life expectancy in this century occurred primarily in infancy and childhood. For men life expectancy at birth increased from 46 to 72 years between 1900 and the present; for women, from 48 to 78 years. But despite improvements in medical care, life expectancy at age 65 has increased by only 3 years in men and 7 years in women since 1900.[1] Thus, the growth of the older population does not reflect an increase in maximal lifespan but the extended lifespan of those individuals who in the past would have died in infancy and childhood.

Influencing factors. Gains in life expectancy have not been equal among all groups. Women can expect to live longer than men and whites can expect to live longer than nonwhites. Increased smoking among women may in future years reduce their life expectancy as death rates from lung cancer continue to increase. Level of education and income that influence accessibility to health care are related to life expectancy and may contribute to the lower life expectancy of nonwhite persons.

Causes of death. The three most common causes of death today are heart disease, cancer, and **cerebrovascular hemorrhage** (stroke). All three causes are related to degenerative changes associated with aging and the environment. In contrast, the leading cause of death in 1900 was infectious disease, for example, pneumonia and influenza, which can now be controlled by antibiotic drugs. A lifestyle based on a diet moderate in sucrose, fat, and sodium; with no smoking; limited or no use of alcohol; and regular exercise can delay the onset of chronic disease and lead to an improvement in health status in the expanding older population.

Socioeconomic Characteristics

The general public associates old age with poor health, illness, and disability. This view often leads to the assumption that the majority of older people live in institutions.

Chronologic age
Age of an individual based on the number of years lived, compared, for example, with *biologic age*, the relative age of a person based on physiologic capacity and measurements.

Life expectancy
The average remaining years a person of a given age may expect to live, based on statistical population averages.

Cerebral hemorrhage
Rupture of an artery in the brain; cerebrovascular accident (CVA), stroke.

In fact 95% of aged persons live within the community, either with a spouse, other family member or friend, or alone. Specific living arrangements are related to the sex of the individual. About three fourths of older men are married. In contrast over half of older women are widows, and over one third of these live alone. Living situation can contribute to food problems of older people. An aged widow who lives in a rural area and cannot drive is dependent on relatives or friends for transportation to a food store.

Older women, minority groups, and those 85 or above are also more vulnerable to poor nutrition because of lower income. Usually couples have a more adequate income than single individuals. Black and Hispanic elderly persons are more likely to be poor. Government programs such as food stamps or **congregate meals** (p. 376) can help those with limited food money.

Congregate meals
Group meals for older adults, served in a social setting in the community and funded by Title III-C of the Older Americans Act.

NUTRITION AND THE LIFESPAN

Since antiquity people have been searching for potions to preserve health and prolong life. Ponce de Leon came to the New World seeking the "fountain of youth." Francis Bacon (1591 to 1626) was the first author to recommend scientific evaluation of diet and longevity. He advocated a frugal diet and encouraged the study of people in various climates and living situations to determine those characteristics that influence lifespan. Unfortunately, Bacon's recommendations for study are only beginning to receive attention.

Animal Studies

Energy restriction. Energy intake controls not only the increase in body size but also the rate of maturation and aging. Animals fed diets restricted in kilocalories, yet adequate in protein, vitamins, and minerals, live 40% longer than those given unlimited access to food; chronic problems such as kidney disease also appear at a later age in these animals. Diet restriction also delays biochemical alterations such as the decline in the immune system.

Rate of growth. Protein, in addition to total energy, influences both rate of growth and survival. In animal models diets high in both energy and protein lead to rapid growth, large body size and weight, and early onset of degenerative disease. The suggestion that rapid growth and increased body weight accelerate the aging process has serious implications for current growth patterns. Children today are both taller and heavier, and reach puberty at earlier ages, compared with previous generations. Regular physical exercise slows the rate of growth, lowers body weight, and increases the lifespan in animal models. Regular physical exercise may be a form of intervention to slow the aging process in humans.

Human Studies

Little information is now available to evaluate the influence of lifelong dietary habits on health and longevity. Studies that did collect detailed information did not follow subjects at regularly scheduled intervals nor did they continue over an extended period of years. Following the same individual over time—a **longitudinal study**—is needed to evaluate the influence of diet and lifestyle on physiologic and biochemical aging.

Longitudinal study
Study of persons or populations over a long period of time to measure effects of specific factors on the aging process and incidence and course of disease.

Body weight and mortality in the aged. Life insurance standards used to evaluate the body weight of individuals in relation to their peers of similar height and sex have been used to predict mortality risk. The general conclusion drawn from these statistics is that the greater the deviation between actual body weight and standard weight (weights of policy holders who lived the longest) the greater the risk of death.

Patterns of overweight, however, differ according to age, sex, and race. National Health and Nutrition Examination Surveys (NHANES) data suggest that overweight is more common in black men than caucasian men between the ages of 35 and 54. Between the ages of 55 and 75 the prevalence of overweight is similar in both groups. In women the situation is quite different. The percentage of white women who are overweight increases from 25% in the 35 to 44 age group to 36% in the 65 to 74 age group. Among black women, the percentage for these age groups is 41% and 60%, respectively.[3]

The association between overweight, chronic disease, and **mortality rate** at older ages remains controversial. Although obese men between the ages of 20 and 45 are at high risk for hypertension, diabetes, and high blood lipids, the hazards of obesity at older ages are less obvious. This perception is due in part to the fact that these problems also increase in prevalence among the nonobese as they get older. Nevertheless, the 30-year follow-up of 5500 men and women in Framingham, Massachusetts, indicates that relative weights from 10% to 30% above standard weights have an adverse effect on longevity.[3] Although women are more resistant to the hazards of overweight, women in the Framingham study who were more than 30% overweight had an increased risk of cardiovascular disease.

The problem in assigning mortality risk to overweight compared with underweight older people is associated with the time of onset. Underweight in persons age 60 and over decreases life expectancy, and mortality is likely to occur within a few years. In contrast, the effects of overweight are delayed, sometimes for 10 years or more, so that short-term follow-up overlooks its effects. Optimal **ideal weights** for older persons are within 10% of average weights for their age, height, and sex. However, average weights at older ages are 10 to 15 pounds heavier than in younger persons of the same sex and height. A major consideration in dietary management for older persons is prevention of inappropriate weight gain.

Longitudinal studies. Longitudinal studies evaluating diet and exercise patterns and subsequent morbidity and mortality indicate that good eating habits and continued physical activity contribute to health and survival in middle age and beyond. Several studies conducted in different parts of the country serve as examples.

Michigan study. Diet quality influenced physical well-being and the length of life in a longitudinal study of 100 Michigan women first evaluated in 1948 when they ranged in age from 40 to 85 years.[4] Over the next 7 years mortality was higher in those consuming diets containing less than 40% of the RDA for one or more nutrients. Nutrients most frequently deficient were calcium, vitamin A, and ascorbic acid.

In 1972 (24 years after the first interview) 28 of the women were located and reinterviewed by this author.[5] Their average age was 75 years. The survivors had reduced the quantity but not the quality of food consumed. Total energy, fat, and carbohydrate decreased by 25% although mean intakes of protein, vitamins, and minerals (with the exception of calcium) met or exceeded 67% of the RDA. Protein, fat, and carbohydrate provided 18%, 35%, and 47% of total energy, respectively. Foods high in simple carbohydrate and fat but providing few other nutrients were deleted from the diet. Fruits, vegetables, milk products, and breads and cereals were emphasized. A decrease in energy intake to prevent weight gain, with continued emphasis on protein, vitamins, and minerals appears to be a dietary model for the transition from middle to advanced age.

California study. An on-going study that began with 7000 adults living in Alameda, California, examined the influence on mortality of the following health practices—adequate sleep, regular meals (including breakfast), desirable body weight, not smoking, limited or no use of alcohol, and regular physical activity.[6] After 5 years it was evident that poor health practices resulted in earlier death, whereas good health habits led to longer life. Men who followed at least five of the health practices had a life expectancy 11 years longer than men who followed three or less. For women the comparable difference in life expectancy was 7 years. The health habits identified above continue to be important as a 17-year follow-up of participants 70 years of age and older indicated that increased

Mortality rate
Total number of deaths in a specific category divided by the total number of deaths in the total population.

Ideal weight
Optimal weight for an individual of a given height, sex, or age in relation to health.

risk of death was related to being male, smoking, having little physical activity, deviating from average weight, and not regularly eating breakfast. These findings were unrelated to age and health status when the study began. This study suggests areas for **nutrition education** and intervention for reducing risk, even among the very old.

Honolulu heart study. This program is evaluating risk factors that may relate to the development of coronary heart disease among 8000 men.[7,8] After 12 years of follow-up, two factors have emerged as risk factors in those older than 64: (1) elevated serum cholesterol levels and (2) lack of physical activity. Older men who remained moderately active had a coronary risk less than half that of the sedentary men. Also, previous studies had suggested that serum cholesterol levels were unrelated to coronary risk in those above age 65 or older. It appears that dietary measures to reduce serum cholesterol levels combined with reasonable physical activity can have a positive effect upon the health of older as well as middle-aged men.

BIOLOGIC ASPECTS OF AGING
The Aging Process

In general terms the study of aging includes all changes in body structure and function that occur throughout the lifespan as a result of growth, maturation, and **senescence.** In our context aging refers to the time-dependent biologic and physiologic changes that begin about age 30 and are degenerative in their effect. The pattern and sequence of the changes in normal aging are always the same although the rate at which these changes occur differ from one person to another. For example muscle mass, which comprises a very small proportion of body weight in the infant and young child, increases steadily throughout early adulthood and declines in middle and old age. Both genetic and environmental factors influence the rate of aging. Individuals with long-lived parents are more likely to survive beyond age 70. Environmental factors such as irradiation or level of nutrition influence lifespan in experimental animals. In humans environmental stress that increases one's vulnerability to either acute or chronic disease increases the rate of aging.

Cellular Level Changes

Although no one knows exactly how the aging process takes place, changes are observed first at the cellular level. Among cell types that continue to divide throughout their normal lifespan, for example, skin cells or mucosal cells lining the gastrointestinal tract, the rate of division slows as the cell nears the end of its normal lifespan and eventually stops. Cells from species having shorter lifespans will undergo fewer divisions than those from species having longer lifespans. Cells from an older donor will undergo fewer divisions than those from a younger donor. Although the older person will always have some cells that are rapidly dividing, they will be fewer in number and the total cell count is reduced. Decreases in gastric acid secretion, observed in some older persons, relates to a reduced number of **parietal cells** within the mucosa.

Organ Level Changes

Highly differentiated cells including brain, kidney, and muscle that do not continue to divide throughout life undergo functional changes with time and some cells die. As a result these organ systems become less efficient as fewer cells remain to carry on normal body functions. The aging cell that has undergone changes in structure and function is less able to synthesize important molecules such as ones required for hormonal or neural control or for the induction of a specific enzyme. As a result, specialized organs and tissues are less able to respond to environmental stimuli and there is a breakdown in the coordination of body systems that may need to work together to carry out a physiologic function.

Nutrition education
The process of helping individuals obtain the knowledge, skills, and motivation needed to make appropriate food choices for positive health throughout life.

Senescence
(L *senescere*, to grow old) Normal process or condition of growing old.

Parietal cells
(L *parietes*, wall) Cells lining the stomach that secrete hydrochloric acid; chief cells.

Theories of Aging

Current theories attempting to explain what happens in aging point to the replication of deoxyribonucleic acid (DNA) within the cell nucleus as the site of control. Aging may occur through a programmed series of events in the life of the organism. An opposing view suggests that aging results from random environmental insults that damage the genetic code.

Programmed aging theory. In later life particular sequences of DNA required for the synthesis of vital proteins may no longer be produced resulting in changes in structure and function of organ systems and leading to inevitable decline. These events may be under the control of the hypothalamus, acting as the biologic clock. Evidence supporting the programmed theory includes the close similarity in age at death of monozygous twins, which is not apparent in dizygous twins or other siblings.

Random environmental error theory. The error theory suggests that aging results from environmental insults such as radiation, pollution, or other harmful substances that damage particular genetic sequences and lead to the production of abnormal proteins. Inappropriate intakes or deficiencies of nutrients might inflict damage on important body tissues. According to this viewpoint lifestyle rather than genetic inheritance holds the key to years of life.

Free radical theory. Many aging changes occurring at the tissue, cellular, and subcellular level can be caused by the actions of free radicals. Free radicals are highly charged molecules that enter into oxidation reactions at sites containing double bonds. This reaction occurs in the lipid components of membranes changing their function and in protein and collagen. These reactions have been implicated in the development of atherosclerosis, cancer, and cataracts. Nutrients that function as **antioxidants** (e.g., vitamins C and E, and selenium) can prevent such reactions. Antioxidants normally found in the diet may play a role in preventing age-related changes.

PHYSIOLOGIC ASPECTS OF AGING
Brain and Neural Control

Functional changes. Both structural and biochemical changes contribute to functional alterations in the aging brain. Although there is general agreement that neurons are lost in advanced age (estimates of losses range as high as 20% to 40%), questions regarding changes in brain weight are still unresolved.[9] Because brain weight is related to body size, smaller brain weights may be a secular effect (one related to outside events) and not indicative of age-related changes within individuals. Neither brain weight nor cell number appears to be related to **Alzheimer-type senile dementia (ATSD).** Blood flow through the aging brain decreases as a result of vascular changes, contributing to a decline in cerebral function.

Neurotransmitters. Decreased synthesis of **neurotransmitters,** such as dopamine, serotonin, or acetylcholine, required for the conduction of nerve impulses, has been observed in older people. The most striking reductions in transmitter levels occur in the hypothalamus and cerebral cortex; these areas of the brain control psychomotor skills and cognitive function, activities that exhibit age-related alterations. **Parkinson's disease,** a disorder of the central nervous system occurring among older persons, is thought to relate to the altered metabolism of dopamine. The muscle rigidity, tremors, and shuffling gait associated with this disease can be improved with treatment with L-dopa.

Organic brain syndrome. Brain disorders that lead to behavior changes and mental deterioration increase with age. Loss of cells, changes in the physical arrangement of cells, or atherosclerosis of the brain blood vessels can lead to progressive and irreversible dementia. Brain disorders increase in prevalence after age 80. ATSD is distinguished by the age of onset—before 65 years of age. Characteristic neurofibrillary tangles with increased

Antioxidant
(Gr *anti*, against; *oxys*, keen) A substance that inhibits oxidation of polyunsaturated fatty acids and formation of free radicals in the cells.

Alzheimer-type senile dementia (ATSD)
A type of senile dementia first described by German physician Alois Alzheimer (1864-1915); progressive, irreversible degenerative changes in the brain, resulting in loss of neuromuscular function and mental capacity.

Neurotransmitter
(Gr *neuron*, nerve; L *trans*, through, across; *missio*, a sending) A large group of some 40 different chemical substances, including compounds as diverse as acetylcholine, various hormones, and several amino acids, which function as essential synaptic transmitters, chemical messengers for sending (or inhibiting) nerve impulses across synapses of connecting nerve endings.

Parkinson's disease
A neurologic disorder, described by English physician James Parkinson (1755-1824), characterized by tremor, muscular rigidity, and abnormally decreased motor function and ability, as well as mobility.

accumulation of aluminum are found at autopsy. High aluminum levels in brain cells are the result, not the cause, of this disorder; use of aluminum cooking utensils is not associated with the development of ATSD. As the disease progresses patients are increasingly unable to care for themselves and will no longer recognize family members or friends. Changes occur in eating behavior as patients first forget how to use eating utensils; for example, they may try to eat soup with a fork. They eventually lose all ability to feed themselves.

Coordination of Physiologic Functions

Response to stimuli. One characteristic of physiologic aging is the decreased ability to respond to changes in the environment. In the older person organ systems respond more slowly to changes in the external environment such as changes in room temperature. The return to homeostasis following a change in the internal environment, such as the rise in blood glucose following a high carbohydrate meal, requires a longer period of time in older persons.

The age-related decline in physiologic function occurring between ages 30 and 80 has been studied in a group of men at the **Gerontology** Research Center of the National Institute on Aging in Baltimore.[10] This study has been on-going for almost 30 years and each subject returns every 2 years for reevaluation. This arrangement makes it possible for researchers to observe at what age changes occur in each individual as well as allowing a comparison among men of different ages. Functional capacity at age 30 (Fig. 9-1) is rated as 100% and a decline in function to **functional disability** is rated accordingly. The degree of loss observed is influenced by the level of coordination required among one or more organ systems. Fasting blood glucose levels exhibit little change whereas resting cardiac output, requiring both neural and muscular control, declines by 30%. Renal function declines by 40%.

Response to added demand. As a system becomes more complex, impairment becomes more apparent. For example an older person may walk with comparative ease on a level surface, but climbing stairs may require much effort. In spite of known decrements in physiologic systems most older persons function quite well on a day-to-day basis. However, when extreme demands, such as heavy exercise or severe illness, are placed on the system or when functional losses are excessive, problems become evident.

Endocrine System

Information is limited regarding age-related changes in hormone levels or the mechanisms involved. Although blood levels of some hormones such as aldosterone decrease, others such as thyroxin (T_4) remain the same. Decreased secretion of hormones can result from either impaired hormone synthesis or release. Reduced hormone utilization or slowed excretion may limit hormone release through homeostatic mechanisms. Current research is looking at hypothalamus-pituitary regulation of hormone secretion, storage, and release. The aged hypothalamus appears to be less sensitive to messages received and may play a role in altered endocrine function.

Cardiovascular System

Functional changes. Age-related changes in the heart and circulatory system involve both structure and function. The work load of the heart increases as a result of increased peripheral resistance caused by atherosclerotic deposition and loss of arterial elasticity. At the same time the effectiveness of the heart muscle as a pump is reduced as the strength of contraction is diminished. Resting **cardiac output** falls measurably as the volume of blood pumped with each stroke decreases. As a result blood flow through the coronary arteries supplying nutrients to the heart muscle itself is compromised. Therefore, the work load on the heart increases as nutrients become less available. As a consequence, the aged

Gerontology
The study of aging including biologic, physiologic, psychologic, and sociologic aspects. Contrast with *geriatrics*, which is the medical specialty dealing with chronic disease, as well as physical health, in older adults.

Functional disability
Disability that interferes with activities of daily living, such as bathing, dressing, shopping, preparing meals, eating.

Cardiac output
Total amount of blood pumped by the heart per minute.

A. Fasting blood glucose
B. Nerve conduction velocity and some cellular enzyme activities
C. Cardiac index (resting)
D. Vital capacity and renal blood flow
E. Maximum breathing capacity
F. Maximum work rate and maximum O_2 uptake

FIG. 9-1 Age-related decline in physiologic function.

From Shock NW: Energy metabolism, caloric intake, and physical activity of the aging. In Carlson LA, editor: Nutrition in old age, Symposia Swedish Nutrition Foundation X, Stockholm, Sweden, 1972, Almqvist & Wiksell. Used by permission.

heart is much less tolerant of either physiologic or emotional stress. This intolerance points to the importance of medical evaluation of older persons before they begin an exercise program.

Hypertension. Changes in cardiovascular function contribute to the age-related rise in blood pressure observed in both sexes. Hypertension is a significant medical and nutritional problem among older persons. Effective management may require weight control and sodium restriction. In a national survey about two thirds of those older than age 64 had systolic pressures above 140 mm Hg or diastolic pressures above 90 mm Hg.[11] The subgroup with the highest incidence was black females. High blood pressure increases the risk of stroke and coronary artery disease.

Renal System

Functional changes. Kidney function deteriorates with age as a result of both a loss of nephrons and a 30% decrease in blood flow, a consequence of reduced cardiac output. Total nephrons decline by 30% to 40%.[9] As the **glomerular filtration rate** is slowed, it takes longer to clear drugs or metabolic wastes from the blood. On that basis excessive protein intakes resulting in high blood urea nitrogen levels, or megadoses of the water-

Glomerular filtration rate
A measure of the amount of blood filtered by the cup-like glomerulus at the head of each kidney nephron per unit of time (ml/min).

soluble vitamins, should be avoided. The aged kidney is less able to form concentrated urine so adequate fluid intake is essential. In the nephron tubule, nutrients including glucose, plasma proteins, and ascorbic acid are less efficiently reabsorbed while drug metabolites and H^+ ions are less efficiently excreted.

Water balance. Fluid regulation and water balance are serious needs to consider in the nutritional management of older people. Dehydration leads to seriously elevated electrolyte levels and is an ever-present danger. A recent study evaluating fluid intake in younger and older persons following 6 hours of fluid deprivation reported a decreased sense of thirst in the older persons.[12] Not only did they experience less feelings of thirst, they also drank considerably less water than was needed for fluid replacement once water became available. At the same time the kidney is less able to respond to **antidiuretic hormone (ADH)** and reduce the amount of fluid lost in the urine. At the other extreme drugs that induce ADH activity can contribute to water intoxication. Therefore, records of fluid intake become very important in the care of older persons, particularly those with limited access to water.

Pulmonary System

Structural changes in the lung result in loss of alveolar surface area and a decrease in elasticity. Although total lung capacity does not change, the proportion of alveolar space ventilated with each breath and thus the total surface area for gas exchange decreases. Gas exchange itself is less efficient because of decreased permeability of the alveolar membranes and reduced blood flow. As a result **oxyhemoglobin** saturation of arterial blood is lowered in advanced age, making oxygen transfer to the tissues more difficult. The reduced ability to effectively increase oxygen intake and maintain an adequate **vital capacity** of the lungs becomes a significant factor in exercise or physiologic stress.

Gastrointestinal Function

Functional changes. At present there is little evidence to support the generally held concept that advancing age results in dysfunction of the stomach, small intestine, and colon. However, gastrointestinal discomforts including nausea, heartburn, and constipation increase in frequency with advancing age. Such symptoms can relate to poor eating and bowel habits, mental anxiety, or side effects of commonly used drugs. Gastrointestinal distress does not necessarily indicate malabsorption. Persons with no discomfort may absorb nutrients poorly, whereas others with persistent distress may absorb nutrients normally.

Eating problems. Changes in muscle innervation and reduced secretion of saliva can lead to difficulty in swallowing, particularly among frail, aged persons. The result may be fear of choking and food may be refused resulting in progressive weight loss. General dehydration or certain drugs causing dry mouth can add to this problem. Older people should eat only when seated in an upright position. Being fed in a supine position increases the risk of food aspiration and pneumonia.

Bowel problems. Constipation, a problem for many older people, is related to low fluid intake, diets low in fiber and bulk, medications, and a general lack of exercise. **Constipation** is more often perception than fact. Many older people have an exaggerated concern with bowel habits and the belief that a daily bowel movement is essential. True constipation is characterized by (1) fewer than two bowel movements per week, (2) persistent difficulty in passing stools, (3) bleeding with bowel movements, or (4) pain with bowel movements. Any bleeding from the rectum should be reported to a physician immediately.

Laxative abuse. Individuals with normal bowel function who do not have a daily bowel movement sometimes turn to laxatives in an effort to relieve the perceived problem. After

Antidiuretic hormone (ADH)
Hormone secreted by the posterior pituitary gland in response to body stress. It acts on the distal tubules of the kidney's nephrons to cause water reabsorption and thus protect vital body water; also called *vasopressin.*

Oxyhemoglobin
Hemoglobin with bound oxygen for transport of oxygen from the lungs to the cells for vital metabolic work.

Vital capacity
Volume of air moved in and out of the lungs with each breath. The residual volume is the amount of air remaining in the lungs after the person has exhaled.

Constipation
(L *constipatio*, a crowding together) Infrequent, sometimes difficult, passage of feces; condition is often a source of anxiety to elderly persons and may be perceived more in mental attitude than in physiologic reality; sometimes called "irritable bowel."

the purging effect of the laxative, normal bowel movements may not resume the following day. This reinforces the idea that the individual is constipated and leads to a vicious cycle. Use of laxatives over a prolonged period results in loss of normal bowel function. Diets generous in whole grain breads and cereals, and fruits and vegetables, along with an adequate fluid intake (1500 to 2000 ml daily) contribute to the formation of large, soft stools and more frequent bowel movements.

Enzyme Secretion for Digestion and Absorption

Digestive enzyme secretion. For the most part, a lack of important digestive enzymes does not impair the absorption of nutrients in healthy older people. Because digestive enzymes are normally secreted at levels substantially above what is required, actual enzyme levels (although sometimes reduced) are still sufficient to break down all food consumed into the forms required for absorption. Significant reductions in salivary enzymes can cause **xerostomia,** thereby making swallowing difficult possibly resulting in serious weight loss in some older people, although this is not widespread. On the other hand both the total volume and the hydrochloric acid concentration of gastric juice, and the volume of pepsin, are decreased in many aged persons. These changes in gastric secretion result from decreases in both the number of parietal cells and the secretory capacity of remaining cells. Other changes in the mucosa can reduce the secretion of intrinsic factor resulting in vitamin B_{12} deficiency. It is estimated that 25% of older people have **achlorhydria** caused by atrophy of the mucosal lining and secretory cells.[13] This alteration in the strongly acid environment of the stomach interferes with the absorption of iron, calcium, vitamin B_{12}, vitamin B_6, and folacin. A rise in pH can permit increased bacterial overgrowth leading to further mucosal damage and malabsorption of carbohydrate and fat. In the small intestine pancreatic enzymes and bile are usually present in sufficient amounts to allow normal breakdown of carbohydrate and fat.

Lactose intolerance. Reduced lactase levels have been evaluated in relation to low milk consumption among some older persons.[14] It appears that psychologic attitudes toward milk are as important, if not more so, than physiologic factors in lactose intolerance. Malabsorption was not related to the incidence of digestive symptoms, as equal numbers of absorbers and malabsorbers reported symptoms following ingestion of a lactose-containing and a lactose-free beverage. These results suggest that a component other than lactose was causing the problem. Over half of the malabsorbers reported drinking more than one glass of milk per day indicating that other factors in addition to lactose malabsorption influence low milk consumption in this age group.

Nutrient Digestion and Absorption

Protein, carbohydrate, and fat. Although the process of digestion and absorption is slowed, there is no evidence to suggest that carbohydrate or protein is handled differently by the older as compared with the younger individual. The absorption of common monosaccharides is evaluated using D-xylose as a test substance. Since this sugar is not metabolized, completeness of absorption is measured by recovery of D-xylose in the urine. Equal amounts of the test substance are recovered in all age groups. Similarly, healthy older people do not lose greater amounts of protein through the gastrointestinal tract than younger people, although completeness of digestion and absorption should be evaluated in physically impaired older persons with elevated protein requirements.

To some extent the absolute amount of fat absorbed does decrease with age. Under normal conditions neutral fat (triglyceride) comprises only a minor portion of fecal fat with fatty acids being the predominant form. Some older individuals, particularly those with extremely high levels of dietary fat, do have higher than usual fecal fat. Existing levels of pancreatic lipase appear to be the limiting factor.

Xerostomia
(Gr *xeros*, dry; *stoma*, mouth) Dryness of the mouth from lack of normal secretions.

Achlorhydria
(L *a-*, negative; *chlorhydria*, hydrochloric acid) Absence or reduced amounts of hydrochloric acid in the gastric secretions.

Vitamins and minerals. Age-related alterations in vitamin and mineral absorption are poorly understood. For the most part these nutrients have been studied in a clinical context considering age-related changes in nutritional status or incidence of deficiency disorders. For this reason absorption of vitamins and minerals will be discussed in later sections.

NUTRIENT REQUIREMENTS OF OLDER PEOPLE
Recommended Dietary Allowances

Limitations. The Recommended Dietary Allowances (RDA) as applied to older adults have many limitations.[15] Because studies of older individuals have been few, the RDA for persons over 50 has been extrapolated from that developed for young adults. For the majority of nutrients, recommended intakes are the same for younger (ages 25 to 50) and older (age 51 and over) adults. There are no adjustments in the recommended intakes of any nutrients beyond age 51.

Older adult differences. The current RDA fails to recognize that 51 year olds differ from 85 year olds in body composition, physiologic function, and metabolic adaptation. Physiologic changes in digestion or absorption could increase the need for a particular nutrient. Estrogen withdrawal following menopause alters calcium absorption and metabolism. Reduced efficiency of the renal system in excreting nitrogenous or other wastes contraindicates excessive intakes of protein or water-soluble vitamins.

Disease interaction. Another issue is the interrelation between nutritional status and degenerative disease. Chronic disorders influence requirements both as a result of the disease process and in relation to drugs prescribed in therapeutic management. Kidney disease can result in excessive loss of albumin in the urine. Diuretics prescribed in the management of hypertension lead to depletion of potassium, pyridoxine, folic acid, or zinc, depending on the particular drug. Munro advocates the development of recommendations for both healthy older persons and those with **chronic disease.**[16] It is important to evaluate each older client as an individual considering general health, level of physical activity, and presence of chronic disease.

Chronic diseases
(Gr *chronos*, time) Diseases of aging or long duration.

Energy Needs

Energy needs decrease with age as the result of changes in basal metabolism and physical activity. Basal needs are not under the individual's control, but energy expended in physical exercise varies according to individual activity patterns. Physical activity can play a major role in maintaining energy balance.

Basal metabolism. Basal oxygen consumption (measured in milliliters per minute) is influenced by sex, age, body size, and body composition, but mainly by lean body mass. Women at all ages have lower basal needs per unit of body height and weight because of their higher proportions of body fat and lower proportions of lean body mass. **Basal oxygen consumption** and associated energy needs decrease about 20% to 25% in men between the ages of 20 and 70 as a result of the loss of lean body mass.[17] Changes in adult body composition have been described in Chapter 3. The metabolic activity of remaining cells, however, appears to be unchanged. Decreases in basal metabolism in later life generally do not result from impaired thyroid function. On the average, basal energy needs of older persons range from 1100 to 1300 kilocalories for women and 1100 to 1400 kilocalories for men. For the sedentary elderly the total energy requirement is very close to the basal need.

Data from the Baltimore study (Fig. 9-1) indicate that basal metabolism continues to decline beyond age 60. Basal energy expenditure was 1541 kcal/day for 60 year olds and 1369 kcal/day for 80 year olds.[17] When basal needs were calculated on the basis of

Basal oxygen consumption
Amount of oxygen intake to meet basal metabolic needs; a means of measuring basal metabolic rate (BMR). Comparative metabolic measures in current use are derived by formula calculation using individual factors of weight, height, age, and sex: basal energy expenditure (BEE), and resting energy expenditure (REE).

TABLE 9-1   Recommended Energy Intakes (Persons Over 50 Years of Age)

	Females	Males
Body weight (kg)	65	77
Body height (cm)	160	173
Kcal/kg	30	30
Kcal/day	1900	2300
Range (variation of 20%)	1520-2280	1840-2760

Body height and weight are reference values for this age group.
Modified from Food and Nutrition Board, National Research Council: Recommended dietary allowances, ed 10, Washington, DC, 1989, National Academy Press.

kilocalories per kilogram per day, however, there was little difference between the two age groups (19.8 versus 18.7 kcal/kg/day). The RDA calculated to include basal and activity needs equals 30 kcal/kg (Table 9-1). These data confirm the idea expressed earlier that differences in basal needs among individuals of differing age are the result of differences in lean body mass and not in the metabolic rate in individual cells.

Physical activity. Physical fitness is the state in which a person's muscular, cardiovascular, and respiratory systems have the ability to respond to physical work with rapid recovery and minimal fatigue. Decreases in fitness occur as a result of smoking, lack of exercise, and age-related deterioration. Regular exercise leads to improved functional capacity that enhances the individual's ability to carry on daily activities and remain independent. Regular walking improves aerobic capacity with decreased fatigue, increases mental alertness and effectiveness, and increases bone strength. No strenuous exercise regimen should be undertaken, however, without a physical examination and professional supervision.

Energy intake and expenditure. An increase in body weight throughout adulthood will result if energy intake continues at the same level as both basal metabolism and physical activity decline. Diaries of food intake and physical activity of 252 healthy men 30 to 80 years old indicated that total energy intake declined on an average of 12.4 kcal a day each year.[10] Physical activity fell more rapidly than basal requirements (7.8 kcal per day per year as compared with 5.2 kcal). The steepest drop in total energy needs (physical activity plus basal needs) occurred between ages 70 and 80.

Other work suggests that the most precipitous decline in physical activity occurs in young adulthood rather than later in life.[18] Daily energy expenditure decreased by 40 kcal between ages 35 and 44, 17 kcal between ages 55 and 74, and 24 kcal between ages 75 and 84. This pattern emphasizes the importance of developing a regular exercise program early in life that with modifications can be continued throughout adulthood.

Problems with low energy intake. Many older individuals, particularly those for whom physical activity may be difficult, have low energy intakes. In a national survey, mean energy intakes were 1961 and 1340 kcal/day, respectively, for men and women 60 to 69 years of age. For men and women age 70 and older, energy intakes dropped to 1734 and 1270 kcal/day. Energy intake affects the intakes of vitamins and minerals as well. In a study of 691 older people in Boston (Table 9-2), those with lower energy intakes were more likely to have inadequate intakes of vitamin B_6, folacin, calcium, and zinc.[20]

Analysis of long-term energy balance suggests that individuals possess a regulatory mechanism that acts to ensure energy homeostasis. Shifts in basal metabolic rate (BMR) will conserve energy when fewer kilocalories are ingested and in some individuals will

TABLE 9-2 *Percent of Older People Consuming Less Than Two Thirds of the RDA of Vitamins and Minerals on High and Low Energy Intakes*

	Males*		Females†	
	Low kcal	High kcal	Low kcal	High kcal
Vitamin A	32	8	13	6
Folic acid	75	27	85	55
Vitamin B_6	83	48	85	62
Vitamin B_{12}	27	12	45	19
Calcium	39	4	60	14
Zinc	65	18	77	56

*Daily energy intakes: low < 21.5 kcal/kg; high > 27.5 kcal/kg.
†Daily energy intakes: low < 20.0 kcal/kg; high > 25.5 kcal/kg.
Modified from McGandy RB: Nutrition and the aging cardiovascular system. In Hutchinson ML and Munro HN, editors: Nutrition and aging, Bristol-Myers Nutrition Symposia, vol 5, New York, 1986, Academic Press, Inc.

dissipate unneeded kilocalories as heat when intake exceeds expenditure. Decreasing energy intake may be necessary to prevent weight gain. However, if energy expenditure declines due to increasing disability, a severe caloric restriction, that results in weakness and further limitation of physical activity, may not accomplish the intended goal. A moderate energy intake balanced by an increase in energy expenditure within the physical capabilities of the older adult is the most effective plan.

Essential Fatty Acids

Linoleic acid deficiency in adults is virtually unknown under normal conditions. However, efforts to control both fat and energy intakes can result in low intakes of linoleic acid, the essential fatty acid. Including one tablespoon of vegetable oil or equivalent in the daily diet will provide both linoleic acid and appropriate amounts of vitamin E.

Protein and Amino Acids

Protein needs of adults. Protein metabolism continues as a dynamic process throughout the adult life. Although physical growth has ceased, sufficient protein must be consumed to replace obligatory nitrogen losses through desquamated cells from the skin or gastrointestinal tract, body secretions, and metabolic end products. When nitrogen excretion exceeds intake, as might occur following surgery, in debilitating illness, or when the diet is poor, protein depletion ensues.

Skeletal muscle
Muscles attached to skeletal bones for control of body movements; major component of lean body mass.

Visceral organs
(L *viscus*, large body organ) Large internal organs of the body, located in the chest and abdomen.

Even well-nourished adults appear to lose body nitrogen as a function of age. It is estimated that total body nitrogen decreases from 1320 g in the young adult to 1070 g in the aged adult. **Skeletal muscle** contributes a major portion of the protein that is lost with lesser amounts coming from vital organs such as the heart or liver. Muscle mass comprises 45% of body weight in the young adult, but only 27% of body weight beyond age 70. As a result body protein turnover—protein breakdown and synthesis—shifts in location from the muscle to the **visceral organs.**[21]

Changes in body nitrogen content have led to different interpretations of protein requirements of older people. First, a decrease in active metabolic tissue and protein synthesis could reduce the need for protein and amino acids. Second, an inadequate intake of nitrogen during adulthood could ultimately lead to the observed loss in body nitrogen. Evaluations of protein metabolism and nitrogen requirements have not resolved this issue.

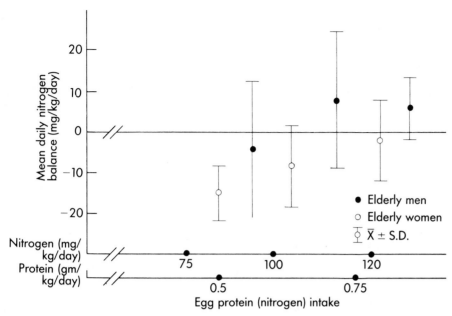

FIG. 9-2 Nitrogen balance in older people given graded levels of egg protein.

From Uauy R, Scrimshaw NS, and Young VR: Human protein requirements: nitrogen balance response to graded levels of egg protein in elderly men and women, Am J Clin Nutr 31:779, 1978. Used by permission.

Evaluating protein requirements. The methods used to evaluate protein requirements in adults are the factorial method and nitrogen balance study. The factorial method involves measuring obligatory nitrogen losses on a protein-free diet and calculating the daily intake required to replace these losses. Nitrogen balance studies evaluate the level of dietary protein that must be fed to replace obligatory losses and achieve nitrogen balance. Unfortunately, in older subjects results obtained by the two methods do not agree.

Total obligatory nitrogen losses do not differ between younger men and older men, when calculated per kilogram of body weight. Differences between men and women relate to the higher proportion of muscle and lower proportion of body fat in men. When calculated on the basis of body cell mass, obligatory nitrogen losses are higher in older than in younger individuals. This reflects the shift in protein turnover from muscle to visceral organs. Despite similar nitrogen losses per kilogram of body weight, protein requirements may still differ between old and young of the same sex if dietary protein is less efficiently used by the older adult.

Factorial estimates of obligatory nitrogen losses, adjusted to allow for efficiency of use and individual variability, predict a safe level of protein intake to be 0.42 g/kg/day for older women and 0.55 g/kg/day for older men. These values are lower than those suggested for young adults (0.52 and 0.57 g/kg/day for women and men, respectively). Older people receiving egg protein, however, cannot maintain nitrogen balance on the "safe" levels of intake suggested for either young or older adults (Fig. 9-2). A study evaluated the current RDA (0.8 g/kg/day), given as egg protein in 15 men and women ranging from 70 to 85 years of age and consuming various prescription drugs.[22] After a balance period of 30 days, nearly half of these subjects were still in negative nitrogen balance. These workers concluded that the recommended level of protein, even high-quality protein, is not adequate to prevent nitrogen loss in many persons above age 70 with chronic disease.

Factors influencing protein requirements. The inability of some older persons to achieve nitrogen balance on the test diets fed may relate to the type and level of protein consumed in the months preceding. On self-selected diets older people can maintain nitrogen balance on lower levels of protein than when fed a test diet. Individuals may over the years adapt to a diet actually considered inadequate by general standards. Then if they maintain reasonable health they retain that accommodation throughout life. Thus, previous diet should be considered when developing a therapeutic regimen for an older person. Emotional and physical stress can increase protein requirements. Inflammation or infection leads to negative nitrogen balance and loss of labile body proteins, mediated in part by the stress response of the adrenal **corticosteroid** hormones.

Factors influencing protein utilization. Classic studies described the protein-sparing action of carbohydrate and pointed to the need for sufficient nonprotein energy intake to support the use of the protein consumed to maintain body protein mass. When kilocalories are limited, protein metabolism is compromised regardless of protein intake. The inability of some older individuals to maintain nitrogen balance on what appear to be adequate levels of protein may relate to the energy value of the diet. Although protein use is maximal at 40 kcal/kg/day, the recommended energy intake for those over 50 is 30 kcal/kg/day. Encouraging physical activity to allow greater flexibility in energy intake should be a priority in nutritional counseling for older persons.

Insulin plays an important part in the metabolism and utilization of carbohydrate and protein. As people age, fat and muscle become less sensitive to insulin in promoting the uptake and utilization of glucose. However, this is not the case with protein and amino acids. Insulin infusions in healthy younger and older volunteers increase protein synthesis and prevent protein breakdown. Thus, a decrease in insulin effectiveness does not explain the impaired protein utilization in some older people.

Evaluating amino acid requirements. The present knowledge of amino acid requirements of older persons is both limited and conflicting. Early studies suggested that older individuals may have higher requirements for some amino acids. But these reports have not been confirmed. Recent work indicates that essential amino acid requirements, calculated on the basis of body weight, may change with age although the direction of change is not consistent. Tryptophan requirements appear to decrease with age, but threonine and valine requirements seem to increase. When estimated on the basis of body cell mass, however, essential amino acid requirements do increase with age.

Protein-energy malnutrition. The older person with a history of debilitating disease and poor diet is likely to have low nutrient reserves and is particularly vulnerable to overt malnutrition. These circumstances no doubt contribute to the poor nutritional status observed in some institutionalized elderly persons. But their condition may relate to energy intake before as well as after admission. Poorly nourished persons may have had a disability before entering the health-care facility and, consequently, had inadequate meals. Protein-energy malnutrition is difficult to identify in this age group because assessment values specific for older persons have not been developed. Measurements such as skinfold thickness and arm circumference or serum albumin and transferrin levels (see Chapter 2) may change as a function of age.

Protein intake. Protein intake for most older Americans appears to be adequate but protein status is income related. Low-income people are more likely to have low intakes. In a national survey about 10% of higher-income women 65 to 74 years of age consumed less than two thirds of the RDA, although 25% of lower-income women consumed less than that amount.[23] At greatest risk are those consuming inadequate levels of both protein and energy. Over 50% of the low-income women had less than two thirds of the recommended level of kilocalories. It is reasonable to expect that some of those low in one nutrient value were also low in the other. Inadequate energy intake results in less efficient

Corticosteroid

(L *corticis*, bark, shell) Any of the steroids affecting carbohydrate, fat, and protein metabolism that are produced in the outer region (cortex) of the adrenal glands in response to stimulus of the adrenocorticotropic hormone (ACTH) from the pituitary gland, or any of their synthetic derivatives. These compounds include *glucocorticoids* affecting glucose metabolism, and mineralocorticoids affecting electrolyte (Na$^+$) concentration and hence fluid-electrolyte balance.

use of the protein that is available. Thus, vulnerability to both infection and chronic disease increases.

Fat-Soluble Vitamins

Absorption of fat-soluble vitamins requires the secretion of pancreatic lipase and bile for breaking down dietary fat and "packaging" it in fat **micelles** for transport. Thus, persons with gallbladder disease might have impaired fat absorption. Decreased intakes of fat could also interfere with this process. Because of competition for binding sites, highly concentrated supplements, particularly vitamin A, can produce imbalances as well as general toxicity.

Micelle
(L *micella*, small body) A microscopic colloid particle of fat and bile formed in the small intestine for initial stage of fat absorption.

Vitamin A and vitamin E. Advancing age does not increase the requirements for these vitamins or hinder their absorption. In fact, vitamin A may be more easily absorbed by older people. When deficient serum levels are detected they usually relate to low intake and respond to dietary improvement. But questions have been raised about the ability of older persons to store and mobilize vitamin A from the liver. These differences are emphasized in a recent report describing use of vitamin A supplements by 562 healthy elderly people and 194 healthy young adults.[24] Long-term use of supplements containing one to two times the RDA resulted in serum vitamin A levels in older persons that were double those in young adults. Older persons using supplements containing more than 10,000 IU of vitamin A over a 5-year period had evidence of liver damage. Many older persons routinely consume vitamin E supplements at levels up to 1000 times the RDA. Although there is currently no evidence of toxicity resulting from such intakes, it appears that high levels of vitamin E enhance vitamin A storage in the liver. This emphasizes the need for caution among those consuming high levels of both vitamins.

Many low-income older persons consume less than 67% of the RDA for vitamin A (5000 IU for men; 4000 IU for women). In a national survey one fourth of those 65 to 74 years of age consumed less than 2000 IU daily. Although Hispanics are thought to be particularly vulnerable to low vitamin A intakes, a recent survey gave little evidence of low serum retinol levels. Dietary deficiency can be influenced by income since dark green and deep yellow vegetables and fruits, which are high in carotene (provitamin A), tend to be expensive, especially in cold winter months. Vitamin E may be less of a problem as reasonably priced vegetable oil is a good source.

Vitamin D. The vitamin D status of older people based on either dietary intake or serum vitamin D metabolite levels is less than optimal. Dietary sources make only a limited contribution to the vitamin D requirement. In older people in Boston the **median** vitamin D intake was about 50% of the RDA in women and 67% in men.[20] Serum vitamin D metabolite levels in older persons are lower in winter, emphasizing the importance of sunlight in meeting the requirement. Older people have a reduced ability to synthesize vitamin D in the epidermis. But this source is important in maintaining adequate vitamin D status.

Because many older people have low serum levels of **calcitriol,** the active vitamin D hormone, attention has been directed to possible problems in the absorption or the conversion of ingested or synthesized vitamin D to the active form. Both healthy and institutionalized older persons can absorb vitamin D in food and supplements. The ability to absorb supplemental vitamin D may be especially important for impaired elderly who are unable to go outdoors. When vitamin D is available in the diet, older persons can maintain adequate serum levels of both 25-OH-D, the intermediate metabolite produced in the liver, and $1,25(OH)_2D$, the active hormone produced in the kidney.

Calcitriol
Activated hormone form of vitamin D, [1,25 (OH)2 D3], 1,25,dihydroxy-cholecalciferol.

Vitamin D status does seem to be involved in the increase in parathyroid hormone (PTH) levels that result in mobilization of calcium and phosphorus from the bones. Postmenopausal women with vitamin D as **cholecalciferol** intakes of 2.8 µg (112 IU)/

day (RDA = 5 μg [200 IU]/day) had elevated PTH levels during the winter months when endogenous vitamin D could not be produced. In contrast, those consuming at least the RDA of 5 μg (200 IU)/day had normal PTH levels. Women suffering hip fractures had lower sunshine scores than healthy control women.[25]

The current trend toward using calcium supplements rather than dairy products as calcium sources contributes to poor dietary intakes of vitamin D. One cup of milk supplying about 300 mg of calcium will also provide 100 IU of vitamin D. Because of the danger of vitamin D toxicity and subsequent hypercalcemia, supplements should be used with caution and those containing more than 400 IU are hazardous.

Water-Soluble Vitamins

Thiamin, riboflavin, and niacin. These three B vitamins are all coenzyme factors in energy metabolism. Thus their requirements are based on energy intake and decrease beyond age 50 in response to lowered energy needs. Poor status usually relates to low dietary intake or excessive alcohol consumption. Surveys suggest that many older persons consume less than the recommended amounts of thiamin and riboflavin. However, little actual biochemical deficiency based on red blood cell enzyme activity is observed. Blacks have lower intakes of riboflavin, possibly related to lower consumption of dairy products.

Vitamin C. Ascorbic acid metabolism differs in older men and older women as men have lower plasma levels despite intakes equal to or higher than those of women. This increased requirement could relate to the higher proportion of lean body mass in men. Women maintained higher plasma levels than men at intakes ranging from 30 to 280 mg/day.[26]

An important factor in ascorbic acid metabolism is the total body pool of the vitamin that is estimated to reach a maximal tissue saturation of 20 mg/kg body weight at a plasma concentration value of about 1.0 mg/dl. Older men require intakes of about 150 mg/day to maintain that plasma level with no further increase in plasma level at higher levels of intake. Older women maintain a plasma concentration of 1.0 mg/dl on intakes of 75 to 80 mg/day, and reach a maximum concentration of 1.3 mg/dl at an intake of 280 mg/day. On intakes that equal the current RDA (60 mg) older men have plasma concentrations below 0.4 mg/dl, the level used to identify individuals at risk for ascorbic acid deficiency. This finding suggests a need for further study of the ascorbic acid requirement of older men.

In older people socioeconomic status relates to ascorbic acid status. Older persons with lower incomes are more likely to have deficient serum ascorbic acid levels. Limited intakes of vitamin C-rich fruits and vegetables may contribute to this problem. Ascorbic acid is lost if cooked vegetables are held at serving temperature for long periods of time, as happen with quantity meal programs. Citrus fruits are better under such circumstances.

Pyridoxine

Chemical name for vitamin B_6, named for its ring-like structure.

Vitamin B_6. Vitamin B_6 **(pyridoxine)** is a problem nutrient for some older persons. Both serum levels of the vitamin and the activity levels of red blood cell enzymes requiring vitamin B_6 as a cofactor tend to be low as compared with younger subjects. Among 198 low-income, community-living elderly, low vitamin B_6 status was attributed in part to low vitamin intakes as 36% of the women and 18% of the men had intakes below 67% of the RDA.[27] The higher intakes of men were due to their increased energy intake and not to increased selection of vitamin B_6-dense foods. Health problems contribute to low vitamin B_6 status. Older individuals reporting two or more health problems are more likely to have marginal serum vitamin levels despite vitamin B_6 intakes of at least 100% of the RDA. Absorption may be impaired in older persons with achlorhydria or those who are consuming high levels of prescription drugs known to interfere with vitamin B_6. Users of vitamin B_6 supplements are likely to have normal serum vitamin levels despite reported health problems.

Decreased intake of meat, poultry, or fish because of chewing problems or financial constraints also influences vitamin B_6 intake. Frail, elderly persons with low energy intakes may not be able to meet requirements through food only and may need a supplement. Because vitamin B_6 can be destroyed by heat processing, prepared foods can be poor sources. Potatoes and other vegetables are good sources of this vitamin.

Folate. Folate deficiency in older persons is associated with poor dietary intake, gastric atrophy resulting in achlorhydria, use of antacids or prescription drugs that interfere with folate absorption or utilization, and alcoholism. Overt deficiency is seldom observed in healthy, financially advantaged older people even on daily intakes of 200 µg. Based on this evidence the 1989 revision of the RDA lowered the recommended daily intake from 400 µg to 200 µg for men and 180 µg for women.[15] Older persons in hospitals or other **long-term care** facilities are at greatest risk of folate deficiency.

Cooking practices can contribute to folate deficiency since boiling vegetables for long periods of time destroys the vitamin. Orange juice and raw dark green leafy vegetables are good sources. Nutrition education and counseling should stress low-cost food sources of folate and cooking practices that retain it.

Vitamin B_{12}. Intrinsic factor found in the gastric secretions is required for the absorption of vitamin B_{12}. Lack of intrinsic factor causes a deficiency of the vitamin and **pernicious anemia.** Eventually, degenerative changes occur in the brain and spinal cord bringing mental deterioration. Impaired vitamin B_{12} absorption does exist in some older people. Various conditions such as **gastrectomy,** achlorhydria, or decreased gastric secretions reduce available intrinsic factor and subsequent vitamin B_{12} absorption. There may be atrophy of the intestinal mucosa, although physical findings may be similar in older people with normal absorption.

The nutritional significance of the observed decrease in serum vitamin B_{12} levels in older individuals (Fig. 9-3) has not been resolved. Although impaired absorption may

Long-term care
Medical, personal, or homemaking services provided within an institution or in the community for older adults who are no longer able to care for their own needs.

Gastrectomy
Surgical removal of all or part of the stomach.

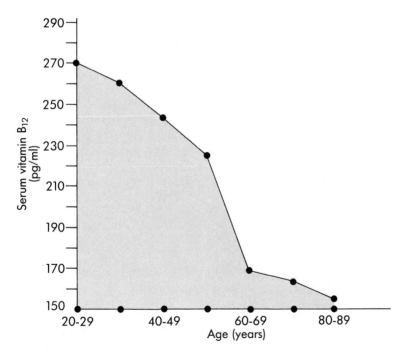

FIG. 9-3   Serum vitamin B_{12} levels according to age.

Data from Gaffney GW et al: Vitamin B_{12} serum concentrations in 528 apparently healthy human subjects of ages 12-94, J Gerontol 12:32, 1957.

play a role, older people may also consume less meat, fish, or poultry because of low incomes or chewing problems and not compensate with increased intakes of milk or cheese. At the same time older persons with normal serum vitamin B_{12} levels have been found to have degenerative changes in nerve tissue and function caused by vitamin B_{12} deficiency. Further evaluation of serum vitamin levels as indicators of vitamin status is essential.

Minerals

Iron. Absorption of iron, a complicated and inefficient process in people of all ages, is even more difficult in older people with gastrointestinal changes. When gastric secretions including hydrochloric acid are reduced or absent, iron absorption is limited. Components of these secretions bind to iron and enhance its absorption, and the hydrochloric acid reduces iron from its ferric form in food to its ferrous form necessary for absorption. Also, the absorbing surface "brush border," microvilli of the small intestine mucosa, undergoes age-related morphologic changes that can modify the rate of absorption. Finally, antacids that raise gastric pH levels and certain drugs (for example, cholestyramine) that bind both inorganic iron and iron complexes can further decrease iron uptake. A liberal intake of fiber to promote normal bowel function may bind trace minerals and decrease iron absorption. However, absorption does not appear to be a problem for many older people who are able to maintain adequate iron status on intakes approximating the RDA.

After menopause and cessation of monthly iron loss in women, and after age 50 in men, body iron stores begin to increase. By age 70 body iron stores average 800 mg in women (increased from 300 mg prior to menopause) and 1200 mg in men.[28] Daily iron losses in the form of desquamated cells have been estimated to be less than 1.0 mg per day in older men and in nonmenstruating women. This loss can be replaced easily by an intake of 10 mg of iron per day. Pathologic conditions such as peptic ulcers, undiagnosed cancer in the gastrointestinal tract, or excessive aspirin use leading to continual blood loss can significantly deplete iron reserves. A low level of blood loss may not be detected in a **guaiac test** of the stools for occult (hidden) blood. Nevertheless, this test should immediately follow any diagnosis of iron deficiency.

Older women are more vulnerable to poor iron intake based on their relatively low energy intakes. As a high proportion of dietary iron can be obtained from fortified cereal products, nutrition education should include combining foods to best advantage for maximum iron absorption. At the same time we must caution older persons to avoid multiple daily servings of cereals fortified to meet the iron requirement of the menstruating female. These products contain 15 mg of iron per serving.

Calcium and phosphorus. Calcium metabolism has important implications for both nutritional and physical health. To ensure normal function of the heart and nervous system, serum calcium must be maintained within very narrow limits (9 to 11 mg/dl). A decrease in serum calcium levels or increase is serum phosphate levels triggers the release of PTH which restores serum calcium levels by (1) releasing calcium from the bone (resorption), (2) increasing calcium absorption in the intestine, and (3) increasing calcium reabsorption in the kidney.

Prior to menopause estrogen exerts a protective effect on bone, although how this happens is not well understood. Estrogen may balance the action of PTH in promoting bone calcium release. Following menopause and estrogen withdrawal, bone becomes increasingly sensitive to PTH and calcium mobilization accelerates. As bone resorption continues to bring about high serum calcium levels, less PTH is released, resulting in lowered intestinal calcium absorption and reduced renal calcium reabsorption. Thus, loss of body calcium is increasing while net absorption is decreasing. If this process continues, eventual loss of bone density and strength increases the susceptibility to fracture. Another

Guaiac test
A laboratory test for occult (unseen) blood in the stool.

possible role for estrogen is stimulating the conversion of vitamin D to its active form to increase calcium absorption in the intestine. When calcium absorption decreases following estrogen withdrawal, more calcium is released from the bone.

Several researchers have proposed that calcium balance in older women can be improved by increasing dietary calcium.[29] Although the percentage of absorption may still be low, the net amount absorbed from a larger intake will be greater. Based on their studies, postmenopausal women can approach calcium balance on intakes of 1500 mg of calcium per day. This is substantially above the current RDA for adult women (800 mg). The NHANES data found median calcium intakes of older women to be 475 mg/day; older men had higher daily intakes (median levels, 597 mg).[23] Based on the recommendations of Heaney and colleagues, postmenopausal women are consuming only 32% of the calcium needed.[29]

Recommendations for a daily calcium intake that will limit calcium loss in postmenopausal women remain controversial. The position of the Food and Nutrition Board is that calcium intakes above the current RDA do not consistently prevent or reverse bone loss.[15] Studies indicating that intakes above 800 mg calcium per day lead to increased bone density in postmenopausal women have also included supplementation with vitamin D to maintain intakes of 10 μg (400 IU) per day. Lower daily intakes of vitamin D among controls may have limited the absorption of available calcium. Dawson-Hughes and coworkers found that calcium intakes below 400 mg/day were associated with lower bone density in older women.[30] In those women calcium supplementation raising intakes to 800 mg per day reduced bone loss.

The differences observed among investigators as to the benefits of calcium supplements could relate to the site selected for bone density measurements. Bone metabolism in **cortical bone** found in the long bones such as the femur may differ from **trabecular bone** found in the vertebrae. Calcium supplements taken at mealtime can interfere with iron absorption and retention. However, supplements in the form of calcium carbonate do not seem to lower the absorption of zinc.

Current research implicates low-calcium intakes with elevated systolic blood pressure levels. Older women consuming less than 800 mg of calcium daily have significantly higher systolic blood pressure.[15] Since high levels of calcium from supplements can interfere with the absorption of other minerals consumed at that meal, a prudent choice is consuming calcium obtained from food sources at a level that at least equals the RDA. Choosing dairy products as calcium sources will also provide the vitamin D necessary for calcium absorption.

Chromium. The suggested daily intake of chromium is 50 to 200 μg. Healthy older persons consuming self-selected diets containing these levels appear to maintain appropriate tissue stores. Age as such does not seem to be a factor in chromium deficiency. Chromium tends to be lost in food processing and can be low in diets made up largely of highly processed items. Whole grains, meats, and cheese are good sources.

Zinc. Dietary zinc is influenced by total energy intake, total money spent for food, and food selection. Older men with an energy intake of 1800 kcal consume about 10.6 mg of zinc. Older women consuming about 1300 kcal take in only 7.2 mg of zinc or 60% of the RDA.[31] In the average American diet about 40% of the zinc is provided by meat, fish, and poultry, relatively expensive items in the food budget. The most common food source is beef. A diet based on dairy products and processed breads and cereals will be limited in zinc. Older people with low intakes from the meat group as a result of limited income or chewing difficulties are at risk.

Both hair and plasma zinc concentrations are used to evaluate zinc status, although both have limitations. Among low-income individuals over 60, only 8% had hair zinc values indicating a deficiency, despite the fact that mean zinc intake was well below the

Cortical bone
(Gr *corticis*, bark, shell) Long bones of the body extremities with heavy outer cortex layer.

Trabecular bone
(L *trabs*, a little beam) General term for small meshwork of bones at ends of long bones forming attached joints, and part of the connecting network between vertebrae.

RDA. In an NHANES report 39% of women 65 and older had serum zinc levels considered to be less than adequate, and levels were consistently lower in poor versus nonpoor groups.[32] Whether the serum levels observed reflect reduced intake or a metabolic response associated with aging requires further study.

Zinc plays an important metabolic role in taste, wound healing, and immune response. These functions are sometimes altered in older people. However, zinc supplementation does not reverse such changes in older persons with adequate zinc status. Zinc status is particularly important in older individuals with decubitus ulcers or recovering from surgery.

Fluid intake. Water is supplied to the body by food, liquids consumed, and water of oxidation. In younger people the thirst mechanism ensures adequate fluid intake. Diminished sensitivity to dehydration can reduce fluid intake in the older person. The disabled individual who cannot drink without help is particularly vulnerable to low fluid intake. Those subject to incontinence may consciously restrict fluid intake to avoid embarrassment. Patients given high protein supplements are subject to dehydration if fluids are limited. Because older persons are less able to concentrate urine, fluid intake becomes more critical. Unless they have cardiac or renal complications, older people should drink six to eight glasses of fluid each day.

NUTRITIONAL DISORDERS IN THE AGED
Carbohydrate Metabolism and Glucose Tolerance

Glucose tolerance, or the ability to metabolize a glucose load, deteriorates with age. In younger individuals abnormal glucose tolerance is associated with the development of diabetes. In older individuals the difference between the pathology of disease and normal aging is less clear.

Fasting blood glucose levels. In older persons fasting blood glucose levels are not significantly higher than in younger individuals. However, 2 hours after administration of glucose under standard conditions, blood glucose levels remain significantly higher in older age groups. Many factors contribute to this alteration in glucose tolerance. The age-related decrease in lean body mass and increase in body fat play a role as excessive fatness in younger people leads to impaired glucose tolerance. Increased physical activity enhances metabolic activity and glucose uptake for fuel in the skeletal muscle. Conversely, bed rest or limited exercise reduces glucose entry into the cell. Finally, potassium depletion resulting from inadequate or prolonged use of particular diuretics can impair glucose tolerance as potassium ions are required for glucose movement into cells.

Comparison with diabetes. In diabetes a major factor is the deficiency of the active form of insulin required to facilitate both the entry and metabolism of glucose into the cell. This is not the case in older persons. In fact, insulin levels may even be higher in older than in younger groups. One problem is that older fat cells are less sensitive to the action of insulin and the rate of glucose entry and metabolism is slowed. Fat cells in older people are larger than those found in normal-weight younger people and have fewer insulin receptors. Older people may also secrete a different form of insulin (proinsulin) with limited effectiveness on fat and muscle cells.

Diet effects. High-carbohydrate (especially complex carbohydrate), high-fiber diets can improve glucose tolerance in older persons. Fiber slows the rate at which glucose is released into the blood from the small intestine, thereby lowering blood glucose levels after eating. Efforts at weight control and exercise throughout adulthood may pay dividends in avoiding deterioration in glucose tolerance.

Bone Metabolism

Loss of bone mineral and matrix, a physiologic effect of aging, has been identified in prehistoric skeletons from the year 2000 BC. **Osteoporosis** (porous bone) is the clinical syndrome resulting when over one third of the bone is lost. Beginning at age 30 to 40, women lose about 10% of their bone mass per decade; men lose about 3%.[29] All people lose bone as a result of aging. However, not all develop osteoporosis. Bone loss can occur in many locations including the spine, hip, or femur. Loss of bone (and bone strength) increases susceptibility to fracture and possible disability. The incidence of spontaneous fractures (resulting from little or no trauma) increases at an accelerating rate among older persons, especially women. The resulting immobility can change one's lifestyle. For example, an older woman may be forced to give up her home after breaking her hip.

Osteoporosis. Osteoporosis is the most common bone disorder among older persons. Decreased bone mass occurs with no change in the chemical ratio of mineral to protein matrix. Existing bone is normal. There is just less of it. In **osteomalacia** (adult rickets) bone density is decreased because of poor mineralization of available matrix. These conditions are illustrated in Fig. 9-4. Relative bone mass at older ages is influenced by the total bone laid down during periods of growth. Men at all ages have greater bone mass than women and lose bone less rapidly. Blacks have more bone than caucasians and are less likely to develop osteoporosis.

Factors influencing bone loss. Many factors affecting bone loss have been identified:

- **Diet**—calcium, protein, vitamin D, fluoride, boron, calcium-phosphorus ratio, alcohol
- **Hormones**—estrogen, parathyroid hormone, **calcitonin**
- **Other**—age, sex, race, physical exercise, smoking

The most obvious predisposing factor to bone loss is being female. Heaney and coworkers have summarized two general theories describing age-related bone loss.[29] The first theory considers bone loss the result of a deficiency of $1,25(OH)_2D$, the active form of vitamin D hormone that, in partnership with PTH, controls body calcium balance. This active metabolite regulates calcium absorption in the intestine and calcium deposit in the bone. The primary problem is reduced production of this metabolic hormone in the kidney, most likely related to estrogen withdrawal. With less calcium absorbed and supplied to the blood, serum calcium falls, resulting in the secretion of PTH, mobilization of bone calcium, and eventual development of osteoporosis.

The second theory proposes that an underlying imbalance exists between bone resorption and bone formation. Bone remains a dynamic tissue throughout life with remodeling occurring at many locations at any given time. When bone resorption occurs

Calcitonin
(L *calx*, lime, calcium; *tonus*, tension, balance) A polypeptide hormone secreted by the thyroid gland in response to hypercalcemia, which acts to lower both calcium and phosphate in the blood.

FIG. 9-4 Normal bone, osteoporosis, and osteomalacia. **A,** Normal bone. **B,** Osteoporosis in which there is a reduced amount of bone of normal composition. **C,** Osteomalacia in which the amount of bone is normal but the composition is abnormal.

at a faster rate than bone replacement as a result of age, estrogen withdrawal, or lack of physical activity, osteoporosis results. Both theories agree that calcium absorption is reduced and production of the active vitamin D hormone is depressed. Both theories may be correct depending on the individual and the severity of bone loss.

Prevention of osteoporosis. No effective treatment now exists for replacing bone that has been lost. For this reason prevention must be the focus, beginning with adolescent girls and younger women (see Chapter 3), to reduce the risk factors involved. Smoking and excessive use of alcohol appear to accelerate bone loss. Regular physical exercise and muscle pull on the bone are necessary to maintain bone tissue. Body weight must be exerted on the bone. In fact, weightlessness as shown by space flights results in rapid loss of bone tissue similar to that experienced in prolonged bed rest, despite normal calcium intakes and efforts to exercise. Even general inactivity contributes to calcium loss. Older persons who exercise only infrequently have significant bone loss in contrast to those who exercise several times a week. Walking is an effective way to preserve bone mass.

Calcium supplements have been shown to preserve bone mass in postmenopausal women *under certain conditions*.[30] First, menopause must have occurred more than 5 years before. In the first 5 years after menopause, estrogen deficiency will prevent any possible benefit of calcium supplementation. Second, women benefiting from supplementation must have had low calcium intakes (<400 mg per day) before supplementation. In this study the supplement of 500 mg per day raised intake to the recommended level of 800 mg per day. Reducing calcium loss in the urine can also be effective in preventing bone loss. Excessive intakes of protein (two to three times the RDA) can increase urinary loss of calcium, although the resulting impact upon the development of osteoporosis is controversial. Older persons being treated for hypertension with thiazide diuretics that reduce urinary excretion of calcium may have reduced bone loss. Boron, which appears to influence bone metabolism and physiologic doses of $1,25(OH)_2D$, and the active vitamin D hormone are being evaluated as measures to reduce the risk of osteoporosis. Fluoride supplements, considered to offer promise as a therapeutic agent to reverse the effects of osteoporosis, have recently been shown to increase fractures in weight-bearing bones as new bone formed is poor in quality.[33]

Calcium supplements. Current publicity regarding the ability of high-calcium intakes to prevent bone loss has led to mass marketing of calcium supplements. Calcium intakes up to 1500 mg daily appear to have no adverse effects in women with no previous history of kidney problems. **Hypercalcemia** has been reported in persons consuming large amounts of both calcium and alkali (sodium bicarbonate) and individuals should check with their physicians before using such combinations. Helping older persons select high-calcium foods that are reasonably low in fat and energy and contain the vitamin D necessary for calcium absorption should be a priority in all nutrition counseling. For those who choose not to consume dairy products because of lactose intolerance or cultural food pattern, calcium supplements in the form of calcium carbonate, lactate, gluconate, or citrate malate (the form used to fortify orange juice) are all reasonably well absorbed. Consider which form or brand will provide the most calcium per tablet at the lowest cost. Large doses above 500 mg per tablet should be avoided as they can result in gastrointestinal discomfort or constipation.

Osteomalacia. Osteomalacia is usually the result of vitamin D deficiency. It is characterized by demineralization of the bone matrix. Among older people this can relate to (1) low vitamin D intake coupled with nonexposure to sunlight, (2) malabsorption of ingested vitamin D, or (3) liver or renal disease that interferes with the conversion of the vitamin to its active form. The active form of vitamin D or an analogue is used in treatment. Daily calcium supplements (1500 mg) in addition to vitamin D therapy may be required.

Hypercalcemia
Elevated level of calcium in the blood.

Nutritional Anemia

Anemia results from changes in either the number or characteristics of the erythrocyte. A decrease in the oxygen-carrying capacity of the blood and the consequent oxygen deficit in the tissues leads to increased heart rate, shortness of breath, and weakness. Unfortunately, such symptoms are often considered typical of older people and may go unnoticed as danger signs of a developing anemia.

Iron-deficiency anemia. The most common cause of anemia in older people is iron deficiency, although vitamin deficiencies may complicate the problem. Blood loss through the gastrointestinal tract is a frequent and critical cause of iron deficiency in older people. Extreme blood losses impart a dark red or black color to the stool, but abnormal losses are frequently not visible (occult) and require chemical analysis for detection. Conditions associated with gastrointestinal bleeding include gastric or duodenal ulcers, diverticulitis, hiatus hernia, hemorrhoids, and cancer. Long-term use of aspirin with irritation of the stomach lining can lead to significant blood loss.

Healthy older people have hemoglobin levels similar to those of younger people, although several trends are apparent with age. Among men hemoglobin levels decrease with age and prevalence of anemia is higher after age 65. Women have lower hemoglobin levels throughout the child-bearing years, but improve in iron status when menstruation ceases. Aged black persons, particularly women, are more likely to have hemoglobin levels below 12 g/dl. Older people in general have reduced numbers of red blood cells compared with established standards. **Mean** cell hemoglobin concentration, however, is relatively unchanged suggesting that red blood cells produced have normal hemoglobin concentration.[32]

Erythropoiesis can be less efficient in advanced age as a result of changes in the bone marrow or a lack of nutrients. Protein-energy malnutrition depresses red blood cell production. Decreased erythropoiesis will result if body iron is not released for hemoglobin synthesis as occurs in infection. Chronic low-grade infection as occurs with fever, inflammation, and renal disease produces an anemia characterized by reduced erythropoiesis, reduced numbers of red blood cells normal in size and hemoglobin content, and low serum iron. Uncomplicated iron deficiency anemia will respond to iron therapy; anemia of chronic disorders is highly resistant to treatment.

Treatment of iron-deficiency anemia must be preceded by careful evaluation. Administering supplemental iron to persons who in fact have **megaloblastic anemia** caused by a lack of folate or vitamin B_{12} has serious consequences since vitamin B_{12} deficiency and neural damage continue. Equally unwise is the shotgun approach of including iron and all necessary cofactors. A healthy nonanemic individual who is not consuming adequate iron should be helped to select iron-rich foods. If the diet cannot be improved, a supplement containing the recommended allowance for iron (10 mg) is a reasonable alternative. Self-medication with iron supplements above the recommended intake is extremely dangerous. It can lead to **hemochromatosis** and liver damage or mask a pathologic condition causing gastrointestinal blood loss.

Megaloblastic anemia. A megaloblastic pernicious anemia occurs in less than 1% of the population, with an average age at onset of 60 years. It was originally given the name "pernicious" anemia before its underlying cause was discovered to be a vitamin B_{12} absorption defect, and because its persistent downward course led to death. A general age-related decline in serum vitamin B_{12} levels has been reviewed in relation to its possible significance as a predictor of vitamin B_{12} deficiency or onset of pernicious anemia. If vitamin B_{12} is poorly absorbed and body stores are systematically being depleted, overt deficiency is imminent. On the other hand, many people with serum levels below normal, observed over time, do not develop overt anemia. The need for a sensitive and specific

Anemia
(Gr *a-*, negative; *haima*, blood) Blood condition marked by a decrease in number of circulating red blood cells, hemoglobin, or both.

Mean
Mathematical term for the average numeric value of a group of numbers.

Megaloblastic anemia
(Gr *mega*, great size; *blastos*, embryo, germ) Anemia due to faulty production of abnormally large immature red blood cells, due to a deficiency of vitamin B_{12} and folate.

Hemochromatosis
(Gr *haima*, blood; *chroma*, color) Disorder of iron metabolism characterized by excess iron deposits in the tissues, especially the liver and pancreas; results from iron overload from prolonged use of iron supplements or from transfusions.

method for detecting B_{12} deficiency is underscored by the report that several older patients with no abnormal blood parameters were found to have neurologic damage resulting from vitamin B_{12} deficiency.

Increasing numbers of older people are being treated with intramuscular injections of vitamin B_{12} as a preventive measure. Those diagnosed and treated for pernicious anemia must be made aware of the need to return periodically for continued treatment to prevent subsequent deterioration.

DRUG-NUTRIENT RELATIONSHIPS
Drug Use by Aged Persons

Older persons comprise about 12% of the general population, but they use about 25% of all prescription drugs. This is not surprising because many chronic diseases associated with aging are managed with prescription drugs. Hypertension, heart disease, and diabetes mellitus are the most commonly diagnosed conditions among older persons. In the very old, those above age 84, arthritis is a common ailment. Over half of older people take at least one medication daily and many take six or more a day for multiple health problems.[34]

Older persons are particularly vulnerable to adverse nutritional effects from drug therapy. Nutritional status may already be jeopardized by physiologic changes and less than optimal nutrient intake influenced by social and economic conditions. Chronic disease necessitates long-term drug therapy that can contribute to gradual depletion of nutrient reserves. Multiple drug intake compounds nutritional problems. Moreover, the effects of most drugs have been tested and validated on younger individuals who have different rates of drug absorption, metabolism, and excretion, based on differences in body composition and renal function.

Mechanisms of Drug-Nutrient Actions

Modes of metabolic interference. Drugs may interfere with nutrients at the point of ingestion, absorption, utilization, or excretion. Food intake may decrease because of drugs that depress appetite or cause nausea or vomiting. Interference with the secretion of digestive enzymes or alterations in pH or transit time by particular drugs can prevent the digestion of foods into the nutrient forms required for absorption. Competition for binding sites on the mucosa may reduce nutrient uptake. Drugs may prevent the metabolic conversion of a vitamin into its active form, thereby negating its physiologic function. Some drugs form insoluble complexes with nutrients that then cannot be metabolized and are therefore eliminated. In general, vitamins and minerals are most affected.

Nutrient depletion. Nutrient depletion is most likely to occur with a drug that inhibits nutrient absorption or with a drug taken for an extended period of time. A drug that acts as a vitamin **antagonist,** or affects a nutrient such as folic acid that participates in a variety of metabolic processes, will result in impaired biochemical function. Finally, nutritional effects of drugs will be more serious in individuals with preexisting subclinical malnutrition. Those with marginal status who consume multiple drugs over periods of years are at greatest risk of nutrient depletion.

Antagonist
(Gr *antagonisma*, struggle) Agent that has an opposite, conflicting, or inhibiting action to another substance.

Nutritional Aspects of Nonprescription Drugs

Analgesic and gastrointestinal drugs. Because over-the-counter (OTC) drugs are easily obtained and commonly used they are often perceived to be without risk. Use of these drugs may not be reported to a physician, creating the possibility of a dangerous interaction with a prescription drug. The person may have increased dosage above that recommended if the desired effect was not achieved.

The analgesic most used by older persons with arthritis, headache, and muscle pain is aspirin (acetylsalicylic acid; ASA). Prolonged use can induce iron-deficiency anemia from irritation of the gastrointestinal mucosa and subsequent blood loss. Among the gastrointestinal drugs, laxative abuse can lead to depletion of sodium and potassium as well as chronic diarrhea. Mineral oil used as a cathartic interferes with the absorption of fat-soluble vitamins. Sodium bicarbonate and other antacids increase gastric pH which inactivates thiamin and hinders the absorption of iron, calcium, and folic acid. Aluminum-hydroxide–containing antacids that bind phosphate have been shown to cause phosphate depletion and accelerate bone loss.[35]

Alcohol. A significant number of older people consume alcoholic beverages regularly, but the number who abuse alcohol is not known. Physical and emotional upset, loneliness, and bereavement all contribute to increased use of alcohol. Among 691 older persons in Boston, 43% of the men and 28% of the women consumed alcohol at least once over the 3-day record period, but alcohol use decreased with age.[20] As persons grow older, tolerance to alcohol decreases and adverse side effects increase, even in chronic alcoholics. The risk of nutritional deficiency arising from use of other drugs is markedly increased by excessive use of alcohol or when prior alcoholism has depleted nutrient stores. Also, alcohol interacts with some drugs and conditions to worsen any negative effects. Both alcohol and aspirin irritate the gastric mucosa and can lead to bleeding; when combined, the anticoagulant effect of aspirin can result in serious hemorrhage. High alcohol intakes decrease serum potassium levels, making the cardiac patient on digitalis at risk of toxicity. The person with insulin-dependent diabetes can become hypoglycemic following high alcohol intakes as the alcohol interferes with **gluconeogenesis.**

Alcohol has both primary and secondary effects on nutritional status. It interferes with the absorption of thiamin by inhibiting the active transport mechanism required to move the vitamin across the mucosal cell and into the blood. Alcohol-induced damage to the intestinal mucosa results in malabsorption of both vitamin B-12 and folate. Excessive zinc excretion is associated with alcohol abuse. Alcohol intake may lead to lower food intake. Among moderate users of alcohol, alcohol kilocalories may be substituted for carbohydrate, fat, and protein, in an effort to limit total energy intake.

Use of vitamin and mineral supplements. Many older persons regularly use vitamin and mineral supplements. However, the specific supplements chosen do not necessarily provide those dietary nutrients that are in shortest supply. Although calcium is frequently the nutrient lowest in intake relative to the RDA, calcium supplements have begun only recently to gain popularity.

Of concern is the excessive use of vitamin-mineral supplements by some older individuals. Among healthy older persons in New Mexico, 95% of those taking a multivitamin preparation daily also used other vitamin or mineral products.[36] The nutrient supplemented at the highest level was vitamin E, with median supplemental intake 18 times the RDA. Supplements did, however, contribute toward meeting the RDA for vitamins B₆ and D and folate. For those not taking supplements, median intakes of these vitamins were less than 67% of the RDA. Some individuals, however, were routinely consuming at least five times the recommended levels of vitamins A and D, intakes that over prolonged periods are potentially toxic.

Some of the **diuretics** prescribed for the management of hypertension result in the loss of potassium in the urine. Serum potassium levels must be maintained within a narrow range as either hypokalemia (low serum potassium levels) or hyperkalemia (high serum potassium levels) interfere with cardiac function and can result in sudden death. To replace daily potassium losses and prevent hypokalemia, some older persons have been given potassium supplements rather than depending on food sources. However, potassium supplements have been associated with development of hyperkalemia and are particularly

Gluconeogenesis
(Gr *gleukos*, sweetness; *neos*, new; *gennan*, to produce) Production of glucose from non-carbohydrate molecules, such as amino acids from protein and the glycerol portion of fatty acids.

Diuretics
(Gr *diouretikos*, promoting urine) Drugs that stimulate urination.

dangerous for those with poor renal function.[35] A more prudent recommendation is daily consumption of foods high in potassium such as orange juice, bananas, or a baked potato.

Effects of prescription drugs. The drugs most frequently prescribed for older persons are diuretics and cardiac drugs to treat cardiovascular disease, antiinflammatory drugs to treat arthritis, and analgesics. Digoxin, a drug that stimulates the heart and is used to treat cardiac failure sometimes causes anorexia and nausea resulting in weight loss. Lipid-lowering drugs carry the risk of vitamin depletion with prolonged use. Particular diuretics that promote the excretion of water and sodium also bring about loss of potassium; others can increase the risk of both hyperglycemia and hyperlipidemia in diabetics.[35] Older persons consuming large amounts of aspirin to alleviate arthritis pain and inflammation may have low serum folate and ascorbic acid levels and be at risk of iron deficiency anemia as discussed earlier. Medicines used to control seizures increase the need for vitamin D. Too high a level of particular vitamins can interfere with the action of certain drugs. Therefore, older individuals should avoid self-medication with high-potency supplements.

FOOD SELECTION PATTERNS OF OLDER PEOPLE
Environmental Factors

Living situation changes. In the older person food patterns reflect lifelong attitudes and habits as influenced by the changing environment. To better understand the influence of lifestyle, health, and economic status on the food choices of older people, review the examples listed in Table 9-3. Many influencing factors have been identified that can act both individually and in combination. The older woman who has prided herself on "cooking from scratch" may have to rely on heat-and-serve items or home-delivered meals if her worsening arthritis makes food preparation difficult. Solving the food problems of older people often involves seeking alternatives as living situations and resources change, and things have to be done differently than before.

Adequate diets. Living alone and having less money to spend on food results in poor nutrient intake in some older people, but this is not true for all older people. The stereotype of an old person who subsists on tea and toast is not substantiated by survey data from the United States or Great Britain. Although there are individuals who do follow this pattern, it is not typical of this age group. The mere fact of their survival indicates their ability to select a reasonably adequate diet over a period of years.

Changes in Lifelong Food Patterns

Decreased energy needs and nutrient density. Normal aging brings about a decrease in energy requirements and the quantity of food consumed. According to NHANES data, mean daily intake decreased by about 900 kcal (2734 to 1829 kcal) in men and 325 kcal (1643 to 1295 kcal) in women between the ages of 25 and 65.[19] Older blacks and Hispanics have lower energy intakes than older caucasians. Older persons appear to compensate for lower energy intakes by choosing their foods more carefully, as shown by the fact that intakes of vitamins A and C and iron per 1000 kcal were higher in the older group. If older persons decrease their energy intakes by consuming less of all foods usually eaten, rather than selectively reducing intakes of items low in nutrient density, the overall quality of the diet will suffer. Among 194 older Canadians, perceived health benefit was a stronger determinant of food choice than convenience, price, or prestige value, supporting the idea that nutrition education can be effective in helping older people modify their food patterns.[37]

Food market changes. Changes in agriculture, food preservation, and food processing over the past 35 years have multiplied the food forms now available to the consumer. Frozen orange juice, unheard of during the early adult years of people now over 60, is a

TABLE 9-3   *Factors Influencing Food Selection Patterns of Older People*

Psychologic
Loneliness
Bereavement
Social isolation
Food aversion
Symbolism of food
Mental awareness
Feelings of self-worth
Food faddism
Nutrition knowledge
Dissatisfaction with family or living situation

Physiologic
Loss of appetite
Loss of taste
Dental problems
Prescribed diets
Chronic disease
Food intolerance
State of health
Physical disability
Degree of physical exercise
Vision problems

Socioeconomic
Age
Sex
Level of income
Cooking facilities
Daily schedule
Retirement/leisure time
Level of education
Distance to food store
Availability of transportation
Availability of familiar foods

common item. Adoption of new food items by older persons suggests that nutritious foods not used previously may be accepted if introduced in a positive way.

Psychologic Aspects of Food Selection

Eating alone. Throughout life eating is a social activity. The birthday party, the wedding breakfast, and family sharing at the table are all social acts. Loss of spouse or friends results in a loss of eating companions for the older individual who may now be eating alone for the first time in life. It is important, however, to differentiate between isolation and desolation. Isolates are content living alone and may have done so most of their lives. Desolates, on the other hand, live alone but are both lonely and unhappy. Depression or need for attention may be expressed in the form of food-related problems and can lead to significant weight loss.

Retirement. Retirement brings a change in lifestyle for older single people and couples. Less money may be available for food. Since both husband and wife are now home both may be involved in meal planning and food preparation. Among one group of retired couples not only did husbands participate in food-related decisions, but their level of participation had nutritional implications.[38] The greater the husband's involvement in meal planning and actual food purchase, the better the diet. Women who expressed dissatisfaction with their traditional role consumed poorer diets and may have had less commitment to meal preparation. Nutrition education programs are often directed toward women, but leaders should make an effort to involve men who may be less bored with food activities and therefore are more receptive and those who strongly influence the food decisions within a retired family.

Mental disorders. Psychologic and mental disorders in the older person can result in confusion, irritability, acute depression, or, in extreme situations, dementia. Those with organic brain syndrome may forget to eat or be unable to differentiate between breakfast, lunch, and dinner. If they are unable to prepare food, meals may consist totally of bread and jam or prepackaged foods, thus limiting nutrient intake both in quantity and quality. Patients with Alzheimer-type senile dementia may not remember how to use a knife and fork or how to lift a cup to the mouth. For these individuals it may be advantageous to have the main meal at noon when they are most alert and attentive to food intake.

Physiologic Aspects of Food Selection

Sensory loss. The majority of older persons living in the community describe their appetite as good, but anorexia is a common side effect of many prescription drugs. Taste and odor also influence the older person's selection and enjoyment of food. Taste thresholds for the four basic tastes—sweet, sour, salty, bitter—have been shown to decline with age although the general ability to taste undergoes little change throughout adulthood. However, even healthy aged persons have a diminished sense of smell, which also plays a role in taste. Some older persons have a mild **dysgeusia** or chronic taste in the mouth, possibly caused by dentures or poor oral hygiene. Prescription drugs can contribute to unpleasant or disordered taste. In practice, the tendency to use generous quantities of salt may be an effort to strengthen flavor when taste has been altered.

Dental problems. Dental problems such as **gingivitis** and tooth loss are often thought to alter dietary patterns in older people, particularly those who are **edentulous** (without any teeth). Economic problems may prevent them from seeking professional services for preparation or repair of dentures. In general, lack of dentures influences the enjoyment of eating more than it does actual nutrient intake. Dairy products, eggs, ground beef, and well-cooked chicken and fish can provide high-quality protein for those with chewing problems. Fruit juices and cooked vegetables are good sources of vitamins A and C and folic acid. Most fresh fruits can be eaten if ripe, peeled, and cut into small pieces.

Physical health. Older persons limited in vision or movement find it difficult to shop for groceries or prepare meals. Moving about the kitchen requires special effort for a person who must grasp a cane or walker. Poor eyesight can preclude reading a nutrition label or package directions for use. Preparing vegetables is painful or in some cases impossible for a person whose hands are crippled with arthritis. All of these problems can result in increased use of heat-and-serve items that tend to be high in sodium and fat, and somewhat low in vitamins and trace minerals. Nutrition education should assist older persons in making healthful choices from the preprepared foods available.

Special diets. Impaired physical health or multiple high-risk factors in a reasonably healthy older person sometimes necessitates a prescribed diet limited in energy, fat, sodium, or cholesterol. Other diets may be self-prescribed such as a diet to prevent or alleviate arthritis. Many older people following a special diet obtain their food information from

Dysgeusia
(Gr *dys*, bad; *geusis*, taste) Abnormally perverted sense of taste, or bad taste in the mouth.

Edentulous
(L *e-*, without; *dens*, tooth) Absence of natural teeth.

someone other than a clinical nutritionist/registered dietitian, nurse, or physician. These diets include low fat, "diabetic," and various weight-loss regimens that in many cases are not appropriate for the individual.

Sociologic Aspects of Food Selection

Living situations. Older people living in their own homes usually have adequate facilities for food storage and preparation including a working stove, oven, and refrigerator. The type and size of appliance can affect its use. With rising utility costs older people may hesitate to heat their conventional oven for one item such as a baked potato. A small toaster-oven or a microwave oven is a wise investment for the person cooking for one or two. Individuals who rent a room with no kitchen facilities are forced to eat in restaurants or elsewhere. They may heat some foods on a hotplate or use a heating coil to heat water for soup or beverages.

Access to food market. Lack of access to a grocery store may present additional problems. In rural areas stores may be at some distance, requiring either a car or a ride. Even in urban settings the older person may be required to ride the bus or walk to the store and carry bundles home (Fig. 9-5). During the winter months icy sidewalks may present special difficulties for the infirm. For inner-city elderly the nearby store may be a convenience store with high prices and poor selection, since supermarkets in such areas are closing because of poor profit margins and the growth of suburban shopping malls. Shopping services would be a valuable program for a volunteer community agency to undertake.

Lifestyle. Some persons eating alone may not feel motivated to prepare adequate meals. But available evidence does not support the generalization that older individuals residing in one-person households have poorer diets than those in households of two or more. Socioeconomic status influences both social participation and nutrition in older people living alone. Those with higher incomes entertain friends in restaurants more frequently and tend to have more nutritionally adequate diets. Low-income older people have few mealtime visitors and those that do serve food items that they usually eat themselves such

FIG. 9-5 Carrying groceries from the store is a difficult task for older people.

as macaroni and cheese or tomato soup. Company at meals can have a positive influence on food intake, particularly among those who may not care to cook for themselves.

Evaluation of dietary data from the National Food Consumption Survey (NFCS) indicates that single older men, especially those over 75, are at higher risk of nutrient intakes below 67% of the RDA than single older women.[39] Lower nutrient intakes in these men did not relate to less money for food or consuming food items lower in nutrient quality. The basis for the lower intakes was that these men consumed less food overall and had lower energy intakes. Single women 65 and over had mean nutrient intakes similar to women residing with a spouse. Single men are less likely to consume fruits and vegetables and have poor intakes of vitamins A and C, although they drink generous quantities of milk providing riboflavin and calcium.

Susceptibility to quackery. The sale of useless and in some cases potentially harmful medical devices, potions, and nutritional supplements for the cure of specific ailments is a $10 billion industry. Unfortunately, older people are particularly vulnerable to exploitation by entrepreneurs promoting such products because they have a strong interest in health and have many physical impairments with no known cure. Thus, promises of miracle cures for chronic problems or the restoration of vitality and well-being appear to warrant attention.

A potentially dangerous practice is the use of high-potency vitamin and mineral supplements or herbal products to cure a physical problem. Such products not only delay appropriate treatment but also can result in toxicity or medical emergency. In younger persons high-potency supplements can result in gastrointestinal upset, confusion, and loss of coordinated movement. Such physical changes in an older person may be overlooked in the belief that they are age-related. Older persons are also susceptible to unvalidated methods of nutritional assessment such as hair or saliva analysis used as a basis for supplement sales. Health personnel must gain the confidence of the older individual and then discuss appropriate use of nutritional products.

Economic Aspects of Food Selection

Food patterns. Women and minority groups are most likely to be poor. This influences food patterns in various ways: (1) the level of income will determine how much money can be spent for food, (2) the low-income individual is less likely to own a car to simplify grocery shopping, and (3) the individual is more likely to live in either the inner city or a rural area where food is more expensive. Therefore the buying power of the money available is reduced. Older households spend a larger proportion of their total income on food but less of their food dollar goes toward food away from home. While younger people eat in restaurants, older people are more likely to eat at each other's homes, congregate meal programs, or "pot luck" socials.

Income and ethnic group. Both income and ethnic group influence food selection and nutrient intake. National survey data reveal that energy levels (kilocalories) decrease with income in both black and white women 65 to 74 years of age, although black women consume less food regardless of income. However, iron intake per 1000 kcal was 8.2 mg in older women in both higher and lower income groups. The nutritional vulnerability of low-income women in general and black women in particular is emphasized by the fact that median intakes were about 75% the RDA for iron and vitamin A.[19] Therefore, half of those surveyed were consuming less than this amount. In a comparison of 254 low-income Mexican American and non-Hispanic older people, food choices were determined by ethnic ties rather than income.[40] Mexican-American older people used more saturated fats, eggs, organ meats, and legumes, and consumed fewer dairy products, fruits, and vegetables. This food pattern resulted in lower intakes of vitamins A and C in the older Mexican-Americans. A better understanding of the food preferences of ethnic groups can help in planning appropriate programs that will support positive health-related behavior.

Implications for Nutrition Education

Food group patterns of older people as recorded in NHANES indicate that bread and ready-to-eat cereals (both enriched and whole grain) are consumed regularly as are whole and low-fat milk.[41] Unfortunately, this evaluation did not include actual quantities, so daily use of milk could reflect small amounts used with coffee, tea, or cereal. Eggs and luncheon meats were the most common foods from the meat or protein group. Orange juice, bananas, lettuce, and potatoes were the fruits and vegetables included most regularly in meal planning.

Immediately apparent is the absence of a dark green leafy vegetable as a source of both folate and vitamin A. Orange juice brings ascorbic acid, folate, and potassium to the diet, and bananas supply both potassium and vitamin B_6. Increased use of milk and other dairy products should be encouraged and whole grain products emphasized. Alternatives to costly luncheon meats, frequently high in fat and sodium and low in other nutrients, should be explored. Such practical approaches as these could be used in nutrition education programs.

NUTRITION PROGRAMS FOR OLDER PEOPLE
Community-Based Long-Term Care

Long-term care refers to the medical and support services, including nutrition services, required to maintain the functionally impaired older person at an optimum level of well-being. Long-term care can take place in an institutional or community setting. In a community setting nutrition support services provided by family members, neighbors, or community agencies can allow the older person to continue to live independently for an extended period of time. Such services may take the form of a ride to the grocery store with a son or daughter or delivery of meals by a community-sponsored home-delivered meals program. Congregate meals providing both a nutritious meal and a social outlet can help to maintain health and well-being in the relatively fit adult.

Food Assistance Programs

Food stamps and the commodity distribution program are available to older people meeting specific income guidelines. Programs that increase food buying power can improve dietary quality. Unfortunately, eligible older persons are less likely to participate in such programs than eligible younger persons. Older persons may be less well informed concerning available programs, may lack transportation to the appropriate office, may be in poor health generally, or may not apply because of pride.

Food stamps. A USDA evaluation of 854 older persons either receiving or eligible to receive food stamps indicated that men over age 64 and both sexes over age 75 benefit most.[42] Intakes of protein, calcium, magnesium, and vitamin A did not differ between participating and nonparticipating women 65 to 74 years of age. Those using food stamps had higher intakes of vitamin B_{12} but all met at least 100% of the RDA. Vitamin B_6 fell to below two thirds the RDA among all women evaluated. Men 75 and over, who were not using food stamps, had less than 67% of the RDA for energy, magnesium, and vitamin B_6, and only 71% of the RDA for vitamin A. Men of similar age who used food stamps met at least three fourths the RDA for all nutrients except vitamin B_6.

Commodity distribution program. This program provides supplemental foods and nutrition education to individuals at least 60 years of age who have low incomes or are at nutritional risk. The monthly food packages contain surplus commodities such as flour, rice, cornmeal, hot cereal, canned and nonfat dry milk, canned meat or poultry, juice, dried beans, peanut butter, and cheese. One report concluded that the commodity package supplied 100% of the RDA for protein, vitamins D and B_{12}, calcium, iron and riboflavin.[43] However, it did little to improve intakes of folate and vitamins B_6 and E. Unfortunately, the commodity distribution program is not available in all regions.

National Nutrition Program for the Elderly (Title III-C)

Title III-C
The statute of the Older Americans Act authorizing congregate and home-delivered meals for people 60 years old and over.

Basic authorization. The Older Americans Act of 1965 as amended is the major piece of legislation providing programs for persons 60 and over. When establishing the nutrition program in 1972 Congress directed attention toward elderly persons who might not eat adequately because:

- They cannot afford to do so.
- They lack the skills to select and prepare nourishing meals.
- They have limited mobility that hinders shopping and cooking.
- They feel rejected and lonely and lack incentive to cook and eat alone.

The congregate meal program, funded under Title III-C of the Older Americans Act, was designed to make available meals at little or no cost in a social setting. It operates through meal sites in community or recreation centers, municipal buildings, public housing, senior citizens centers, or churches. Meals are served 5 days per week in urban settings but often only 2 to 3 days per week in rural locations. Important criteria in selecting a location are accessibility and familiarity to the older people in the community. See box on p. 377 that describes a potential client for such a meal program in an urban community. Close to 150 million congregate meals are served each year.

Since the congregate meal program was developed, the older population has changed both in age and general characteristics. There are more persons 75 and over and these individuals are more likely to be frail, chronically ill, and homebound. To meet this emerging need, recent amendments to the Older Americans Act have authorized increasing funds for home-delivered meals. About 40% of the meals now funded under Title III-C are home-delivered.

Home-Delivered Meals

General organization. Meal delivery programs have been developed by community nonprofit organizations and health and social service agencies such as hospitals, churches, nursing homes, and visiting nurses associations. Most receive some funding through Title III-C. Within community-sponsored programs meals are usually delivered by volunteers who pay their own transportation costs. People who deliver meals for a Title III-C program administered by a government agency are usually reimbursed for both time and mileage.

Meal delivery programs operate Monday through Friday. A hot meal is delivered at noon, sometimes accompanied by a cold meal to be eaten later. Some programs include additional cold lunches on Friday or before a holiday to provide for days when meals are not delivered. Delivery of cold lunches requires that the recipient have a refrigerator to safely store the additional food. No program provides meals on all days or for all meals of the day.

Eligibility requirements. Older people can request meal delivery directly or be referred by a family member, physician, visiting nurse, dietitian or nutritionist, outreach worker, or social worker. Programs receiving Title III-C funding require that (1) recipients be age 60 or over, although spouses younger than 60 can be served, and (2) recipients must be unable to leave their homes because of disability or other extenuating circumstances.

When meal delivery is not appropriate, the client should be assisted in exploring other options. If the individual can leave home, transportation to a Title III-C meal site provides an opportunity for both food and social activity. A two-person household may be in need

CASE STUDY

The Needs of an Elderly Woman Living Alone

Miss Evans has just celebrated her 80th birthday. She is 65 inches tall, weighs 158 pounds, and has no major health problems other than arthritis. She uses aspirin regularly for pain. Miss Evans lives in a subsidized high-rise apartment complex for senior citizens. She has a four-burner stove and small refrigerator, but very limited storage space for frozen or self-stable items. She prepares all her own meals and eats alone. She usually has toast and coffee for breakfast and either a bowl of cereal or a peanut butter sandwich for lunch. She does not drink any milk except with her cereal but is fond of cheese. She makes a lot of stew-type meals, often buying chicken when it is on sale. She likes all fruits and vegetables but uses mostly canned because they are cheaper than fresh. She finds the amount of money she can spend for food very limited. She likes whole wheat bread and usually selects it although her favorite brand is higher in cost than other breads. Miss Evans had shopped about twice a week at a supermarket located about 1 mile from her apartment. After a recent fall, she is afraid to ride the bus alone and now her nephew shops for her once every 2 weeks. In between she buys necessary items at a convenience store about one city block from her apartment, but the prices there are much higher. She has not been feeling hungry lately although she has well-fitting dentures and is able to eat anything she wishes. She weighs herself every week and noticed that she lost 5 pounds over the past month.

Questions for analysis
1. What are the socioeconomic or lifestyle factors that influence Miss Evans's food intake?
2. What are the physiologic factors that may influence her food intake?
3. Which nutrients appear to be lacking in her dietary pattern?
4. What would you recommend to improve her food situation?
5. What are some food programs that would assist Miss Evans in remaining independent?

of home-delivered meals if one person is so burdened caring for an invalid partner that he or she has little time, incentive, or energy to prepare adequate meals. Implementation of **diagnosis-related group (DRG)** guidelines, resulting in earlier release of older patients from medical facilities for extended convalescence at home, has led to a dramatic increase in requests for home-delivered meals.

Innovative approaches to food delivery. As the number of home-bound elderly continues to escalate, the cost of daily meal delivery is becoming prohibitive. Meal delivery in rural areas is especially burdensome in relation to both cost and the added problem of maintaining foods at appropriate temperatures over an extended delivery time. One alternative to daily delivery of hot meals is weekly delivery of several frozen meals. This allows recipients to choose what they want to eat on a particular day and at what time. Supplementing one or two home-delivered meals each week with several frozen meals presents another option. Milk, fruit, and canned or freeze-dried items could accompany the frozen meals. However, recipients must have freezer space for storing meals as well as an oven for reheating.

For homebound persons able to move about within their homes, groceries can supplement either frozen or hot meals. Canned, dehydrated, and freeze-dried foods could

Diagnosis-related group (DRG)
A US government cost-containment management classification scheme for predesignation of Medicare payments based on specific diagnosis categories of disease.

replace either a congregate or home-delivered meals program. They are also appropriate as a supplementary food source for weekends or other nondelivery days. Analysis of the relative cost-effectiveness and cost-benefit of alternative food delivery systems should be a priority for community-based long-term care.

Nutrition Standards for Meals Programs

Meals are expected to provide one third of the RDA for this age group. Proposed standards would require that nutrient content be determined by calculation based on the nutrient content of individual food items. When two or three meals are provided, the total for the day should equal 67% or 100% of the RDA, respectively, allowing some flexibility within individual meals.

Menu planning. The method currently used by many programs for planning menus is the Title III-C Meal Pattern (Table 9-4). Maximal nutrient quality of the meals can be maintained by the selection of foods with high **nutrient density.** Bread products prepared from enriched flour are acceptable, but whole-grain items increase intakes of fiber, vitamins, and trace minerals. Whole-grain breads and pasta might be introduced gradually to improve acceptance among those not accustomed to these items.

Because rising food costs limit the frequency of meat, fish, or poultry, the use of other sources of iron, zinc, and important vitamins needs to be emphasized. One alternative is legumes including lentils. If cheese or other dairy product is the primary protein source, iron could be provided in the form of a whole-grain bread and a dessert containing eggs or iron-rich fruit. Milk consumption may increase if there is a choice of lowfat, nonfat, or buttermilk. Nonfat dried milk or grated cheese can fortify soups or sauces, increasing the calcium, protein, and riboflavin content.

Dessert should be a significant source of nutrients as well as a pleasant climax to the meal. Fruit desserts such as a baked apple or apple crisp contribute important nutrients, particularly if made with whole grains. Pudding, custard, or ice cream provide calcium as well as high-quality protein for those who do not drink milk. Moist, flavorful baked products prepared with whole grains, oatmeal, raisins, applesauce, pumpkin, carrots, or banana add iron, B-complex vitamins, provitamin A, and trace minerals. Recipes containing sugar, fat, and little else are generally avoided.

Limited funding and lack of professionally trained personnel make modified diets impractical in most locations. For persons with diabetes or those limiting energy intake, the Title III-C pattern is likely to be acceptable if portion size is controlled, skim milk is available, and fruit is offered as an alternative to a high caloric dessert. General modifications limiting sodium, sugar, and fat are of potential benefit to all participants.

Nutrient density
The protein, vitamin, or mineral content of a food expressed in relation to its energy (caloric) content.

TABLE 9-4 Title III-C Meal Pattern Meeting Federal Guidelines

Food Type	Recommended Portion Size*
Meat or meat alternate	3 oz cooked edible portion
Vegetables and fruits	Two ½ cup servings
Enriched white or whole grain bread or alternate	One serving (one slice bread or equivalent)
Butter or margarine	1 teaspoon
Dessert	½ cup
Milk	½ pint (1 cup)

*A vitamin C–rich fruit or vegetable is to be served each day; a vitamin A–rich fruit or vegetable is to be served at least three times per week.

From United States Department of Health, Education and Welfare: Guide to effective site operations: the Nutrition Program for the Elderly, Corvallis, 1973, Oregon State University.

Program Evaluation

Congregate meals. Kohrs and coworkers evaluated the impact of Title III-C congregate meals on the nutritional status of 466 rural elderly persons.[44] They reported that menus provided considerably more than one third of the RDA for all nutrients calculated. For women the meals contained at least 80% of the RDA for protein, vitamins A and C, and riboflavin, and at least 40% of the RDA for energy, calcium, iron, and the B vitamins. For men the levels provided of protein, vitamins A and C, and energy were between 40% and 67% of the RDA. It cannot be assumed, however, that all food served is consumed, including the cup of milk. Both men and women received about half of their daily intakes of protein, calcium, iron, vitamin A, and vitamin C from the Title III-C meal. Women who live alone and individuals with limited education and lower incomes consume a greater share of their daily nutrient intakes at the meal site.

A national evaluation of Title III-C concluded that participants consume better diets on days that include a site meal and consume better diets than nonparticipating neighbors of similar age and socioeconomic background.[43] Also, diets of participants are in some cases higher on days not including a site meal. Nutrition education received at the meal site may improve food selection or the fact that fewer meals have to be provided from personal resources may have a positive effect upon the overall food pattern. For those with the poorest economic status, the negative impact of a low income on diet quality was ameliorated by the Title III-C meal. Calcium and vitamin A, the nutrients in shortest supply in the diets of older people, were most influenced by participation. This suggests that older people consume less milk and dark green and deep yellow fruits and vegetables at home.

Home-delivered meals. Evaluation of the impact of home-delivered meals on the diet quality of recipients is urgently needed. In general, recipients find that delivered meals allow them to eat a greater variety of food. However, one delivered meal per day will not bring individual intakes to within two thirds of the RDA for most important nutrients. Greater attention is also needed concerning the maintenance of appropriate food temperatures to guarantee food safety.

Summary

People above age 60 are increasing in number faster than any other segment of the population. The control of infectious diseases has reduced the number of early deaths. The major causes of death are now heart disease, cancer, and stroke. The aging process with loss of cells results in declining heart, renal, and pulmonary function. Both structural and functional alterations in the brain and target organs contribute to the changes observed.

For the most part the RDAs for older persons have been extrapolated from those for younger adults. Energy requirements decrease with age due to the decline in basal metabolic rate and physical activity. Protein needs may be increased among those older persons with serious chronic disease, but a wider problem may be the inefficient use of ingested protein because of inadequate energy intakes. Vitamin needs do not increase in the healthy elderly population. Biochemical deficiencies more likely relate to low intake or use of prescription drugs that interfere with nutrient absorption and utilization. Trace mineral intake tends to be low among older people who rely on highly processed food items or who have low energy intakes. Iron-deficiency anemia is most often due to occult blood loss. Age-related bone loss may be retarded by increased calcium intake, an adequate supply of vitamin D, and regular exercise.

Loneliness, physical disability, and poverty contribute to inadequate nutrient intakes. Individuals over age 75, older men living alone, and the homebound are most vulnerable to poor dietary intake. Government and community programs including food stamps, congregate meals, and home-delivered meals make positive contributions to the nutritional status of older persons.

Review Questions

1. What factors have led to the significant increase in life expectancy that has occurred since 1900? Why has life expectancy at age 65 not changed over this period?
2. Describe several physiologic changes that occur with normal aging. What is a nutritional implication of each?
3. What are some limitations of the current RDAs for older persons? How do the RDAs for persons over 50 differ from those for younger adults?
4. Low serum levels of folic acid, vitamin B_6, and vitamin B_{12} have been reported in some older people. What might be the causes of these lowered levels?
5. Explain the difference between osteoporosis and osteomalacia. What are the physiologic and dietary factors that are associated with the development of osteoporosis? What recommendations would you give to a postmenopausal woman who is concerned about her bone health?
6. What are some nutritional implications of commonly used over-the-counter drugs and prescription drugs? Describe the mechanisms by which drugs can adversely affect nutritional status.
7. How do age, sex, loneliness, physical disability, poverty, and living alone influence nutrient intake in older people? Who is most vulnerable?
8. Describe several types of community nutrition programs that serve older people. What levels of nutrient intake are provided by each?
9. You receive a telephone call from a woman who is concerned about her elderly mother who appears to have an inadequate diet. The daughter has asked you to recommend a vitamin-mineral supplement. How would you respond?

References

1. US Senate Special Committee on Aging: Aging America: trends and projections, 1987-88 ed, Washington, DC, 1988, US Government Printing Office.
2. US Department of Health and Human Services: Health promotion and aging: Proceedings of the Surgeon General's Workshop, Washington, DC, 1988, US Government Printing Office.
3. Van Itallie TB and Lew EA: Health implications of overweight in the elderly. In Prinsley DM and Sandstead HH, editors: Nutrition and aging, Progress in clinical and biological research, vol 326, New York, 1990, Alan R Liss, Inc.
4. Kelley L, Ohlson MA, and Harper LJ: Food selection and well-being of aging women, J Am Diet Assoc 33:466, 1957.
5. Schlenker ED: Nutritional status of older women, PhD dissertation, Michigan State University, East Lansing, Mich, 1976.
6. Kaplan GA et al: Mortality among the elderly in the Alameda County study: behavioral and demographic risk factors, Am J Public Health 77:307, 1987.
7. Donahue RP et al: Physical activity and coronary heart disease in middle-aged and elderly men: the Honolulu Heart Program, Am J Public Health 78:683, 1988.
8. Benfante R and Reed D: Is elevated serum cholesterol level a risk factor for coronary heart disease in the elderly, JAMA 263:393, 1990.
9. Kenney RA: Physiology of aging: a synopsis, Chicago, 1982, Year Book Medical Publishers, Inc.

10. Shock NW: Energy metabolism, caloric intake and physical activity of the aging. In Carlson LA, editor: Nutrition in old age, Symposia Swedish Nutrition Foundation X, Stockholm, 1972, Almqvist & Wiksell.

11. US Department of Health and Human Services, US Department of Agriculture: Nutrition monitoring in the United States. A progress report from the Joint Nutrition Monitoring Evaluation Committee, DHHS Publication No (PHS) 86-1255, Washington, DC, 1986, US Government Printing Office.

12. Rolls BJ and Phillips PA: Aging and disturbances of thirst and fluid balance, Nutr Rev 48:137, 1990.

13. Kemp JA and Russell RM: Nutritional consequences of disorders of gastric secretion, Nutrition & the MD 16(12):1, 1990.

14. Rorick MH and Scrimshaw NS: Comparative tolerance of elderly from differing ethnic backgrounds to lactose-containing and lactose-free dairy drinks: a double-blind study, J Gerontol 34:191, 1979.

15. Food and Nutrition Board: Recommended dietary allowances, ed 10, Washington, DC, 1989, National Academy of Sciences.

16. Munro HN: Major gaps in nutrient allowances: the status of the elderly, J Am Diet Assoc 76:137, 1980.

17. James WPT, Ralph A, and Ferro-Luzzi A: Energy needs of the elderly: a new approach. In Munro HN and Danford DE, editors: Nutrition, aging, and the elderly, Human nutrition, A comprehensive treatise, vol 6, New York, 1989, Plenum Press.

18. Elahi VK and others: A longitudinal study of nutritional intake in men, J Gerontol 38:162, 1983.

19. US Department of Health and Human Services, US Department of Agriculture: Nutrition monitoring in the United States. An update report on nutrition monitoring, DHHS Publication No (PHS) 89-1255, Washington, DC, 1989, US Government Printing Office.

20. McGandy RB et al: Nutritional status survey of healthy noninstitutionalized elderly: nutrient intakes from three-day diet records and nutrient supplements, Nutr Res 6:785, 1986.

21. Munro HN: Protein nutriture and requirements of the elderly. In Munro HN and Danford DE, editors: Nutrition, aging, and the elderly, Human nutrition, A comprehensive treatise, vol 6, New York, 1989, Plenum Press.

22. Gersovitz M et al: Human protein requirements: assessment of the adequacy of the current Recommended Dietary Allowance for dietary protein in elderly men and women, Am J Clin Nutr 35:6, 1982.

23. US Department of Health and Human Services: Dietary intake source data: United States 1976-80, DHHS Publication No (PHS) 83:1681, Washington, DC, 1983, US Government Printing Office.

24. Krasinski SD et al: Relationship of vitamin A and vitamin E intake to fasting plasma retinol, retinol-binding protein, retinyl esters, carotene, α-tocopherol, and cholesterol among elderly people and young adults: increased plasma retinyl esters among vitamin A-supplement users, Am J Clin Nutr 49:112, 1989.

25. Krall EA et al: Effect of vitamin D intake on seasonal variations in parathyroid hormone secretion in postmenopausal women, N Engl J Med 321:1777, 1989.

26. VanderJaqt DJ, Garry PJ, and Bhagavan HN: Ascorbic acid intake and plasma levels in healthy elderly people, Am J Clin Nutr 46:290, 1987.

27. Manore MM, Vaughan LA, Carroll SS, and Leklem JE: Plasma pyridoxal 5-phosphate concentration and dietary vitamin B-6 intake in free-living, low-income elderly people, Am J Clin Nutr 50:339, 1989.

28. Herbert V: Nutritional anemias in the elderly. In Prinsley DM and Sandstead HH, editors: Nutrition and aging, Progress in clinical and biological research, vol 326, New York, 1990, Alan R Liss, Inc.

29. Heaney RP et al: Calcium nutrition and bone health in the elderly, Am J Clin Nutr 36:986, 1982.

30. Dawson-Hughes B et al: A controlled trial of the effect of calcium supplementation on bone density in postmenopausal women, N Engl J Med 323:878, 1990.
31. Sandstead H et al: Zinc nutriture in the elderly in relation to taste acuity, immune response, and wound healing, Am J Clin Nutr 36:1046, 1982.
32. US Department of Health and Human Services: Hematological and nutritional biochemistry reference data for persons 6 months to 74 years of age: United States, 1976-80, DHHS Publication No (PHS) 83-1682, Hyattsville, Md, 1982, US Government Printing Office.
33. Riggs BL et al: Effect of fluoride treatment on the fracture rate in postmenopausal women with osteoporosis, N Engl J Med 322:802, 1990.
34. Lecos CW: Diet and the elderly. Watch out for food-drug mismatches, FDA Consumer 18(10):7, 1984-85.
35. Roe DA: Handbook on drug and nutrient interactions. A problem-oriented reference guide, ed 4, Chicago, 1989, American Dietetic Association.
36. Garry PJ et al: Nutritional status in a healthy population: dietary and supplemental intakes, Am J Clin Nutr 36:319, 1982.
37. Krondl M et al: Food use and perceived food meanings of the elderly, J Am Diet Assoc 80:523, 1982.
38. Schafer RB and Keith PM: Social-psychological factors in the dietary quality of married and single elderly, J Am Diet Assoc 81:30, 1982.
39. Davis MA, Murphy SP, Neuhaus JM, and Lein D: Living arrangements and dietary quality of older U.S. adults, J Am Diet Assoc 90:1667, 1990.
40. Bartholomew AM, Young EA, Martin HW, and Hazuda H: Food frequency intakes and sociodemographic factors of elderly Mexican Americans and non-Hispanic whites, J Am Diet Assoc 90:1693, 1990.
41. Fanelli MT and Stevenhagen KJ: Characterizing consumption patterns by food frequency methods: core foods and variety of foods in diets of older Americans, J Am Diet Assoc 85:1570, 1985.
42. US Department of Agriculture: Food and nutrient intakes of individuals in 1 day, low-income households, November 1979 to March 1980. Nationwide Food Consumption Survey 1977-1978, preliminary report no 13, Washington, DC, 1982, US Government Printing Office.
43. Ponza M and Wray L: Final results of the elderly programs study. Evaluation of the food assistance needs of the low-income elderly and their participation in USDA programs, US Department of Agriculture, Food and Nutrition Service, Alexandria, Va, 1990.
44. Kohrs MB, O'Hanlon P, and Eklund D: Title VII Nutrition Program for the Elderly, I. Contribution to one day's dietary intake, J Am Diet Assoc 72:487, 1978.

Further Reading

D'Urso-Fischer E, Heller K, Netterville L, and Storey M: Reaching out to the elderly, Nutr Today 25:20, 1990.
This article describes several successful nutrition education projects that can be adapted to local situations.
Fischer J and Johnson MA: Low body weight and weight loss in the aged, J Am Diet Assoc 90:1697, 1990.
Physiologic and psychologic factors relating to involuntary weight loss in older adults including anorexia arising from medications, gastrointestinal distress, and depression are described. This article stresses the importance of monitoring body weight.
Goodwin JS: Social, psychological, and physical factors affecting the nutritional status of elderly subjects: separating cause and effect, Am J Clin Nutr 50(suppl):1201, 1989.
Cognitive function, alcoholism, and institutionalization can influence nutritional status in older persons. This article provides a framework for evaluating available evidence.

Patlak M: Older adults examine health-care options, FDA Consumer 25(1):1991.
   This article provides an overview of options for health care at home, including home improvements to accommodate the older individual with disabilities, home helpers, and medical equipment.
Ranno BS, Wardlaw GM, and Geiger CJ: What characterizes elderly women who overuse vitamin and mineral supplements, J Am Diet Assoc 88:347, 1988.
   This article provides insight toward identifying those older persons who may be vulnerable to overuse of supplements and providing appropriate nutrition education.
Seeman E et al: Reduced bone mass in daughters of women with osteoporosis, N Engl J Med 320:554, 1989.
   Daughters whose mothers have osteoporosis tend to have less bone than other women of similar age. This article discusses related genetic and environmental issues and need for screening.

10

Nutrition Education

Eleanor D. Schlenker

Basic Concepts

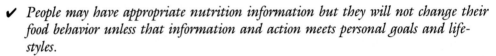

✔ *People may have appropriate nutrition information but they will not change their food behavior unless that information and action meets personal goals and life-styles.*

✔ *An effective nutrition education program must first identify audience communication goals and lifestyles.*

✔ *Nutrition education for all ages includes a variety of strategies according to need.*

✔ *Programs providing a served meal present opportunities for immediate practical nutrition education.*

Nutrition education can be defined as the process of helping individuals develop the knowledge, skills, and motivation needed to make appropriate food choices throughout life. Although simple in definition, this task is complex in application.

Consumers are confused by conflicting views on nutrition issues that appear in the popular press and on television. Changing skills are needed for good food selection as a person moves through the life cycle. The teenager eats on the run. The older widow prepares all her meals at home and eats alone. Peer pressure and persuasive advertising compete with personal concerns about health. Increasing recognition of the effect that appropriate nutrition has on lifetime health and well-being has led to more attention to nutrition education by community health agencies, government agencies, and the food industry. Nutrition counseling is emerging as a professional focus for registered dietitians and nutritionists working in clinical, community, and educational settings.

This chapter explores personal and environmental forces that affect individual food choices. It reviews educational strategies that can be developed to influence these choices. Appropriate settings and programs for delivery of nutrition information to target groups are also considered.

NUTRITION, KNOWLEDGE, MOTIVATION, AND FOOD BEHAVIOR
Basis of Nutrition Behavior

Establishing food patterns. What, when, where, and with whom one eats is determined mainly by personal, psychosocial, and cultural needs, rather than by physiologic ones. Ethnic background, religious teaching, or geographic region can be strong determinants of food preferences. Food habits are learned in childhood. Yet the adult may continue to choose homemade pasta or greens with salt pork long after leaving the family home. Refugees from southeast Asia and Mexican-Americans often retain accustomed food patterns as symbols of their cultural heritage even though particular foods may be expensive or difficult to obtain. The success of nationally advertised fast food chains may be due in part to the sense of security related to a standard food and common experience.

Not only the kinds of food eaten as a child but also the way parents handled food behavior make lasting impressions. Foods used as rewards or special treats can continue to serve as comfort foods throughout life. Noting the time or passing a favorite restaurant can trigger feelings of hunger. Boredom, loneliness, or guilt can lead to eating, often to excess. This interaction of factors contributing to development of personal food behavior is described in Fig. 10-1.

Changing food patterns. Changing food behavior requires both direct and structural interventions.[1] Direct intervention includes such strategies as publications, public service announcements, and individual counseling to provide consumers with the knowledge to help motivate them to make appropriate dietary changes. Ultimately, the **motivation** must come from within, but sound knowledge at the right time, when an individual is highly receptive, can provide a basic stimulus. An individual who has just been informed that his blood pressure level is putting him at risk of a stroke may be motivated to consider ways of decreasing his sodium intake or increasing his exercise level to bring about weight loss.

Motivation
Forces that affect individual goal-directed behavior toward satisfying needs or achieving personal goals.

Structural intervention involves such strategies as changing food production methods or the economic environment to improve accessibility to nutritious food. Distributing food stamps to low-income families, developing prepared foods low in sodium, or genetically producing leaner meat are examples of structural interventions. Although nutrition educators traditionally have focused on direct intervention, structural intervention is becoming increasingly important in solving contemporary nutrition problems.

Nutrition knowledge and behavior change. A common belief is that acquiring nutrition knowledge will in itself lead to improved diet practices. This is rooted in the idea that it is lack of nutrition information that prevents people from making better food choices. Although practical knowledge is a necessary tool, it is of use only if and when one makes a conscious decision to use it. Hochbaum hypothesizes that a person must be emotionally "ready" to make a behavioral change for factual knowledge to be effective.[2]

Optimum health or disease prevention has been considered to be a primary motivator. Some people value health for its own sake and will deliberately select a lifestyle that will contribute to this end. The majority of individuals, however, select behaviors consistent with their personal goals regardless of their health-promoting qualities. Even people with a strong health orientation experience conflicts relating to taste, cost, convenience, or peer acceptance of food items. Among women who regularly purchased food products fortified with vitamins and minerals such as breakfast cereals or fruit drinks, the major reason given was to ensure meeting nutrient requirements.[3] However, 77% indicated that a strong consideration in their choice was taste.

Food behavior is extremely complex. It frequently involves group as well as individual

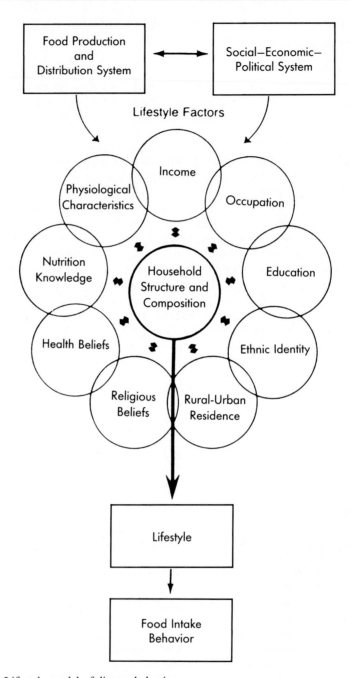

FIG. 10-1   Lifestyle model of dietary behavior.

From Pelto GH: Anthropological contributions to nutrition education research, J Nutr Educ 13(suppl):2, 1981. © Society for Nutrition Education. Used by permission.

decisions. A child may not have the option of selecting a cereal lower in sugar if siblings favor a high-sugar brand. A working mother may choose prepared items although she considers fresh ingredients better nutritionally, because short-term goals at that moment take precedence over long-term advantages. Positive approaches that relate to practical concerns such as time, cost, and taste should be emphasized in nutrition education. The box on pp. 388-389 provides basic conceptual guidelines to assist in selecting essential food and nutrition information for all age groups.

Nutrition Knowledge and Attitudes

Children and youth. Nutrition education in school settings has traditionally included the Basic Four Food Groups guide (p. 37), with limited emphasis on specific nutrients. However, current nutritional concerns require a more sophisticated approach regarding the composition of processed foods and the influence of particular nutrients in maintaining lifelong health. A study of over 5000 students from grades 1 to 12 indicated a general awareness that fiber was health-promoting.[4] Foods identified as "good for you"—apples, whole milk, and broccoli—were thought to contain fiber. "Bad" foods, including soda, sugar, and ice cream were expected to be high in fat and cholesterol. The problem of selecting curricula for nutrition education that will provide young people with the necessary skills to select a healthy diet throughout their lifetime is still unsolved.

Adults. Among adults nutrition knowledge is related to both age and level of education. Younger individuals and those with more years of formal education score higher on nutrition knowledge tests. Men are more likely to be interested in nutrition information as related to health. Food selection and preparation are usually the responsibility of the woman in the family. In two-parent households younger men sometimes help with the cooking but seldom with food selection. In retired families men tend to be more involved in food shopping and food budget decisions.[5] The increasing numbers of single males and single parent households headed by males, and the increasing interest of men in sharing food preparation suggests a need to target nutrition information to male audiences.

Current Trends in Consumer Attitudes

Food quality, safety, and relation to health are growing concerns of the general public. Among supermarket shoppers surveyed by the Food Marketing Institute, 96% indicated that nutrition was somewhat or very important when purchasing food. However, 65% of shoppers admitted that their diet needed some degree of improvement.[6] The nutrient of greatest concern was fat, followed closely by cholesterol. According to a poll conducted by the National Restaurant Association, 39% of the adult population base their food choices on good nutrition.[6]

Consumer attention to health has raised concerns about the use of health claims in food advertising. Current regulations allow such claims if they are truthful, based upon reliable scientific evidence, and presented within the context of a healthy diet. The majority of food advertisements do not promote either a general or specific health claim. Nevertheless, nutrition educators should alert consumers to the need to carefully evaluate health claims associated with food products (see box on p. 390).

THE LEARNING PROCESS
Teaching versus Learning

The terms teaching and learning are sometimes confused. A teacher may assume that a learner has acquired knowledge or skill simply because information has been provided.

ONE STEP FURTHER

Concepts for Food and Nutrition Education

Nutrition

Nutrition is the process by which food is selected and becomes part of the human body.

Food and its handling

A. Food contains nutrients that work together and interact with body chemicals to serve the needs of the body.

B. No one food by itself contains all the nutrients in the appropriate amounts and combinations needed for optimal growth and health.

C. Many different combinations of food can provide the needed nutrients in appropriate amounts.

D. Food contains important nonnutritive components, such as dietary fiber, which are needed for healthy functioning of the body.

E. Toxicants, additives, contaminants, and other nonnutritive factors in food affect its saftey and quality.

F. The way food is grown, processed, stored, and prepared for eating influences the amount of nutrients in the food and its safety, appearance, taste, cost, and waste.

G. Varying amounts of energy and other resources are required to produce, process, package, and deliver food to the consumer.

Nutrients and dietary components

A. Nutrients in the food that we eat enable us to live, grow, keep healthy and well, and be active.

B. Each nutrient—carbohydrates, protein, fats, vitamins, minerals, and water—has specific functions in the body.

C. Nutrients must be obtained from outside the body on a regular basis because the body cannot produce them in sufficient amounts.

D. Most healthy people can obtain all the nutrients, in the amounts needed, from a variety of foods.

E. Nutrients are distributed to and used by all parts of the body.

F. Nutrient interactions may affect the amounts of nutrients needed and their functioning.

G. The body stores some nutrients and withdraws them for use as needed.

H. Nutrients are found in varying amounts, proportions, and combinations in the plant and animal sources that serve as food.

I. Ongoing scientific research determines nutrients, their functions, and the amounts needed.

J. Both dietary excesses and nutrient deficiencies affect health.

K. Optimum intakes of nutrients and dietary components have both upper and lower limits.

L. All persons throughout life have need for the same nutrients, but the amounts of nutrients needed are influenced by age, sex, size, activity, specific activity, specific conditions of growth, state of health, pregnancy, lactation, and environmental stress.

Nutrition and physical activity

A. Balancing energy intake and energy expenditure is important for achieving and maintaining desirable body weight.

B. There is a synergistic relationship between nutrition and physical activity that affects health and well-being.

ONE STEP FURTHER

Concepts for Food and Nutrition Education—cont'd

Food selection

A. Food (that is, what people consider edible) is culturally defined.
B. Physiologic, cultural, social, economic, psychologic, and geographic factors influence food selection.
C. Knowledge, attitudes, and beliefs about food and nutrition affect food selection.
D. Food availability and merchandising influence food choices.

National and international food policy

A. Food plays an important role in the physical, psychologic, and economic health of a society.
B. Food production, distribution, and merchandising systems have economic, social, political, and ecologic consequences.
C. Effective utilization of individual and community resources is beneficial for the economic and nutritional well-being of the individual, family, and society.
D. The availability of food and maintenance of nutritional well-being is a matter of public policy.
E. Knowledge of food and nutrition combined with social consciousness enables citizens to understand and participate in the development and adoption of public policy affecting the nutritional well-being of societies.

From Society for Nutrition Education: SNE concepts for food and nutrition education, J Nutr Educ 14:1, 1982. © Society for Nutrition Education. Concepts developed by the membership and approved by the Board of Directors. Used with permission.

Also, the learner's interpretation of what has been said may differ from what the teacher intended. Emphasis on the importance of vitamins and minerals may motivate a mother to purchase a vitamin-mineral supplement for her child if it was not made clear that nutrient requirements are best met by the selection of appropriate food. To develop programs that not only provide useful information but also lead to appropriate behavior, we need to understand how people learn.

Stages in the Learning Process

Personal nature of learning. Learning is a highly personal process. It relates directly to the personal needs and goals of the learner. Learning may take place to satisfy either a conscious or subconscious need or to avoid a loss of privilege or a punishment. Current interests, ambitions, satisfactions from new activities, and past experiences all influence the learning process.

Stages of learning. For all of us, new ideas take time to grow. Actually, individuals adopt new ideas through several merging stages:

• Becoming aware of a new idea or practice
• Developing an interest and seeking more information
• Evaluating advantages and disadvantages of the practice
• Trying the practice to test its usefulness
• Accepting or rejecting the practice for further use

Different types of information sources are more or less important depending on the stage in the adoption process.[7] Mass media—radio, television, or newspapers—are most

ONE STEP FURTHER

Nutrition Education and Food Marketing

Emphasis on the influence of healthy food choices toward prevention of chronic disease has resulted in nutrition educators directing consumers' attention to the total fat content and degree of saturation, sodium content, and nutrient density of particular food items. Some foods such as meat products, dairy products, or frozen entrees have been cited as items high in fat, saturated fat, or sodium.

Food marketing groups have responded by joining with nutritionists or dietitians to promote healthy food choices among their products. These cooperative nutrition education efforts have emphasized the role of particular food items within a healthy diet pattern, for example, suggesting that a food moderate in fat but high in other nutrients can make a positive contribution to the diet when used in appropriate amounts. Beef, pork, and dairy commodity groups and processors of fats and oils have participated in such collaborative programs.

Community nutrition programs have cooperated with the meat industry in promoting heart healthy eating by educating consumers regarding lean cuts of meat, appropriate portion size, and low fat methods of preparation. Programs that provide information regarding specific choices within a food group are more healpful to consumers than the mixed messages that can arise when food categories are promoted by producers for their nutritive value while their use is discouraged by health professionals because of particular nutrient components.

When developing such a collaborative program, consider the following guidelines:

1. Develop educational criteria for evaluating the food products and the consumer education materials to be provided. Be sure that these criteria are stated in writing.
2. Ensure that all parties are knowledgeable about the nutrition content, as well as the production and marketing of the product.
3. Develop a working relationship with food producers based on mutual respect; producers can provide resources and helpful communication strategies to ensure program success.
4. Seek cooperation from other health care professionals in the community; provide information regarding the goals of your programs and the information to be presented.

By working together nutrition professionals and food producers can better serve the nutrition information needs of the consumer.

Adapted from Mullis RM and Pixie P: Lean meats make the grade—a collaborative nutrition intervention program, J Am Diet Assoc 88:191, 1988.

important in the first two stages; making people aware of new ideas and helping them obtain more information about them. Friends, neighbors, or professional sources, less important in early stages of the adoption process, exert the greatest influence in later stages as an individual evaluates, tests, and finally accepts or rejects the idea. Personal experience is the most important factor influencing the continued use of an idea or practice. **Implications for nutrition education.** The relative importance of information sources has implications for nutrition education at all ages. A child may be required to learn nutrition facts, but his choice of an after-school snack will likely depend on what his friend or sibling chooses to have. An overweight adult may be interested in a weight-loss program described in a newspaper article or leaflet from a local health agency, but long-term adherence to a weight-control program requires support from famiy or friends. Media impact in promoting initial recognition of an idea or problem points to our need to make more effective use of radio, television, and printed materials.

Sources of Nutrition Information

Types of sources. Eating behavior is influenced by both the source of nutrition information and the frequency of its use. Nutrition information is obtained from three main sources: (1) casual sources—articles or advertising read or seen or heard as a result of another activity such as watching television or reading; (2) selective sources—government pamphlets or special nutrition programs; and (3) significant persons—persons in the immediate environment, such as family, friends, or neighbors.[5]

Sources used by children. For children and youth, casual sources are the most common. Television is usually the most frequent source of nutrition information. On the average, children watch television 30 hours per week and see numerous food commercials.[8] Children also receive food and nutrition information from their parents, but their peer group is an extremely important source of nutrition attitudes. Although nutrition education still receives only limited attention in the classroom, this setting has strong potential for a graded, systematic treatment of essential information.

Sources used by adults. Information sources used by adults relate to age, sex, place of residence, and stage in the family life cycle.[5] Young families in the process of developing appropriate food patterns are more likely to seek information from classes, government sources, and relatives, and less likely to use advertisements and university extension programs. Older persons, especially those in rural areas, use television and newspaper advertisements as sources of nutrition information. The 867 adult participants in a health survey mentioned physicians most frequently as sources of credible nutrition information, followed by books, newspapers, and magazines.[9] Only 12% read nutrition labels.

Unfortunately, many consumers do not know where to find reliable nutrition information, so they depend on media sources that may present a biased point of view. Voluntary health organizations and government agencies need to cooperate in making appropriate information available to the public.

FOOD GUIDANCE AND NUTRITION EDUCATION
Need for Food Guides

The ultimate goal of nutrition education is to provide consumers of all ages with the information they need to plan, purchase, prepare, and consume wholesome, economic diets. Reaching this goal requires a food-selection guidance system that can be used as a model for planning and evaluating daily food intake. Several **food guides** have been developed as described in Chapter 2. These guides include the basic four good groups, the food exchange lists, and the dietary guidelines for Americans. However, all have limitations that raise questions about their usefulness (see p. 37).

Food guide
A model for planning and evaluating a daily diet.

Basis for Development

Historically, food guidance systems were developed to translate dietary standards into simple and reliable tools that would be useful in planning day-to-day food intake. Several criteria must be considered in their development and evaluation:
- They must be consistent with known nutrition needs and provide adequate levels of protein, vitamins, and minerals without exceeding energy requirements.
- They must address current diet-health issues.
- They must be easily used and understood.
- They must be adaptable to a wide variety of cultural, religious, and regional food preferences and economic situations.
- They must be consistent with general food availability and, to the extent possible, generally accepted food patterns.

Food guides based on common food items rather than on abstract nutrient calculations are more easily used. Similarly, the closer the guide to current food intake the more likely it is to be adopted by consumers. A food guide requiring radical dietary changes is of limited use, if it is used at all.

Nutrition labeling. Nutrition labeling guidelines, established by the Food and Drug Administration (FDA) in 1973, were developed to provide consumers with information regarding the nutrient content of food products. At present a food product is not required to carry a **nutrition label** unless (1) it makes a nutrition claim of some type; or (2) nutrients have been added to the product, as is the case with enriched or fortified items. Although the nutrition label is not required on most food products, many now carry one.

Nutrition label
Food product label providing nutrition information concerning nutrient and energy values per designated size portion.

Mandatory components of the nutrition label include an indication of serving size and the number of servings in the container. Nutrients that must be defined include (1) energy in kilocalories; (2) fat, carbohydrate, and protein in grams; and (3) protein, vitamins A and C, thiamin, riboflavin, niacin, calcium, and iron as percentages of the U.S. RDA. The law was extended in 1985 to include categories for stating sodium content. Nutrition labeling enables consumers to evaluate the nutrient content of processed foods or compare the nutrient content of different products.

Debate as to the usability and ease of understanding of the information currently included on the nutrition label has led to proposals for revision of the current labeling regulations.[10] When implemented these proposals would require (1) nutrition labeling on most packaged foods and nutrition information at point of purchase for fresh produce, meats, seafood, and poultry; (2) designation of percentage of kilocalories from fat and number of grams of saturated and unsaturated fats and dietary fiber; and (3) ingredient definition of terms such as "lite" or "no cholesterol." A carefully designed nutrition label, easily read and understood, is a vital component of a comprehensive nutrition education program.

DEVELOPING NUTRITION EDUCATION PROGRAMS

Communication is the transfer of ideas from one person to another. It can occur without speech or language. A smile, nod, or frown can convey a message of trust, understanding, or doubt. Although human beings learn to communicate at an early age, the effort to transfer ideas is not always successful. Many misunderstandings occur even when ethnic and educational backgrounds are the same and are even more common between persons of different backgrounds.

A Communication Model

Communication
Process of giving or interchanging information, thoughts, or feelings by writing, speaking, signing, discussing, listening, responding.

A model that identifies important components in the **communication** process and describes how those components relate to each other can aid in planning and implementing nutrition education programs (Fig. 10-2). The first step is defining communication goals for the program, handout, or media message. What do you want to happen as a result of your nutrition message? You may have several goals in mind, both immediate and long term, as you plan.

One component in the communication model is the *source* of the nutrition message. If you are a community nutritionist you may be the source, working directly with individuals and families. Within a work-site fitness program you may be training and supervising workshop leaders who will be the source of nutrition information for their peers. The *message* component of the model is not only what you say but how you say it. The *medium* could be a face-to-face class or workshop, a handout to send by mail, or a radio message. Finally, the *receiver* is the audience. What do you know about your audience? What are their needs? Before making any decisions, you must examine carefully each component in relation to your communication goals.

FIG. 10-2   A communication model for nutrition education.

Developed with MG Ashman, Office of Information, College of Agriculture and Life Sciences, University of Vermont, Burlington.

Selecting Communication Goals

The general goal of nutrition education is to improve or enhance personal nutritional status, health, and well-being. When defining specific goals for a particular program or message, you must consider communication outcomes on three levels—cognitive, affective, and behavioral.[11]

Cognitive goals. Cognitive goals relate to thinking skills and acquisition of knowledge. A cognitive goal for both children and adults could be learning to use nutrition labels to identify foods high in sodium and limiting their use in the daily meal plan.

Affective goals. Affective goals relate to values and attitudes toward food, and whether proposed changes are good or desirable. A teenager may recognize that french fries are high in fat but not desire to reduce intake.

Behavioral goals. Behavioral goals relate to actual change in eating behavior. They are the most difficult to achieve. People are resistant to change, particularly in the short term. Repeated exposure to the same message over a long period of time is usually required for behavioral change unless motivation is extraordinary. A woman who does not like milk may consume generous quantities during pregnancy but revert to her former habits

Cognitive goal
(L *cognito*, to know) Communications goal related to the process of knowing and learning; mental processes of thinking and remembering.

Affective goal
Communication goal related to processes of feelings and desires, attitudes and values.

Behavioral goal
Communication goal related to processes of changing behavior.

following the birth. Eppright and associates, in their classic work on nutrition education, pointed out that changing the way people think about food may be less important than changing the way they feel about it.[12]

Selecting the Source

The source or apparent sender of the nutrition message influences the success of the message in several ways. First, the communication skills of the individual preparing the media presentation, written materials, or workshop will determine the technical quality of the presentation. A second factor is the sender's depth of knowledge or familiarity with the subject area. This will affect the accuracy and appropriateness of the information presented. A final issue is the credibility of the source with the population to be reached. An organization such as a hospital, government food program, or university extension service, or someone who works for one of these agencies, is usually recognized as a valid source of nutrition information.

Selecting the Message

For a message to be successful it must focus on the real-life situation of the audience. It must consider income, housing, accessibility to different types of food, and lifestyle. In a school or work-site program, the nutrition information should be consistent with the choices available in the school lunchroom or employee cafeteria. A message developed for low-income mothers must be based on food that they can purchase. A message must also be reasonable in length and complexity. People soon lose interest in material that is difficult to understand. On the other hand, messages can be too simplistic and, consequently, misleading. For example, not all green vegetables are equally good sources of carotene, the precursor of vitamin A. Before developing a nutrition message, educators may benefit from "putting themselves in the receivers' shoes," becoming familiar with their neighborhood, shopping in their local food stores, and eating their suggested diet for several days.[13]

Selecting the Medium

The medium for nutrition education depends on what you have to say and to whom. Interpersonal or face-to-face communication is ideal for small, well-defined groups. For reaching large numbers of persons, mass media (radio, television, newspapers) or printed materials are both efficient and cost-effective. A further consideration is the educational level of the audience. For persons with poor reading ability a face-to-face format with visual aids, radio, or television would be a logical choice. For teenagers radio messages scheduled after school on music stations are appropriate. The Social Security office is a good location for reaching large numbers of older persons with a nutrition message.

Both children and adults learn more easily if several senses are stimulated simultaneously. A film followed by discussion, or a presentation describing the nutritional importance of dairy foods followed by tasting of milk-based recipe products, are examples of combinations that can lead to behavioral change. Table 10-1 describes some activity-oriented experiences that can be adapted for different age or educational levels.

Attracting the Audience

People are being constantly bombarded with messages. They selectively choose those to which they will give attention. This selection process requires interaction between the audience, the message sender, and the message itself. The interactive process is depicted on the model (Fig. 10-2) by the arrows going in both directions. If no interaction occurs, attention is lost.

TABLE 10-1   *Learning Activities for Nutrition Education*

Type of Activity	Example
Demonstration	Prepare a "new" food or low-cost or low-kilocalorie food for tasting with directions or recipe handout for children or adults to try at home; lead the group in exercises that can be done at home.
Skits; role playing	Have children write and perform skits of social situations relating to food such as selecting a fast food meal or snack; volunteers in a work-site weight control support group may role play graciously refusing second helpings at a party.
Problem solving	Using newspapers with weekly food specials, select groceries for a week considering both nutritional adequacy and cost; keep diet diaries and evaluate using a food guide or computer program.
Field trip	Visit a grocery store, food cooperative, or dairy (this may be a special treat for both children or adults who lack personal transportation).
Panel	Have several "experts" (group members or visitors) discuss or debate a topic, then continue discussion with the entire group. With adults topics might be food buying, use of food stamps, or child-feeding problems; children might present a panel describing exercise games they enjoy; high school students might organize a debate on the benefits versus the risks of food additives.
Group activity	Develop and duplicate a "cookbook" applicable to the group (e.g., snack book or cooking for one or two); plant a vegetable garden outside or vegetables in containers under lights; prepare an exhibit for the school lunchroom, employee cafeteria, WIC center, or senior center (such an activity provides a way for participants to get to know each other).

Attention to the message depends on the extent to which it appears to meet an identified need. As Gillespie pointed out, people who are not involved in meal-planning or food preparation may not realize that they can benefit from nutrition information.[11] Attention-getting cues pointing to the importance or relevance of the message must precede or accompany it. Getting the most for your money or time, weight control, or pleasurable food experiences may be topics for such cues. An effective strategy for assessing the needs of the target audience in ongoing nutrition education programs is forming an advisory board. Members would include representatives of the target audience and professionals with knowledge and experience in the field.

When developing goals, consider a measure by which you can evaluate the outcome of your program. Did you bring about a change in nutrition knowledge (cognitive), nutrition attitudes (affective), or food selection (behavioral)? Examples of different types of evaluation are given in the following section.

EVALUATING NUTRITION EDUCATION PROGRAMS

Evaluation procedures must be developed as an integral component when the program is being planned. Accomplishments should be measured against specific objectives. Did a greater number of children select whole-grain rather than white bread following the classroom or lunchroom nutrition education program? Did participants in the weight-control support group maintain their weight loss over a 6-month period? Has the employee

Evaluation
Process of determining the value of an educational or clinical program in terms of its initial identified objectives.

cafeteria reported increased sales of broiled versus fried chicken portions? Such **evaluation** requires, however, that goals be stated in measurable terms.

Types of Evaluation

Evaluation is appropriate at many stages in a nutrition education program. *Continuous evaluation* provides ongoing information indicating whether or not changes are needed and, if so, what kinds. *Periodic evaluation* monitors progress and effectiveness. *Follow-up evaluation* conducted some time after completion of a project evaluates the extent to which desired outcomes were achieved or continued.

In addition to the desired or anticipated effects of an education program, there may be side effects or unanticipated results that are equally important. A nutrition education program in an elementary school may lead to increased consumption of milk with the school lunch. If, however, this is accompanied by reduced consumption of the bread and vegetable items, the behavior change, although intended, is not of benefit. Also, the characteristics of those who did not exhibit the behavior change are as important as those who did. The teaching method, communication medium, or message presented may not have been suitable for that segment of the audience.

Methods of Evaluation

Nutrition knowledge. The most common evaluation procedure in nutrition education is testing nutrition knowledge. Although children are accustomed to being tested, adults may resent the traditional pre-test, post-test approach. With adults a pre-test can serve as a teaching tool if class members keep their tests as a basis for a discussion to follow. If the knowledge tests are used for formal evaluation, they must be pre-tested with individuals of similar age and background so that misunderstandings can be avoided.

Nutrition attitudes. Another method is evaluating attitudes toward the information presented. Attitudes regarding the relative importance of nutrition and food choices have been strongly correlated with nutrition knowledge. An evaluation of workshops for adults might include such questions as "Will the information presented today be of use to you (for example, in your food shopping, in controlling your weight)? If not, why not?" With children, true-false items could focus on food likes and dislikes or food behavior patterns (for example: I like to try new foods).

Food record
A 3 to 7 day record of all food consumed, detailed with portion sizes, amounts, and preparation, for nutrition analysis as part of a total nutrition assessment process for planning nutrition care and education.

Nutritional status. If nutrition education is one component of a broad nutrition intervention program, an evaluation of **nutritional status** using dietary, clinical, and biochemical measurements may be possible. Because of the many uncontrollable factors influencing both the dietary intake and biochemical status of all age groups, however, it is often difficult to draw conclusions regarding the success of a nutrition intervention program.

Dietary practices. The most desirable criterion for evaluating the effectiveness of a nutrition education program, although the most difficult, is food-related behavior. Behavior change can be evaluated through use of **food records** or **food frequency questionnaires**. Participants can be asked to provide a record of food consumed for one or more days prior to beginning the nutrition education and during or following the program. Guidelines and problems related to the use of food intake records can be found in Chapter 2. One inherent problem is the tendency for program participants to record what they think they should be eating rather than what they are eating.

Food frequency questionnaire (FFQ)
A tool for collecting nutrition information about food habits. Consists of a comprehensive list of foods and a scale for checking frequency of use over a period of time.

In a group feeding situation such as a school lunch program or employee cafeteria, plate waste or sale of particular food items provides measures of program outcomes. The use of computer scanning devices in supermarkets permits evaluation of food choices as influenced by a community education program.

Guidelines for Program Evaluation

Evaluations of nutrition education programs should provide information relating to both program impact upon participants as well as effectiveness of program delivery. This information will assist program planners in improving the present program or developing a new one. There are three components of this evaluation model: (1) program delivery, (2) program outcome, and (3) learner characteristics.[14]

Program delivery. A successful nutrition education program must reach the target audience. Thus, evaluation should include a comparison of the socioeconomic or behavioral characteristics of the actual participants with the criteria established for the intended audience. The effectiveness of the instruction methods and materials can be reviewed using participants' and instructors' evaluations. Use of all program resources including staff time, money, and materials should be monitored for effectiveness in meeting the program objectives.

Program outcome. The purpose of this analysis is to understand how program inputs or resources contributed to the achievement of program objectives. Program outcome can be measured using changes in nutrition knowledge or behavior, as described above, or participants' satisfaction with the program. Participants' ratings of instructional materials or methods can be used as indicators of program success.

Learner characteristics. The health-related values, attitudes, and **sociodemographic** characteristics that a participant brings to the learning environment will influence receptivity to and understanding of the nutrition information presented. Analysis of program outcomes according to the characteristics of individual participants will indicate what changes, if any, are required to allow for individual differences within the target audience.

Sociodemographic
Relating to social and cultural values, geographic distribution, and physical environments of persons and populations.

SELECTING NUTRITION EDUCATION MATERIALS
Sources of Materials

A nutrition educator may have neither the time nor the resources to prepare original materials. Instead existing materials must be adapted for the client group. Although a wide range of materials are available for school-age children and youth, and for pregnant women, nutrition resources for other ages or target groups are limited. Professionals working with Spanish-speaking populations of all ages, preschoolers, the developmentally disabled, low literacy groups, or the aged may have difficulty finding materials appropriate to the teaching level, income level, ethnic group, or topic of choice. Attractive, well-designed materials are often available free from companies or trade associations selling particular food products. But in some cases these materials are biased to promote the organization's products to best advantage. Government agencies at the local, state, and federal level are good sources of informative nutrition and health education materials and curriculum. Professional voluntary associations such as the American Heart Association or American Dietetic Association also develop materials for use by professionals and the general public.

Criteria for Evaluating Content

Materials from any source should be examined carefully as to content and presentation. The following criteria should be included in the evaluation:

- **Do they present a favorable image of all types of individuals?** Persons of all nationalities, ethnic groups, ages, and physical status deserve to be described in a positive light. **Stereotypic** images (for example, an obese individual sitting before a plate heaped with food) or illustrations that are unrealistic in light of population

Stereotype
Oversimplified and generalized conception or image held by persons or groups that has distorted or unreal meaning, but influences attitudes and behavior of persons holding such views.

trends, such as presenting all food budgets based on two-parent households, can alienate the group being taught.

- **Are they appropriate for the particular group?** Both subject matter and visual content enter into the evaluation of nutrition materials. Cartoons or stick figures, acceptable for a school age group, can be insulting to an adult audience. Nutritional needs and problems also differ among age and sex groups. A pamphlet describing dairy products low in kilocalories will be most appealing to weight-conscious young women who should increase their calcium intake.

- **Is the information presented with a positive approach?** Individuals of all ages are more receptive to learning principles that are positive in tone. Negative or unpleasant associations are shut out and are more likely to be forgotten. Food choices should be presented as options within the individual's control, not as edicts that should be feared.

- **Is the information accurate?** Extravagant claims regarding the nutrient contribution of any one food or food group is misleading. Generalizations that present only part of the picture lead to inaccurate conclusions. The comment that "high-calorie foods should be eliminated from a weight reduction diet" does not deal with the issue of serving size or the fact that a food such as lean meat is a source of many important nutrients.

- **Is the information practical?** Food guidance is of no value unless it can be put into practice. Cost, time, cooking skills, and available cooking facilities must be considered when selecting both lesson content and materials. Emphasis on the nutritional quality of fresh green leafy vegetables has little value for the low-income homemaker dependent on an inner-city convenience store that sells no fresh produce.

Criteria for Evaluating Format

Materials that are dull, drab, or difficult to read will neither attract nor hold attention. A common mistake in preparing materials is including too many details and too many pictures. As a result, posters or handouts look crowded and confused. Keep wording as brief as possible and illustrations simple. Use real objects whenever practical.

Need for Preview

Regardless of source, do not distribute materials or show audiovisuals that have not been previewed carefully. Your use of a material implies that you endorse the facts or ideas presented. Although you might point out a specific inaccuracy, your clarification can be forgotten when your handout is read later at home. Your standards as a professional are reflected in the general appearance and quality of the materials. A copy that is so light or dark that it is barely legible or text that abounds in spelling or typographical errors suggests that you do not really care about the audience or the accuracy of the material being presented.

Selecting Materials for Low Literacy Audiences

Nutrition is a complex science and effective written communication is especially difficult when clients or patients have reading skills at or below the sixth grade level. Lack of problem-solving skills may further hinder understanding. A nationwide study conducted by the FDA indicated that less than half of consumers could correctly answer a question dealing with percentages and thus were hindered in reading and understanding food labels.[15] Reader comprehension is enhanced when material is presented in a conversational style. Whenever possible, use words that can be visualized or associated with a familiar situation or object. Limiting the number of concepts presented to three or less allows the reader to concentrate on the main points. Readability formulas that can be used to estimate grade reading level are the Fry graph and SMOG index. (See Reference 15 for further readings on writing for low literacy audiences.)

CURRENT STRATEGIES IN NUTRITION EDUCATION

Increasing emphasis on preventive health has brought about the development and implementation of innovative educational strategies to meet the needs of particular individuals and programs. Efforts to reach greater numbers of people have led to the use of mass media and locations included in the normal daily pattern such as the work site or grocery store. Nutrition intervention programs with individuals at risk because of body weight or serum lipid or blood pressure measurements have expanded the role of the nutrition counselor as a nutrition educator.

Guidelines for Nutrition Counseling

Nutrition **counseling** provides individualized instruction to assist a person in adjusting daily food intake to meet health or personal needs. Although diet counseling has been most commonly applied to patients assigned to a therapeutic regimen for treatment of a chronic disease, this mode of nutrition education is now being used in preventive care and health-fitness programs. Health or exercise clubs may provide nutrition counseling as one of their services to members. Nutrition counseling is being used with both children and adults and is an integral component of the National Cholesterol Education Program and the Special Supplemental Foods Program for Women, Infants, and Children (WIC). These programs are described in Chapters 6 and 7.

Counseling
Dynamic process of communication that is client-centered, where the role of the counselor is to guide the client to identify problems and priorities and to set goals and possible solutions.

Goal. The goal of diet counseling is to develop a diet strategy that will meet nutrition and health objectives and be consistent with the individual's lifestyle, ethnic food pattern, food preferences, and socioeconomic realities. Diet counseling can enable clients to evaluate a problem, make decisions about their needs, and set goals for the desired behavior change.[16] Clients should be active participants in this process and eventually become self-sufficient in monitoring their day-to-day dietary behavior.

Process. Dietary counseling should be client-centered. An individual cannot be helped by merely listening to basic information about a diet. Counseling deals with both content and feelings.

The counseling process consists of five stages[16]:

1. **Involving**—developing a trusting relationship between client and counselor; helping the client feel comfortable with the process
2. **Exploring**—identifying the problem; allowing the client to present specific details and related issues.
3. **Resolving**—examining alternatives; helping the client to identify and establish goals
4. **Concluding**—selecting a plan of action; reviewing the plan to make certain that both the client and counselor understand what is to be done
5. **Following-up**—providing continued support; modifying the plan as needed; setting new goals based on progress made

A critical component in making a change in eating behavior is the compatibility of the suggested diet with the client's lifestyle. A worker who must carry lunch and has no access to a refrigerator at the work site needs foods that both meet diet recommendations and are safely held at room temperature. Also, for the recommended diet to be implemented, appropriate food must be available. Nutrition educators should be familiar with local food distribution programs that can provide assistance as needed.

Group versus Individual Counseling

The type of counseling to be provided is a decision related in part to the professional setting. In a clinic or hospital, when nutrition counseling focuses on a therapeutic regimen mandated by medical considerations, individual counseling is usually employed. In a work-site program or voluntary weight-control program, group counseling is more common. Group counseling is considered to be advantageous in weight-control programs as it provides social support to the clients and reduces costs. On the other hand, the group process can be less effective if one member who is experiencing less success is negative in attitude or extremely vocal. The importance of social support should not be underestimated, as those who continue in a support group for 1 year are more likely to *sustain* their weight loss than those who discontinue attendance after the initial instruction period.[17]

Family Counseling

Success with a diet plan is influenced by the support a client receives from family or friends. Involving the individual who does the shopping and cooking in the counseling session contributes to successful implementation of the diet plan. Family nutrition counseling should include others in the client's household whether or not they are related.[18] All members sharing the environment can keep a daily record to identify general eating patterns and allow the counselor to target less healthy habits. Each household member should be encouraged to make a personal commitment to one dietary change. This could involve substituting unsalted popcorn for high-salt, high-fat snack foods while watching television or playing games. Even one change by family members provides support for the individual with the health problem while improving the general fitness of all.

Nutrition Education at the Work Site

Escalating health care costs plus the expense of lost work time have led to the development of work-site health-promotion programs. Work-site programs offer particular advantages for nutrition educators. In the first place, workers are at the program location so attending class or obtaining materials is convenient. Secondly, since most work sites have lunch facilities, principles can be reinforced by the food options available.

Approaches to work-site programs. Corporate wellness programs promote nutrition through direct and environmental approaches.[19] Direct approaches include nutrition classes or discussion groups, individual counseling, or distribution of printed materials. Environmental approaches that facilitate participation or awareness include released time for attending classes, appropriate food choices in cafeterias or vending machines, and nutrition information where food is served or consumed. Successful programs have combined both approaches. A government agency distributed healthy recipes and nutrition handouts, encouraged employees to walk on their coffee breaks and awarded prizes such as a jar of low-sodium seasoning for the person walking the farthest each month, and sponsored "Nutrabreaks," at which healthy snacks were available at low cost.[20] If employees develop habits of exercising and eating healthy snacks at the workplace, they are more likely to continue these behaviors at home.

Nutrition topics for work-site programs. Work-site programs may target individuals identified as high risk based on blood cholesterol level, elevated blood pressure level, or body fat. The emphasis may also be on general nutrition principles with all employees invited to participate. Usually programs are developed around weight control or dietary patterns to reduce cardiovascular risk. A work-site program directed to farm workers reported that 50% of the participants were found to have elevated blood pressure when entering the program.[21] Improvement was observed in 68% of the hypertensive individuals following the group classes. Participants reported increasing their levels of exercise and decreasing their intakes of fat, cholesterol, and sodium. Long-term evaluations are needed to determine whether such changes in health behavior are continued following completion of the formal classes.

Television and Mass Media

The average American spends more time watching television than doing anything else except sleeping. Much has been written about the negative impact that television commercials for high-sugar cereals and snacks have on children. On the other hand, the mass media is an untapped resource for spreading positive nutrition information. Expanding cable and satellite networks and home videocassette recorders offer increasing opportunities.

One effective use of television is the short sequence, 1 minute or less, inserted as a public service announcement. Such a message demands neither interest nor motivation. It reaches its objective through repetition over days and weeks. Public service announcements are most useful for simple messages such as announcing a cholesterol screening program, promoting a school lunch program, or giving a number to call for information about food stamps or the WIC program.

Television cooking shows attract many viewers and can provide important nutrition information in an entertaining format. Although nutritionists may wish to deemphasize "cooking," the fact remains that persons not interested in nutrition may be attracted to such a program. Recipes low in fat, sugar, and sodium, and rich in vitamins and minerals could bring a significant change in nutrient intake if incorporated in the diet as replacements for less nutrient-dense food items.

Nutrition education has traditionally been presented in a face-to-face format. However, in a recent comparison, adults had higher nutrition knowledge scores 3 weeks following a nutrition education program presented on videocassette than following a program presented by a lecturer with visual materials.[22] Participants' ranking of both programs according to clarity of information presented and enjoyment of session did not differ between the two formats.

Commercial television stations are required to provide time for nonprofit programming and public television stations seek educational programming. Health agencies and community groups should consider pooling resources to make possible the development of media materials.

Point-of-Choice Nutrition Information

Food service approaches. A growing concept in nutrition education is providing food product information at the point of purchase. In a cafeteria serving either children or adults visual aids can highlight the nutrient content of one food choice as compared to another. Nutrient content information in a cafeteria appears to be more effective if directed toward the health benefit of a food such as one lower in fat or sodium. A trend in point-of-choice nutrition education has been the movement from public programs such as school food service to the private business sector and upscale dining facilities. Nutrition education for restaurants has involved classes for chefs and featured menu items consistent with the Dietary Guidelines for Americans. Programs for chefs focus on food safety and high quality food with reduced amounts of saturated fat, sodium, and cholesterol. Such classes have been approved for continuing education credits for professional chefs. Menu inserts and a heart-healthy logo beside designated menu items resulted in a 15% increase in the number of customers choosing a healthy lunch or requesting that sauces or dressings be served on the side.[23] As growing segments of the population who eat regularly at restaurants become concerned about healthy food choices, restaurant owners and chefs will represent a growing audience for nutrition education.

Supermarket approaches. Several approaches have been used to provide nutrition information in supermarkets. About one third of supermarket chains now have some form of in-store nutrition education program.[24] The most common technique is shelf labeling indicating fat, cholesterol, sugar, and sodium content. However, a major problem with shelf labeling is the lack of uniformity regarding the standards used for product evaluation. Although some programs use the FDA criteria for such terms as "low sodium" or "low calorie," others developed their own standards. Other in-store activities include taste-testing booths focusing on heart-healthy food items or supermarket tours conducted by nutritionists/dietitians who point out more appropriate food choices and emphasize label reading and product evaluation. Although some reports suggest that shelf labels and similar programs have influenced customers to make more appropriate food choices, findings are inconsistent. Nevertheless, these programs do provide an opportunity to reach consumers who otherwise may not seek out nutrition information.

Nutrition Education by Mail

As costs of face-to-face nutrition education programs have increased, sending materials by mail has been found to be an effective alternative. Individuals can read the materials at their leisure, including evenings and weekends. For households in which both adults are employed, single parents with many responsibilities and busy lifestyles, or older persons who lack transportation, written materials provide a valuable resource. Among young families materials to be read at home or posted on the refrigerator door were highly preferred over evening meetings.[25] It is possible to further contain costs by including materials in other mailings such as pension checks or utility bills.

Computers in Nutrition Education

The rapid proliferation of microcomputers and nutrient-related software has made computer-assisted nutrition instruction a valuable tool in elementary and secondary class-rooms and with adults. Computer programs for children evaluate diets according to servings from the various food groups. Older students and adults can calculate the nutrient content of their diets and compare the totals with recommended levels for their age, sex, and level of physical activity. Interpretation of the findings, however, requires professional input. *Individuals must be reminded that nutrient intakes calculated are estimates, not absolute values.* It must be made clear that persons consuming less than recommended levels are not necessarily deficient. Individuals must not assume that intakes below the RDA require the use of vitamin and mineral supplements for improvement.

Advances in technology for interactive video or applications in which the learner "touches the screen" for further information offer promise for effective nutrition learning by children and adults. Such equipment has been used in schools and supermarkets to facilitate learning.

FOOD PROGRAMS AND NUTRITION EDUCATION

Food programs developed and funded by the USDA and the Administration on Aging reach pregnant and lactating mothers, children of all ages, low-income adults, and older adults. These programs provide a framework for nutrition education in population groups who can benefit from practical information on food selection and meal management.

National School Lunch Program

The National School Lunch Program, begun in 1946, was developed for two purposes: (1) to safeguard the health and well-being of the nation's children by providing them with nutritious food and (2) to support farm income by encouraging the use of agricultural commodities. Cash reimbursements and donated commodity foods from the federal government meet about half the cost of the served lunch. The remaining cost is met by local sources including the price paid by students. Children falling under poverty guidelines are eligible for free or reduced-cost lunches. In recent years a school breakfast program was added to serve children in need of this meal.

Nutritional impact. Under federal guidelines the school lunch is expected to provide one third of the required nutrients for the day. Portion sizes vary according to the age of the child with the exception of milk, with all receiving 1 cup. The food items in a Type A school lunch include:

- Protein-rich food (one of the following or a combination thereof)—meat, fish, poultry, egg, peanut butter, or cooked dry beans or peas
- Two or more vegetables or fruits
- Whole-grain or enriched bread or alternate (for example, rice, corn, waffle, or tortilla)
- Milk (whole, low-fat, skim, or buttermilk)

Children who participate in the school lunch program meet a higher percentage of their RDA for energy, protein, vitamin A, the vitamin B complex, and magnesium than nonparticipants similar in age and socioeconomic status.[26] Milk is an important contributor of nutrients, and students who consume a school lunch are more likely to meet the RDA for calcium.

Potential in nutrition education. The school lunch is a valuable tool in nutrition education although this was not a major objective when it began. It provides an example of a basic meal pattern that includes foods from all the major food groups. Children can also be introduced to new foods that they have not eaten at home. Nutrition education activities promoting good food choices, when integrated with the school lunch program, can increase not only participation in the program but also the amount of food in the lunch actually consumed.

Nutrition Education and Training Program

A 1977 amendment to the Child Nutrition Act established the Nutrition Education and Training Program (NET). It was designed to encourage teaching scientifically valid food and nutrition information to children participating or eligible to participate in the school lunch program. Funds were made available to states to develop and implement nutrition education programs that would incorporate the school lunch program as a learning activity and integrate food and nutrition information with other subject areas such as health and physical education, science, social studies, or home economics. School nutrition education programs have resulted in increases in students' nutrition knowledge and improvement in attitudes toward nutrition. However, changes in food selection are not always observed.

Expanded Food and Nutrition Education Program

The Expanded Food and Nutrition Education Program (EFNEP) helps low-income persons acquire the knowledge, skills, and attitudes necessary to select nutritionally sound diets. The primary audiences are low-income households, particularly those with young children, and 4-H youth in both urban and rural areas.

A unique concept in EFNEP is the use of **paraprofessionals** who work one-on-one with the individual in the household who is responsible for planning and preparing the family's food. These paraprofessionals, usually called nutrition or program aides, are selected from the target audience. They are given instruction in planning an adequate diet; food preparation, safety, and presentation; and family food budgeting and financial management. Emphasis is placed on practical applications that can be carried out by a person with limited income, equipment, and skills. Although the one-on-one teaching

Paraprofessional
(Gr *para-*, along side) A nonprofessional person, often from the community being served and thus having valuable insights concerning needs, who is trained to assist the professional community or clinical nutrition specialist in carrying out the nutrition program.

method has proven to be highly successful with multi-problem families, it is extremely expensive, limiting the number of families who can be helped.

Special Supplemental Food Program for Women, Infants, and Children

The Special Supplemental Food Program for Women, Infants, and Children (WIC) was established in 1972 to improve the diets of low-income pregnant and lactating mothers, and infants and children up to age 5 who because of poor nutritional patterns or inadequate health care are at high risk.

Foods provided to WIC recipients represent all four major food groups and include:
- Milk (skim, low-fat, whole, or buttermilk), infant formula, and cheese
- Eggs and peanut butter
- Juice (orange, grapefruit, pineapple, tomato, or apple with vitamin C)
- Cereal (iron-fortified infant cereal; others for children, mothers)

The amounts of food provided are designed to include 3½ servings from the milk group, 1 serving from the meat group, 2 servings of fruit, and 1 to 2 servings of cereal per participant per day. Although all WIC programs must provide foods from each major food group, there is some flexibility at the local level. For example, a program may choose to exclude sugar-coated cereals.

Although nutrition education is required, the level provided depends on the local program. In many situations nutrition education occurs only at the clinic visit required once every 6 months for recertification. A national study indicated that WIC families made better food choices with the money available for food than did non-WIC families of similar income.[27] This could reflect nutrition education focusing on wise buying practices.

Congregate and Home-Delivered Meals for the Aged (Title III-C)

Congregate meal programs (see Chapter 9) and senior centers provide excellent opportunities for nutrition education in a group setting. Some form of nutrition education is available at most meal sites, but the actual time spent and the type of instruction presented are quite varied. Distribution of printed materials or posting of visual materials is most common. Group discussion, tasting of recipe products, or market trips provide informal opportunities for older people to talk and learn about nutrition. Such activities are more successful than "lecture" sessions in teaching older adults. For those receiving home-delivered meals, printed materials that suggest healthy snacks, or easy-to-prepare meals for use when no meals are delivered, would be helpful. With older age groups, materials with large print that can be read easily are most appropriate.

Summary

Food habits are learned behaviors based on psychologic and cultural rather than physiologic needs, and tend to resist change. Nutrition knowledge alone will not result in improved food patterns unless the individual is motivated by personal goals or health concerns to initiate such a change. Nutrition educators seeking to help people make appropriate food choices must recognize the need to define such choices within the chosen lifestyle.

Whether or not an individual implements nutrition information may depend on the source or sender, the media through which it is presented, and the ability of the message to meet identified personal needs. Mass media including radio, television, or newspapers are effective in making people aware of new ideas. But individuals are more likely to implement information received from a professional or reinforced by a friend or relative. Limited resources for nutrition education make evaluation of such programs extremely important in development and implementation. Both the impact upon the target audience as well as the cost-effectiveness of the strategies used should be considered. Tests of nutrition knowledge are sometimes used to evaluate the effectiveness of nutrition education. An observed change in food behavior, although more difficult to measure, is the desired goal.

Increasing emphasis on health promotion has led to the development of innovative strategies to reach consumers at the point of purchase (restaurant or supermarket), the work site, or at home through television. Nutrition counseling on an individual, group, or family basis is effective in helping individuals adjust to therapeutic regimens, manage weight loss, or improve general dietary patterns. School lunch programs, meals for the aged, or food distribution programs such as WIC provide excellent opportunities to present practical nutrition information.

Review Questions

1. What is the basis for the food behavior of most individuals? Does nutrition information lead to changes in food behavior? Explain.
2. What are the stages leading to the adoption of new ideas? How does the type of media interact at each stage?
3. Develop a nutrition education program for a group of your choice. Briefly describe your (1) communication goals; (2) message; (3) medium; (4) audience; and (5) method of evaluation.
4. Describe three government-sponsored programs that provide meals or supplementary foods and nutrition education to target populations. Give an example of a nutrition education topic or activity that would be appropriate for each.

References

1. Glanz K: Social psychological perspectives and applications to nutrition education, J Nutr Educ 13(suppl):66, 1981.
2. Hochbaum GM: Strategies and their rationale for changing people's eating habits, J Nutr Educ 13(suppl):59, 1981.
3. Subar AF and Bowering J: Fortified food: Considerations in purchase, awareness of nutrient addition, and reasons for usage, J Nutr Educ 21:133, 1989.
4. Resnicow K and Reinhardt J: What do children know about fat, fiber, and cholesterol. A survey of 5116 primary and secondary school students, J Nutr Educ 23:65, 1991.
5. Schafer RB and Keith PM: Influences on food decisions across the family life cycle, J Am Diet Assoc 78:144, 1981.
6. Strategies for implementing dietary guidance, Dairy Council Digest 61(4):19, 1990.
7. Yarbrough P: Communication theory and nutrition education research, J Nutr Educ 13(suppl):16, 1981.
8. Gortmaker SL, Dietz WH, and Cheung LWY: Inactivity, diet, and the fattening of America, J Am Diet Assoc 90:1247, 1990.
9. Kunkel ME, Cody MM, Davis RJ, and Wheeler FC: Nutrition information sources used by South Carolina adults, J Am Diet Assoc 86:371, 1986.
10. Earl R, Porter DV, and Wellman NS: Nutrition labeling: issues and directions for the 1990s, J Am Diet Assoc 90:1599, 1990.
11. Gillespie AH: Planning and evaluating nutrition education programs: A communications ap-

proach. In Professional Perspectives, Division of Nutritional Sciences, Cornell University, January-February 1983.

12. Eppright E, Pattison M, and Barbour H: Teaching nutrition, ed 2, Ames, 1963, Iowa State University Press.
13. Achterberg C: Factors that influence learner readiness, J Am Diet Assoc 88:1426, 1988.
14. Edwards PK, Mullis RM, and Clarke B: A comprehensive model for evaluating innovative nutrition education programs, J Nutr Educ 18:10, 1986.
15. Nitzke S: Improving the effectiveness of nutrition education materials for low literacy clients, Nutr Today 24:17, 1989.
16. Holli BB and Calabrese RJ: Communication and education skills. The dietitian's guide, ed 2, Philadelphia, 1991, Lea and Febiger.
17. Visocan BJ, Dworkin MF, and Klein LW: Effect of long-term group support on weight-loss maintenance, J Nutr Educ 17:3, 1985.
18. Dwyer J: Focus on family nutrition counseling. New ways to reinforce and extend eating behavior changes, Nutrition Update 1:1, Spring 1991.
19. Glanz K and Seewald-Klein T: Nutrition at the worksite: An overview, J Nutr Educ 18(suppl):1, 1986.
20. Courtney A and Dennis C: Nutrition and fitness education in the workplace, J Nutr Educ 19:168B, 1987.
21. Masur-Levy P, Tavres DR, and Elsey-Pica L: Cardiovascular risk changes in a work-site health promotion program, J Am Diet Assoc 90:1427, 1990.
22. Byrd-Bredbenner C, Martin R, Lewis CJ, and Shannon B: The effectiveness of two methods of delivering nutrition information to the general public, J Nutr Educ 20:63, 1988.
23. Forster-Coull L and Gillis D: A nutrition education program for restaurant patrons, J Nutr Educ 20:22B, 1988.
24. Pennington JAT, Wisniowski LA, and Logan GB: In-store nutrition information programs, J Nutr Educ 20:5, 1988.
25. Crockett JJ, Perry CL, and Pirie P: Nutrition intervention strategies preferred by parents: results of a marketing survey, J Nutr Educ 21:90, 1989.
26. Hanes S, Vermeersch J, and Gale S: The national evaluation of school nutrition programs: program impact on dietary intake, Am J Clin Nutr 40(suppl):390, 1984.
27. Rush D: National WIC evaluation, Public Health Currents 26(4):1, 1986.

Further Reading

US Department of Agriculture:
> Preparing foods and planning menus using the Dietary Guidelines, Home and Garden Bulletin No. 232-8
> Making bag lunches, snacks and desserts using the Dietary Guidelines, Home and Garden Bulletin No. 232-9
> Shopping for food and making meals in minutes using the Dietary Guidelines, Home and Garden Bulletin No. 232-10
> Eating better when eating out using the Dietary Guidelines, Home and Garden Bulletin No. 232-11

Washington, DC, 1989, US Government Printing Office.
> This colorful, attractive set of booklets provides excellent practical advice for the consumer regarding food selection and preparation that will limit intakes of energy, fat, and sodium and increase intakes of fiber and complex carbohydrates.

Weinstock CP: The grazing of America: a guide to healthy snacking, FDA Consumer 23(2):8, 1989.
> Snacking throughout the day is for some people replacing the traditional three meals a day. This article gives recommendations for appropriate snack choices.

Cohen BC: Food security and hunger policy for the 1990s, Nutr Today 25:23, 1990.

> A review of the causes of hunger in America, the psychosocial impact of hunger upon children and adults, and intervention strategies to assure food security for all individuals and families.

Parham ES: Applying a philosophy of nutrition education to weight control, J Nutr Educ 22:194, 1990.

> A sensitive discussion of considerations and strategies for working with weight control clients.

Hill LA, Harveywebster MJ, Usinger-Lesquereux J, and St. Jeor ST: The use of voice mail in a nutrition and cancer information telephone service, J Am Diet Assoc 91:347, 1991.

> A description of how this new telephone technology can be used to provide answers to nutrition questions of patients in the community.

McMurry MP, Hopkins PN, Gould R, et al: Family-oriented nutrition intervention for a lipid clinic population, J Am Diet Assoc 91:57, 1991.

> A description of a family counseling program for lowering serum cholesterol that could be adapted to a variety of counseling situations.

Granzin KL and Bahn KD: The role of consumers' attitudes toward nutrition in restaurant patronage, J Nutr Educ 20:56, 1988.

> A discussion of the attitudes of various types of consumers toward the importance of nutritionally appropriate foods when selecting a restaurant and applications for developing nutrition education programs.

APPENDIX

Physical Growth
NCHS Percentiles

GIRLS: BIRTH TO 36 MONTHS
PHYSICAL GROWTH
NCHS PERCENTILES*

NAME _____ RECORD # _____

*Adapted from: Hamill PVV, Drizd TA, Johnson CL, Reed RB, Roche AF, Moore WM: Physical growth: National Center for Health Statistics percentiles. AM J CLIN NUTR 32-607-629, 1979. Data from the Fels Research Institute, Wright State University School of Medicine, Yellow Springs, Ohio.
© 1982 ROSS LABORATORIES

Ross
Growth &
Development
Program

DATE	AGE	LENGTH	WEIGHT	HEAD CIRC.	COMMENT
	BIRTH				

MOTHER'S STATURE _____
FATHER'S STATURE _____
GESTATIONAL AGE _____ WEEKS

BOYS: BIRTH TO 36 MONTHS
PHYSICAL GROWTH
NCHS PERCENTILES*

NAME _____ RECORD # _____

Ross
Growth &
Development
Program

*Adapted from: Hamill PVV, Drizd TA, Johnson CL, Reed RB,
Roche AF, Moore WM. Physical growth: National Center for Health
Statistics percentiles. AM J CLIN NUTR 32:607-629, 1979. Data
from the Fels Research Institute, Wright State University School of
Medicine, Yellow Springs, Ohio.
© 1982 ROSS LABORATORIES

MOTHER'S STATURE _____ GESTATIONAL

FATHER'S STATURE _____ AGE _____ WEEKS

DATE	AGE	LENGTH	WEIGHT	HEAD CIRC.	COMMENT
	BIRTH				

**GIRLS: BIRTH TO 36 MONTHS
PHYSICAL GROWTH
NCHS PERCENTILES***

NAME _____ RECORD # _____

*Adapted from: Hamill PVV, Drizd TA, Johnson CL, Reed RB, Roche AF, Moore WM. Physical growth: National Center for Health Statistics percentiles. AM J CLIN NUTR 32:607-629, 1979. Data from the Fels Research Institute, Wright State University School of Medicine, Yellow Springs, Ohio.

© 1982 ROSS LABORATORIES

DATE	AGE	LENGTH	WEIGHT	HEAD CIRC.	COMMENT

Recommend the formulation you prefer with the name you trust

**SIMILAC®
SIMILAC® WITH IRON
SIMILAC® WITH WHEY**
Infant Formulas

The **ISOMIL®** System of
Soy Protein Formulas

ADVANCE®
Nutritional Beverage

ROSS LABORATORIES
COLUMBUS, OHIO 43216
Division of Abbott Laboratories, USA

G106/JUNE 1983   LITHO IN USA

BOYS: BIRTH TO 36 MONTHS
PHYSICAL GROWTH
NCHS PERCENTILES*

NAME_____ RECORD #_____

DATE	AGE	LENGTH	WEIGHT	HEAD CIRC.	COMMENT

GIRLS: 2 TO 18 YEARS
PHYSICAL GROWTH
NCHS PERCENTILES*

NAME_____ RECORD #_____

MOTHER'S STATURE _____	FATHER'S STATURE _____			
DATE	AGE	STATURE	WEIGHT	COMMENT

*Adapted from: Hamill PVV, Drizd TA, Johnson CL, Reed RB, Roche AF, Moore WM. Physical growth: National Center for Health Statistics percentiles. AM J CLIN NUTR 32:607-629, 1979. Data from the National Center for Health Statistics (NCHS) Hyattsville, Maryland.

© 1982 ROSS LABORATORIES

Ross
Growth &
Development
Program

BOYS: 2 TO 18 YEARS
PHYSICAL GROWTH
NCHS PERCENTILES*

* Adapted from: Hamill PVV, Drizd TA, Johnson CL, Reed RB, Roche AF, Moore WM: Physical growth: National Center for Health Statistics percentiles. AM J CLIN NUTR 32:607-629, 1979. Data from the National Center for Health Statistics (NCHS) Hyattsville, Maryland.

© 1982 ROSS LABORATORIES

Ross
Growth &
Development
Program

**GIRLS: PREPUBESCENT
PHYSICAL GROWTH
NCHS PERCENTILES***

NAME _____ RECORD # _____

*Adapted from: Hamill PVV, Drizd TA, Johnson CL, Reed RB, Roche AF, Moore WM. Physical growth: National Center for Health Statistics percentiles. AM J CLIN NUTR 32:607-629, 1979. Data from the National Center for Health Statistics (NCHS) Hyattsville, Maryland.

© 1982 ROSS LABORATORIES

Recommend the formulation you prefer with the name you trust

SIMILAC®
SIMILAC® WITH IRON
SIMILAC® WITH WHEY
Infant Formulas

The ISOMIL® System of
Soy Protein Formulas

ADVANCE®
Nutritional Beverage

ROSS LABORATORIES
COLUMBUS, OHIO 43216
Division of Abbott Laboratories, USA

G108/JUNE 1983   LITHO IN USA

**BOYS: PREPUBESCENT
PHYSICAL GROWTH
NCHS PERCENTILES***

NAME_____ RECORD #_____

B

Weight-Height of Youths 12 to 17 Years of Age

Weight-Height of Youths at 12 Years (kg/cm)

| Sex and Height | n | N | X̄ | s | $s_{\bar{x}}$ | \multicolumn{7}{c}{Percentile} |
| | | | | | | \multicolumn{7}{c}{IN KILOGRAMS} |
						5th	10th	25th	50th	75th	90th	95th
MALE												
Under 130 cm	5	15	*	*	*	*	*	*	*	*	*	*
130.0-134.9 cm	4	8	*	*	*	*	*	*	*	*	*	*
135.0-139.9 cm	34	111	32.50	3.741	0.727	26.6	27.6	30.2	31.6	34.7	37.7	39.4
140.0-144.9 cm	80	241	34.28	3.635	0.601	28.1	30.0	31.8	34.1	36.5	38.6	40.7
145.0-149.9 cm	123	386	39.27	6.243	0.615	32.1	33.2	35.7	38.2	40.9	46.1	52.5
150.0-154.9 cm	156	513	42.90	6.314	0.480	34.9	36.1	38.2	42.1	46.0	51.6	56.3
155.0-159.9 cm	135	432	47.35	7.551	0.769	38.3	39.4	41.9	46.2	50.5	57.4	61.9
160.0-164.9 cm	65	201	50.82	8.735	1.388	42.1	42.7	44.9	48.4	56.0	61.1	67.1
165.0-169.9 cm	29	88	55.75	8.811	2.031	43.3	46.4	49.0	54.4	59.9	68.3	76.6
170.0-174.9 cm	8	21	62.37	4.503	1.993	54.0	58.1	60.1	61.0	66.0	69.1	69.5
175.0-179.9 cm	3	10	*	*	*	*	*	*	*	*	*	*
180.0-184.9 cm	1	2	—	—	—	—	—	—	—	—	—	—
185.0-189.9 cm	—	—	—	—	—	—	—	—	—	—	—	—
190.0-194.9 cm	—	—	—	—	—	—	—	—	—	—	—	—
195.0 cm and over	—	—	—	—	—	—	—	—	—	—	—	—
FEMALE												
Under 130 cm	—	—	—	—	—	—	—	—	—	—	—	—
130.0-134.9 cm	3	10	*	*	*	*	*	*	*	*	*	*
135.0-139.9 cm	12	44	29.41	3.372	0.914	25.0	25.0	26.4	28.9	32.1	34.1	34.2
140.0-144.9 cm	32	116	38.30	7.314	1.194	28.8	30.6	33.3	36.8	41.4	49.2	55.1
145.0-149.9 cm	72	258	39.78	6.205	0.975	31.8	32.8	35.5	38.5	42.8	48.3	50.6
150.0-154.9 cm	147	517	44.00	7.421	0.677	34.4	35.8	38.9	42.8	47.4	52.9	57.4
155.0-159.9 cm	144	525	48.74	8.369	0.714	37.9	39.2	43.0	46.8	53.8	60.7	63.5
160.0-164.9 cm	95	336	53.06	8.010	0.658	42.5	43.9	47.2	51.1	57.2	65.6	69.6
165.0-169.9 cm	31	117	54.89	7.022	1.384	43.9	47.1	50.4	53.1	59.7	64.5	71.3
170.0-174.9 cm	11	42	63.66	14.501	6.214	48.7	50.1	50.8	56.7	82.2	86.0	86.1
175.0-179.9 cm	—	—	—	—	—	—	—	—	—	—	—	—
180.0-184.9 cm	—	—	—	—	—	—	—	—	—	—	—	—
185.0-189.9 cm	—	—	—	—	—	—	—	—	—	—	—	—
190.0-194.9 cm	—	—	—	—	—	—	—	—	—	—	—	—
195.0 cm and over	—	—	—	—	—	—	—	—	—	—	—	—

n, sample size; *N*, estimated number of youths in population in thousands; X̄, mean; *s*, standard deviation; $s_{\bar{x}}$, standard error of the mean.
From National Center for Health Statistics: Height and weight of youths 12-17 years, United States. In Vital and health statistics, series 11, no 124, Health Services and Mental Health Administration, Washington, DC, 1973, US Government Printing Office.

Weight-Height of Youths at 13 Years (kg/cm)

Sex and Height	n	N	$\bar{X}$	s	$s_{\bar{x}}$	Percentile IN KILOGRAMS						
						5th	10th	25th	50th	75th	90th	95th
MALE												
Under 130 cm	—	—	—	—	—	—	—	—	—	—	—	—
130.0-134.9 cm	2	5	*	*	*	*	*	*	*	*	*	*
135.0-139.9 cm	6	25	32.62	5.624	7.716	27.2	27.6	28.9	31.0	34.9	43.1	43.2
140.0-144.9 cm	18	56	36.54	5.852	1.607	30.0	30.5	32.1	36.1	39.2	41.7	53.2
145.0-149.9 cm	65	204	39.03	5.270	0.662	32.4	33.9	36.1	37.9	41.2	44.5	46.4
150.0-154.9 cm	99	312	42.58	6.724	0.865	34.8	36.2	37.9	41.0	45.5	49.4	61.0
155.0-159.9 cm	131	421	47.27	7.482	0.717	37.8	39.2	41.7	45.8	51.1	58.7	61.7
160.0-164.9 cm	125	393	53.01	9.324	0.916	41.5	43.7	46.9	50.4	58.2	64.4	72.5
165.0-169.9 cm	91	285	55.92	8.560	0.833	46.3	47.5	49.3	53.6	59.4	69.0	75.0
170.0-174.9 cm	63	215	62.01	10.362	1.033	51.2	51.6	53.7	60.1	67.0	76.0	85.0
175.0-179.9 cm	19	68	67.92	12.085	3.428	56.3	57.9	60.1	63.3	70.3	88.3	89.0
180.0-184.9 cm	5	15	*	*	*	*	*	*	*	*	*	*
185.0-189.9 cm	—	—	—	—	—	—	—	—	—	—	—	—
190.0-194.9 cm	—	—	—	—	—	—	—	—	—	—	—	—
195.0 cm and over	—	—	—	—	—	—	—	—	—	—	—	—
FEMALE												
Under 130 cm	—	—	—	—	—	—	—	—	—	—	—	—
130.0-134.9 cm	1	3	*	*	*	*	*	*	*	*	*	*
135.0-139.9 cm	—	—	—	—	—	—	—	—	—	—	—	—
140.0-144.9 cm	15	51	37.13	7.317	2.259	26.6	27.5	30.5	36.7	40.1	44.5	56.1
145.0-149.9 cm	47	165	42.23	6.880	0.888	34.7	35.6	38.2	40.5	44.2	53.6	57.6
150.0-154.9 cm	98	329	44.32	7.029	0.787	35.6	36.5	39.2	42.9	47.3	53.7	57.9
155.0-159.9 cm	152	499	49.75	8.757	0.699	39.1	39.9	43.8	48.4	53.8	61.0	65.9
160.0-164.9 cm	156	515	53.16	8.399	0.522	41.2	43.9	47.7	52.2	57.0	63.8	68.5
165.0-169.9 cm	86	284	58.17	9.125	0.921	46.2	47.4	52.2	58.1	61.5	69.3	76.2
170.0-174.9 cm	24	87	58.11	13.209	2.343	46.2	47.1	48.4	52.9	65.3	68.6	96.8
175.0-179.9 cm	3	10	*	*	*	*	*	*	*	*	*	*
180.0-184.9 cm	—	—	—	—	—	—	—	—	—	—	—	—
185.0-189.9 cm	—	—	—	—	—	—	—	—	—	—	—	—
190.0-194.9 cm	—	—	—	—	—	—	—	—	—	—	—	—
195.0 cm and over	—	—	—	—	—	—	—	—	—	—	—	—

Weight-Height of Youths at 14 Years (kg/cm)

Sex and Height	n	N	$\bar{X}$	s	$s_{\bar{x}}$	Percentile						
						5th	10th	25th	50th	75th	90th	95th
						IN KILOGRAMS						
MALE												
Under 130 cm	—	—	—	—	—	—	—	—	—	—	—	—
130.0–134.9 cm	—	—	—	—	—	—	—	—	—	—	—	—
135.0–139.9 cm	2	7	*	*	*	*	*	*	*	*	*	*
140.0–144.9 cm	3	13	*	*	*	*	*	*	*	*	*	*
145.0–149.9 cm	11	42	40.51	1.829	0.644	36.9	38.6	39.6	40.6	42.0	42.5	42.7
150.0–154.9 cm	45	135	43.63	6.277	1.182	36.2	37.0	39.0	41.4	48.0	51.7	55.3
155.0–159.9 cm	83	261	47.42	7.822	0.872	37.7	38.7	41.8	46.1	51.2	58.0	62.7
160.0–164.9 cm	96	299	52.28	6.785	0.584	42.5	44.0	47.5	52.1	56.3	61.5	65.1
165.0–169.9 cm	134	432	58.07	9.416	1.054	47.7	49.3	51.6	55.4	62.3	70.6	75.7
170.0–174.9 cm	144	435	62.37	11.516	1.095	49.7	51.0	55.0	59.4	65.6	79.2	86.3
175.0–179.9 cm	71	228	65.54	9.704	1.306	50.9	55.1	58.5	64.7	69.9	74.5	84.0
180.0–184.9 cm	25	81	72.44	13.014	2.298	59.6	60.0	65.1	69.4	77.0	83.0	94.3
185.0–189.9 cm	3	9	*	*	*	*	*	*	*	*	*	*
190.0–194.9 cm	1	3	*	*	*	*	*	*	*	*	*	*
195.0 cm and over	—	—	—	—	—	—	—	—	—	—	—	—
FEMALE												
Under 130 cm	—	—	—	—	—	—	—	—	—	—	—	—
130.0–134.9 cm	—	—	—	—	—	—	—	—	—	—	—	—
135.0–139.9 cm	1	2	*	*	*	*	*	*	*	*	*	*
140.0–144.9 cm	2	6	*	*	*	*	*	*	*	*	*	*
145.0–149.9 cm	17	52	42.00	5.879	1.683	32.0	35.3	36.3	42.3	47.5	49.5	51.1
150.0–154.9 cm	64	196	48.26	6.797	0.926	37.7	39.2	42.5	47.9	53.3	55.9	58.8
155.0–159.9 cm	157	508	51.35	7.705	0.520	42.1	43.4	46.3	49.6	55.6	62.2	64.3
160.0–164.9 cm	186	603	54.59	8.810	0.707	43.0	45.0	48.4	53.0	59.7	66.7	70.7
165.0–169.9 cm	114	372	58.46	10.185	0.955	45.9	47.5	52.1	56.8	61.8	70.5	76.4
170.0–174.9 cm	36	121	64.37	15.821	2.814	49.2	52.1	56.2	59.8	70.5	72.9	99.4
175.0–179.9 cm	7	28	61.33	5.496	2.620	51.7	52.0	57.7	59.8	64.6	70.2	70.6
180.0–184.9 cm	2	7	*	*	*	*	*	*	*	*	*	*
185.0–189.9 cm	—	—	—	—	—	—	—	—	—	—	—	—
190.0–194.9 cm	—	—	—	—	—	—	—	—	—	—	—	—
195.0 cm and over	—	—	—	—	—	—	—	—	—	—	—	—

Weight-Height of Youths at 15 Years (kg/cm)

| | | | | | | | | | Percentile IN KILOGRAMS | | | | |
Sex and Height	n	N	$\overline{X}$	s	$s_{\bar{x}}$	5th	10th	25th	50th	75th	90th	95th
MALE												
Under 130 cm	—	—	—	—	—	—	—	—	—	—	—	—
130.0-134.9 cm	—	—	—	—	—	—	—	—	—	—	—	—
135.0-139.9 cm	—	—	—	—	—	—	—	—	—	—	—	—
140.0-144.9 cm	1	2	*	*	*	*	*	*	*	*	*	*
145.0-149.9 cm	10	30	45.72	8.582	3.550	35.7	39.2	42.6	44.7	46.0	48.7	76.1
150.0-154.9 cm	34	99	52.81	10.552	1.695	40.3	43.1	46.7	49.2	56.7	69.6	76.3
155.0-159.9 cm	71	206	53.01	8.417	0.986	42.7	44.1	46.9	51.5	56.3	65.3	68.8
160.0-164.9 cm	132	404	57.72	8.503	0.819	48.0	48.8	53.1	56.4	61.3	67.1	73.3
165.0-169.9 cm	176	574	62.88	8.464	0.633	51.6	53.4	56.7	61.9	67.2	72.9	78.1
170.0-174.9 cm	118	374	65.80	9.457	1.045	53.1	55.6	59.7	64.3	69.5	80.2	89.2
175.0-179.9 cm	51	144	72.00	11.928	1.724	54.6	60.3	64.4	70.2	68.4	84.4	96.6
180.0-184.9 cm	14	48	74.21	15.035	5.200	58.3	58.5	62.9	70.7	84.6	92.4	110.8
185.0-189.9 cm	6	15	83.39	16.431	10.332	66.4	66.7	69.6	73.8	103.0	105.7	106.2
190.0-194.9 cm	—	—	—	—	—	—	—	—	—	—	—	—
195.0 cm and over	—	—	—	—	—	—	—	—	—	—	—	—
FEMALE												
Under 130 cm	—	—	—	—	—	—	—	—	—	—	—	—
130.0-134.9 cm	—	—	—	—	—	—	—	—	—	—	—	—
135.0-139.9 cm	—	—	—	—	—	—	—	—	—	—	—	—
140.0-144.9 cm	2	5	*	*	*	*	*	*	*	*	*	*
145.0-149.9 cm	15	51	47.91	7.875	3.623	36.0	39.4	42.1	45.4	52.7	55.7	66.3
150.0-154.9 cm	69	242	49.69	8.895	1.190	39.1	40.6	44.3	48.1	52.8	60.5	68.3
155.0-159.9 cm	111	400	51.52	8.473	0.934	41.4	43.5	46.3	50.8	55.1	59.8	65.2
160.0-164.9 cm	137	509	57.03	10.828	0.875	45.1	47.3	50.2	55.0	60.2	71.7	77.7
165.0-169.9 cm	109	398	60.71	10.357	1.053	47.5	49.3	55.1	58.4	65.7	74.1	81.0
170.0-174.9 cm	49	188	65.27	10.730	1.880	49.7	53.6	57.2	61.2	71.6	85.3	86.4
175.0-179.9 cm	7	23	63.30	8.872	4.807	49.7	49.9	53.8	62.4	71.1	71.9	79.2
180.0-184.9 cm	3	26	*	*	*	*	*	*	*	*	*	*
185.0-189.9 cm	1	3	*	*	*	*	*	*	*	*	*	*
190.0-194.9 cm	—	—	—	—	—	—	—	—	—	—	—	—
195.0 cm and over	—	—	—	—	—	—	—	—	—	—	—	—

Weight-Height of Youths at 16 Years (kg/cm)

Sex and Height	n	N	$\bar{X}$	s	$s_{\bar{x}}$	IN KILOGRAMS						
						5th	10th	25th	50th	75th	90th	95th
MALE												
Under 130 cm	—	—	—	—	—	—	—	—	—	—	—	—
130.0-134.9 cm	—	—	—	—	—	—	—	—	—	—	—	—
135.0-139.9 cm	—	—	—	—	—	—	—	—	—	—	—	—
140.0-144.9 cm	1	1	*	*	*	*	*	*	*	*	*	*
145.0-149.9 cm	4	12	*	*	*	*	*	*	*	*	*	*
150.0-154.9 cm	11	33	49.89	7.323	3.572	42.0	42.2	44.7	46.8	54.4	59.8	67.2
155.0-159.9 cm	32	108	53.09	6.459	1.273	44.2	44.9	48.2	51.4	58.0	60.9	66.1
160.0-164.9 cm	87	275	59.39	9.178	0.981	48.5	49.8	52.7	58.0	63.9	69.3	75.9
165.0-169.9 cm	166	552	62.66	7.556	0.629	51.6	53.8	57.5	61.6	67.1	73.1	78.0
170.0-174.9 cm	149	511	67.33	9.018	0.856	56.3	58.2	61.0	65.4	72.5	80.1	83.8
175.0-179.9 cm	72	227	72.38	12.485	1.993	58.3	59.3	64.4	68.9	76.5	90.2	96.9
180.0-184.9 cm	29	95	81.06	14.268	3.265	63.7	66.6	69.7	78.4	90.3	97.0	111.4
185.0-189.9 cm	3	10	*	*	*	*	*	*	*	*	*	*
190.0-194.9 cm	2	7	*	*	*	*	*	*	*	*	*	*
195.0 cm and over	—	—	—	—	—	—	—	—	—	—	—	—
FEMALE												
Under 130 cm	—	—	—	—	—	—	—	—	—	—	—	—
130.0-134.9 cm	—	—	—	—	—	—	—	—	—	—	—	—
135.0-139.9 cm	—	—	—	—	—	—	—	—	—	—	—	—
140.0-144.9 cm	2	5	*	*	*	*	*	*	*	*	*	*
145.0-149.9 cm	10	33	52.58	8.198	3.191	43.9	44.1	44.9	51.0	54.5	72.0	72.1
150.0-154.9 cm	57	178	51.79	10.457	1.053	41.4	42.0	45.8	48.9	54.1	61.5	83.3
155.0-159.9 cm	117	354	53.20	7.766	0.734	44.0	45.6	48.4	51.6	56.4	61.9	69.0
160.0-164.9 cm	160	547	57.71	11.129	1.246	46.1	47.3	51.5	55.5	61.2	69.5	75.1
165.0-169.9 cm	122	450	61.72	11.998	0.802	47.1	48.8	53.3	59.1	67.3	78.7	86.7
170.0-174.9 cm	53	170	63.61	8.734	1.126	52.9	53.8	58.1	62.1	66.8	73.8	84.2
175.0-179.9 cm	14	45	72.55	15.012	5.224	58.6	58.8	61.7	65.9	80.6	99.1	105.5
180.0-184.9 cm	1	2	*	*	*	*	*	*	*	*	*	*
185.0-189.9 cm	—	—	—	—	—	—	—	—	—	—	—	—
190.0-194.9 cm	—	—	—	—	—	—	—	—	—	—	—	—
195.0 cm and over	—	—	—	—	—	—	—	—	—	—	—	—

Percentile

Weight-Height of Youths at 17 Years (kg/cm)

Sex and Height	n	N	X̄	s	$s_{\bar{x}}$	Percentile 5th	10th	25th	50th	75th	90th	95th
						IN KILOGRAMS						
MALE												
Under 130 cm	—	—	—	—	—	—	—	—	—	—	—	—
130.0-134.9 cm	—	—	—	—	—	—	—	—	—	—	—	—
135.0-139.9 cm	—	—	—	—	—	—	—	—	—	—	—	—
140.0-144.9 cm	—	—	—	—	—	—	—	—	—	—	—	—
145.0-149.9 cm	—	—	—	—	—	—	—	—	—	—	—	—
150.0-154.9 cm	1	3	*	*	*	*	*	*	*	*	*	*
155.0-159.9 cm	11	39	54.63	9.397	3.414	43.8	46.4	48.2	49.7	57.8	69.9	73.2
160.0-164.9 cm	25	81	57.75	6.503	1.355	49.7	51.1	52.5	56.9	61.6	70.1	70.8
165.0-169.9 cm	63	248	62.57	8.344	1.224	50.2	53.2	56.4	61.5	66.9	72.7	77.3
170.0-174.9 cm	115	396	67.06	11.163	0.704	53.3	55.5	59.5	64.6	71.9	80.9	91.6
175.0-179.9 cm	151	537	68.37	9.907	0.831	56.9	58.9	61.5	66.5	73.6	79.4	88.4
180.0-184.9 cm	80	297	73.31	12.454	1.335	59.6	61.0	65.1	71.2	78.4	91.8	102.7
185.0-189.9 cm	36	133	76.03	9.171	1.301	62.4	66.3	70.5	75.3	80.8	90.3	92.9
190.0-194.9 cm	7	25	81.40	10.985	7.588	62.9	62.9	67.8	87.3	90.3	90.6	90.6
195.0 cm and over	—	—	—	—	—	—	—	—	—	—	—	—
FEMALE												
Under 130 cm	—	—	—	—	—	—	—	—	—	—	—	—
130.0-134.9 cm	—	—	—	—	—	—	—	—	—	—	—	—
135.0-139.9 cm	—	—	—	—	—	—	—	—	—	—	—	—
140.0-144.9 cm	2	5	*	*	*	*	*	*	*	*	*	*
145.0-149.9 cm	8	26	43.49	3.939	1.604	38.6	38.8	40.1	45.1	45.7	51.1	51.2
150.0-154.9 cm	43	151	49.96	6.508	0.827	41.6	42.3	44.6	48.9	53.5	59.2	64.1
155.0-159.9 cm	103	385	54.71	9.903	0.775	44.4	45.5	48.7	53.2	57.7	61.6	76.2
160.0-164.9 cm	133	506	57.79	10.620	1.028	46.8	48.0	50.2	55.4	61.5	72.3	82.3
165.0-169.9 cm	116	433	60.63	10.117	1.182	47.9	50.3	55.1	59.3	65.1	69.4	71.6
170.0-174.9 cm	51	186	62.18	9.132	1.407	50.6	52.9	55.5	60.2	65.7	76.1	82.7
175.0-179.9 cm	12	47	65.76	8.405	2.229	54.9	56.7	60.1	61.7	75.2	75.9	83.0
180.0-184.9 cm	1	2	*	*	*	*	*	*	*	*	*	*
185.0-189.9 cm	—	—	—	—	—	—	—	—	—	—	—	—
190.0-194.9 cm	—	—	—	—	—	—	—	—	—	—	—	—
195.0 cm and over	—	—	—	—	—	—	—	—	—	—	—	—

Weight-Height of Youths at 12 Years (lb/in)

Sex and Height	n	N	$\bar{X}$	s	$s_{\bar{x}}$	Percentile IN POUNDS 5th	10th	25th	50th	75th	90th	95th
MALE												
Under 51.18 in	5	15	*	*	*	*	*	*	*	*	*	*
51.18-53.15 in	4	8	*	*	*	*	*	*	*	*	*	*
53.15-55.12 in	34	111	71.65	8.248	1.603	54.6	60.8	66.6	69.7	76.5	83.1	86.9
55.12-57.09 in	80	241	75.57	8.014	1.325	61.9	66.1	70.1	75.2	80.5	85.1	89.7
57.09-59.06 in	123	386	86.58	13.764	1.356	70.8	73.2	78.7	84.2	90.2	101.6	115.7
59.06-61.02 in	156	513	94.58	13.920	1.058	76.9	79.6	84.2	92.8	101.4	113.8	124.1
61.02-62.99 in	135	433	104.39	16.647	1.695	84.4	86.9	92.4	101.9	111.3	126.5	136.5
62.99-64.96 in	65	201	112.04	19.257	3.060	92.8	94.1	99.0	106.7	123.5	134.7	147.9
64.96-66.93 in	29	88	122.91	19.425	4.478	95.5	102.3	108.0	119.9	132.1	150.6	168.9
66.93-68.90 in	8	21	137.50	9.927	4.394	119.0	128.1	132.5	134.5	145.5	152.3	153.2
68.90-70.87 in	3	10	*	*	*	*	*	*	*	*	*	*
70.87-72.83 in	1	2	*	*	—	*	*	*	*	*	*	—
72.83-74.80 in	—	—	—	—	—	—	—	—	—	—	—	—
74.80-76.77 in	—	—	—	—	—	—	—	—	—	—	—	—
76.77 in and over	—	—	—	—	—	—	—	—	—	—	—	—
FEMALE												
Under 51.18 in	—	—	—	—	—	—	—	—	—	—	—	—
51.18-53.15 in	3	10	*	*	*	*	*	*	*	*	*	*
53.15-55.12 in	12	44	64.84	7.434	2.015	55.1	55.1	58.2	63.7	70.8	75.2	75.4
55.12-57.09 in	32	116	84.44	16.125	2.632	63.5	67.5	73.4	81.1	91.3	108.5	121.5
57.09-59.06 in	72	258	87.70	13.680	2.150	70.1	72.3	78.3	78.9	94.4	106.5	111.6
59.06-61.02 in	147	517	97.00	16.361	1.493	75.8	78.9	85.8	94.4	104.5	116.6	126.5
61.02-62.99 in	144	525	107.45	18.451	1.574	83.6	86.4	94.8	103.2	118.6	133.8	140.0
62.99-64.96 in	95	336	117.00	17.659	1.451	93.7	96.8	104.1	112.7	126.1	144.6	153.4
64.96-66.93 in	31	117	121.01	15.481	3.051	96.8	103.8	111.1	117.1	131.6	142.2	157.2
66.93-68.90 in	11	42	140.35	31.969	13.700	107.4	110.5	112.0	125.0	181.2	189.6	189.8
68.90-70.87 in	—	—	—	—	—	—	—	—	—	—	—	—
70.87-72.83 in	—	—	—	—	—	—	—	—	—	—	—	—
72.83-74.80 in	—	—	—	—	—	—	—	—	—	—	—	—
74.80-76.77 in	—	—	—	—	—	—	—	—	—	—	—	—
76.77 in and over	—	—	—	—	—	—	—	—	—	—	—	—

Weight-Height of Youths at 13 Years (lb/in)

Sex and Height	n	N	$\bar{X}$	s	$s_{\bar{x}}$	Percentile (IN POUNDS)						
						5th	10th	25th	50th	75th	90th	95th
MALE												
Under 51.18 in	—	—	—	—	—	—	—	—	—	—	—	—
51.18-53.15 in	2	5	*	*	*	*	*	*	*	*	*	*
53.15-55.12 in	8	25	71.91	12.399	17.011	60.0	60.8	63.7	68.3	76.9	95.0	95.2
55.12-57.09 in	18	56	80.56	12.902	3.543	66.1	67.2	70.8	79.6	86.4	91.9	117.3
57.09-59.06 in	65	204	86.05	11.618	1.460	71.4	74.7	79.6	83.6	90.8	98.1	102.3
59.06-61.02 in	99	312	93.87	14.824	1.907	76.7	79.8	83.6	90.4	100.3	108.9	134.5
61.02-62.99 in	131	421	104.21	16.495	1.581	83.3	86.4	91.9	101.0	112.7	129.4	136.0
62.99-64.96 in	125	393	116.87	20.556	2.019	91.5	96.3	103.4	111.1	128.3	142.0	159.8
64.96-66.93 in	91	285	123.28	18.872	1.837	102.1	104.7	108.7	118.2	131.0	152.1	165.3
66.93-68.90 in	63	215	136.71	22.844	2.277	112.9	113.8	118.4	132.5	147.7	167.6	187.4
68.90-70.87 in	19	68	149.72	26.643	7.557	124.1	127.6	132.5	139.6	155.0	194.7	196.2
70.87-72.83 in	5	15	*	*	*	*	*	*	*	*	*	*
72.83-74.80 in	—	—	—	—	—	—	—	—	—	—	—	—
74.80-76.77 in	—	—	—	—	—	—	—	—	—	—	—	—
76.77 in and over	—	—	—	—	—	—	—	—	—	—	—	—
FEMALE												
Under 51.18 in	—	—	—	—	—	—	—	—	—	—	—	—
51.18-53.15 in	1	3	*	*	*	*	*	*	*	*	*	*
53.15-55.12 in	—	—	—	—	—	—	—	—	—	—	—	—
55.12-57.09 in	15	51	81.86	16.131	4.980	58.6	60.6	67.2	80.9	88.4	98.1	123.7
57.09-59.06 in	47	165	93.10	15.168	1.958	76.5	78.5	84.2	89.3	97.4	118.2	127.0
59.06-61.02 in	98	329	97.71	15.496	1.735	78.7	80.5	86.4	94.6	104.3	118.4	127.6
61.02-62.99 in	152	499	109.68	19.306	1.541	86.2	88.0	96.6	106.7	118.6	134.5	145.3
62.99-64.96 in	156	515	117.20	18.517	1.151	90.8	96.8	105.2	115.1	125.7	140.7	151.0
64.96-66.93 in	86	284	128.24	20.117	2.031	101.9	104.5	115.1	128.1	135.6	152.8	168.0
66.93-68.90 in	24	87	128.11	29.121	5.165	101.9	103.8	106.7	116.6	144.0	151.2	213.4
68.90-70.87 in	3	10	*	*	*	*	*	*	*	*	*	*
70.87-72.83 in	—	—	—	—	—	—	—	—	—	—	—	—
72.83-74.80 in	—	—	—	—	—	—	—	—	—	—	—	—
74.80-76.77 in	—	—	—	—	—	—	—	—	—	—	—	—
76.77 in and over	—	—	—	—	—	—	—	—	—	—	—	—

Weight-Height of Youths at 14 Years (lb/in)

Sex and Height	n	N	$\bar{X}$	s	$s_{\bar{x}}$	Percentile (IN POUNDS)						
						5th	10th	25th	50th	75th	90th	95th
MALE												
Under 51.18 in	—	—	—	—	—	—	—	—	—	—	—	—
51.18-53.15 in	—	—	—	—	—	—	—	—	—	—	—	—
53.15-55.12 in	2	7	*	*	*	*	*	*	*	*	*	*
55.12-57.09 in	3	13	*	*	*	*	*	*	*	*	*	*
57.09-59.06 in	11	42	89.31	4.032	1.420	81.4	85.1	87.3	89.5	92.6	93.7	94.1
59.06-61.02 in	45	135	96.19	13.838	2.606	79.8	81.6	86.0	91.3	106.8	114.0	121.9
61.02-62.99 in	83	261	104.54	17.245	1.922	83.1	85.3	92.2	101.6	112.9	127.9	138.2
62.99-64.96 in	96	299	115.26	14.958	1.288	93.7	97.0	104.7	114.9	124.1	135.6	143.5
64.96-66.93 in	134	432	128.02	20.759	2.324	105.2	108.7	113.8	122.1	137.4	155.6	166.9
66.93-68.90 in	144	435	137.50	25.388	2.414	109.6	112.4	121.3	131.0	145.0	165.2	185.2
68.90-70.87 in	71	228	144.49	21.394	2.879	112.2	121.5	129.0	142.6	154.1	174.1	190.3
70.87-72.83 in	25	81	159.70	28.691	5.066	131.4	132.3	143.5	153.0	170.9	183.0	207.9
72.83-74.80 in	3	9	*	*	*	*	*	*	*	*	*	*
74.80-76.77 in	1	3	*	*	*	*	*	*	*	*	*	*
76.77 in and over	—	—	—	—	—	—	—	—	—	—	—	—
FEMALE												
Under 51.18 in	—	—	—	—	—	—	—	—	—	—	—	—
51.18-53.15 in	—	—	—	—	—	—	—	—	—	—	—	—
53.15-55.12 in	1	2	*	*	*	*	*	*	*	*	*	*
55.12-57.09 in	2	6	*	*	*	*	*	*	*	*	*	*
57.09-59.06 in	17	52	92.59	12.961	3.710	70.5	77.8	80.0	93.3	104.7	109.1	112.7
59.06-61.02 in	64	196	106.40	14.985	2.042	83.1	86.4	93.7	105.6	117.5	123.2	129.6
61.02-62.99 in	157	508	113.21	16.987	1.146	90.8	95.7	102.1	109.3	122.6	137.1	141.8
62.99-64.96 in	186	603	120.35	19.423	1.559	94.8	99.2	106.7	116.8	131.6	147.0	155.0
64.96-66.93 in	114	372	128.88	22.454	2.105	101.2	104.7	114.9	125.2	136.2	155.4	168.4
66.93-68.90 in	36	121	141.91	34.879	6.204	108.5	114.9	123.9	131.8	155.4	160.7	219.1
68.90-70.87 in	7	28	135.21	12.117	5.776	114.0	114.6	127.2	131.8	142.4	154.8	155.6
70.87-72.83 in	2	7	*	*	*	*	*	*	*	*	*	*
72.83-74.80 in	—	—	—	—	—	—	—	—	—	—	—	—
74.80-76.77 in	—	—	—	—	—	—	—	—	—	—	—	—
76.77 in and over	—	—	—	—	—	—	—	—	—	—	—	—

Weight-Height of Youths at 15 Years (lb/in)

Sex and Height	n	N	$\bar{X}$	s	$s_{\bar{x}}$	Percentile — IN POUNDS						
						5th	10th	25th	50th	75th	90th	95th
MALE												
Under 51.18 in	—	—	—	—	—	—	—	—	—	—	—	—
51.18-53.15 in	—	—	—	—	—	—	—	—	—	—	—	—
53.15-55.12 in	—	—	—	—	—	—	—	—	—	—	—	—
55.12-57.09 in	1	2	*	*	*	*	*	*	*	*	*	*
57.09-59.06 in	10	30	100.80	18.920	7.826	78.7	86.4	93.9	98.5	101.4	107.4	167.8
59.06-61.02 in	34	99	116.43	23.263	3.737	88.8	95.0	103.0	108.5	125.0	153.4	168.2
61.02-62.99 in	71	206	116.87	18.556	2.174	94.1	97.2	103.4	113.5	124.1	144.0	151.7
62.99-64.96 in	132	404	127.25	18.746	1.806	105.8	107.6	117.1	124.3	135.1	147.9	161.6
64.96-66.93 in	176	574	138.63	18.660	1.396	113.8	117.7	125.0	136.5	148.2	160.7	172.2
66.93-68.90 in	118	374	146.06	20.849	2.304	117.1	122.6	131.6	141.8	153.2	176.8	196.7
68.90-70.87 in	51	144	158.73	26.297	3.801	120.4	132.9	142.0	154.8	172.8	186.1	213.0
70.87-72.83 in	14	48	163.61	33.147	11.464	128.5	129.0	138.7	155.9	186.5	203.7	244.3
72.83-74.80 in	6	15	183.84	36.224	22.778	146.4	147.0	153.4	162.7	227.1	233.0	234.1
74.80-76.77 in	—	—	—	—	—	—	—	—	—	—	—	—
76.77 in and over	—	—	—	—	—	—	—	—	—	—	—	—
FEMALE												
Under 51.18 in	—	—	—	—	—	—	—	—	—	—	—	—
51.18-53.15 in	—	—	—	—	—	—	—	—	—	—	—	—
53.15-55.12 in	—	—	—	—	—	—	—	—	—	—	—	—
55.12-57.09 in	2	5	*	*	*	*	*	*	*	*	*	*
57.09-59.06 in	15	51	105.62	17.361	7.987	79.4	86.9	92.8	100.1	116.2	122.8	146.2
59.06-61.02 in	69	242	109.55	19.610	2.624	86.2	89.5	97.7	106.0	116.4	133.4	150.6
61.02-62.99 in	111	400	113.58	18.680	2.059	91.3	95.9	102.1	121.0	121.5	131.8	143.7
62.99-64.96 in	137	509	125.73	23.872	1.929	99.4	104.3	110.7	121.3	132.7	158.1	171.3
64.96-66.93 in	109	398	133.84	22.833	2.322	104.7	108.7	121.5	128.8	144.8	163.4	178.6
66.93-68.90 in	49	188	143.90	23.656	4.145	109.6	118.2	126.1	134.9	157.9	188.1	190.5
68.90-70.87 in	7	23	139.55	19.559	10.598	109.6	110.0	118.6	137.6	156.1	158.5	174.6
70.87-72.83 in	3	26	*	*	*	*	*	*	*	*	*	*
72.83-74.80 in	1	3	*	*	*	*	*	*	*	*	*	*
74.80-76.77 in	—	—	—	—	—	—	—	—	—	—	—	—
76.77 in and over	—	—	—	—	—	—	—	—	—	—	—	—

Weight-Height of Youths at 16 Years (lb/in)

Sex and Height	n	N	$\bar{X}$	s	$s_{\bar{x}}$	5th	10th	25th	50th	75th	90th	95th
								IN POUNDS — Percentile				
MALE												
Under 51.18 in	—	—	—	—	—	—	—	—	—	—	—	—
51.18-53.15 in	—	—	—	—	—	—	—	—	—	—	—	—
53.15-55.12 in	—	—	—	—	—	—	—	—	—	—	—	—
55.12-57.09 in	1	1	*	—	—	*	*	*	*	*	*	*
57.09-59.06 in	4	12	*	*	*	*	*	*	*	*	*	*
59.06-61.02 in	11	33	109.99	16.145	7.875	92.6	93.0	98.5	103.2	119.9	131.8	148.2
61.02-62.99 in	32	108	117.04	14.240	2.807	97.4	99.0	106.3	113.3	127.9	134.3	145.7
62.99-64.96 in	87	275	130.93	20.234	2.163	106.9	109.8	116.2	127.9	140.9	152.8	167.3
64.96-66.93 in	166	552	138.14	16.658	1.387	113.8	118.6	126.8	135.8	147.9	161.2	172.0
66.93-68.90 in	149	511	148.44	19.881	1.887	124.1	128.3	134.5	144.2	159.8	176.6	184.7
68.90-70.87 in	72	227	159.57	27.525	4.394	128.5	130.7	142.0	151.9	168.7	198.9	213.6
70.87-72.83 in	29	95	178.71	31.456	7.198	140.4	146.8	153.7	172.8	199.1	213.8	245.6
72.83-74.80 in	3	10	*	*	*	*	*	*	*	*	*	*
74.80-76.77 in	2	7	*	*	*	*	*	*	*	*	*	*
76.77 in and over	—	—	—	—	—	—	—	—	—	—	—	—
FEMALE												
Under 51.18 in	—	—	—	—	—	—	—	—	—	—	—	—
51.18-53.15 in	—	—	—	—	—	—	—	—	—	—	—	—
53.15-55.12 in	—	—	—	—	—	—	—	—	—	—	—	—
55.12-57.09 in	2	5	*	*	*	*	*	*	*	*	*	*
57.09-59.06 in	10	33	115.92	18.074	7.035	96.8	97.2	99.0	112.4	120.2	158.7	158.9
59.06-61.02 in	57	178	114.18	23.054	2.322	91.3	92.6	101.0	107.8	119.3	135.6	183.6
61.02-62.99 in	117	354	117.29	17.121	1.618	97.0	100.5	106.7	113.8	124.3	136.5	152.1
62.99-64.96 in	160	547	127.23	24.535	2.747	101.6	104.3	113.5	122.4	134.9	153.2	165.6
64.96-66.93 in	122	450	136.07	26.451	1.768	103.8	107.6	117.5	130.3	148.4	173.5	191.1
66.92-68.90 in	53	170	140.24	19.255	2.482	116.6	118.6	128.1	136.9	147.3	173.7	185.6
68.90-70.87 in	14	45	159.95	33.096	11.517	129.2	129.6	136.0	145.3	177.7	218.5	232.6
70.87-72.83 in	1	2	*	*	*	*	*	*	*	*	*	*
72.83-74.80 in	—	—	—	—	—	—	—	—	—	—	—	—
74.80-76.77 in	—	—	—	—	—	—	—	—	—	—	—	—
76.77 in and over	—	—	—	—	—	—	—	—	—	—	—	—

Weight-Height of Youths at 17 Years (lb/in)

Sex and Height	n	N	$\bar{X}$	s	$s_{\bar{x}}$	5th	10th	25th	50th	75th	90th	95th
						IN POUNDS						
MALE												
Under 51.18 in	—	—	—	—	—	—	—	—	—	—	—	—
51.18-53.15 in	—	—	—	—	—	—	—	—	—	—	—	—
53.15-55.12 in	—	—	—	—	—	—	—	—	—	—	—	—
55.12-57.09 in	—	—	—	—	—	—	—	—	—	—	—	—
57.09-59.06 in	—	—	—	—	—	—	—	—	—	—	—	—
59.06-61.02 in	1	3	*	*	*	*	*	*	*	*	*	*
61.02-62.99 in	11	39	120.44	20.717	7.527	96.6	102.3	106.3	109.6	127.4	154.1	161.4
62.99-64.96 in	25	81	127.32	14.337	2.987	109.6	112.7	115.7	125.4	135.8	154.5	156.1
64.96-66.93 in	63	248	137.94	18.395	2.699	110.7	117.3	124.3	135.6	147.5	160.3	170.4
66.93-68.90 in	115	396	147.84	24.610	1.552	117.5	122.4	131.2	142.4	158.5	178.4	202.2
68.90-70.87 in	151	537	150.73	21.841	1.832	125.4	129.9	135.6	146.6	162.3	175.0	194.9
70.87-72.83 in	80	297	161.62	27.456	2.943	131.4	134.5	143.5	157.0	172.8	202.4	226.4
72.83-74.80 in	36	133	167.62	20.219	2.868	137.6	146.2	155.4	166.0	178.1	199.1	204.8
74.80-76.77 in	7	25	179.46	24.218	16.729	138.7	138.7	149.5	192.5	199.1	199.7	199.7
76.77 in and over	—	—	—	—	—	—	—	—	—	—	—	—
FEMALE												
Under 51.18 in	—	—	—	—	—	—	—	—	—	—	—	—
51.18-53.15 in	—	—	—	—	—	—	—	—	—	—	—	—
53.15-55.12 in	—	—	—	—	—	—	—	—	—	—	—	—
55.12-57.09 in	2	5	*	*	*	*	*	*	*	*	*	*
57.09-59.06 in	8	26	95.88	8.684	3.536	85.1	85.5	88.4	99.4	100.8	112.7	112.9
59.06-61.02 in	43	151	110.14	14.348	1.823	91.7	93.3	98.3	107.8	117.9	130.5	141.3
61.02-62.99 in	103	385	120.61	21.832	1.709	97.9	100.3	107.4	117.3	127.2	135.8	168.0
62.99-64.96 in	133	506	127.41	23.413	2.266	103.2	105.8	110.7	122.1	127.2	159.4	181.4
64.96-66.93 in	116	433	133.67	22.304	2.606	105.6	110.9	121.5	130.7	143.5	153.0	157.9
66.93-68.90 in	51	186	137.08	20.133	3.102	111.6	116.6	122.4	132.7	144.8	167.8	182.3
68.90-70.87 in	12	47	144.98	18.530	4.914	121.0	125.0	132.5	136.0	165.8	167.3	183.0
70.87-72.83 in	1	2	*	*	*	*	*	*	*	*	*	*
72.83-74.80 in	—	—	—	—	—	—	—	—	—	—	—	—
74.80-76.77 in	—	—	—	—	—	—	—	—	—	—	—	—
76.77 in and over	—	—	—	—	—	—	—	—	—	—	—	—

Percentile

Andres Age-Specific Weight-Height Table for Adults and the Elderly*

Height	Weight Range for Men and Women by Age (Years) in Pounds†				
	25	35	45	55	65
ft—in					
4—10	84-111	92-119	99-127	107-135	115-142
4—11	87-115	95-123	103-131	111-139	119-147
5—0	90-119	98-127	106-135	114-143	123-152
5—1	93-123	101-131	110-140	118-148	127-157
5—2	96-127	105-136	113-144	122-153	131-163
5—3	99-131	108-140	117-149	126-158	135-168
5—4	102-135	112-145	121-154	130-163	140-173
5—5	106-140	115-149	125-159	134-168	144-179
5—6	109-144	119-154	129-164	138-174	148-184
5—7	112-148	122-159	133-169	143-179	153-190
5—8	116-153	126-163	137-174	147-184	158-196
5—9	119-157	130-168	141-179	151-190	162-201
5—10	122-162	134-173	145-184	156-195	167-207
5—11	126-167	137-178	149-190	160-201	172-213
6—0	129-171	141-183	153-195	165-207	177-219
6—1	133-176	145-188	157-200	169-213	182-225
6—2	137-181	149-194	162-206	174-219	187-232
6—3	141-186	153-199	166-212	179-225	192-238
6—4	144-191	157-205	171-218	184-231	197-244

*Values in this table are in pounds for height without shoes and weight without clothes. To convert inches to centimeters, multiply by 2.54, to convert pounds to kilograms, multiply by 0.455.

†Data from Andres R: Gerontology Research Center, National Institute of Aging, Baltimore, Md.

D Mid–Upper Arm Circumference Percentiles (cm)

Age (years)	Female					Male				
	5th	25th	50th	75th	95th	5th	25th	50th	75th	95th
1	13.8	14.8	15.6	16.4	17.7	14.2	15.0	15.9	17.0	18.3
2	14.2	15.2	16.0	16.7	18.4	14.1	15.3	16.2	17.0	18.5
3	14.3	15.8	16.7	17.5	18.9	15.0	16.0	16.7	17.5	19.0
4	14.9	16.0	16.9	17.7	19.1	14.9	16.2	17.1	18.0	19.2
5	15.3	16.5	17.5	18.5	21.1	15.3	16.7	17.5	18.5	20.4
6	15.6	17.0	17.6	18.7	21.1	15.5	16.7	17.9	18.8	22.8
7	16.4	17.4	18.3	19.9	23.1	16.2	17.7	18.7	20.1	23.0
8	16.8	18.3	19.5	21.4	26.1	16.2	17.7	19.0	20.2	24.5
9	17.8	19.4	21.1	22.4	26.0	17.5	18.7	20.0	21.7	25.7
10	17.4	19.3	21.0	22.8	26.5	18.1	19.6	21.0	23.1	27.4
11	18.5	20.8	22.4	24.8	30.3	18.6	20.2	22.3	24.4	28.0
12	19.4	21.6	23.7	25.6	29.4	19.3	21.4	23.2	25.4	30.3
13	20.2	22.3	24.3	27.1	33.8	19.4	22.8	24.7	26.3	30.1
14	21.4	23.7	25.2	27.2	32.2	22.0	23.7	25.3	28.3	32.3
15	20.8	23.9	25.4	27.9	32.2	22.2	24.4	26.4	28.4	32.0
16	21.8	24.1	25.8	28.3	33.4	24.4	26.2	27.8	30.3	34.3
17	22.0	24.1	26.4	29.5	35.0	24.6	26.7	28.5	30.8	34.7
18	22.2	24.1	25.8	28.1	32.5	24.5	27.6	29.7	32.1	37.9
19-25	21.1	24.7	26.5	29.0	34.5	26.2	28.8	30.8	33.1	37.2
25-35	23.3	25.6	27.7	30.4	36.8	27.1	30.0	31.9	34.2	37.5
35-45	24.1	26.7	29.0	31.7	37.8	27.8	30.5	32.6	34.5	37.4
45-55	24.2	27.4	29.9	32.8	38.4	26.7	30.1	32.2	34.2	37.6
55-65	24.3	28.0	30.3	33.5	38.5	25.8	29.6	31.7	33.6	36.9
65-75	24.0	27.4	29.9	32.6	37.3	24.8	28.5	30.7	32.5	35.5

Data derived from the Health and Nutrition Examination Survey data of 1971-1974, using same population samples as those of the National Center for Health Statistics (NCHS) growth percentiles for children. Adapted from Frisancho AR: New norms of upper limb fat and muscle areas for assessment of nutritional status, Am J Clin Nutr 34:2540, 1981.

Triceps Skinfold Percentiles (mm)

Age (years)	Female					Male				
	5th	25th	50th	75th	95th	5th	25th	50th	75th	95th
1	6	8	10	12	16	6	8	10	12	16
2	6	9	10	12	16	6	8	10	12	15
3	7	9	11	12	15	6	8	10	11	15
4	7	8	10	12	16	6	8	9	11	14
5	6	8	10	12	18	6	8	9	11	15
6	6	8	10	12	16	5	7	8	10	16
7	6	9	11	13	18	5	7	9	12	17
8	6	9	12	15	24	5	7	8	10	16
9	8	10	13	16	22	6	7	10	13	18
10	7	10	12	17	27	6	8	10	14	21
11	7	10	13	18	28	6	8	11	16	24
12	8	11	14	18	27	6	8	11	14	28
13	8	12	15	21	30	5	7	10	14	26
14	9	13	16	21	28	4	7	9	14	24
15	8	12	17	21	32	4	6	8	11	24
16	10	15	18	22	31	4	6	8	12	22
17	10	13	19	24	37	5	6	8	12	19
18	10	15	18	22	30	4	6	9	13	24
19-25	10	14	18	24	34	4	7	10	15	22
25-35	10	16	21	27	37	5	8	12	16	24
35-45	12	18	23	29	38	5	8	12	16	23
45-55	12	20	25	30	40	6	8	12	15	25
55-65	12	20	25	31	38	5	8	11	14	22
65-75	12	18	24	29	36	4	8	11	15	22

Data derived from the Health and Nutrition Examination Survey data of 1971-1974, using same population samples as those of the National Center for Health Statistics (NCHS) growth percentiles for children. Adapted from Frisancho AR: New norms of upper limb fat and muscle areas for assessment of nutritional status, Am J Clin Nutr 34:2540, 1981.

Mid–Upper Arm Muscle Circumference Percentiles (cm)

Age (years)	Female 5th	Female 25th	Female 50th	Female 75th	Female 95th	Male 5th	Male 25th	Male 50th	Male 75th	Male 95th
1	10.5	11.7	12.4	13.9	14.3	11.0	11.9	12.7	13.5	14.7
2	11.1	11.9	12.6	13.3	14.7	11.1	12.2	13.0	14.0	15.0
3	11.3	12.4	13.2	14.0	15.2	11.7	13.1	13.7	14.3	15.3
4	11.5	12.8	13.8	14.4	15.7	12.3	13.3	14.1	14.8	15.9
5	12.5	13.4	14.2	15.1	16.5	12.8	14.0	14.7	15.4	16.9
6	13.0	13.8	14.5	15.4	17.1	13.1	14.2	15.1	16.1	17.7
7	12.9	14.2	15.1	16.0	17.6	13.7	15.1	16.0	16.8	19.0
8	13.8	15.1	16.0	17.1	19.4	14.0	15.4	16.2	17.0	18.7
9	14.7	15.8	16.7	18.0	19.8	15.1	16.1	17.0	18.3	20.2
10	14.8	15.9	17.0	18.0	19.7	15.6	16.6	18.0	19.1	22.1
11	15.0	17.1	18.1	19.6	22.3	15.9	17.3	18.3	19.5	23.0
12	16.2	18.0	19.1	20.1	22.0	16.7	18.2	19.5	21.0	24.1
13	16.9	18.3	19.8	21.1	24.0	17.2	19.6	21.1	22.6	24.5
14	17.4	19.0	20.1	21.6	24.7	18.9	21.2	22.3	24.0	26.4
15	17.5	18.9	20.2	21.5	24.4	19.9	21.8	23.7	25.4	27.2
16	17.0	19.0	20.2	21.6	24.9	21.3	23.4	24.9	26.9	29.6
17	17.5	19.4	20.5	22.1	25.7	22.4	24.5	25.8	27.3	31.2
18	17.4	19.1	20.2	21.5	24.5	22.6	25.2	26.4	28.3	32.4
19-25	17.9	19.5	20.7	22.1	24.9	23.8	25.7	27.3	28.9	32.1
25-35	18.3	19.9	21.2	22.8	26.4	24.3	26.4	27.9	29.8	32.6
35-45	18.6	20.5	21.8	23.6	27.2	24.7	26.9	28.6	30.2	32.7
45-55	18.7	20.6	22.0	23.8	27.4	23.9	26.5	28.1	30.0	32.6
55-65	18.7	20.9	22.5	24.4	28.0	23.6	26.0	27.8	29.5	32.0
65-75	18.5	20.8	22.5	24.4	27.9	22.3	25.1	26.8	28.4	30.6

Values derived by formula calculation. Data derived from the Health and Nutrition Examination Survey data of 1971-1974, using same population samples as those of the National Center for Health Statistics (NCHS) growth percentiles for children. Adapted from Frisancho AR: New norms of upper limb fat and muscle areas for assessment of nutritional status, Am J Clin Nutr 34:2540, 1981.

APPENDIX

Clinical Signs and Symptoms of Various Nutrient Deficiencies

Area of Examination	Sign/Symptom	Potential Nutrient Deficiency
Hair	Alopecia	Zinc, essential fatty acids
	Easy pluckability	Protein, essential fatty acids
	Lackluster	Protein, zinc
	"Corkscrew" hair	Vitamin C, vitamin A
	Decreased pigmentation	Protein, copper
Eyes	Xerosis of conjunctiva	Vitamin A
	Corneal vascularization	Riboflavin
	Keratomalacia	Vitamin A
	Bitot's spots	Vitamin A
Gastrointestinal tract	Nausea, vomiting	Pyridoxine
	Diarrhea	Zinc, niacin
	Stomatitis	Pyridoxine, riboflavin, iron
	Cheilosis	Pyridoxine, iron
	Glossitis	Pyridoxine, zinc, niacin, folate, vitamin B_{12}
	Magenta tongue	Riboflavin
	Swollen, bleeding gums	Vitamin C
	Fissured tongue	Niacin
	Hepatomegaly	Protein
Skin	Dry and scaling	Vitamin A, essential fatty acids, zinc
	Petechiae/ecchymoses	Vitamin C, vitamin K
Skin — cont'd	Follicular hyperkeratosis	Vitamin A, essential fatty acids
	Nasolabial seborrhea	Niacin, pyridoxine, riboflavin
	Bilateral dermatitis	Niacin, zinc
Extremities	Subcutaneous fat loss	Kilocalories
	Muscle wastage	Kilocalories, protein
	Edema	Protein
	Osteomalacia, bone pain, rickets	Vitamin D
	Arthralgia	Vitamin C
Hematologic	Anemia	Vitamin B_{12}, iron, folate, copper, vitamin E, vitamin K
	Leukopenia, neutropenia	Copper
	Low prothrombin, prolonged clotting time	Vitamin K
Neurologic	Disorientation	Niacin, thiamin
	Confabulation	Thiamin
	Neuropathy	Thiamin, pyridoxine, chromium
	Paresthesia	Thiamin, pyridoxine, vitamin B_{12}
Cardiovascular	Congestive heart failure, cardiomegaly, tachycardia	Thiamin
	Cardiomyopathy	Selenium

From Ross Laboratories.

Normal Biochemical Levels for Nutrients and Test Measurements

Biochemical Indicators of Good Nutrition Status

Nutrient or Measurement	Test	Normal or Acceptable Levels	
		Men	Women
Iron	Hemoglobin (g/100 ml)	≥14.0	≥12.0
	Infants (under 2 years)	≥10.0	≥10.0
	Children (6-12 years)	≥11.5	≥11.5
	Pregnancy (2nd trimester)		≥11.0
	(3rd trimester)		≥10.5
Protein	Serum albumin (g/100 ml)	≥3.5	≥3.5
Normal lipid metabolism	Serum cholesterol (mg/100 ml)	<200	<200
	Serum triglyceride (mg/100 ml)	<250	<250
Normal carbohydrate metabolism	Serum glucose (mg/100 ml)	75-110	75-110
Sodium	Serum sodium (mEq/L)	130-150	130-155
Potassium	Serum potassium (mEq/L)	3.5-5.3	3.5-5.3
Vitamin A	Plasma vitamin A (μg/100 ml)	>20	>20
Vitamin C	Serum vitamin C (mg/100 ml)	≥0.3	≥0.3
Riboflavin	Erythrocyte glutathione peroxidase (% stimulation of activity by added riboflavin cofactor)	<20	<20
Vitamin B$_6$	Tryptophan load test—increase in excretion of xanthurenic acid (mg/day)	<25	<25
Folate	Serum folate (nanogram/ml)	>6.0	>6.0
Thiamin	Urinary thiamin (μg/g creatinine)	>65	>65
Zinc	Plasma zinc (μg/100 ml)	80-115	80-115

Some information obtained from Roe DA: Drug-induced nutritional deficiencies, Westport, Conn, 1976, AVI Press; and Sauberlich HE, Skala HH and Dowdy RP: Laboratory tests for the assessment of nutritional status, Cleveland, 1974, CRC Press, Inc.

I

Recommended Nutrient Intakes for Canadians

Age	Sex	Energy (kcal)	Thiamin (mg)	Riboflavin (mg)	Niacin NE	n-3 PUFA (g)	n-6 PUFA (g)
0-4 months	Both	600	0.3	0.3	4	0.5	3
5-12 months	Both	900	0.4	0.5	7	0.5	3
1 year	Both	1100	0.5	0.6	8	0.6	4
2-3 years	Both	1300	0.6	0.7	9	0.7	4
4-6 years	Both	1800	0.7	0.9	13	1.0	6
7-9 years	M	2200	0.9	1.1	16	1.2	7
	F	1900	0.8	1.0	14	1.0	6
10-12 years	M	2500	1.0	1.3	18	1.4	8
	F	2200	0.9	1.1	16	1.2	7
13-15 years	M	2800	1.1	1.4	20	1.5	9
	F	2200	0.9	1.1	16	1.2	7
16-18 years	M	3200	1.3	1.6	23	1.8	11
	F	2100	0.8	1.1	15	1.2	7
19-24 years	M	3000	1.2	1.5	22	1.6	10
	F	2100	0.8	1.1	15	1.2	7
25-49 years	M	2700	1.1	1.4	19	1.5	9
	F	1900	0.8	1.0	14	1.1	7
50-74 years	M	2300	0.9	1.2	16	1.3	8
	F	1800	0.8*	1.0*	14*	1.1*	7*
75+ years	M	2000	0.8	1.0	14	1.1	7
	F†	1700	0.8*	1.0*	14*	1.1*	7*
Pregnancy (additional)							
1st Trimester		100	0.1	0.1	0.11	0.05	0.3
2nd Trimester		300	0.1	0.3	0.22	0.16	0.9
3rd Trimester		300	0.1	0.3	0.22	0.16	0.9
Lactation (additional)		450	0.2	0.4	0.33	0.25	1.5

NE, niacin equivalents; PUFA, polyunsaturated fatty acids.
*Level below which intake should not fall.
†Assumes moderate physical activity.
From Scientific Review Committee: Nutrition recommendations, Ottawa, 1990, Health and Welfare.

Summary Examples of Recommended Nutrient Intake Based on Age and Body Weight Expressed as Daily Rates

Age	Sex	Weight (kg)	Protein (g)	Vitamin A RE	Vitamin D (μg)	Vitamin E (mg)	Vitamin C (mg)	Folate (μg)	Vitamin B_{12} (μg)	Calcium (mg)	Phosphorus (mg)	Magnesium (mg)	Iron (mg)	Iodine (μg)	Zinc (mg)
0-4 months	Both	6.0	12*	400	10	3	20	25	0.3	250†	150	20	0.3‡	30	2‡
5-12 months	Both	9.0	12	400	10	3	20	40	0.4	400	200	32	7	40	3
1 year	Both	11	13	400	10	3	20	40	0.5	500	300	40	6	55	4
2-3 years	Both	14	16	400	5	4	20	50	0.6	550	350	50	6	65	4
4-6 years	Both	18	19	500	5	5	25	70	0.8	600	400	65	8	85	5
7-9 years	M	25	26	700	2.5	7	25	90	1.0	700	500	100	8	110	7
7-9 years	F	25	26	700	2.5	6	25	90	1.0	700	500	100	8	95	7
10-12 years	M	34	34	800	2.5	8	25	120	1.0	900	700	130	8	125	9
10-12 years	F	36	36	800	2.5	7	25	130	1.0	1100	800	135	8	110	9
13-15 years	M	50	49	900	2.5	9	30	175	1.0	1100	900	185	10	160	12
13-15 years	F	48	46	800	2.5	7	30	170	1.0	1000	850	180	13	160	9
16-18 years	M	62	58	1000	2.5	10	40¶	220	1.0	900	1000	230	10	160	12
16-18 years	F	53	47	800	2.5	7	30¶	190	1.0	700	850	200	12	160	9
19-24 years	M	71	61	1000	2.5	10	40¶	220	1.0	800	1000	240	9	160	12
19-24 years	F	58	50	800	2.5	7	30¶	180	1.0	700	850	200	13	160	9
25-49 years	M	74	64	1000	2.5	9	40¶	230	1.0	800	1000	250	9	160	12
25-49 years	F	59	51	800	2.5	6	30¶	185	1.0	700	850	200	13	160	9
50-74 years	M	73	63	1000	5	7	40¶	230	1.0	800	1000	250	9	160	12
50-74 years	F	63	54	800	5	6	30¶	195	1.0	800	850	210	8	160	9
75+ years	M	69	59	1000	5	6	40¶	215	1.0	800	1000	230	9	160	12
75+ years	F	64	55	800	5	5	30¶	200	1.0	800	850	210	8	160	9
Pregnancy (additional)															
1st Trimester			5	0	2.5	2	0	200	1.2	500	200	15	0	25	6
2nd Trimester			20	0	2.5	2	10	200	1.2	500	200	45	5	25	6
3rd Trimester			24	0	2.5	2	10	200	1.2	500	200	45	10	25	6
Lactation (additional)			20	400	2.5	3	25	100	0.2	500	200	65	0	50	6

RE, retinol equivalents.
*Protein is assumed to be from breast milk and must be adjusted for infant formula.
†Infant formula with high phosphorus should contain 375 mg of calcium.
‡Breast milk is assumed to be the source of the mineral.
¶Smokers should increase vitamin C by 50%.
From Scientific Review Committee: Nutrition recommendations, Ottawa, 1990, Health and Welfare.

J

Food Guide: Exchange Lists for Meal Planning (1986 Revision)

The *exchange system of dietary control,* developed by two professional organizations—the American Dietetic Association and the American Diabetes Association—is based on a simple grouping of common foods according to generally equivalent nutritional values. This system may be used for any situation requiring caloric and food value control.

The foods are divided into six basic groups (with subgroups), called the "exchange lists." Each food item within a group or subgroup contains about the same food value as other food items in that group, allowing for exchange within groups, thus providing for variety in food choices as well as food value control. Hence the term *food exchanges* is sometimes used to refer to food choices or servings. The total number of "exchanges" per day depends on individual nutritional needs, based on normal nutrition standards. Although there is some variation in the composition of foods within the exchange groups, for simplicity the following values for carbohydrate, protein, fat, and kilocalories are used.

Exchange Lists

Food Groups	Carbohydrate (g)	Protein (g)	Fat (g)	Kcal
Starch/Bread	15	3	Trace	80
Meat				
Lean	—	7	3	55
Medium-fat	—	7	5	75
High-fat	—	7	8	100
Vegetable	5	2	—	25
Fruit	15	—	—	60
Milk				
Skim	12	8	Trace	90
Low-fat	12	8	5	120
Whole	12	8	8	150
Fat	—	—	5	45

List 1: Starch/Bread List

Whole grain foods have about 2 g fiber per serving. Foods containing 3 g fiber per serving or more are marked with the symbol *.

Cereals/grains/pasta

*Bran cereals, concentrated	⅓ cup
*Bran cereals, flaked (such as Bran Buds, All Bran)	½ cup
Bulgur (cooked)	½ cup
Cooked cereals	½ cup
Cornmeal (dry)	2½ tbsp
Grapenuts	3 tbsp
Grits (cooked)	½ cup
Other ready-to-eat unsweetened cereals	¾ cup
Pasta (cooked)	½ cup
Puffed cereal	1½ cup
Rice, white or brown (cooked)	⅓ cup
Shredded Wheat	½ cup
*Wheat germ	3 tbsp

Dried beans/peas/lentils

*Beans and peas (cooked; such as kidney, white, split, black-eyed)	⅓ cup
*Lentils (cooked)	⅓ cup
*Baked beans	¼ cup

Starchy vegetables

*Corn	½ cup
*Corn on cob, 6 inches long	1
*Lima beans	½ cup
*Peas, green (fresh, frozen, or canned)	½ cup
*Plantain	½ cup
Potato, baked	1 small (3 oz)
Potato, mashed	½ cup
Squash, winter (acorn, butternut)	¾ cup
Yam, sweet potato, plain	⅓ cup

Bread

Bagel	½ (1 oz)
Bread sticks, crisp (4 inches long × ½ inch)	2 (⅔ oz)
Croutons, low fat	1 cup
English muffin	½
Frankfurter bun or hamburger bun	½ (1 oz)
Pita (6 inches across)	½
Plain roll, small	1 (1 oz)
Raisin, unfrosted	1 slice (1 oz)
*Rye, pumpernickel	1 slice (1 oz)
Tortilla, 6 inches across	1
White (including French, Italian)	1 slice (1 oz)
Whole wheat	1 slice (1 oz)

Crackers/snacks

Animal crackers	8
Graham crackers (2½ inches square)	3
Matzoth	¾ oz
Melba toast	5 slices
Oyster crackers	24
Popcorn (popped, no fat added)	3 cups
Pretzels	¾ oz
Rye crisp (2 inches × 3½ inches)	4
Saltine-type crackers	6
Whole wheat crackers, no fat added (crisp breads, such as Finn, Kavli, Wasa)	2-4 slices (¾ oz)

Starch foods prepared with fat (count as 1 starch/bread serving + 1 fat)

Biscuit (2½ inches across)	1
Chow mein noodles	½ cup
Corn bread (2 inch cube)	1 (2 oz)
Cracker, round butter type	6
French fried potatoes (2 to 3½ inches long)	10 (1½ oz)
Muffin, plain, small	1
Pancake (4 inches across)	2
Stuffing, bread (prepared)	¼ cup
Taco shell (6 inches across)	2
Waffle (4½ inch square)	1
Whole wheat crackers, fat added (such as Triscuits)	4-6 (1 oz)

List 2: Meat and Meat Substitutes List

To reduce fat intake, choose items mainly from the lean and medium-fat groups, using more fish and poultry (with skin removed) as meat choices, and trimming fat from all meats. Items having 400 mg sodium or more per exchange are marked with the symbol **. None of the items on this list contributes fiber to the diet. One exchange is equal to the amount listed for each item. In the case of meat, for example, a serving may be 2-3 exchanges (2-3 oz).

Lean meat and substitutes

Beef	USDA Good or Choice grades of lean beef, such as round, sirloin, and flank steak; tenderloin; and chipped beef**	1 oz
Pork	Lean pork, such as fresh ham; canned, cured, or boiled ham**; Canadian bacon**; tenderloin	1 oz
Veal	All cuts except for veal cutlets (ground or cubed)	1 oz
Poultry	Chicken, turkey, Cornish hen (without skin)	1 oz
Fish	All fresh and frozen fish	1 oz
	Crab, lobster, scallops, shrimp, clams (fresh or canned in water**)	2 oz
	Oysters	6 medium
	Tuna** (canned in water)	¼ cup
	Herring (uncreamed or smoked)	1 oz
	Sardines (canned)	2 medium
Wild game	Venison, rabbit, squirrel	1 oz
	Pheasant, duck, goose (without skin)	1 oz
Cheese	Any cottage cheese	¼ cup
	Grated parmesan	2 tbsp
	Diet cheeses** (less than 55 kcal/oz)	1 oz
Other	95% fat-free luncheon meat	1 oz slice
	Egg whites	3 whites
	Egg substitutes (less than 55 kcal/¼ cup)	¼ cup

Medium-fat meat and substitutes

Beef	Ground beef, roast (rib, chuck, rump), steak (cubed, Porterhouse, T-bone), and meatloaf (most beef products are in this category)	1 oz
Pork	Chops, loin roast, Boston butt, cutlets (most pork products fall into this category)	1 oz
Lamb	Chops, leg, and roast (most lamb products fall into this category)	1 oz
Veal	Cutlet (ground or cubes, unbreaded)	1 oz
Poultry	Chicken (with skin), domestic duck or goose (well-drained of fat), ground turkey	1 oz
Fish	Tuna** (canned in oil and drained)	¼ cup
	Salmon** (canned)	¼ cup
Cheese	Skim or part-skim cheeses, such as:	
	Ricotta	¼ cup
	Mozzarella	1 oz
	Diet cheeses** (56-80 kcal/oz)	1 oz
Other	86% fat-free luncheon meat**	1 oz
	Egg (high in cholesterol, limit to 3/week)	1
	Egg substitutes (56-80 kcal per ¼ cup)	¼ cup
	Tofu (2½ × 2¾ × 1 inch)	4 oz
	Liver, heart, kidney, sweetbreads (high in cholesterol, limit use)	1 oz

High-fat meat and substitutes (these items are high in saturated fat, cholesterol, and kilocalories; limit to 3 times/week)

Beef	USDA Prime cuts, ribs; corned beef**	1 oz
Pork	Spareribs, ground pork, pork sausage**	1 oz
Lamb	Ground lamb patties	1 oz
Fish	Any fried fish product	1 oz
Cheese	Regular cheeses**, such as American, Blue, Swiss	1 oz
Other	Luncheon meat**, such as bologna, salami, pimento loaf	1 oz slice
	Sausage**, such as Polish, Italian	1 oz
	Knockwurst, smoked	1 oz
	Bratwurst**	1 oz
	Frankfurter** (turkey or chicken)	1 frank (10/lb)
	Frankfurter** (beef, pork, or combination) (count as 1 high-fat meat + 1 fat)	1 frank (10/lb)
	Peanut butter	1 tbsp

List 3: Vegetable List

Unless otherwise noted, one vegetable exchange is 1 cup raw vegetable or ½ cup cooked vegetable or vegetable juice. Vegetables containing 400 mg sodium or more per serving are marked with the symbol **. Fresh and frozen vegetables have less added salt. Canned vegetables contain more salt, but rinsing will help remove much of it. In general, vegetables contain 2-3 g dietary fiber per serving. Starchy vegetables are found in the Starch/Bread List. Other free vegetables are in the Free Food List.

Artichoke (½ medium)	Mushrooms, cooked
Asparagus	Okra
Beans (green, wax, Italian)	Onions
Bean sprouts	Pea pods
Beets	Peppers (green)
Broccoli	Rutabaga
Brussels sprouts	Sauerkraut**
Cabbage	Spinach
Carrots	Summer squash (crookneck)
Cauliflower	Tomato (1 large)
Eggplant	Tomato/vegetable juice
Greens (collard, mustard, turnip)	Turnips
Kohlrabi	Water chestnuts
Leeks	Zucchini

List 4: Fruit List

Fruits containing 3 g dietary fiber or more per serving are marked with the symbol *. Portions are usual serving sizes of commonly eaten fruits.

Fresh, unsweetened frozen, and unsweetened canned fruit

Apple (raw, 2 inches across)	1 apple
Applesauce (unsweetened)	½ cup
Apricots (medium, raw)	4 apricots
Apricots (canned)	½ cup or 4 halves
Banana (9 inches long)	½ banana
*Blackberries (raw)	¾ cup
*Blueberries (raw)	¾ cup
Canteloupe (5 inches across)	⅓ melon
Canteloupe (cubes)	1 cup
Cherries (large, raw)	12 cherries
Cherries (canned)	½ cup
Figs (raw, 2 inches across)	2 figs
Fruit cocktail (canned)	½ cup

Grapefruit (medium)	½ grapefruit
Grapefruit (segments)	¾ cup
Grapes (small)	15 grapes
Honeydew melon (medium)	⅛ melon
Honeydew melon (cubes)	1 cup
Kiwi fruit (large)	1 kiwi fruit
Mandarin oranges (segments)	¾ cup
Mango (small)	½ mango
*Nectarine (1½ inches across)	1 nectarine
Orange (2½ inches across)	1 orange
Papaya (small cubes or balls)	1 cup
Peach (2¾ inches across)	1 peach
Peach (slices)	¾ cup
Peaches (canned)	½ cup or 2 halves
Pear	½ large pear or 1 small
Pears (canned)	½ cup or 2 halves
Persimmon (medium, native)	2 persimmons
Pineapple (raw, cubes)	¾ cup
Plum (raw, 2 inches across)	2 plums
*Pomegranate	½ pomegranate
*Raspberries (raw)	1 cup
*Strawberries (raw, whole)	1¼ cups
Tangerine (2½ inches across)	2 tangerines
Watermelon (cubes or balls)	1¼ cup

Dried fruit

*Apples	4 rings
*Apricots	7 halves
Dates	2½ medium
*Figs	1½
*Prunes	3 medium
Raisins	2 tbsp

Fruit juice

Apple juice or cider	½ cup
Cranberry juice cocktail	⅓ cup
Grapefruit juice	⅓ cup
Grape juice	⅓ cup
Orange juice	½ cup
Pineapple juice	½ cup
Prune juice	⅓ cup

List 5: Milk List

Milk may be used alone or in combination with other foods. See the Combination Foods List.

Skim and very lowfat milk

Skim or nonfat milk	1 cup
½% milk	1 cup
1% milk	1 cup
Lowfat buttermilk	1 cup
Evaporated skim milk	½ cup
Dry nonfat milk	⅓ cup
Plain nonfat yogurt	8 oz

Lowfat milk

2% milk	1 cup
Plain lowfat yogurt (with added nonfat milk solids)	8 oz

Whole milk (more than 3¼% butterfat; limit use)

Whole milk	1 cup
Evaporated whole milk	½ cup
Whole plain yogurt	8 oz

List 6: Fat List

Measure carefully; use mainly unsaturated fats. Sodium content varies widely, so check labels.

Unsaturated fats

Avocado	⅛ medium
Margarine	1 tsp
Margarine, diet	1 tbsp
Mayonnaise	1 tsp
Mayonnaise, reduced kcal	1 tbsp
Nuts and seeds	
Almonds, dry roasted	6 whole
Cashews, dry roasted	1 tbsp
Pecans	2 whole
Peanuts	20 small or 10 large
Walnuts	2 whole
Other nuts	1 tbsp
Seeds, pine nuts, sunflower (shelled)	1 tbsp
Pumpkin seeds	1 tsp
Oil (corn, cottonseed, safflower, soybean, sunflower, olive, peanut)	1 tsp
Olives	10 small or 5 large
Salad dressing, mayonnaise type	2 tsp
Salad dressing, mayonnaise type, low kcal	1 tbsp
Salad dressing (all varieties)	1 tbsp
Salad dressing, low kcal	2 tbsp
(2 tbsp low-calorie salad dressing is a free food)	

Saturated fats

Butter	1 tsp
Bacon	1 slice
Chitterlings	½ oz
Coconut, shredded	2 tbsp
Coffee whitener, liquid	2 tbsp
Coffee whitener, powder	4 tsp
Cream (light, coffee, table)	2 tbsp
Cream, sour	2 tbsp
Cream (heavy, whipping)	1 tbsp
Cream cheese	1 tbsp
Salt pork	¼ oz

FREE FOODS

Any food or drink containing less than 20 kcal/serving is "free." If a serving size is given, 2-3 servings per day are sufficient. Higher fiber* and sodium** foods are indicated. Use *nonstick pan spray* for cooking as desired.

Drink

Bouillon** or broth, fat-free	
Bouillon, low sodium	
Carbonated drinks, sugar-free	
Carbonated water	
Club soda	
Cocoa powder, unsweetened	1 tbsp
Coffee/Tea	
Drink mixes, sugar-free	
Tonic water, sugar-free	

Condiments

Catsup	1 tbsp
Horseradish	
Mustard	
Pickles**, dill, unsweetened	
Salad dressing, low kcal	2 tbsp
Taco sauce	1 tbsp
Vinegar	

Seasonings

Basil (fresh)	
Celery seeds	
Cinnamon	
Chili powder	
Chives	
Curry	
Dill	
Flavoring extracts (vanilla, almond, walnut, butter)	
Garlic, fresh and powder	
Herbs, spices	
Hot pepper sauce and flakes	
Lemon, juice and zest (outer skin)	
Lemon pepper	
Lime, juice and zest	
Mint, fresh leaves	
Onion powder	
Oregano	
Paprika	
Parsley	
Pepper	
Pimento	
Soy sauce**	
Soy sauce, low sodium—"lite"	
Wine, used in cooking	¼ cup
Worcestershire sauce	

Fruits

Cranberries, unsweetened	½ cup
Rhubarb, unsweetened	½ cup

Vegetables

Cabbage	
Celery	
Chinese cabbage*	
Cucumber	
Green onion	
Hot peppers	
Mushrooms	
Radishes	
Zucchini*	

Salad greens

Endive	
Escarole	
Lettuce	
Romaine	
Spinach	

Sweet substitutes

Candy, hard, sugar-free	
Gelatin dessert, sugar free	
Gum, sugar-free	
Jam/Jelly, sugar-free	2 tsp
Pancake syrup, sugar-free	1-2 tbsp
Sugar substitutes (saccharin, aspartame)	
Whipped topping	2 tbsp

Combination Foods

Check the *American Dietetic Association/American Diabetes Association Family Cookbooks* and the *American Diabetes Association Holiday Cookbook* for many recipes and much information, including combination foods.

Food	Amount	Exchanges
Casseroles, homemade	1 cup (8 oz)	2 starch, 2 medium-fat meat, 1 fat
Cheese pizza**, thin crust	¼ of 10 inch	2 starch, 1 medium-fat meat, 1 fat
Chili beans* **	1 cup (8 oz)	2 starch, 2 medium-fat meat, 2 fat
Chow mein* ** (without noodles or rice)	2 cups	1 starch, 2 vegetables, 2 lean meat
Macaroni and cheese**	1 cup	2 starch, 1 medium-fat meat, 2 fat
Spaghetti and meatballs (canned)	1 cup	2 starch, 1 medium-fat meat, 1 fat
Sugar-free pudding (made with skim milk)	½ cup	1 starch

Soup

Food	Amount	Exchanges
Bean* **	1 cup	1 starch, 1 vegetable, 1 lean meat
Chunky, all varieties**	10¾ oz can	1 starch, 1 vegetable, 1 medium-fat meat
Cream** (made with water)	1 cup	1 starch, 1 fat
Vegetable** or broth**	1 cup	1 starch

Beans used as a meat substitute

Food	Amount	Exchanges
Dried beans*, peas*, lentils* (cooked)	1 cup	2 starch, 1 lean meat

Foods for Occasional Use

Food	Amount	Exchanges
Angel food cake	1/12 cake	2 starch
Plain cake, no icing	1/12 cake or 3 in square	2 starch, 2 fat
Cookies	2 small (¾ in across)	1 starch, 1 fat
Frozen fruit yogurt	⅓ cup	1 starch
Gingersnaps	3	1 starch
Granola	¼ cup	1 starch, 1 fat
Granola bars	1 small	1 starch, 1 fat
Ice cream, any flavor	½ cup	1 starch, 2 fat
Ice milk, any flavor	½ cup	1 starch, 1 fat
Sherbet, any flavor	¼ cup	1 starch
Snack chips**, all varieties	1 oz	1 starch, 2 fat
Vanilla wafers	6 small	1 starch, 1 fat

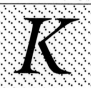

Dietary Fiber and Kilocalorie Values for Selected Foods

Foods	Serving	Dietary fiber (g)	Kcal
Breads and cereals			
All Bran	⅓ cup	8.5	70
Bran (100%)	½ cup	8.4	75
Bran Buds	⅓ cup	7.9	75
Corn Bran	⅔ cup	5.4	100
Bran Chex	⅔ cup	4.6	90
Cracklin' Oat Bran	⅓ cup	4.3	110
Bran Flakes	¾ cup	4.0	90
Air-popped popcorn	1 cup	2.5	25
Oatmeal	1 cup	2.2	144
Grapenuts	¼ cup	1.4	100
Whole-wheat bread	1 slice	1.4	60
Legumes, cooked			
Kidney beans	½ cup	7.3	110
Lima beans	½ cup	4.5	130
Vegetables, cooked			
Green peas	½ cup	3.6	55
Corn	½ cup	2.9	70
Parsnip	½ cup	2.7	50
Potato, with skin	1 medium	2.5	95
Brussels sprouts	½ cup	2.3	30
Carrots	½ cup	2.3	25
Broccoli	½ cup	2.2	20
Beans, green	½ cup	1.6	15
Tomato, chopped	½ cup	1.5	17
Cabbage, red & white	½ cup	1.4	15
Kale	½ cup	1.4	20
Cauliflower	½ cup	1.1	15
Lettuce (fresh)	1 cup	0.8	7
Fruits			
Apple	1 medium	3.5	80
Raisins	¼ cup	3.1	110
Prunes, dried	3	3.0	60
Strawberries	1 cup	3.0	45
Orange	1 medium	2.6	60
Banana	1 medium	2.4	105
Blueberries	½ cup	2.0	40
Dates, dried	3	1.9	70
Peach	1 medium	1.9	35
Apricot, fresh	3 medium	1.8	50
Grapefruit	½ cup	1.6	40
Apricot, dried	5 halves	1.4	40
Cherries	10	1.2	50
Pineapple	½ cup	1.1	40

Adapted from Lanza E and Butrum RR: A critical review of food fiber analysis and data, J Am Diet Assoc 86:732, 1986.

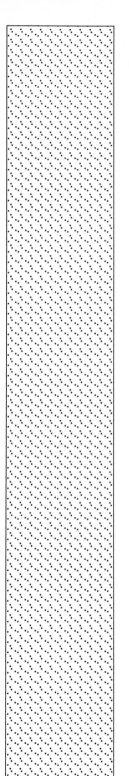

Glossary

Abscissa   (L *ab*, from; *scindere*, to cut) Usually the horizontal X line used as a base of reference in graphing relative data. When suitable values are assigned to both of the two lines of the graph, the horizontal X axis or ordinates and the bisecting vertical Y axis or abscissas, corresponding data with reference to the other can be plotted.

Achlorhydria   (L *a-*, negative; *chlorhydria*, hydrochloric acid) Absence or reduced amounts of hydrochloric acid in the gastric secretions.

Acne   (Gr *achne*, chaff) Common inflammation *(acne vulgaris)* of the pilosebaceous (L *pilus*, hair; *sebum*, suet; thick semifluid secretion composed of fat and epithelial cell debris) glands of the skin, mainly on the face, chest, and back. Precise cause unknown, but suggested factors include hormones, stress, heredity, and bacteria; usually self-limiting after the physiologic stress of puberty.

Acrocyanosis   (Gr *akron*, extremity; *kyanos*, blue) Condition due to excessive concentration of reduced hemoglobin in the blood, resulting in arterial unsaturation with oxygen; marked by cyanosis of extremities with mottled blue or red discoloration of skin on fingers, wrists, toes, and ankles, accompanied by coldness of the fingers and toes.

Addiction   (L *addictio*, a giving over, surrender, being enslaved to) State of being enslaved to some undesirable practice that is physically or psychologically habit-forming to the extent that its cessation causes severe trauma.

Adenoidal pad   (Gr *adenos*, gland; *eidos*, form) Normal lymphoid tissue in the nasopharynx of children.

Adenosine triphosphate (ATP)   The high energy compound formed in the cell, called the "energy currency" of the cell due to the binding of energy in its high-energy phosphate bonds for release for cell work as these bonds are split.

Adipocytes   (L *adipis*, fat; *kytos*, hollow vessel, cell) Fat cells.

Adipose tissue   (L *adipis*, fat, lard) Loose connective tissue in which fat cells (adipocytes) accumulate and are stored.

Affective goal   Communication goal related to processes of feelings and desires, attitudes and values.

Alopecia   (Gr *alopekia*, disease in which hair falls out) Baldness; absence of hair from skin areas of the body where it normally is present.

Alveoli   (L *alveus*, hollow) Small sac-like formations; thin-walled chambers in the lungs surrounded by networks of capillaries through whose walls exchange of carbon dioxide and oxygen takes place.

Alveoli   (L *alveus*, hollow) Small sac-like outpouching areas in the mammary gland, secretory units that produce and secrete milk.

Alzheimer-type senile dementia (ATSD)   A type of senile dementia first described by German physician Alois Alzheimer (1864-1915); progressive, irreversible degenerative changes in the brain, resulting in loss of neuromuscular function and mental capacity.

Amenorrhea   (Gr *a-*, negative; *men*, month; *rhoia*, flow) Absence of menses. Nutritional amenorrhea results from extreme weight loss and malnutrition, as in eating disorders such as anorexia nervosa.

Amino acids   (*amino*, the monovalent chemical group -NH2) Carriers of the essential element nitrogen; structural units of protein, specific amino acids being linked in specific sequence by peptide chains to form specific proteins.

Amylase   (Gr *amylon*, starch; *-ase*, enzyme suffix) Group name for enzymes that act on starch to render successively smaller and smaller molecules of dextrins and maltose, for example, salivary amylase (ptyalin) and pancreatic amylase (amylopsin). The generic group name amylase is now more widely used for any starch-splitting enzyme.

Anabolic steroids (Gr *anabole,* a building or construction) Any of a group of synthetic derivatives of testosterone, the male sex hormone, having pronounced anabolic (tissue building) properties; a drug used in clinical medicine to promote growth and repair of tissues in debilitating illness. Widespread illegal abuse of the drug by some athletes and body builders harms their health.

Anabolism Metabolic process by which body tissues are built.

Anemia (Gr *a-,* negative; *haima,* blood) Blood condition marked by a decrease in number of circulating red blood cells, hemoglobin, or both.

Anorexia nervosa (Gr *anorektos,* without appetite; L *nervosa,* nervous or emotional disorder) A severe psychophysiologic eating disorder, usually seen in girls and young women, in which the person does not lack appetite, as the label would indicate, but is psychologically unable to eat and refuses food, becoming extremely emaciated; a form of self-starvation.

Antagonist (Gr *antagonisma,* struggle) Agent that has an opposite, conflicting, or inhibiting action to another substance.

Antepartum (L, *anto,* before; *partum,* parting, a separate part) Period of gestation before onset of maternal labor and birth of the infant.

Anthropometry (Gr *anthropos,* man, human; *metron,* measure) The science and procedures that deal with measurement of the size, weight, and proportional dimensions of the human body.

Antibodies Immune system components, specific immunoglobulins, especially secretory IgA in the bowel and upper respiratory mucosa that destroy invading antigens.

Antidiuretic hormone (ADH) Hormone secreted by the posterior pituitary gland in response to body stress. It acts on the distal tubules of the kidney's nephrons to cause water reabsorption and thus protect vital body water; also called *vasopressin.*

Antigen (antibody + Gr *gennan,* to produce) Any disease agent such as toxins, bacteria, viruses, and other foreign substances, whose presence stimulates the production of antibodies of the immune system to combat and destroy them.

Antioxidant (Gr *anti-,* against; *oxys,* keen) A substance that inhibits oxidation of polyunsaturated fatty acids and formation of free radicals in the cells.

Antirachitic (Gr *anti-,* against; *rachitis,* a spinal disorder) An agent that is therapeutically effective against rickets, a nutritional deficiency disease affecting childhood bone development, in which vitamin D is lacking.

Aorta Main large trunk blood vessel from the heart, leading down the center of the body through the chest and upper abdomen from which the systemic arterial blood system proceeds.

Apgar score A scale developed by American anesthesiologist Virginia Apgar (1909-1974), by which an infant's condition is defined 1 minute after birth by scoring the heart rate, respiratory effort, muscle tone, reflex irritability, and color.

Apocrine (Gr *apokrinesthai,* to be secreted) A type of glandular secretion in which the end portion of the secreting cell is removed with the secretory product.

Areola (L *areola,* area, space) Pigmented area surrounding the nipple of the human breast.

Ascorbic acid Chemical name for vitamin C, based on its antiscorbutic function in prevention of the deficiency disease scurvy.

Atherosclerosis (Gr *athere,* gruel; *skleros,* hard) Condition characterized by gradual formation, beginning in childhood in genetically predisposed individuals, of fatty cheese-like streaks that develop into hardened plaques in the intima or inner lining of major blood vessels such as coronary arteries, eventually in adulthood cutting off blood supply to the tissue served by the vessel; the underlying pathology of coronary heart disease.

Atherosclerotic lesions Characteristic lesions, called athromas, the fatty raised streaks and plaques that signal atherosclerosis, the underlying cardiovascular disease associated with elevated levels of serum lipids, especially cholesterol, and related risk factors such as smoking, obesity, and hypertension.

Autonomy   (Gr *autos,* self; *nomos,* law) State of functioning independently; self-determination.

Axis   (L *axis,* axle, central line) One of two coordinates (the other called abscissa) used as a frame of reference between values in graphing data; usually the vertical Y axis, also called ordinate axis.

Basal oxygen consumption   Amount of oxygen intake to meet basal metabolic needs; a means of measuring basal metabolic rate (BMR). Comparative metabolic measures in current use are derived by formula calculation using individual factors of weight, height, age, and sex: basal energy expenditure (BEE), and resting energy expenditure (REE).

Basic four food groups   A simple general food guide issued by the U.S. Department of Agriculture, using a grouping of commonly used foods and agricultural products for planning a day's balanced meals: breads/cereals, vegetables/fruits, milk and dairy products, and meat, with recent suggested food item revisions to reduce fats and sugars.

Behavioral goal   Communication goal related to processes of changing behavior.

Bile   (L *bilis,* bile) A fluid secreted by the liver and transported to the gallbladder for concentration and storage; released into duodenum upon entry of fat to facilitate enzymatic fat digestion by acting as an emulsifying agent.

Bioavailability   Amount of a nutrient ingested in food that is absorbed and thus available to the body for metabolic use.

Blastocyst   (Gr *blastos,* germ; *kystis,* sac, bladder) A stage in the development of the embryo in which the cells are arranged in a single layer to form a hollow sphere.

Body compartment   The collective quantity of a particular vital substance in the body, for example, the mineral compartment, composed mainly of the skeletal bone mass.

Body composition   The relative sizes of the four body compartments that make up the physical body—lean body mass, fat, water, and mineral mass.

Body mass index   A calculated assessment of body mass based on weight and height: BMI = [weight (kg) divided by height (m)]^2.

Botulism   A serious, often fatal, form of food poisoning from ingesting food contaminated with the powerful toxins of the bacteria *Clostridium botulinum.* The toxin blocks transmission of neural impulses at the nerve terminals, causing gradual paralysis and death when affecting respiratory muscles. Most cases result from eating carelessly home-canned food, so that all such foods should be boiled at least 10 minutes before eating. Cases reported in infants have been related to eating spore-containing honey, so honey should not be fed to infants.

Bradycardia   (Gr *bradys,* slow; *kardia,* heart) A slow heart beat, evidenced by slowing of the pulse rate to less than 60 beats/min.

Brush border   Vast array of microvilli covering each villus on the absorptive surface of the small intestine, holding nutrients ready for absorption within an unstirred layer of water and facilitating their absorption with a greatly expanded surface area. So named because they appear as the bristles of a brush when viewed with an electron microscope.

Buffering capacity   Function of the body's main buffer system, composed of two balancing partners, an acid partner (carbonic acid) and a base partner (sodium bicarbonate), that act together to buffer or neutralize any incoming acid or base to maintain the necessary degree of acidity and alkalinity in the body fluids that is compatible with life and health.

Bulimia nervosa   (L *bous,* ox; *limos,* hunger; *nervosa,* nervous or emotional condition) A psychophysiologic eating disorder, seen mainly in girls and young women, marked by alternate gorging on large amounts of food followed by self-induced vomiting and purging with laxative; weight usually remains fairly stable at a normal amount.

Cachexia   (Gr *kakos,* bad, ill; *hexia,* habit) A profound and grave state of body disorder and deterioration, as seen in cases of advanced malignant disease or starvation, causing gross body weight loss to cadaverous proportions as a result of disorder metabolism.

Calcitonin   (L *calx,* lime, calcium; *tonus,* balance) A polypeptide hormone secreted by the thyroid gland in response to hypercalcemia, which acts to lower both calcium and phosphate in the blood.

Calcitriol   Activated hormone form of vitamin D $[1,25(OH)_2D_3]$—1,25,dehydroxycholecalciferol.

Candida albicans   (L *candidus,* glowing white) Most frequent agent of *candidiasis,* a yeast-like fungus infecting moist tissue areas of the body, involving skin, vaginal, and oral mucosa.

Carbohydrate fuel   Basic organic carbon compound in food (starches and sugars) that is the primary and most efficient form of body fuel for energy, especially for building body muscles.

Carboxypeptidase   (L *carbo-,* coal, carbon—fundamental element in all organic compounds) The chemical group *carboxyl*—COOH—at the end of the carbon chain identifies the compound as an organic acid. The end of this term, *-peptidase,* indicates a protein-splitting enzyme, which together with the first part means that this is an enzyme that acts on the peptide bond of the terminal amino acid having a free-end carboxyl group.

Cardiac output   Total amount of blood pumped by the heart per minute.

Carnitine   A naturally occurring amino acid $(C_7H_{15}NO_3)$ formed from methionine and lysine, required for transport of long-chain fatty acids across the mitochondrial membrane where they are oxidized as fuel substrate for metabolic energy.

Carotenemia   Condition associated with excess intake or impaired metabolism of carotenoid pigments, especially beta-carotene, resulting in excess carotene in the blood, sometimes to the extent of producing a yellowing of the skin resembling jaundice.

Carotenoids   Any of a group of red and yellow pigments chemically similar to and including carotene found in dark green and yellow vegetables and fruits.

Casein hydrolysate formula   Infant formula with base of hydrolyzed casein, major milk protein, produced by partially breaking down the casein of cow's milk into smaller peptide fragments, making a product that is more easily digested.

Catabolism   Metabolic process by which body tissue is broken down.

Catalyst   (Gr *katalysis,* dissolution) A substance, such as enzymes and their component trace elements, that control specific cell metabolism reactions but are not changed or consumed themselves in the reaction as are their specific substrates on which they work.

Celiac disease   (Gr *koilia,* belly) A malabsorption diarrheal disease of intestinal mucosa caused by an abnormal reaction to gluten in certain grains such as wheat; infantile form marked by extreme wasting, growth retardation, and celiac crisis.

Cephalopelvic disproportion   (Gr *kephale,* head; *pyelos,* an oblong trough, pelvis) Relationship of fetal head to size of the maternal pelvis.

Cerebral hemorrhage   Rupture of an artery in the brain; cerebrovascular accident (CVA), stroke.

Cheilosis   (Gr *cheilos,* lip) A general symptom of tissue inflammation and breakdown producing swelling and reddening of the lips, a chapped appearance, and fissures at the corners of the mouth; associated with general malnutrition, especially a deficiency of riboflavin.

Cholecalciferol   Chemical name for vitamin D in its inactive dietary form (D_3). Formerly measured in terms of International Units (IU), a concept based on the "biologic activity" of a vitamin as measured in rats according to its ability to forestall the development of a disease associated with a deficiency of that specific vitamin. Now, instead, vitamin recommendations are given in direct quantity (mg or μg) needed for health based on current population studies. In the case of vitamin D, 10 μg as cholecalciferol equals 400 IU. When the inactive cholecalciferol is consumed, it is then activated first in the liver and then completed in the kidney to its active vitamin D hormone form *calcitriol* (1,25-dihydroxycholecalciferol $[1,25(OH)_2D_3]$). Additional amounts of D_3 are generated by effect of sunlight on 7-dehydrocholesterol in the skin, a precursor cholesterol compound.

Chronic diseases   (Gr *chronos,* time) Diseases of aging or long duration.

Chronologic age   Age of an individual based on the number of years lived, compared, for example, with *biologic age,* the relative age of a person based on physiologic capacity and measurements.

Chymotrypsin   (Gr *chymos,* chyme, creamy gruel-like material produced by gastric digestion of food) One of the protein-splitting and milk-curdling pancreatic enzymes, activated in the intestine from precursor chymotrypsinogen; breaks peptide linkages of the amino acids phenylalanine and tyrosine.

Cineradiographs   (Gr *cine-, kineisis,* movement; L *radius,* ray; Gr *graphein,* to write) Fluoroscopic motion film records of internal structures and functions.

Citric acid cycle   Final energy production pathway in the cell mitochondria that transforms the ultimate fuel acetyl CoA from carbohydrate and fat, capturing this energy in the cell's metabolic enzyme cycle production of high-energy phosphate bonds of ATP.

Clinical care process   An interactive process between health care professional and client of planning personal health care through five phases of assessment and data collection, analysis of findings, planning care according to a written individual care plan, implementing the plan, and evaluating and recording results.

Cobalamin   Chemical name for vitamin B_{12}, from its structure as a complex red crystalline compound of high molecular weight, with a single cobalt atom at its core. Its food sources are of animal origin, but the ultimate source is from colonies of synthesizing microorganisms inhabiting the gastrointestinal tract of herbiverous animals.

Coefficient of variation   Change or effect produced by the variation in certain factors, or the ratio between two different quantities.

Coenzyme factors   A major metabolic role of the micronutrients, vitamins and minerals, as essential partners with cell enzymes in a variety of reactions in both energy and protein metabolism.

Cognitive goal   (L *cognito,* to know) Communications goal related to the process of knowing and learning; mental processes of thinking and remembering.

Colostrum   (L *colostrum,* bee sting swelling and secretions) Thin yellowish milky liquid, mother's initial breast secretion before and immediately after birth of her baby; rich in immune factors and nutrition, especially protein and minerals; foremilk.

Communication   Process of giving or interchanging information, thoughts, or feelings by speaking, writing, signing, discussing, listening, responding.

Community care process   Program planning to meet defined community health needs through assessment procedures, objectives, program plan, and evaluation.

Complement   Series of enzymatic proteins that interact with an antigen-antibody complex to promote phagocyte activity or destroy other cells; component of the body's immune system.

Complementary amino acids   Combinations of amino acids from a variety of combined protein foods that complete one another according to their relative amounts of individual amino acids, in order to meet growth requirements for the nine essential amino acids that the body does not sufficiently synthesize.

Complete protein   A protein food containing all of the essential amino acids, animal food sources are milk, cheese, meat, eggs. Plant proteins alone are incomplete, but complementary combinations may be planned to make a complete protein mix, as a vegetarian would do.

Complex carbohydrates   Main dietary carbohydrate, the polysaccharide starch in varied foods such as legumes, grains, breads, pasta, cereals, and potatoes.

Condom   (L *condus,* a receptacle) A penile sheath serving not only as a barrier method of contraception but also as a means of preventing the spread of sexually transmitted diseases.

Congregate meals   Group meals for older adults, served in a social setting in the community and funded by Title III-C of the Older Americans Act.

Constipation (L *constipation,* a crowding together) Infrequent, sometimes difficult, passage of feces; condition is often a source of anxiety to elderly persons and may be perceived more in mental attitude than in physiologic reality; sometimes called "irritable bowel."

Corpus luteum (Gr *corpus,* body; *luteum,* yellow) Mass of estrogen and progesterone secretory cells; produced monthly from the ovarian follicle in the postovulation phase of the female sexual cycle.

Cortical bone (Gr *corticis,* bark, shell) Long bones of the body extremities with heavy outer cortex layer, giving strength to body movements.

Corticosteroid (L *corticis,* bark, shell) Any of the steroids affecting carbohydrate, fat, and protein metabolism, that are produced in the outer region (cortex) of the adrenal glands in response to stimulus of the adrenocorticotropic hormone (ACTH) from the pituitary gland, or any of their synthetic derivatives. These compounds include *glucocorticoids* affecting glucose metabolism, and *mineralocorticoids* affecting electrolyte (Na^+) concentration and hence fluid-electrolyte balance.

Counseling A dynamic process of communication that is client-centered; the role of counselor is to guide the client to identify problems and priorities and to set goals and possible solutions.

Crohn's disease Inflammatory disease first described by New York physician Bernard Crohn (born 1884), involving any part of the gastrointestinal tract, but commonly affecting the lower small intestine and colon.

Cushing's syndrome A condition first described by Boston surgeon Harvey Cushing (1869-1939), due to hypersecretion of adrenocorticotropic hormone (ACTH) or excessive intake of glucocorticoids, characterized by rapidly developing fat deposits of face, neck, and trunk, giving an enlarged and rounded "moon-face" or cushingoid appearance.

Cytoplasm (Gr *kytos,* hollow vessel; *plasma,* anything formed or molded) The protoplasm of the cell outside the nucleus, a continuous gel-like aqueous solution in which the cell organelles are suspended; site of major cell metabolism.

Deamination Process by which the nitrogen radical (NH_4) is split off from amino acids, important in maintaining nitrogen balance.

De novo (L *anew,* from the beginning) To make new product afresh from the beginning with the principal components; akin to "from scratch" as in cooking.

Dental caries (L *caries,* "rottenness") Molecular decay or death of hard tissue; disease of the calcified tissues of the teeth resulting from action of microorganisms on carbohydrate producing acid erosion of the tooth surface; characterized by disintegration of hard outer enamel, followed by breakdown of softer inner dentin material, leaving cavities and exposed soft tissue.

Dentin (L *dens,* tooth) Chief substance of the tooth, which surrounds the innermost tooth pulp and is covered by the enamel of the crown and the cementum on the roots.

Depot fat Body fat stored in adipose tissue.

Desquamation (L *de-,* from; *squama,* scale) The shedding of epithelial tissue, mainly from the skin and oral mucosa, in scales or small sheets.

Diagnosis-related groups (DRGs) A U.S. government cost-containment management classification scheme for predesignation of Medicare payments based on specific diagnosis categories of disease.

Dietary fiber Nondigestible form of carbohydrate, of nutritional importance in gastrointestinal disease such as diverticulosis, and in management of serum lipid and glucose levels in risk-reduction related to chronic conditions such as heart disease and diabetes.

Dietary guidelines for Americans Diet and health guidelines for planning a healthy diet and reducing disease risks.

Diuresis (Gr *diourein,* to urinate) Increased excretion of urine.

Diuretics (Gr *diouretikos,* promoting urine) Drugs that stimulate urination.

Docosahexanoic acid (DHA) (Gr *docosa*, 22; *hexa*, 6) Long chain polyunsaturated omega-3 fatty acid, having a 22 carbon chain with 6 double bonds; a metabolic product of omega-3 eicosapentanoic (*eicosa*, 20; *penta*, 5)—EPA, long-chain fatty acid with 20 carbon atoms and 5 double bonds. Both are found in fatty fish. The body also synthesizes both EPA and DHA from the essential fatty acid linoleic and its product linolenic acid.

Dysgeusia (Gr *dys*, bad; *geusis*, taste) Abnormally perverted sense of taste, or bad taste in the mouth.

Ectoderm (Gr *ektos*, outside; *derma*, skin) The outermost of the three primitive cell layers of the embryo.

Edema (Gr *oidema*, swelling) An unusual accumulation of fluid in the intercellular tissue spaces of the body.

Edentulous (L *e-*, without; *dens*, tooth) Absence of natural teeth.

Eicosapentanoic acid (EPA) (Gr *eicosa*, 20; *penta*, 5) Long-chain polyunsaturated fatty acid composed of a chain of 20 carbon atoms with 5 double (unsaturated) bonds; one of the omega-3 fatty acids found in fatty fish and fish oils.

Electrolyte (Gr *electron*, amber [which emits electricity when rubbed]; *lytos*, soluble) A chemical element or compound, which in solution dissociates as ions carrying a positive or negative charge, for example, H^+, Na^+, K^+, Ca^{++}, Mg^{++}, and Cl^-, HCO_3^-, HPO_4^{--}, SO_4^{--}. Electrolytes constitute a major force controlling fluid balances within the body through their concentrations and shifts from one place to another to restore and maintain balance—*homeostasis*.

Elemental formula Infant formula produced with elemental, ready to be absorbed, components of free amino acids and carbohydrate as simple sugars.

Enamel The very hard white surface substance that covers and protects the soft inner dentin of a tooth.

Endoderm (Gr *endon*, within; *derma*, skin) The innermost of the three primitive embryonic cell layers.

Endometrium (Gr *endon*, within; *metra*, uterus) The inner mucous membrane of the uterus.

Endoplasmic reticulum (Gr *endon*, within; *plassein*, to form; L *rete*, net) A protoplasmic network in cells of flattened double membrane sheets; important metabolic cell organelles, some with rough surfaces bearing ribosomes for protein synthesis and other smooth surfaces synthesizing fatty acids.

Energy (Gr *energeia*, energy) The power to overcome resistance, to do work.

Energy balance Physiologic aspect of weight management, based on balance between energy intake in food and energy output in physical activity and internal metabolic work.

Energy intake Energy value of the three energy-yielding macronutrients in food—carbohydrate, fat, and protein in food, measured in kilocalories, abbreviated kcalories or kcal.

Enmeshed To catch, as in a net, and entangle; intertwined family relationships that capture and diminish individual autonomy or self-regard.

Epidemiology (Gr *epidemios*, prevalent; *-ology*, study) The study of factors determining the frequency, distribution, and strength of diseases in population groups.

Epiglottis (Gr *api-*, on; *glottis*, vocal apparatus of the larynx) Lid-like cartilaginous structure overhanging the entrance to the larynx and preventing food from entering the larynx and trachea while swallowing.

Epipharynx (Gr *epi-*, on; *pharynx*, throat) Nasopharynx that lies above the level of the soft palate.

Episiotomy (Gr *epision*, pubic region; *tome*, a cutting) Surgical incision into the peritoneum and vagina for obstetrical purposes.

Epithelium (Gr *epi-*, on, upon, over; *thele*, nipple) The covering tissue of internal and external surfaces of the body, including linings of vessels and other small cavities.

Erythrocyte   (Gr *erythro-,* red; *cyte,* hollow vessel) Red blood cell.

Erythropoiesis   (Gr *erythros,* red; *poiesis,* making) The production of erythrocytes, red blood cells.

Essential amino acid   Any one of nine amino acids that the body cannot synthesize at all or in sufficient amounts to meet body needs, so it must be supplied by the diet, hence a *dietary* essential for these nine specific amino acids: histidine, isoleucine, leucine, lysine, methionine, phenylalanine, threonine, tryptophan, and valine.

Esterification   Chemical process of converting an acid into an *ester,* catalyzed by the enzyme *esterase.* An ester is any compound formed from an alcohol and an acid by removal of water, for example, cholesterol esterification by attaching a fatty acid to the sterol base.

Estrogen   Generic group name for the ovarian hormones—beta-estradiol (the most potent), estrone, and estriol, which function to develop and maintain the female sexual organs and to stimulate bone growth.

Ethanol   Chemical name for beverage alcohol.

Evaluation   Process of determining the value of an educational or clinical program in terms of its initial identified objectives.

Extracellular fluid (ECF)   The total body water compartment composed of the collective water outside of cells.

Extracellular water   Alternate term for collective body water or fluids outside of cells.

18:2 fatty acid   Naming system for fatty acids according to structure: carbon chain length and number of double (unsaturated) bonds. Thus, an 18:2 fatty acid would have a long chain of 18 carbon atoms with 2 double bonds. This is the chemical shorthand for linoleic acid, the essential fatty acid.

Ferrous sulfate   Iron fortification compound in infant formulas used as needed to prevent anemia.

Flatulence   (L *flatus,* a blowing) Excessive formation and expulsion of gases in the gastrointestinal tract.

Follicle   (L *follis,* leather bag) Sac-like secretory cavity encasing an ovum and nourishing its growth.

Food abuse   Misuse and excessive eating of food as a reflection of underlying personal needs or problems, rather than in normal amount and nature as an essential part of good health and enjoyment.

Food exchange lists (groups)   A meal-planning food guide of six food exchange lists, with indicated portion sizes and equivalent food values for each item in a group, hence items may be exchanged within each group to maintain both variety and food values. The six food groups are bread/cereal, vegetable, fruit, milk, meat, and fat. Easily used for nutrient and energy calculations for management of diabetes and weight.

Food frequency questionnaire (FFQ)   A tool for collecting nutrition information about food habits. Consists of a comprehensive list of foods and a scale for checking frequency of use over a period of time.

Food guide   A model for planning and evaluating a daily diet.

Food record   A 3 to 7 day record of all food consumed, detailed with portion sizes, amounts, and preparation methods or recipes, for nutrition analysis as part of a total nutrition assessment process for planning nutrition care and education, or as an ongoing tool for monitoring nutritional therapy.

Fortified cereal   Cereal food products enriched by additions of minerals such as iron and zinc, and vitamins such as thiamin, riboflavin, niacin, folate B_6, and B_{12}.

Frontal bossing   (ME *boce,* lump, growth) A rounded protuberance of the forehead. In general terms, a boss is a knob-like rounded protuberance on the body or some body organ.

Functional disability   Disability that interferes with activities of daily living, such as bathing, dressing, shopping, preparing meals, eating.

Galactosemia   A rare genetic disease in newborns caused by a missing enzyme (galactose-1-phosphate uridyltransferase-G-1-PUT) required for conversion of galactose to glucose for metabolic use in the body. Untreated, galactose (from lactose) accumulates in the blood, causing extensive tissue damage and potential death. Normal growth and development now follows mandatory newborn screening and immediate initiation of a galactose-free diet with a special soy-based formula.

Gastrectomy   Surgical removal of all or part of the stomach.

Gastric pH   (Gr *gaster,* stomach; *pH,* power of the hydrogen ion—H⁺) Chemical symbol relating to H⁺ concentration or activity in a solution; expressed numerically as the negative logarithm of H⁺ concentration: pH 7.0 is neutral—above it alkalinity increases, and below it acidity increases. The hydrochloric acid (HCl) gastric secretions maintain a gastric pH of about 2.0.

Generativity   (L *generatio,* generation) The dynamic psychosocial process of renewing a society's values from one generation to the next.

Gerontology   The study of aging including biologic, physiologic, psychologic, and sociologic aspects. Contrast with *geriatrics,* which is the medical specialty dealing with chronic disease, as well as physical health, in older adults.

Gestation   (L *gestare,* to bear) Intrauterine fetal growth period (40 weeks) from conception to birth.

Gestational age   Period of embryonic-fetal growth and development from ovum fertilization to birth, varying from preterm development of a premature infant to a full-term mature newborn.

Gingivitis   (L *gingiva,* "gum of the mouth") Inflammation of the gum tissue surrounding the base of the teeth.

Glomerular filtration rate   A measure of the amount of blood filtered by the cup-like glomerulus at the head of each kidney nephron, per unit of time (ml/min).

Gluconeogenesis   (Gr *gleukos,* sweetness; *neos,* new; *gennan,* to produce) Production of glucose from keto-acid carbon skeleton from deaminated amino acids and the glycerol portion of fatty acids.

Glucose   Simple sugar, basic refined body fuel, circulated in the blood to cells for energy production.

Glycogen   A briefly stored form of carbohydrate in the liver and muscle tissues, available for energy fuel during brief fasting periods of sleep; built up in larger storage amounts by high starch meals prior to endurance athletic events for sustained energy.

Glycogen loading   Practice among athletes in endurance events of increasing intake of complex carbohydrates in days before the event to increase glycogen storage for energy reserve fuel during the event.

Glycolysis   Initial energy production enzyme pathway outside the mitochondria, by which 6-carbon glucose is changed to active 3-carbon fragments of acetyl CoA, the fuel ready for final energy production in the mitochondria to the high-energy phosphate bond compound adenosine triphosphate (ATP).

Goitrogens   Natural substances in certain foods such as soybeans that cause hypothyroidism and a compensatory enlargement of the thyroid gland, producing symptoms of iodine-deficiency goiter; effect diminished by adequate heating of the soy meal and adding iodine supplementation.

Golgi apparatus   A complex cup-like structure of membranes with associated vesicles, first described by Italian Nobel prize-winning histologist Camillo Golgi (1843-1926); site for synthesis of numerous carbohydrate metabolic products such as lactose, glycoproteins, and mucopolysaccharides.

Granulosa cells   Cells surrounding the primitive ovarian follicle and forming its outer layer and the mature ovary.

Grazing Informal descriptive label for food pattern of frequent small snacks throughout the day rather than more formal regular meals. Term taken from animal pattern of constant eating in a pastureland.

Growth acceleration Period of increased speed of growth at different points of childhood development.

Growth channel The progressive regular growth pattern of children, guided along individual genetically controlled channels, influenced by nutritional and health status.

Growth deceleration Period of decreased speed of growth at different points of childhood development.

Growth grid Chart indicating weight-height growth rates of infants and children by percentiles of a representative population, on which an individual child's growth may be plotted for comparison and monitoring over time.

Growth velocity (L *velocitas*, speed) Rapidity of motion or movement; rate of childhood growth over normal periods of development, as compared with a population standard.

Guaiac test A laboratory test for occult (unseen) blood in the stool.

Gynecologic age (Gr *gynaikos*, women) Length of time from onset of menses to present time of conception.

Hematocrit (Gr *haima*, blood; *krinein*, to separate) The volume percentage of red blood cells in whole blood, showing ratio of RBC volume to total blood volume, normally about 35% in women; abbreviated HCT.

Heme iron Dietary iron from animal sources, from heme portion of hemoglobin in red blood cells. More easily absorbed and transported in the body than nonheme iron from plant sources, but supplying the smaller portion of the body's total dietary iron intake.

Hemochromatosis (Gr *haima*, blood; *chroma*, color) Disorder of iron metabolism characterized by excess iron deposits in the tissues, especially the liver and pancreas; results from iron overload from prolonged use of iron supplements or from transfusions.

Hemoglobin (Gr *haima*, blood; L *globus*, a ball) Oxygen-carrying pigment in red blood cells; a conjugated protein containing 4 heme groups combined with iron and 4 long polypeptide chains forming the protein globin, named for its ball-like form; made by the developing RBC in bone marrow.

Hemolytic anemia (Gr *haima*, blood; *lysis*, dissolution) An anemia (reduced number of red blood cells) caused by breakdown of red blood cells and loss of their hemoglobin.

Hemorrhoids (Gr *haima*, blood; *rhoia*, to flow) Enlarged veins in the mucous membranes inside or outside of the rectum; causes pain, itching, discomfort, and bleeding.

Heterozygote (Gr *hetero*, other; *zygotos*, yoked together) An individual possessing different *alleles* (gene forms occupying corresponding chromosome sites) in regard to a given character trait.

Hirsutism (L *hirsutus*, shaggy hair) A condition marked by abundant and excessive hair; abnormal hairiness, especially an adult male pattern of body hair distribution in women.

Homeostasis (Gr *homoios*, like, unchanging; *stasis*, standing, steady) The life-sustaining relative dynamic equilibrium within the body's internal environment; a biochemical and physiologic balance achieved through the constant operation of numerous interrelated homeostatic mechanisms.

Homogenization (Gr *homos*, same; *genos*, kind) Process of forming a permanent emulsion by breaking up fat portion into fine globules and dispersing them equally throughout the milk for uniform quality.

Hydrocephalus (Gr *hydro-*, water; *kephale*, head) A condition characterized by enlargement of the cranium caused by abnormal accumulation of fluid.

Hydrolysis   (Gr *hydro-*, water; *lysis*, dissolution) Process by which a chemical compound is split into other simpler compounds by taking up the elements of water, as in the manufacture of infant formulas to produce easier-to-digest derivatives of the main protein casein in the cow's milk base; process occurs naturally in digestion.

Hydroscopic   (Gr *hydro-*, water; *skopein*, to measure or examine) Possessing tendency to take up and hold water readily.

Hydroxyapatite   The inorganic compound of calcium and phosphorus found in the matrix of bones and teeth, giving rigidity and strength to the structure.

Hypercalcemia   Elevated level of calcium in the blood.

Hyperlipidemia   (Gr *hyper*, above; *lipos*, fat; *haemia*, blood) General term for elevated concentrations of any or all of the lipids in the blood plasma.

Hypernatremic dehydration   An abnormally high sodium ion (Na^+) concentration in the extracellular fluid, due to water loss or restriction, drawing cell water to restore osmotic balance, causing dangerous cell dehydration. Compare with *hyponatremia*.

Hyperplasia   (Gr *hyper*, above; *plasis*, formation) Enlargement of tissue due to a process of rapidly increasing cell number. Compare with *hypertrophy*.

Hypertrophy   (Gr *hyper*, above; *trophe*, nutrition) Enlargement of an organ or part due to the process of increasing cell size.

Hyperventilation   (Gr *hyper*, above; L *ventilatio*, ventilation) Increased respiration with larger intake and consequent oxygen-carbon dioxide exchange in the lungs above the normal amount.

Hypogeusia   (Gr *hypo-*, under; *geusis*, taste; *aisthesis*, perception) An abnormally diminished acuteness of the sense of taste.

Hyponatremia   Abnormally low levels of sodium (Na^+) in the blood; can be easily caused by excess water intake to point of water intoxication, with resulting dilution of the major electrolyte (Na^+) in extracellular circulating fluids.

Hypothalamus   (Gr *hypo-*, under; *thalamus*, inner chamber) A small gland adjacent to the pituitary in the midbasal brain area; serves as a collection and dispatching center for information about the internal well-being of the body, using much of this neuroendocrine information to stimulate and control many widespread important pituitary hormones.

Hypovolemia   (Gr *hypo-*, under; ME *volu-me*, volume; Gr *haima*, blood) Low blood volume.

Ideal weight   Optimal weight for an individual of a given height, sex, or age in relation to personal health.

Immunoglobulins   (L *immunis*, free, exempt; *globulus*, globule, ball) Special components of the body's immune system, proteins synthesized by lymphocytes and plasma cells that have specific antibody activity.

Infant mortality   Number of infant deaths during the first year of life (1 month to 1 year) per 1000 live births.

Insensible water loss   Daily water loss through the skin and respiration, so named because a person is not aware of it. An additional smaller amount is lost in normal perspiration, the amount varying with the surrounding temperature.

Interpolation   (L *interpolare*, to make new) Process of injecting new interpretation or application of data to expand meaning or use, as in deriving data from one age group and applying it to another.

Intracellular water   Collective body water or fluids inside of cells; in body composition measures a large portion assigned to total lean body mass, a vital component in cell metabolism.

Involution   (L *involutio: in*, into; *volvere*, to roll) A process of rolling or turning inward, shrinking an organ to its normal size, as the uterus after childbirth.

Ions (Gr *ion*, wanderer) Activated form of certain minerals, such as sodium (Na^+), potassium (K^+), and chloride (Cl^-), that carry an electrical charge and perform a variety of essential metabolic tasks.

Iron absorption Degree of iron absorption, relativity small at best, depends upon its acid reduction, either by accompanying food such as orange juice or by the gastric HCl secretions, from the ferric form (Fe^{+++}) in foods to the ferrous form (Fe^{++}) required for absorption. After absorption (about 30% of the total intake) it is oxidized back to the ferric form required for incorporation in body metabolism.

Isomaltase (Gr *isos*, equal; L *maltum*, grain) Enzyme of the intestinal mucosa that splits isomaltose, an *isomer* of maltose (an isomer is a compound like another compound capable of behaving in a similar manner), a digestive product of starch in grains.

Juxtaglomerular apparatus (L *juxta*, near; *glomus*, ball) A complex of special cells located near or adjoining the cup-like glomerulus at the head of each kidney nephron; responsible for sensing the level of sodium in the blood.

Ketones Class of organic compounds, including three keto-acid basis that occur as intermediate products of fat metabolism: acetoacetate, hydroxybutyrate, and acetone; excess production, as in the initial stages of starvation from burning body fat for energy fuel, leads to ketoacidosis, which if continued uncontrolled can bring coma and death.

Kilocalorie (kcalorie, kcal) Unit of measure for energy produced in the body by the energy-yielding macronutrients carbohydrate, fat, and protein.

Kwashiorkor Classic protein-deficiency disease, frequently encountered in children in developing countries, but also seen in developed countries such as the United States in poverty areas and in metabolically stressed and debilitated hospitalized patients.

Lactation (L *lactare*, to suckle) The process of milk production and secretion in the mammary glands.

Lactiferous ducts (L *lac*, milk; *ferre*, to bear; *ducere*, to lead or draw) Vessels conducting milk from producing cells to storage and release areas of the breast; tube or passage for secretions.

Lactobacillus bifidus (*L. bifidus*) A predominant fermentative lactobacillus in the intestinal flora of breast-fed infants.

Lactoferrin (L *lac*, milk; *ferrum*, iron) An iron-binding protein found in human milk.

Lactoperoxidase Enzyme found in human milk that catalyzes the oxidation of organic substrate, including harmful microorganisms, thereby protecting the infant.

Lacunae (L *lacuna*, small pit or hollow cavity) Blood spaces of the placenta in which the fetal villi are found.

Lanolin (L *lana*, wool) Fatty substance extracted from wool, used in ointments and salves.

Larynx (Gr *larynx*, upper part of windpipe) Structure of muscle and cartilage lined with mucous membrane, connected to top part of the trachea and to the pharynx; essential sphincter muscle guarding the entrance to the trachea and functioning secondarily as the organ of the voice.

Laws of thermodynamics (Gr *therme*, heat; *dynamis*, power) Basic three laws of physics relating to heat-energy balance: (1) energy-like matter is neither created nor destroyed, only constantly transformed and recycled, thus conserving energy in any process; (2) there is always an increase in *entropy* (Gr *entrope*, a turning inward), a measure of the part of heat or other energy form in a system that is not available to perform work, thus entropy increases in all natural (spontaneous and irreversible) processes; and (3) absolute zero in energy balance is unattainable.

Lean body mass Collective fat-free mass of body composition; most metabolically active portion of body tissues.

Life expectancy The average remaining years a person of a given age may expect to live, based on statistical population averages.

Lifestyle   A person's unique pattern of living which, depending on its form, can be negative or positive in its health result.

Linear growth   (L *linearis,* a line) Linear measure of growing body length; height.

Linoleic acid   The ultimate essential fatty acid for humans.

Lipase   (Gr *lipos,* fat; *-ase,* as, ending indicating an enzyme, attached to a stem that indicates the substrate upon which it works) Group name for enzymes that work on lipids (fats), splitting fatty acids from the glycerol base.

Lipids   Chemical group name for fats and fat-related compounds such as cholesterol, lipoproteins, and phospholipids; general group name for organic substances of a fatty nature, including fats, oils, waxes, and related compounds.

Lipolysis   (Gr *lipos,* fat; *lysis,* dissolution) The breakdown of fat; fat digestion.

Lobule   (L *lobus,* lobe, a well-defined area) A small lobe, one of the primary divisions of a larger lobe; smaller branching vessels or subdivisions that make up a lobe of the mammary gland.

Locus of control   (L *locus,* place, site) A person's perceived control center over his life.

Long-term care   Medical, personal, or home-making services provided within an institution or in the community for older adults who are no longer able to care for their own needs.

Longitudinal study   Study of persons or populations over a long period of time to measure effects of specific factors on the aging process and incidence and course of disease.

Low birth weight   Birth weight less than 2500 g (5.4 lb); very low birth weight, less than 1500 g (3.2 lb).

Lymphoblasts   (L *lympha,* water; Gr *blastos,* germ) The immature stage of the mature lymphocyte.

Lymphocytes   Mature leukocytes, special lymphoid white blood cells, T cells and B cells, major components of the body's immune system; found in human milk.

Lymphoid tissue   (L *lympha,* water) Tissues related to the body system of lymphatic fluids; body tissues giving rise to lymphocytes of the immune system, such as intestinal mucosa and lymph gland.

Lyophilization   (Gr *lyein,* to dissolve; *philein,* to love, having an affinity for a stable solution) Process of rapid freezing and dehydration of the frozen product under high vacuum to stabilize or preserve a biologic substance.

Lysozyme   (Gr *lysis,* dissolution; *zyme,* leaven) A crystalline basic enzyme in many body fluids such as saliva, tears, and human milk; an antibacterial agent.

Macronutrients   (Gr *makros,* large; L *nutriens,* nourishment) Group name for the three large energy-yielding nutrients—carbohydrate, fat, and protein—all organic compounds of large molecular size.

Macrophage   (Gr *makros,* large; *phagein,* to eat) Large phagocytes, cells of the immune system that engulf and consume microorganisms, other cells, or foreign particles, and interact with T cells and B cells to produce inflammatory process and antibodies.

Major minerals   Minerals that occur in relatively large quantities in the body and hence have greater dietary requirements.

Maltase   Enzyme acting on the disaccharide maltose, from starch breakdown, into its two component monosaccharides, two units of glucose.

Mammalian   Any vertebrate animal belonging to the class *Mammalia,* or humans, who give birth to live young and nourish them with milk from the female mammary glands.

Mammary glands   (Gr *mamme,* mother's milk) Milk-producing glands in females of all mammalian species, humans and animals, who are distinguished from all other life by bearing live young and producing milk to nourish them.

Marsupial   (L *marsupium,* a pouch) A member of the animal class of mammals who bear undeveloped young, which they carry in an abdominal pouch and nourish with their milk until development is complete; includes such animals as kangaroos and koala bears.

Mastitis (Gr *mastos,* breast; *-itis,* inflammation) Breast infection; inflammation of the mammary gland.

Maturation (L *maturus,* mature) The process or stage of attaining one's full physical, psychosocial, and mental development. Individual genetic potential guides physical and mental development, which in turn bears the imprint of environmental, psychosocial, and cultural influence.

Mean Mathematical term for the average numerical value of a group of numbers.

Median (L *medianus,* middle) The middle value in a distribution of numbers, with half of the values falling above and half falling below.

Megaloblastic anemia (Gr *mega,* great size; *blastos,* embryo, germ) Anemia due to faulty production of abnormally large immature red blood cells, due to a deficiency of vitamin B_{12} and folate.

Menarche (Gr *men,* month; *arche,* beginning) Onset of menses.

Menopause (Gr *meno-,* month; *pausis,* cessation) Cessation of menses, occurring in North American women at approximately 50 years of age.

Menses Monthly menstrual periods.

Menstruation The monthly discharge of blood and mucosal tissue from the nonpregnant uterus; final phase of the female sexual cycle.

Mesoderm (Gr *mesos,* middle; *derma,* skin) An intermediate layer of embryonic cells developing between the ectoderm (outer layer) and endoderm (inner layer).

Metabolic acidosis Abnormal rise in acid partner of the carbonic acid-base bicarbonate buffer system by excess of organic acids, which displace part of the base bicarbonate in the buffer system and cause the H^+ concentration (acidity) to rise.

Metabolic activity Sum of biochemical actions and reactions in the body that builds and maintains tissue, regulates body functions, and requires a constant energy source. The most metabolically active tissue is the lean body mass.

Metabolism (Gr *metaballein,* to change) Sum of all the various biochemical and physiologic processes by which the body grows and maintains itself (anabolism) and breaks down and reshapes tissue (catabolism), transforming energy to do its work.

Micelle (L *micella,* small body) A microscopic colloid particle of fat and bile formed in the small intestine for initial stage of fat absorption.

Microcephaly (Gr *mikros,* small; *kephate,* head) Small size of the head in relation to the rest of the body.

Micronutrients (Gr *mikros,* small; L *nutriens,* nourishing) Group name for the nonenergy-yielding nutrients, the vitamins, organic compounds of small molecular size, and minerals, single inert elements; essential coenzyme factors in metabolism and tissue structure.

Microphthalmia (Gr *micro,* small; *ophthalmos,* eye) Abnormal smallness of one or both eyes.

Mid–upper arm muscle circumference (MAMC) Indirect measure of the body's skeletal muscle mass based on mid–arm muscle circumference (MAMC) and triceps skinfold (TSF): MAMC (cm) = MAC (cm) − [0.314 × TSF (mm)].

Milieu (Fr *milieux,* surroundings) Environment, social or physical; an important concept in nutrition, referring to both external sociophysical setting and internal biochemical environments, and interacting balances between them.

Milliosmoles (mOsm/L) Osmole (Gr *osme,* small), standard unit of osmotic pressure; equal to the gram molecular weight of solute divided by the number of particles (ions) into which a substance dissociates in solution. Thus milliosmole would be a much smaller unit of measure of osmotic pressure—$1/1000$ of an osmole, equal to $1/1000$ gram molecular weight of a substance divided by the number of ions into which a substance dissociates in 1 liter (L) of solution. The term *osmolality* refers to this concentration of solutes per unit of solvent.

Mineral compartment Smallest part of the body composition, found mainly in the skeletal bone mass.

Mitochondria (Gr *mitos,* thread; *chondrion,* granule) Cells' "powerhouse," small elongated organelles located in the cell cytoplasm; principal site of energy generation (ATP synthesis); contains enzymes of the final energy cycle (citric acid cycle) and cell respiration, as well as ribonucleic acid (RNA) and deoxyribonucleic acid (DNA) for some synthesis of protein.

Mortality rate Total number of deaths in a specific category divided by the total number of deaths in the total population.

Morula (L *morus,* mulberry) A solid mass of cells resembling a mulberry, formed by cleavage of a fertilized ovum.

Motivation Forces that affect individual goal-directed behavior toward satisfying needs or achieving personal goals.

Multigravida (L *multus,* many; *gravida,* pregnant) A woman who has had two or more pregnancies.

Multiparous (L *multus,* many, much; *parere,* to bring forth) Women who have had two or more pregnancies resulting in live births.

Myelin (Gr *myelos,* marrow) High lipid-to-protein substance forming sheath to insulate and protect neuron axons and facilitate their neuromuscular impulses.

Myocardial infarction (MI) (Gr *mys,* muscle; L *infarcire,* to stuff it; Gr *kardia*) Death of heart muscle tissue resulting from blockage of blood flow to or through the coronary arteries, usually caused by fatty plaques and blood clot formation from their tissue irritation to the surrounding blood vessel, effectively "stuffing" the vessel at that point and cutting off blood supply to the heart muscle tissue served by the vessel. This event is commonly called a heart attack.

Myocardium (Gr *mys,* muscle; *kardia,* heart) Heart muscle; middle and thickest layer of heart wall.

Myoepithelial cells (Gr *mys,* muscle; *epi-,* on; *thele,* nipple) Tissue composed of contractile epithelial cells surrounding the alveoli and duct system of the lactating breast.

Narcissism Self-love; from Narcissus, a character in Greek mythology who saw his image mirrored in a pool of water and fell in love with his own reflection.

Necrotizing enterocolitis (Gr *nekrosis,* deadness; *enterion,* intestine) An infectious tissue destroying intestinal disease of the small intestine and the colon; acute inflammation of intestinal mucosa.

Neonatal (Gr *neos,* new; L *natus,* born) The period surrounding birth; especially the first four weeks after birth when the infant is called a neonate.

Neonatal mortality Number of newborn deaths during the neonatal period (birth to 1 month postpartum) per 1000 live births.

Neonate A newborn infant; term usually refers to the first 4 weeks of life.

Nephron Functional unit of the kidneys, constantly filtering the blood, selectively reabsorbing its components as needed to maintain normal blood values, and excreting the remainder in a concentrated urine. At birth, each kidney has about a million of these minute units, far more than actually needed.

Neuromotor (Gr *neuron,* nerve; L *motorium,* movement center) Movement involving nerve impulses to muscles.

Neurotransmitter (Gr *neuron,* nerve; L *trans,* through, across; *missio,* sending) Large group of some 40 different chemical substances, including compounds as diverse as acetylcholine, various hormones, and several amino acids, which function as essential synaptic transmitters, chemical messengers for sending (or inhibiting) nerve impulses across synapses of connecting nerve endings.

Nanogram (abbreviated ng) (Gr *nano-,* dwarf) One billionth gram; also called millimicrogram.

Niacin equivalent (NE) Current international measure for recommended amounts of B vitamin niacin, that accounts for both the preformed vitamin and the amino acid precursor tryptophan, from which the vitamin can be synthesized. Thus 1 NE equals 1 g niacin or 60 mg dietary tryptophan.

Nitrogen balance The metabolic balance between nitrogen intake in dietary protein and output in urinary nitrogen compounds such as urea and creatinine. For every 6.25 g dietary protein consumed 1 g nitrogen is excreted.

Nanomole (abbreviated nmole) (Gr *nanos,* dwarf; *molekul,* molecule) Metric system unit for measuring very small amounts. Prefix *nano-* used in naming very small amounts to indicate one billionth of the unit with which it is combined. *Mole* is chemical term for the molecular weight of a substance expressed in grams—gram molecular weight.

Nonheme iron The larger portion of dietary iron, including all the plant food sources and 60% of the animal food sources, which lacks the more easily absorbed and bioavailable heme iron in the remaining 40% of the animal food sources that contain hemoglobin residues of iron-containing heme.

Normochromic Normal red blood cell color.

Normocytic Normal cell size.

Nulliparity (L *nullus,* none; *parere,* to bring forth) Reproductive status of a woman who has never borne a viable child.

Nutrient density The protein, vitamin, or mineral content of a food expressed in relation to its energy (caloric) content.

Nutrition assessment (L *nutritio,* nourishment; *assessare,* to assess, to estimate property or income value for purposes of taxation) Process of determining individual or group nutritional status as a basis for identifying needs and goals and planning personal health care or community programs to meet these identified goals.

Nutrition care plan The person-centered care plan, based on nutritional assessment data and evaluation, for individual nutritional care and education to promote health and prevent or treat disease.

Nutrition education The process of helping individuals obtain the knowledge, skills, and motivation needed to make appropriate food choices for positive health throughout life.

Nutrition environment (L *nutritio,* nourishment; Fr *environner,* to surround, encircle) The sum of substances, materials, and processes involved in taking in food and nutrients and assimilating and using them for body health and strength.

Nutrition label Food product label providing nutrition information concerning nutrient and energy values per designated size portion.

Nutritional status (L *status,* condition, situation) Condition of an individual's body tissues and health, especially as related to the nutrients that are essential to the structure, function, and maintenance of body tissues.

Odd-numbered carbon-chain fatty acids Most fatty acid carbon chains in the human diet are even numbered, broken down by beta oxidation, successively clipping off 2-carbon fragments of *acetyl-CoA* to feed into the final energy production pathway, the citric acid cycle. A few odd-numbered ones do exist, however. When they do occur, they go through the same beta-oxidation process, clipping off 2-carbon fragments until the final 3-carbon residue remains, *proprionyl-CoA,* which is also an intermediate metabolic product of the essential amino acid threonine. These 3-carbon fragments from both sources are converted to *succinyl-CoA,* a 4-carbon compound in the citric acid cycle, so they feed into the final energy production cycle at this point.

Oligosaccharides   (Gr *oligos,* little; *saccharide,* sugar) Intermediate products of polysaccharide carbohydrate breakdown, containing a small number (from 4 to 10) of single sugar units of the monosaccharide glucose.

Omega-3 fatty acids   Group of long chain polyunsaturated fatty acids having important precursor roles in producing highly active hormone-like substances, the *eicosanoids,* involved in critical metabolic activities such as vascular muscle tone and blood clotting.

Omnivorous   (L *omnia,* all; *vorare,* to eat) Eating all kinds of foods, from both animal and plant sources.

Organohalides   (Gr *organon,* organ; Chem *halides,* compounds of fluorine, chlorine, bromine, or iodine) Chemical compounds used as pesticides or in industrial processes, for example, DDT and PCBs.

Orofacial muscles   (L *os, oris,* mouth) Adjoining muscles of the mouth and face.

Osmolality   (Gr *osmos,* impulsion through a membrane) Property of a solution that depends on the concentration of the particles (solutes) in solution per unit of solvent base; measured as milliosmoles per liter (mOsm/L).

Osteomalacia   (Gr *osteon,* bone; *malakia,* softness) Condition marked by softening of the bones due to impaired mineralization with excess accumulation of osteoid (immature young bone matrix that has not had mineralization to harden it); results from deficiency of vitamin D and calcium.

Osteoporosis   (Gr *osteon,* bone; *poros,* passage, pore) Abnormal thinning of bone, producing a porous fragile lattice-like bone tissue of enlarged spaces, prone to fracture or deformity.

Ovulation   Monthly process in female sexual cycle of secreting a mature ovum for transport through the fallopian tubes to the uterus.

Ovum   (L *ovum,* egg) The female reproductive cell (egg) capable of fertilization and development into a new organism.

Oxalic acid   A compound in a variety of foods, including green leafy vegetables, corn, soy products such as tofu, and wheat germ, that binds calcium in the food mix and hinders its absorption.

Oxyhemoglobin   Hemoglobin with bound oxygen for transport by the red blood cells from the lungs to the body tissue cells for vital metabolic work.

Oxytocin   (Gr *oxys,* sharp, sour; *tokos,* birth) Pituitary hormone causing uterine contractions and milk ejection.

Palate   (L *palatum,* palate) The partition separating the nasal and oral cavities, with a hard bony front section and a soft fleshy back section.

Palmar grasp   Early grasp of the young infant, clasping an object in the palm and wrapping the whole hand around it.

Paraprofessional   (Gr *para-,* along side) A nonprofessional person, often from the community being served and thus having valuable insights concerning needs, who is trained to assist the professional community or clinical nutrition specialist in carrying out the nutrition program.

Parenteral nutrition   (Gr *para,* beyond, beside; *enteron,* intestine) Nourishment received not through the gastrointestinal tract but rather by an alternate route such as injection into a vein; intravenous feeding of elemental nutrients.

Parietal cells   (L *parietes,* wall) Cells lining the stomach that secrete hydrochloric acid; chief cells.

Parity   (L *parere,* to bring forth, produce) Number of pregnancies a woman has had producing viable offspring.

Parkinson's disease   A neurologic disorder, described by English physician James Parkinson (1755-1824), characterized by tremor, muscular rigidity, and abnormally decreased motor function and ability, affecting mobility.

Parturition   (L *parturitio,* to give birth) Act or process of childbirth; maternal labor and delivery.

Pattern for daily food choices   Expanded accompaniment to dietary guidelines to apply them to practical meal planning.

Percentile   (L *per,* through; *centrum,* a hundred, "by the hundred") Rate or proportion per hundred; statistical term indicating status of a value in relation to 100 equal parts of a series of values in order of their measurable magnitude. For example, a value at the 60th percentile would mean that 60% of all the values in the distribution of the population studies lie at or below the 60th percentile, 40% above it.

Perinatal mortality   (Gr *peri-,* around; L *natus,* born) Infant deaths in the perinatal period, shortly before and after birth, approximately from week 20-28 of gestation to 1-4 weeks postpartum, per 1000 live births.

Pernicious anemia   A chronic macrocytic anemia occurring most commonly after age 40; caused by absence of the intrinsic factor normally present in the gastric juices and necessary for the absorption of cobalamin (B_{12}); controlled by intramuscular injections of vitamin B_{12}.

Periodontal disease   (Gr *peri,* around; L *dens,* tooth) General term for disease of tissues surrounding the tooth, affecting its integrity and stability, and contributing to tooth loss.

Peristalsis   (Gr *peri,* around; *stalsia,* contraction) A wave-like progression of alternate contraction and relaxation of the muscle fibers of the gastrointestinal tract.

Phagocytosis   (Gr *phagein,* to eat; *-cyte,* hollow vessel, anything that contains or covers) The engulfing of microorganisms, other cells, or foreign particles by phagocytes.

pH   Power of the hydrogen ion (H^+), a measure indicating degree of acidity or alkalinity of solutions. A pH of 7.0 indicates neutrality, with numbers above it indicating increasing alkalinity and those below, increasing acidity.

Pharynx   (Gr *pharynx,* throat) The muscular membranous passage between the mouth and the posterior nasal passages and the larynx and esophagus.

Phenylketonuria (PKU)   A genetic disease caused by a missing enzyme, phenylalanine hydroxylase, required for the metabolic conversion of the essential amino acid phenylalanine to the amino acid tyrosine. Untreated, profound mental retardation occurs. Normal growth and development now follows current mandatory newborn screening and immediate initiation of a low phenylalanine diet with special low-phe formula such as Lofenalac.

Physiologic age   Rate of biologic maturation in individual adolescents which varies widely and accounts, far more than does chronologic age, for wide and changing differences in their metabolic rates, nutritional needs, and food requirements.

Phytic acid   A compound in certain grains, such as wheat, that binds calcium and hinders its absorption.

Pincer grasp   Later digital grasp of the older infant, usually picking up smaller objects with a precise grip between thumb and forefinger.

Pinocytosis   (Gr *pinein,* to drink; *kytos,* cell) The uptake of fluid nutrient material by a living cell by means of incupping and invagination of the cell membrane, which closes off and forms free cell vacuoles.

Placebo   (L "I will please") An inactive substance or preparation used in controlled drug or nutrient studies to determine the efficacy of an agent under study.

Placenta   (L *placentas,* a flat cake) A characteristic organ of mammals during pregnancy joining mother and offspring, providing supportive nourishment and endocrine secretions for embryonic-fetal development and growth.

Polymer   (Gr *poly-,* many; *meros,* part) A large compound formed by chains of simpler repeating molecules, for example, the glucose polymer oligosaccharide.

Postpartum   (L *post,* after; *partum,* separate part) Period following childbirth or delivery.

Precursor   A substance from which another substance is produced.

Preeclampsia   (Gr *pre-*, before; *eklampein*, to shine forth) Abnormal condition of late pregnancy marked by rather sudden hypertension and increased edema, usually accompanied by protein-uria; may progress to eclampsia with convulsions and coma; better prevented by good prenatal care and optimal nutrition throughout the pregnancy.

Preterm milk   Milk produced by mothers of premature infants.

Preventive approach   Positive health care that seeks to identify and reduce risk factors for disease.

Primigravida   (L *prima*, first; *gravida*, pregnant) A woman pregnant for the first time.

Primiparous   (L *prima*, first; *parere*, to bring forth) State of a woman bearing or having borne only one child.

Primordial follicle   Primitive ovarian follicle (*follis*, a leather bag), formed during fetal life; a sac- or pouch-like cavity, a small secretory sac or gland; an ovarian follicle, ovum surrounded by specialized epithelial cells.

Primordial ova   (L *primordia*, the beginning; *ovum*, egg) Primitive ova cells produced in large life-supply numbers in the female fetal ovaries before birth.

Progesterone   Ovarian hormone that regulates secretory function of the mucosal linings of the uterus and fallopian tubes, and stimulates development of milk-producing structures of the breast.

Prolactin   (Gr *pro-*, before; L *lac*, milk) A hormone of the anterior pituitary gland that stimulates and maintains lactation in postpartum mothers.

Prophylactic   (Gr *prophylassein*, to keep guard before) Preventive treatment to avoid disease, for example, vitamin K for newborns to prevent the formerly widespread hemorrhagic disease of newborns, since they are born with a sterile gastrointestinal tract and lack the microorganisms that synthesize vitamin K.

Proprietary   (L *proprietarius*, owner) Referring to commercial products, such as infant formulas and medical items, which are designed, manufactured, and sold for profit only by the owner of the patent, formula, brand name, or trademark associated with the product.

Prostaglandins   Highly active hormone-like eicosanoid substances produced from essential fatty acid precursors and acting locally in various body tissues with many physiologic effects.

Proteolytic   (Gr *protos*, first, protein; *lysis*, dissolution) Protein-splitting by a series of enzymes through hydrolysis of the peptide bonds into smaller peptides and amino acids.

Prothrombin   (Gr *pro-*, before; *thrombos*, clot) Blood-clotting factor (number II), synthesized in the liver from glutamic acid and CO_2, catalyzed by vitamin K.

Protocol   (Gr *protokollon*, leaf or tag attached to a rolled papyrus manuscript containing notes as to its contents) A set of governing rules; the plan and procedures for carrying out a scientific study or a person's treatment regimen.

Pubertal development   The rapid physical growth and sexual development of puberty.

Pyridoxine   Chemical name for vitamin B_6, derived from its ring-like structure. In its active form, pyridoxal phosphate, it acts as a coenzyme factor in many types of transamination and decarboxylation reactions in amino acid metabolism.

Radioimmunoassay   (L *radius*, ray; *immunis*, free, exempt; *assay*, examine, analyze) Technique using radioactive labeling of the material being studied, for measuring minute quantities of antigen or antibody, hormones, certain drugs, and other substances.

Recommended Dietary Allowances (RDAs)   U.S. nutrient and energy standards for healthy population groups by age and sex, updated every 4-5 years by expert committees of scientists to reflect current research, and issued by the National Research Council of the National Institutes of Health.

Renal solute load   Collective number and concentration of solute particles in solution, carried by the blood to the kidney nephrons for excretion in the urine, usually nitrogenous products from protein metabolism, and the electrolytes Na^+, K^+, Cl^-, and HPO_4^-.

Resting energy expenditure (REE)   Energy expended by a person at rest in a neutral surrounding temperature, neither hot nor cold; similar to other measures of energy needs, such as the classic test of basal metabolic rate (BMR) and the calculated basal energy expenditure (BEE). The three values are often used interchangeably.

Retinol   Chemical name for vitamin A derived from its function relating to the retina of the eye and light-dark adaptation. Daily RDA standards are stated in retinol equivalents (RE) to account for sources of the preformed vitamin A and its precursor provitamin A beta-carotene.

Retinol equivalent (RE)   Unit of measure for dietary sources of vitamin A, both preformed vitamin, retinol, and the precursor provitamin, beta-carotene. 1 RE = 1 μg retinol or 6 μg beta-carotene.

Reverse peristalsis   (Gr *peri-,* around; *stalsis,* contraction) Wave-like contractions of longitudinal and circular muscles of the gastrointestinal tract that normally propel the food mass forward, but may act in reverse in upper GI tract of young infants causing easy spitting up of milk.

Salicylates   Compound salts of salicylic acid, found in certain plants and in drugs such as common aspirin (acetylsalicylic acid—ASA).

Senescence   (L *senescere,* to grow old) Normal process or condition of growing old.

Sexual maturity ratings   Scale defining stages of sexual maturation during puberty.

Simple carbohydrates   The monosaccharides glucose, fructose, and galactose, and the disaccharides sucrose, maltose, and lactose.

Skeletal muscle   Muscles attached to skeletal bones for control of body movements; major component of lean body mass.

Sociodemographic   Relating to the characteristic social and cultural values, geographic distribution, and physical environments of persons and populations.

Solutes   (Gr *solvere,* to dissolve) Particles of a substance in solution; a solution consists of solutes and a dissolving medium (solvent), usually a liquid.

Stereotype   An oversimplified and generalized conception or image held by persons and groups that have distorted or unreal meaning, but influences attitudes and behavior of persons holding such views.

Stress   Sum of biologic reactions to adverse stimuli, physical, mental, or emotional, internal or external, that disturbs the state of homeostasis and sense of well-being.

Sucrase   Intestinal enzyme that splits the disaccharide sucrose into its two component monsaccharides glucose and fructose.

Tactile   (L *tactio,* to touch) Sense of touching, perception by the touch.

Tannic acid   Compound of certain plants such as tea leaves, giving an astringent taste and having astringent properties that promote local tissue healing; an herbal remedy.

Tetany   (Gr *teinein,* to stretch) Condition caused by decrease in ionized serum calcium, marked by intermittent spastic muscle contractions and muscular pain; manifest by characteristic carpopedal spasm of the arm muscles causing flexion of the wrist and thumb with extension of the fingers, called *Trousseau's sign.* A so-called "milk tetany" has been reported in young infants fed undiluted cow's milk, due to the greater ratio of phosphorus to calcium in cow's milk than in human milk, and these infants could not clear the phosphate load, which then accumulated in the blood and caused a compensatory decrease in the serum calcium, resulting in the typical muscular spasms of tetany.

Tidal volume   The amount of gases, oxygen and carbon dioxide, passing into and out of the lungs in each respiratory cycle.

Title III-C   The statute of the Older Americans Act authorizing congregate and home-delivered meals for people age 60 and over.

Tocopherol   (Gr *tokos,* childbirth; *pherein,* to carry) Chemical name for vitamin E, so named by early investigators because their initial work with rats indicated a reproductive function, which did not turn out later to be the case with humans, in whom it functions as a strong antioxidant to preserve structural membranes such as cell walls.

Tonsils   (L *tonsilla,* tonsil) Small rounded mass of lymphoid tissue in the roof and posterior wall of the nasopharynx.

Trabeculae   (L *trabs,* a little beam) Small bones at the ends of long bones at joints such as wrist, vertebrae, and hips.

Trabecular bone   General term for small meshwork of bones at ends of long bones forming attached joints, and part of the connecting network between vertebrae.

Trace elements   Minerals that occur in small amounts or traces in the body, and hence are required in very small amounts.

Tretinoin   A form of retinoic acid, a vitamin A derivative, used as a drug in the medical treatment of chronic acne as a topical keralytic agent (Gr *keras,* horn; *lysis,* dissolution). Keratin is a hard protein; it is the principal constituent of skin, hair, nails, and scar tissue.

Triglyceride   Chemical name for fat, indicating structure: attachment of three fatty acids to a glycerol base. A neutral fat, synthesized from carbohydrate, stored in adipose tissue. It releases free fatty acids into the blood when hydrolyzed by enzymes.

Trophoblast   (Gr *trophe,* nutrition; *blastos,* embryo, germ) Extraembryonic ectodermal tissue on the surface of the cleaving, fertilized ovum, which is responsible for contact with the maternal circulation and supply of nutrients to the embryo.

Trypsin   (Gr *trypein,* to rub; *pepsis,* digestion) A protein-splitting enzyme formed in the intestine by action of enterokinase on the inactive precursor trypsinogen.

Trypsin inhibitor   A natural substance in raw soybeans that is responsible for a toxin in the bean. Fortunately this substance is destroyed by heat and rendered inactive.

U.S. dietary guidelines   A set of 7 statements to guide food choices that reflect current health promotion and disease prevention national health objectives.

U.S. RDA   A condensed food-labeling version of the regular National Research Council's Recommended Dietary Allowances, not to be confused with the regular NRC standards. This U.S. RDA, set up by the FDA in 1974 to replace the old minimum daily requirements (MDA), was compiled at the time from the 1968 regular RDAs using the highest value within age/sex categories. Cost of label changing prevents updating with revised RDA editions, causing confusion to consumers.

Vascular spaces   Spaces within fluid vessels in the body, blood vessels and lymph vessels; contain body fluids in transit, greater amount in blood and remainder in the interconnecting lymphatic system.

Vasodilation   (L *vas,* vessel; *dilatare,* to spread out) Expansion or stretching of a blood vessel.

Vasopressin   Hormone formed in the hypothalamus and stored in the posterior pituitary gland. Stimulates muscle contraction of capillaries and arterioles to maintain blood pressure, and acts on the epithelial cells of the distal tubule of the nephron to cause water reabsorption, producing a concentrated urine and preventing water loss. Thus it is also called the antidiuretic hormone (ADH).

Vegan diet   Strict vegetarian diet allowing no animal protein; requires careful food combinations of incomplete plant proteins to complement one another and achieve an overall adequacy of essential amino acids for growth needs.

Venous stasis   (L *venosus,* vein; Gr *stasis,* standing still) A stoppage, or decreased flow, of blood in the veins draining an organ causing engorgement of the affected vessels and tissues.

Vesicle   (L *vesica,* bladder) A small bladder or sac containing liquid; secretory transport sacs that move out into the cell cytoplasm to aid metabolism.

Visceral organs (L *viscus,* large body organ) Large internal organs of the body, located in the chest and abdomen.

Vital capacity Volume of air moved in and out of the lungs with each breath. The residual volume is the amount of air remaining in the lungs after the person has exhaled.

Vitamin A non–energy-yielding micronutrient required in very small amounts for specific metabolic tasks, but cannot be synthesized by the body so must be supplied in the diet.

Wellness approach An approach to health care that promotes the planning of a healthy positive lifestyle for maintaining physical and mental well-being.

Whey The thin liquid of milk remaining after the curd, containing the major protein casein, and the cream have been removed; contains other milk proteins lactalbumin and lactoferrin.

Xerostomia (Gr *xeros,* dry; *stoma,* mouth) Dryness of the mouth from lack of normal secretions.

Index

t indicates table; f indicates figure

Median Heights and Weights and Recommended Energy Intake

Category	Age (years) or Condition	Weight (kg)	Weight (lb)	Height (cm)	Height (in)	FEE[a] (kcal/day)	Average Energy Allowance (kcal)[b] Multiples of REE	Per kg	Per day[c]
Infants	0.0–0.5	6	13	60	24	320		108	650
	0.5–1.0	9	20	71	28	500		98	850
Children	1–3	13	29	90	35	740		102	1,300
	4–6	20	44	112	44	950		90	1,800
	7–10	28	62	132	52	1,130		70	2,000
Males	11–14	45	99	157	62	1,440	1.70	55	2,500
	15–18	66	145	176	69	1,760	1.67	45	3,000
	19–24	72	160	177	70	1,780	1.67	40	2,900
	25–50	79	174	176	70	1,800	1.60	37	2,900
	51 +	77	170	173	68	1,530	1.50	30	2,300
Females	11–14	46	101	157	62	1,310	1.67	47	2,200
	15–18	55	120	163	64	1,370	1.60	40	2,200
	19–24	58	128	164	65	1,350	1.60	38	2,200
	25–50	63	138	163	64	1,380	1.55	36	2,200
	51 +	65	143	160	63	1,280	1.50	30	1,900
Pregnant	1st Trimester								+ 0
	2nd Trimester								+ 300
	3rd Trimester								+ 300
Lactating	1st 6 months								+ 500
	2nd 6 months								+ 500

[a] Resting energy expenditure (REE); calculation based on FAO equations, then rounded.

[b] In the range of light to moderate activity, the coefficient of variation is ±20%.

[c] Figure is rounded.